W9-AYK-711

THE GENETICS
OF ASTHMA

LUNG BIOLOGY IN HEALTH AND DISEASE

Executive Editor

Claude Lenfant
Director, National Heart, Lung and Blood Institute
National Institutes of Health
Bethesda, Maryland

THE GENETICS
OF ASTHMA

Edited by

Stephen B. Liggett

University of Cincinnati
College of Medicine
Cincinnati, Ohio

Deborah A. Meyers

Johns Hopkins University
School of Medicine
Baltimore, Maryland

Marcel Dekker, Inc.   **New York • Basel • Hong Kong**

ISBN: 0-8247-9729-9

The publisher offers discounts on this book when ordered in bulk quantities. For more information, write to Special Sales/Professional Marketing at the address below.

This book is printed on acid-free paper.

Marcel Dekker, Inc.
270 Madison Avenue, New York, New York 10016

Current printing (last digit):
10 9 8 7 6 5 4 3 2 1

Printed in the United States of America

INTRODUCTION

The first time the title of a monograph in the Lung Biology in Health and Disease series included the word *genetic* was when Volume 11 appeared, in 1978. The monograph in question was *Genetic Determinants of Pulmonary Disease*, edited by Stephen D. Litwin. It touched on many of the issues that are today in the vanguard of our search to uncover and understand the mechanisms of action of genetic factors.

Of course, the notion that genetic determinants exist was not new even then, especially with regard to asthma. Indeed, in his 1882 edition of *On Asthma: Its Pathology and Treatment*, Henry Salter asked the question "Is asthma heredi-tary?" His response was:

> I think there is no doubt that it is.... [T]he kind of inheritance differs very much; sometimes it is direct, sometimes lateral; sometimes immediate, sometimes re-mote....

This statement is rich with meaning in light of today's appreciation that genetic determinants are modulated or expressed in different ways depending on environmental factors.

Since the publication of *Genetic Determinants of Pulmonary Disease*, many major events have occurred. Foremost is the fact that molecular biology and

iii

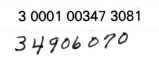

molecular genetics have reached a new maturity and are now commonly used in most research laboratories. Then, too, our understanding that many conditions or diseases are the result of an interplay between genetic and environmental factors has greatly increased. This has led to the concept of *complex diseases*, which is now actively being investigated.

During the past few years, research on the causes of hypertension has set an example because investigators interested in this disease have recognized a situation elegantly stated by Lifton (1):

> The complex interplay of different physiological systems regulating blood pressure has made it difficult to determine whether physiological abnormalities found in hypertensive patients are primary contributors to the hypertensive process, or mere secondary consequences of the true, and elusive, primary causes. A consequence of this ignorance is that our therapeutic approach to this disease is necessarily empiric and not directed toward underlying primary abnormalities.

If the reference to blood pressure were replaced by asthma, the problems confronting asthma researchers would be well described. But, of course, asthma researchers already know what the problems are, and they are now at the forefront of research to try to solve them.

This new volume, *The Genetics of Asthma*, is proof of that. Drs. Stephen B. Liggett and Deborah A. Meyers present a rich panoply of ideas and findings that bring us to the threshold of better asthma control. The field of asthma is a busy one, generating many discoveries from which clinicians, and thus patients, have benefited the world over. To my knowledge, this volume is the first on the genetics of asthma. Its completion is a great tribute to its editors and contributors. I am privileged that they chose the Lung Biology in Health and Disease series as the venue for this remarkable and innovative book.

Claude Lenfant, M.D.
Bethesda, Maryland

Reference

1. Lifton RP. Molecular genetics of human hypertension. In: Mockrin SC, ed. Molecular Genetics and Gene Therapy of Cardiovascular Diseases. New York: Marcel Dekker. 1996: 111–134.

PREFACE

Asthma affects 150 million or more individuals worldwide. In the United States, asthma is one of the most common and economically burdensome chronic diseases. Despite substantial increases in our understanding of the pathophysiology of this disease, only a few new therapeutic agents based on novel mechanisms of action have been developed over the last two decades. In addition, there is no evidence that morbidity and mortality are decreasing.

Over the last five years, an intense global effort has been under way to delineate the genetic basis of asthma. Knowing the precise genetic defect(s) would result in a quantum leap in our understanding of the molecular and cellular mechanisms of asthma. From such information, a major opportunity for the development of new therapeutics will be at hand. Even though asthma has long been recognized as having a significant heritable component, genetic studies have been difficult to perform and the results have been difficult to interpret.

There are several reasons for these problems. First, a clear definition of the disease (or syndrome) termed "asthma" has been more elusive than the casual reader might expect. No single symptom, physical finding, or laboratory test identifies the entity. In addition, asthma can develop at different ages within the population. Thus, defining affected and nonaffected individuals, which is an important aspect of genetic studies, requires careful consideration. Since asthma is often triggered by an allergic response, the environmental milieu of patient populations can play a significant role in expression of the disease. The varied clinical presentations of asthma have led to the concept that there may be multiple asthmatic phenotypes, which adds to the complexity of genetic studies. Finally, it may well be that the genetic component of asthma is due to multiple gene defects. All these difficulties significantly differentiate asthma from diseases such as cystic fibrosis, which has a clearly defined phenotype, has a well-established clinical test, is not substantially affected by the environment, is not easily confused with other diseases, and, as it turns out, is due to mutations in one gene for virtually all patients.

Nevertheless, over the past few years substantial progress has been made in the mapping of genes linked to atopy, elevated IgE levels, bronchial hyperresponsiveness, and asthma. In this book we have approached the genetics of asthma in four sections. In the first, pathways considered critical for the development of asthma that are potentially subject to genetic variability are discussed. From the outset, we recognized that this section was not going to be all-inclusive; indeed, a discussion of basic mechanisms of asthma would fill an entire volume. Rather, we chose some well-established pathways as well as those that are more speculative. The absence of a chapter on a given mechanism/pathway should not be construed to imply that we place any less importance on such than on what is included in this section. In the second section, chapters on traditional animal models of asthma, inbred animal models of hyperreactivity, and genetically altered mice are provided. Transgenic and gene-ablated mice are a powerful tool for probing the mechanisms of disease. As candidate genes for asthma are identified, new mouse models using these techniques will be invaluable in assessing the role of a given pathway in the pathogenesis of asthma.

As published genetic studies of asthma begin to accumulate, the reader must be aware of the issues surrounding how the data are obtained and analyzed. For this reason, the third section was included, in which the techniques for carrying out genetic studies of complex diseases are presented and critiqued. The chapters describe molecular approaches as well as the statistical and analytical methods commonly employed. In the fourth section, the genetics of human asthma are presented. The chapters cover broad issues such as the epidemiology of asthma, phenotyping asthmatic subjects, and study design. In addition, the results of specific genetic studies of the allergic response, serum IgE, bronchial hyperresponsiveness, and asthma are presented in detail.

We would like to thank our families for their patience during preparation of this volume, our contributors and staff, and Dr. Claude Lenfant, for his support and assistance.

Stephen B. Liggett
Deborah A. Meyers

CONTRIBUTORS

Hans Albertsen, Ph.D.   Huntsman Cancer Institute, Eccles Institute of Human Genetics, University of Utah, Salt Lake City, Utah

Pamela J. Amelung, M.D.   Assistant Professor, Department of Medicine, University of Maryland School of Medicine, Baltimore, Maryland

Eugene R. Bleecker, M.D.   Professor, Department of Medicine, University of Maryland School of Medicine, Baltimore, Maryland

Malcolm N. Blumenthal, M.D.   Director, Section of Allergy, Department of Medicine, Medical School, University of Minnesota, Minneapolis, Minnesota

William W. Busse, M.D.   Professor, Department of Medicine, University of Wisconsin Medical School, Madison, Wisconsin

William J. Calhoun, M.D.   Associate Professor of Medicine, Department of Pulmonary, Allergy, and Critical Care Medicine, University of Pittsburgh, Pittsburgh, Pennsylvania

William O. C. M. Cookson, M.D., Ph.D.   Wellcome Senior Clinical Research Fellow, Nuffield Department of Medicine, John Radcliffe Hospital, Oxford, England

Primal de Lanerolle, Ph.D. Associate Professor, Department of Physiology and Biophysics, College of Medicine, University of Illinois at Chicago, Chicago, Illinois

Jeffrey M. Drazen, M.D. Chief, Department of Pulmonary and Critical Care Medicine, Brigham and Women's Hospital, and Professor of Medicine, Harvard Medical School, Boston, Massachusetts

Susan L. Ewart, D.V.M., Ph.D. Assistant Professor, Large Animal Clinical Sciences, Michigan State University, East Lansing, Michigan

Claire M. Fraser, Ph.D. Institute for Genomic Research, Gaithersburg, Maryland

Erwin W. Gelfand, M.D. Chairman, Department of Pediatrics, National Jewish Center for Immunology and Respiratory Medicine, Denver, Colorado

James E. Gern, M.D. Assistant Professor, Department of Pediatrics, University of Wisconsin Medical School, Madison, Wisconsin

Stephen W. Glasser, Ph.D. Associate Professor, Division of Pulmonary Biology, Department of Pediatrics, Children's Hospital Medical Center, Cincinnati, Ohio

Stuart A. Green, M.D. Assistant Professor of Medicine, Division of Pulmonary and Critical Care Medicine, University of Cincinnati College of Medicine, Cincinnati, Ohio

Joanna Groden, Ph.D. Assistant Professor, Department of Molecular Genetics, University of Cincinnati College of Medicine, Cincinnati, Ohio

Thomas R. Korfhagen, M.D., Ph.D. Associate Professor, Division of Pulmonary Biology, Department of Pediatrics, Children's Hospital Medical Center, Cincinnati, Ohio

Gary L. Larsen, M.D. Senior Faculty Member, Department of Pediatrics, National Jewish Center for Immunology and Respiratory Medicine, and Professor and Head, Section of Pediatric Pulmonary Medicine, University of Colorado School of Medicine, Denver, Colorado

Roy Clifford Levitt, M.D. Director, Magaining Institute of Molecular Medicine, Plymouth Meeting, Pennsylvania

Stephen B. Liggett, M.D. Professor of Medicine, Molecular Genetics, and Pharmacology, and Chief, Division of Pulmonary and Critical Care Medicine, University of Cincinnati College of Medicine, Cincinnati, Ohio

Deborah A. Meyers, Ph.D. Associate Professor of Medicine and Epidemiology, Center for Medical Genetics, Johns Hopkins University School of Medicine, Baltimore, Maryland.

Newton E. Morton, Ph.D. CRC Genetic Epidemiology Research Group, and Department of Child Health, University of Southampton and Princess Anne Hospital, Southampton, England

Philip Padrid, D.V.M. Assistant Professor of Medicine, Immunology, and Comparative Medicine and Pathology, Department of Medicine, University of Chicago, Chicago, Illinois

Carolien I. M. Panhuysen, M.D. Postdoctoral Fellow, Department of Medicine, University of Maryland School of Medicine, Baltimore, Maryland

Richard J. Paul, Ph.D. Professor, Department of Molecular and Cellular Physiology, University of Cincinnati College of Medicine, Cincinnati, Ohio

D. S. Postma, M.D., Ph.D. Professor, Department of Pulmonary Medicine, University Hospital, Groningen, The Netherlands

Stephen S. Rich, Ph.D. Professor, Department of Public Health Sciences (Epidemiology), Bowman Gray School of Medicine, Winston-Salem, North Carolina

Lanny J. Rosenwasser, M.D. Head, Allergy–Clinical Immunology, Department of Medicine, National Jewish Center for Immunology and Respiratory Medicine, Denver, Colorado

Jonathan M. Samet, M.D., M.S. Professor and Chairman, Department of Epidemiology, School of Hygiene and Public Health, Johns Hopkins University, Baltimore, Maryland

Alan F. Scott, Ph.D. Associate Professor, Department of Medicine and Center for Medical Genetics, Johns Hopkins University School of Medicine, Baltimore, Maryland

Richard L. Stevens, Ph.D. Associate Professor, Department of Medicine, Harvard Medical School, Boston, Massachusetts

Donata Vercelli, M.D. Chief, Molecular Immunoregulation Unit, San Raffaele Scientific Institute, Milan, Italy

Scott T. Weiss, M.D., M.S. Associate Professor of Medicine, Channing Laboratory, Boston, Massachusetts

Jeffrey A. Whitsett, M.D. Professor of Pediatrics, and Director, Divisions of Neonatology and Pulmonary Biology, Department of Pediatrics, Children's Hospital Medical Center, Cincinnati, Ohio

Denise G. Wiesch, M.P.H.   Research Associate, Department of Epidemiology, School of Hygiene and Public Health, Johns Hopkins University, Baltimore, Maryland

Jianfeng Xu, Dr.P.H.   Johns Hopkins University School of Medicine, Baltimore, Maryland

CONTENTS

Part One

CRITICAL PATHWAYS IN ASTHMA:
POTENTIAL FOR GENETIC REGULATION

1

Potential Genetic Alterations in the 5-Lipoxygenase Pathway in Asthma

JEFFREY M. DRAZEN

Brigham and Women's Hospital
and Harvard Medical School
Boston, Massachusetts

I. Introduction

Among the biochemical pathways that produce substances thought to be of importance in modulating airway tone in patients with asthma is the 5-lipoxygenase pathway [1–3]. This is the series of biochemical reactions that result in the production of the leukotrienes (LTs) from arachidonic acid liberated from membrane phospholipids. In this chapter we review the biochemical pathways leading to the formation of both the cysteinyl LTs (LTC$_4$, LTD$_4$, and LTE$_4$) and the dihydroxy LT (LTB$_4$); why the 5-lipoxygenase pathway is important in asthma; and what we know about potential allelic polymorphisms in the enzymes of this pathway that can alter enzyme function so as to influence asthma. Although *the potential for genetic modification of the 5-lipoxygenase pathway exists* in asthma, polymorphisms in the various components of the pathway or its control elements that lead to altered function or activity of the pathway have not yet been identified.

II. Biosynthesis of the Leukotrienes

Specific details of the synthetic pathways for the LTs have been provided in authoritative reviews [4,5]; only a brief outline is given here. The unique structural requirements for LT action [6,7] make it unlikely that there are significant, genetically based differences in the structure of the leukotrienes per se that could contribute to the biology of asthma.

A. Release of Arachidonic Acid

The first step in the formation of the LTs is the liberation of the biochemical substrate from which the LTs are derived, namely, arachidonic acid, from membrane phospholipids [4,8,9], Fig. 1. Arachidonic acid (5,8,11,14-*cis*-eicosatetraenoic acid) is a fatty acid commonly found esterified in the *sn*-1 and *sn*-2 positions of membrane phospholipids. In the course of cellular activation, such as transmembrane signaling [9,10], antigen–antibody reactions [11], or the action of inflammatory enzymes [12–16], arachidonic acid is released from membrane phospholipids, most likely in perinuclear membranes [15,17], by the action of phospholipases. These enzymes cleave arachidonic acid esterified in the *sn*-2 position from the triglyceride backbone of membrane phospholipids. Once arachi-

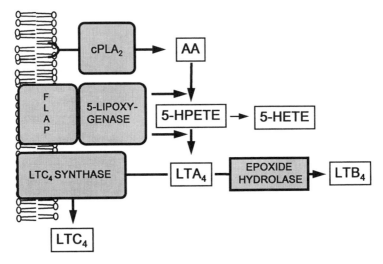

Figure 1 Schematic diagram of the enzymes involved in the formation of the cysteinyl leukotrienes. cPLA$_2$ = cytosolic phospholipase A$_2$, FLAP = 5-lipoxygenase activating protein, AA = arachidonic acid, LTA$_4$ = leukotriene A$_4$, LTC$_4$ = leukotriene C$_4$. The perinuclear membrane is represented schematically by the bilayered structure.

donic acid is liberated, LTs are produced by cells with the necessary enzymatic capacity needed to produce these products. Such cells possess a number of critical enzymes and co-factors including 5-lipoxygenase (5-LO), 5-lipoxygenase-activating protein (FLAP), LTC_4 synthase, LTA_4 epoxide hydrolase, and a specific membrane transport system for the LTs.

B. Synthesis of Leukotrienes from Arachidonic Acid

The biosynthesis of the dihydroxy or cysteinyl leukotrienes results from the repeated action of 5-LO on arachidonic acid, to yield first 5-hydroperoxy eicosatetraenoic acid (5-HPETE) and second the unstable epoxide known as LTA_4 (5,6-oxido-7,9-*trans*-11,14-*cis*-eicosatetraenoic acid; Fig. 1). In the presence of LTC_4 synthase, glutathione is adducted at the C-6 position of the eicosanoid backbone to yield the molecule known as LTC_4 [5(S)-hydroxy, 6(R)-gluta-thionyl-7,9-*trans*-11,14-*cis*-eicosatetraenoic acid]. The LTC_4 so formed is ex-ported from the cytosol to the extracellular microenvironment, where the glutamic acid moiety is cleaved by γ-glutamyl transpeptidase to form LTD_4 [5(S)-hydroxy, 6(R)-cysteinyl-glycyl-7, 9-*trans*-11,14-*cis*-eicosatetraenoic acid]. LTD_4 exerts its effects through action at a specific receptor known as the $cysLT_1$ receptor, which can transduce a variety of biological actions including constriction of airway smooth muscle. The removal of the glycine moiety from LTD_4 by a variety of dipeptidases results in the formation of LTE_4 [5(S)-hydroxy, 6(R)-cysteinyl-7, 9-*trans*-11,14-*cis*-eicosatetraenoic acid], a molecule with a spectrum of biologic activities similar to that of LTD_4, but which is diminished in biopotency by 30- to 100-fold. As will be reviewed later, there is reason to believe that the cysteinyl LTs play an important role in the asthmatic response [18,19].

LTB$_4$ is derived from LTA_4 through the action of a bifunctional enzyme known as epoxide hydrolase. In the intracellular microenvironment, water and molecular oxygen are adducted to LTA_4 to form LTB_4 [5(S),12(R)-dihydroxy-6, 14-*cis*-8,10-*trans*-eicosatetraenoic acid]. LTB_4 exerts its biochemical actions pre-dominantly as a proinflammatory chemotactic molecule at specific receptors.

III. Biological Role of the Leukotrienes in Asthma

Interest in the importance of the leukotrienes as potential mediators of the asth-matic response derives from the observation that the cysteinyl leukotrienes are potent airway contractile agonists and can promote the leakage of intravascular tracers into the extravascular space [20–24]. The potential of LTB_4 as an asthmatic mediator derives from its capacity to function as a chemotactic moiety [18]. Detailed reviews of these biological properties have been published [25,26]; specific aspects of leukotriene biology related to asthma are reviewed below.

A. Evidence for In-Vivo Production of the Leukotrienes

Among the four major lines of evidence implicating the cysteinyl leukotrienes in the biology of asthma (see Table 1), one of the most important pieces of evidence is that LTE_4 can be recovered from the urine in enhanced amounts after induced asthmatic responses. Since it has been established [27–29] that 5–15% of exogenously administered cysteinyl leukotriene is LTE_4, urinary LTE_4 excretion is considered an index of endogenous cysteinyl leukotriene production. Taylor and co-workers recovered increased amounts of LTE_4 from the urine in the early phase after inhalational antigen challenge [30]. This finding has been replicated by a number of other investigative groups [30–36]. In some cases investigators show a positive correlation between the magnitude of the airway responses to antigen challenge and the amount of LTE_4 recovered in the urine [31]. In patients with aspirin-induced asthma, the baseline urinary LTE_4 excretion rates are high, and aspirin challenge results in a substantial increase in urinary LTE_4 excretion [34,37–41]. Urinary LTE_4 excretion is elevated in about two-thirds of patients seeking emergency treatment of asthma and in all with reversible airway narrowing [42]. These data clearly indicate endogenous production of the leukotrienes during induced or spontaneous asthma.

B. Evidence for Leukotrienes as Endogenous Biomolecules Regulating Airway Tone

Patients with moderate to severe asthma develop airway obstruction if their regular treatment with bronchodilator medications is withheld. Investigators interested in the role of leukotrienes in spontaneous airway narrowing in asthma have used the strategy of inducing airway obstruction in asthmatic patients by withholding treatment and then administering agents that can either prevent the action of LTD_4 at its receptor or prevent the formation of the leukotrienes by inhibition of 5-LO [43–47]. In each case, interference with the action of 5-LO products resulted

Table 1   Evidence of a Role for Leukotrienes in Asthma

1. Eosinophils and mast cells, found in high numbers in asthmatic airways, can synthesize cysteinyl leukotrienes.
2. Leukotrienes have a spectrum of biological effects consistent with mediation of abnormalities in asthma.
3. Leukotrienes can be recovered in biological fluids during induced and spontaneous asthma.
4. Agents that can block action of leukotrienes at their receptors or inhibit formation of leukotrienes ameliorate induced or spontaneous asthma.

in an improvement in airway function. This effect occurs only in patients with asthma of moderate or greater severity; normal subjects or individuals with mild asthma do not exhibit such an effect.

In patients with mild, chronic, stable asthma, inhibition of the action of LTD_4 at the $cysLT_1$ receptor or of the formation of leukotrienes results in improvement in airway function and asthma symptoms [47,48]. Therefore spontaneous airway narrowing in asthma derives, in part, from the endogenous production of leukotrienes, which may possibly reflect upregulation of one or more of the enzymes in this pathway. Given these observations, there is good reason to investigate possible genetic variations in the components of the pathway that are responsible for leukotriene biosynthesis.

IV. Enzymes Involved in Leukotriene Biosynthesis: Review of Their Molecular Structure and Evidence for Genetic Variance

A. Cytosolic Phospholipase A_2

Among the forms of phospholipase A_2 that are potentially involved in the synthesis of leukotrienes [9,10,49–51], the cytosolic form ($cPLA_2$) is most likely to be of importance. The importance of this form of PLA_2 derives from the fact that it functions in the cytosol rather than in the extracellular microenvironment. Indeed, studies of the protein derived from expression of a cDNA containing the enzyme's coding sequence demonstrate that $cPLA_2$ contains structural elements homologous to the C2 region of protein kinase C, that it selectively cleaves arachidonic acid from membrane vesicles, and that it translocates from cytosolic fractions to membrane vesicular fractions in the presence of the concentrations of calcium found intercellularly after cell activation [15,16]. Indeed, $cPLA_2$ phosphorylation, initiated by transmembrane signaling events, results in an upregulation of the catalytic activity of the enzyme [14,52]. Additional evidence for the uniqueness of this enzyme, distinct from other forms of PLA_2 such as secretory PLA_2 ($sPLA_2$), derives from the comparison of the responses of Chinese hamster ovary (CHO) cells transfected with either a cDNA-encoding $cPLA_2$ or a cDNA-encoding $sPLA_2$. Activation of these transfected cells by ATP or thrombin results in enhanced catalytic activity for arachidonic acid only in the CHO cells transfected with the $cPLA_2$ cDNA [16]. Furthermore, recent studies have shown that $cPLA_2$ is translocated to the perinuclear membrane upon cellular activation [15], which is of particular importance because, as outlined below, FLAP and LTC_4 synthase are both integral perinuclear membrane proteins and probably act in concert to promote the biosynthesis of LTs.

$cPLA_2$ is a 100- to 110-kDa protein (by SDS-PAGE) originally purified from the human monocytic cell line U937; it is distinguished from secretory forms of PLA_2 by its molecular size, its dithiothreitol resistance, and its activity at calcium concentrations consistent with the intracellular microenvironment [53,54]. The enzyme has been molecularly cloned, and the cDNAs isolated encode a 749-amino acid protein with a putative molecular mass of 85.2 kDa [55,56]. The genomic structure of $cPLA_2$ is not known, nor is it known whether more than one form of this enzyme exists in the genome; evidence for genetic variation in this enzyme has not been obtained.

B. 5-Lipoxygenase

5-LO (EC 1.13.11.34) is the enzyme responsible for the first two steps of biosynthesis of LTs. It is a calcium-, ATP-, and non-heme iron-requiring enzyme. Complementary DNAs for this enzyme, on the order of 2.7 kb in molecular size, are known to encode a 674-amino acid protein with a calculated molecular mass of approximately 78,000 [57,58]. Messenger RNA encoding for 5-LO is found in leukocytes in the lung as well as in a variety of other organs. In isolated cell lines, the enzyme and its mRNA are present only when the cells are stimulated, a fact consistent with the hypothesis that 5-LO activity is transcriptionally regulated. Upon cellular activation, 5-LO and the cytosolic form of phospholipase A2 can translate from the cytosol to the perinuclear membrane [59,60].

The 5-LO gene has been isolated and spans a region of the genome encompassing approximately 85 kb [61,62]. The coding sequence for 5-LO is contained within 14 exons, the longest of which is 613 base pairs. Primer extension analysis indicates that the transcription start site is at a thymidine residue 65 base pairs upstream from the initiation codon. The gene promoter region has no TATA or CCAAT elements but does have GC-rich region. Studies using chloramphenicol acetyltransferase assays show regions within the gene promoter sequence with both positive and negative regulatory effects.

To date, polymorphisms in the 5-LO gene have not been reported. However, because of the critical nature of the histidines found at locations 357, 372, and 550, and the glutamic acid found at 376, genetic regulation of enzyme activity is possible [63,64].

C. 5-Lipoxygenase-Activating Protein (FLAP)

Although 5-LO is a cytosolic enzyme, it had to be translocated from the cytosol to a membrane fraction to be catalytically active, yet the mechanism by which this activation occurred was not clarified until the isolation of FLAP [65]. FLAP is an 18-kDa integral membrane protein that binds 5-LO in the presence of Ca^{2+}; since intracellular Ca^{2+} concentrations increase with cellular activation, the binding of 5-LO by FLAP provides a mechanism by which leukotriene synthesis can be initiated [66].

The critical importance of FLAP in regulating the synthesis of the leukotrienes was first demonstrated in osteogenic sarcoma cells in culture. These cells possess neither 5-LO nor FLAP and hence are not capable of producing leukotrienes when activated. When these cells are transfected with a cDNA that encodes only 5-LO and are stimulated with the calcium ionophore A23187, they do not produce leukotrienes. However, when cells are transfected with both FLAP and 5-LO, they acquire the capacity to synthesize leukotrienes with appropriate stimulation [65,67].

FLAP, by virtue of its three hydrophobic membrane-spanning domains, integrates into plasma membranes [68,69]. Immunoelectron microscopic localization studies have shown that FLAP is localized to the perinuclear membrane of human leukocytes; when cells containing 5-LO and FLAP are activated, 5-LO also localizes to the perinuclear membrane [15,17]. FLAP's specific binding of a radio- and photoaffinity-labeled analog of arachidonic acid, L-739,059, is inhibited by arachidonic acid, a finding consistent with the hypothesis that FLAP binds arachidonic acid [68]. Studies using proteolytic fragments of FLAP have localized the binding of inhibitors of FLAP action to a site in the hydrophilic loop between the first and second transmembrane domains. The co-localization of $cPLA_2$ and FLAP to the perinuclear membrane and the ability of FLAP to bind arachidonic acid provide a physical locus where arachidonic acid can be cleaved from phospholipids by $cPLA_2$ and subsequently transferred to 5-LO.

Since FLAP is present in all cell types known to synthesize leukotrienes and is absent from cells without this capacity [70], FLAP is a potential site for genetic variation in the capacity to activate the LT pathway. The FLAP gene, spanning greater than 31 kb of genomic DNA, contains five small exons and four large introns; analysis of restriction maps of the FLAP gene are consistent with the hypothesis that there is only a single FLAP gene. Although an allelic polymorphism, in intron II of the FLAP gene, is present at high frequency in the normal population [66], allelic polymorphisms in FLAP related to asthmatic conditions have not been identified.

D. LTC$_4$ Synthase

LTC_4 synthase, the enzyme that catalyzes the adduction of glutathione to the C6 position of LTA_4, was the last of the enzymes in the cysteinyl leukotriene pathway to have its molecular structure elucidated [71]. It is a small, ~17-kDa, highly hydrophobic integral membrane protein [72–74] with substantial homology to FLAP. The cDNA for LTC_4 synthase contains a 450-base pair open reading frame encoding a putative protein of 150 amino acids with a deduced molecular mass of 16.5 kDa [71]. At present the gene structure for LTC_4 synthase is not known, nor have the regulatory elements upstream of the transcription start site been delineated. Furthermore, the presence of allelic polymorphism within the population for LTC_4 synthase is not known.

E. LTA_4 Hydrolase

LTA_4 Hydrolase (EC 3.3.2.6) catalyzes conversion of LTA_4 to LTB_4 in the intracellular microenvironment [75]. In conditions found in the extracellular microenvironment, this enzyme can also function as an amino peptidase, although its endogenous substrates are not known [76–78]. LTA_4 hydrolase is a 50-kDa (by SDS-PAGE) enzyme that requires zinc for catalytic hydrolase activity. The mRNA for LTA_4 hydrolase has been found in cells retrieved from human lung by bronchoalveolar lavage [79].

Genetic control of cytosolic LTA_4 hydrolase activity has been studied in unstimulated lymphocytes from normal human subjects [80]. Activity was measured in cells obtained from six sets of monozygotic twins, six sets of dizygotic twins, 100 unrelated male subjects, and six families. The variability in activity, defined as the coefficient of variance, was least in the monozygotic twins, over 22-fold higher in the dizygotic twins, and 40-fold higher in the 100 unrelated male subjects. A member of one of the families had extremely high LTA_4 hydrolase activity; hence other members of that family were phenotyped. Segregation analysis of the data was consistent with single-gene, autosomal-dominant transmission of this activity. However, analysis of LTA_4 hydrolase activity in the other five families, which was not as high to begin with, and in the 12 sets of twins, was unable to distinguish between a monogenic and a polygenic inheritance pattern for LTA_4 hydrolase activity. The molecular basis of this difference in hydrolase action, and its importance in asthma, have yet to be established.

F. γ-Glutamyl Transpeptidase

Once LTC_4 is transported from the intracellular to the extracellular microenvironment [81], the glutamic acid moiety is cleaved by γ-glutamyl transpeptidase (EC 2.3.2.2.; γ-GT) to form LTD_4. LTD_4 is the preferred ligand for the $CysLT_1$ receptor in guinea pigs [20] and human U937 cells [82], although both LTC_4 and LTD_4 can activate this receptor in human lung tissues [83]. There is a distinct form of γ-GT in human lung [84], but its role in cysteinyl leukotriene processing is not known. Current data suggest that there are multiple copies of γ-GT in the human genome [85]. Although allelic polymorphism in γ-GT is likely [84], its importance relative to asthma is not known.

V. Leukotriene Receptors

At present, leukotriene receptors have been categorized functionally but not on a molecular level. Data from studies using pharmacological antagonists suggest that there may be two distinct receptors for cysteinyl [86] LTs and one receptor for LTB_4 [87]. These receptors are known as the $CysLT_1$, $CysLT_2$, and BLT receptors, respectively. Studies in tissues isolated from normal and asthmatic subjects have not suggested differences in the sensitivity, affinity, or reversibility of bronchoconstriction elicited by activation of leukotriene receptors from either normal or asthmatic subjects [83,88,89]. It seems unlikely, based on current information, that variations in leukotriene receptor activity are responsible for variations in biological responses to leukotrienes, but we can make no definitive statement until molecular cloning of these receptors allows specific review of receptor structure and potential polymorphisms.

VI. Summary

Interest in the importance of the leukotrienes as mediators of asthma evolves from a number of distinct lines of evidence. Although a role for the leukotrienes in the biology of asthma is well established, we do not know whether genetic alterations in the control of the enzymatic pathway are involved in asthma. Only minimal information on allelic polymorphism among the leukotriene-forming enzymes in normal and asthmatic subjects is available; this may prove a fruitful area for investigative work.

References

1. Kaliner M. Asthma and mast cell activation. J Allergy Clin Immunol 1989; 83: 510–520.
2. Holgate S. Mediator and cytokine mechanisms in asthma. Thorax 1993; 48:103–109.
3. Busse WW, Gaddy JN. The role of leukotriene antagonists and inhibitors in the treatment of airway disease. Am Rev Respir Dis 1991; 143:S103–S107.
4. Samuelsson B. Leukotrienes: mediators of immediate hypersensitivity reactions and inflammation. Science 1983; 220:568–575.
5. Lewis RA, Austen KF, Soberman RJ. Leukotrienes and other products of the 5-lipoxygenase pathway. Biochemistry and relation to pathobiology in human diseases. N Engl J Med 1990; 323:645–655.
6. Lewis RA, Drazen JM, Austen KF, et al. Contractile activities of structural analogs of leukotrienes C and D: role of the polar substituents. Proc Natl Acad Sci USA 1981; 78:4579–4583.
7. Drazen JM, Lewis RA, Austen KF, et al. Contractile activities of structural analogs of leukotrienes C and D: necessity of a hydrophobic region. Proc Natl Acad Sci USA 1981; 78:3195–3198.
8. Samuelsson B, Dahlen SE, Lindgren JA, Rouzer CA, Serhan CN. Leukotrienes and lipoxins: structures, biosynthesis, and biological effects. Science 1987; 237: 1171–1176.

9. Dennis EA, Rhee SG, Billah MM, Hannun YA. Role of phospholipase in generating lipid second messengers in signal transduction. FASEB J 1991; 5:2068–2077.

10. Ferguson JE, Hanley MR. The role of phospholipases and phospholipid-derived signals in cell activation. Curr Opin Cell Biol 1991; 3:206–212.

11. Peters SP, MacGlashan DW Jr, Schleimer RP, Hayes EC, Adkinson NF Jr, Lichtenstein LM. The modulation of the release of arachidonic acid metabolites from purified human lung mast cells. Am Rev Respir Dis 1985; 132:367–373.

12. Weiss J, Wright G. Mobilization and function of extracellular phospholipase A_2 in inflammation. Adv Exp Med Biol 1990; 275:103–113.

13. White SR, Strek ME, Kulp GVP, et al. Regulation of human eosinophil degranulation and activation by endogenous phospholipase-A_2. J Clin Invest 1993; 91:2118–2125.

14. Kramer RM, Roberts EF, Manetta JV, Hyslop PA, Jakubowski JA. Thrombin-induced phosphorylation and activation of CA(2+)-sensitive cytosolic phospholipase A2 in human platelets. J Biol Chem 1993; 268:26796–26804.

15. Peters-Golden M, McNish RW. Redistribution of 5-lipoxygenase and cytosolic phospholipase A2 to the nuclear fraction upon macrophage activation. Biochem Biophys Res Commun 1993; 196:147–153.

16. Lin LL, Lin AY, Knopf JL. Cytosolic phospholipase A2 is coupled to hormonally regulated release of arachidonic acid. Proc Natl Acad Sci USA 1992; 89:6147–6151.

17. Woods JW, Evans JF, Ethier D, et al. 5-Lipoxygenase and 5-lipoxygenase activating protein are localized in the nuclear envelope of activated human leukocytes. J Exp Med 1993; 178:1935–1946.

18. Lewis RA, Goetzl EJ, Drazen JM, Soter NA, Austen KF, Corey EJ. Functional characterization of synthetic leukotriene B and its stereochemical isomers. J Exp Med 1981; 154:1243–1248.

19. Miki I, Watanabe T, Nakamura M, et al. Solubilization and characterization of leukotriene B4 receptor-GTP binding protein complex from porcine spleen. Biochem Biophys Res Commun 1990; 166:342–348.

20. Drazen JM, Austen KF, Lewis RA, et al. Comparative airway and vascular activities of leukotrienes C-1 and D in vivo and in vitro. Proc Natl Acad Sci USA 1980; 77: 4354–4358.

21. Dahlen SE, Hedqvist P, Hammarstrom S, Samuelsson B. Leukotrienes are potent constrictors of human bronchi. Nature 1980; 288:484–486.

22. Holroyde MC, Altounyan RE, Cole M, Dixon M, Elliott EV. Bronchoconstriction produced in man by leukotrienes C and D. Lancet 1981; 2:17–18.

23. Weiss JW, Drazen JM, Coles N, et al. Bronchoconstrictor effects of leukotriene C in humans. Science 1982; 216:196–198.

24. Hui KP, Lotvall J, Chung KF, Barnes PJ. Attenuation of inhaled allergen-induced airway microvascular leakage and airflow obstruction in guinea pigs by a 5-lipoxygenase inhibitor (A-63162). Am Rev Respir Dis 1991; 143:1015–1019.

25. Piper PJ. Formation and actions of leukotrienes. Physiol Rev 1984; 64:744–761.

26. Piper PJ. Leukotrienes and the airways. Eur J Anaesthesiol 1989; 6:241–255.

27. Orning L, Kaijser L, Hammarstrom S. In vivo metabolism of leukotriene C4 in man: urinary excretion of leukotriene E4. Biochem Biophys Res Commun 1985; 130: 214–220.

28. Sala A, Voelkel N, Maclouf J, Murphy RC. Leukotriene E4 elimination and metabolism in normal human subjects. J Biol Chem 1990; 265:21771–21778.
29. Maclouf J, Antoine C, Decaterina R, et al. Entry rate and metabolism of leukotriene C-4 into vascular compartment in healthy subjects. Am J Physiol 1992; 263:H244–H249.
30. Taylor GW, Taylor I, Black P, et al. Urinary leukotriene E4 after antigen challenge and in acute asthma and allergic rhinitis. Lancet 1989; 1:584–588.
31. Sladek K, Dworski R, Fitzgerald GA, et al. Allergen-stimulated release of thromboxane A2 and leukotriene E4 in humans. Effect of indomethacin. Am Rev Respir Dis 1990; 141:1441–1445.
32. Tagari P, Rasmussen JB, Delorme D, et al. Comparison of urinary leukotriene E4 and 16-carboxytetranordihydro leukotriene E4 excretion in allergic asthmatics after inhaled antigen. Eicosanoids 1990; 3:75–80.
33. Manning PJ, Rokach J, Malo JL, et al. Urinary leukotriene E4 levels during early and late asthmatic responses. J Allergy Clin Immunol 1990; 86:211–220.
34. Kumlin M, Dahlen B, Bjorck T, Zetterstrom O, Granstrom E, Dahlen SE. Urinary excretion of leukotriene-E4 and 11-dehydro-thromboxane-B2 in response to bronchial provocations with allergen, aspirin, leukotriene-D4, and histamine in asthmatics. Am Rev Respir Dis 1992; 146:96–103.
35. Westcott JY, Smith HR, Wenzel SE, et al. Urinary leukotriene-E4 in patients with asthma—effect of airways reactivity and sodium cromoglycate. Am Rev Respir Dis 1991; 143:1322–1328.
36. Smith CM, Christie PE, Hawksworth RJ, Thien F, Lee TH. Urinary leukotriene-E4 levels after allergen and exercise challenge in bronchial asthma. Am Rev Respir Dis 1991; 144:1411–1413.
37. Christie PE, Tagari P, Fordhutchinson AW, et al. Urinary leukotriene-E4 concentrations increase after aspirin challenge in aspirin-sensitive asthmatic subjects. Am Rev Respir Dis 1991; 143:1025–1029.
38. Knapp HR, Sladek K, Fitzgerald GA. Increased excretion of leukotriene-E4 during aspirin-induced asthma. J Lab Clin Med 1992; 119:48–51.
39. Israel E, Fischer AR, Rosenberg MA, et al. The pivotal role of 5-lipoxygenase products in the reaction of aspirin-sensitive asthmatics to aspirin. Am Rev Respir Dis 1993; 148:1447–1451.
40. Lee TH, Smith CM, Arm JP, Christie PE. Mediator release in aspirin-induced reactions. J Allergy Clin Immunol 1991; 88:827–829.
41. Dahlen B, Margolskee DJ, Zetterstrom O, Dahlen SE. Effect of the leukotriene receptor antagonist MK-0679 on baseline pulmonary function in aspirin sensitive asthmatic subjects. Thorax 1993; 48:1205–1210.
42. Drazen JM, Obrien J, Sparrow D, et al. Recovery of leukotriene-E4 from the urine of patients with airway obstruction. Am Rev Respir Dis 1992; 146:104–108.
43. Gaddy JN, Margolskee DJ, Bush RK, Williams VC, Busse WW. Bronchodilation with a potent and selective leukotriene D4 (LTD4) antagonist (MK-571) in patients with asthma. Am Rev Respir Dis 1992; 146:358–363.
44. Hui KP, Barnes NC. Lung Function improvement in asthma with a cysteinyl-leukotriene receptor antagonist. Lancet 1991; 337:1062–1063.

45. Impens N, Reiss TF, Teahan JA, et al. Acute bronchodilation with an intravenously administered leukotriene-D(4) antagonist, MK-679. Am Rev Respir Dis 1993; 147: 1442–1446.

46. Lammers JW, Van Daele P, Van den Elshout FM, et al. Bronchodilator properties of an inhaled leukotriene D4 antagonist (verlukast—MK-0679) in asthmatic patients. Pulm Pharmacol 1992; 5:121–125.

47. Israel E, Rubin P, Kemp JP, et al. The effect of inhibition of 5-lipoxygenase by zileuton in mild to moderate asthma. Ann Intern Med 1993; 119:1059–1066.

48. Cloud ML, Enas GC, Kemp J, et al. A specific LTD4/LTE4-receptor antagonist improves pulmonary function in patients with mild, chronic asthma. Am Rev Respir Dis 1989; 140:1336–1339.

49. Waite M. Phospholipases, enzymes that share a substrate class. Adv Exp Med Biol 1990; 279:1–22.

50. van den Bosch H, Aarsman AJ, van Schaik RH, Schalkwijk CG, Neijs FW, Sturk A. Structural and enzymological properties of cellular phospholipases A2. Biochem Soc Trans 1990; 18:781–785.

51. Kaiser E, Chiba P, Zaky K. Phospholipases in biology and medicine. Clin Biochem 1990; 23:349–370.

52. Lin LL, Wartmann M, Lin AY, Knopf JL, Seth A, Davis RJ. cPLA2 is phosphorylated and activated by MAP kinase. Cell 1993; 72:269–278.

53. Kramer RM, Roberts EF, Manetta J, Putnam JE. The $Ca_2(+)$-sensitive cytosolic phospholipase A2 is a 100-kDa protein in human monoblast U937 cells. J Biol Chem 1991; 266:5268–5272.

54. Clark JD, Milona N, Knopf JL. Purification of a 110-kilodalton cytosolic phospholipase A2 from the human monocytic cell line U937. Proc Natl Acad Sci USA 1990; 87:7708–7712.

55. Sharp JD, White DL, Chiou XG, et al. Molecular cloning and expression of human CA(2+)-sensitive cytosolic phospholipase A2. J Biol Chem 1991; 266:14850–14853.

56. Clark JD, Lin LL, Kriz RW, et al. A novel arachidonic acid-selective cytosolic PLA2 contains a Ca(2+)-dependent translocation domain with homology to PKC and GAP. Cell 1991; 65:1043–1051.

57. Matsumoto T, Funk CD, Radmark O, Hoog JO, Jornvall H, Samuelsson B. Molecular cloning and amino acid sequence of human 5-lipoxygenase [published erratum appears in Proc Natl Acad Sci USA 1988 May; 85(10):3406]. Proc Natl Acad Sci USA 1988; 85:26–30.

58. Dixon RA, Jones RE, Diehl RE, Bennett CD, Kargman S, Rouzer CA. Cloning of the cDNA for human 5-lipoxygenase. Proc Natl Acad Sci USA 1988; 85:416–420.

59. Coffey M, Petersgolden M, Fantone JC, Sporn PHS. Membrane Association of active 5-lipoxygenase in resting cells—evidence for novel regulation of the enzyme in the rat alveolar macrophage. J Biol Chem 1992; 267:570–576.

60. Malaviya R, Jakschik BA. Reversible translocation of 5-lipoxygenase in mast cells upon IgE/antigen stimulation. J Biol Chem 1993; 268:4939–4944.

61. Funk CD, Hoshiko S, Matsumoto T, Rdmark O, Samuelsson B. Characterization of the human 5-lipoxygenase gene. Proc Natl Acad Sci USA 1989; 86:2587–2591.

62. Hoshiko S, Radmark O, Samuelsson B. Characterization of the human 5-lipoxygenase gene promoter. Proc Natl Acad Sci USA 1990; 87:9073–9077.
63. Zhang YY, Lind B, Radmark O, Samuelsson B. Iron content of human 5-lipoxygenase, effects of mutations regarding conserved histidine residues. J Biol Chem 1993; 268:2535–2541.
64. Ishii S, Noguchi M, Miyano M, Matsumoto T, Noma M. Mutagenesis studies on the amino acid residues involved in the iron-binding and the activity of human 5-lipoxygenase. Biochem Biophys Res Commun 1992; 182:1482–1490.
65. Dixon RA, Diehl RE, Opas E, et al. Requirement of a 5-lipoxygenase-activating protein for leukotriene synthesis. Nature 1990; 343:282–284.
66. Kennedy BP, Diehl RE, Boie Y, Adam M, Dixon RA. Gene characterization and promoter analysis of the human 5-lipoxygenase-activating protein (FLAP). J Biol Chem 1991; 266:8511–8516.
67. Miller DK, Gillard JW, Vickers PJ, et al. Identification and isolation of a membrane protein necessary for leukotriene production. Nature 1990; 343:278–281.
68. Mancini JA, Abramovitz M, Cox ME, et al. 5-Lipoxygenase-activating protein is an arachidonate binding protein. FEBS Lett 1993; 318:277–281.
69. Abramovitz M, Wong E, Cox ME, Richardson CD, Li C, Vickers PJ. 5-Lipoxygenase-activating protein stimulates the utilization of arachidonic acid by 5-lipoxygenase. Eur J Biochem 1993; 215:105–111.
70. Reid GK, Kargman S, Vickers PJ, et al. Correlation between expression of 5-lipoxygenase-activating protein, 5-lipoxygenase, and cellular leukotriene synthesis. J Biol Chem 1990; 265:19818–19823.
71. Lam BK, Penrose JF, Freeman GJ, Austen KF. Expression cloning of a cDNA for human leukotriene C4 synthase, a novel integrated membrane protein conjugating reduced glutathione to leukotriene A4. Proc Natl Acad Sci USA 1994; 91(16):7663–7667.
72. Penrose JF, Gagnon L, Goppeltstruebe M, et al. Purification of human leukotriene-C(4) synthase. Proc Natl Acad Sci USA 1992; 89:11603–11606.
73. Soderstrom M, Mannervik B, Garkov V, Hammarstrom S. On the nature of leukotriene-C4 synthase in human platelets. Arch Biochem Biophys 1992; 294:70–74.
74. Nicholson DW, Ali A, Klemba MW, Munday NA, Zamboni RJ, Fordhutchinson AW. Human leukotriene-C(4) synthase expression in dimethyl sulfoxide-differentiated U937 cells. J Biol Chem 1992; 267:17849–17857.
75. Medina JF, Radmark O, Funk CD, Haeggstrom JZ. Molecular cloning and expression of mouse leukotriene-A4 hydrolase cDNA. Biochem Biophys Res Commun 1991; 176:1516–1524.
76. Orning L, Gierse JK, Fitzpatrick FA. The bifunctional enzyme leukotriene-A(4) hydrolase is an arginine aminopeptidase of high efficiency and specificity. J Biol Chem 1994; 269:11269–11273.
77. Wetterholm A, Haeggstrom JZ. Leukotriene-A4 hydrolase—an anion activated peptidase. Biochim Biophys Acta 1992; 1123:275–281.
78. Wetterholm A, Medina JF, Radmark O, et al. Recombinant mouse leukotriene-A4 hydrolase—a zinc metalloenzyme with dual enzymatic activities. Biochim Biophys Acta 1991; 1080:96–102.

79. Munafo DA, Shindo K, Baker JR, Bigby TD. Leukotriene A(4) hydrolase in human bronchoalveolar lavage fluid. J Clin Invest 1994; 93:1042–1050.
80. Norris KK, DeAngelo TM, Vesell ES. Genetic and environmental factors that regulate cytosolic epoxide hydrolase activity in normal human lymphocytes. J Clin Invest 1989; 84:1749–1756.
81. Lam BK, Owen WF Jr, Austen KF, Soberman RJ. The identification of a distinct export step following the biosynthesis of leukotriene C4 by human eosinophils. J Biol Chem 1989; 264:12885–12889.
82. Wetmore LA, Gerard NP, Herron DK, et al. Leukotriene receptor on U-937 cells: discriminatory responses to leukotrienes C4 and D4. Am J Physiol 1991; 261:L164–L171.
83. Buckner CK, Krell RD, Laravuso RB, Coursin DB, Bernstein PR, Will JA. Pharmacological evidence that human intralobar airways do not contain different receptors that mediate contractions to leukotriene C4 and leukotriene D4. J Pharmacol Exp Ther 1986; 237:558–562.
84. Wetmore LA, Gerard C, Drazen JM. Human lung expresses unique gamma-glutamyl transpeptidase transcripts. Proc Natl Acad Sci USA 1993; 90:7461–7465.
85. Pawlak A, Lahuna O, Bulle F, et al. Gamma-glutamyl transpeptidase: a single copy gene in the rat and a multigene family in the human genome. J Biol Chem 1988; 263:9913–9916.
86. Snyder DW, Krell RD. Pharmacological evidence for a distinct leukotriene D4 receptor in guinea-pig trachea. J Pharmacol Exp Ther 1984; 231:616–622.
87. Herron DK, Goodson T, Bollinger NG, et al. Leukotriene-B4 receptor antagonists—the LY255283-series of hydroxyacetophenones. J Med Chem 1992; 35:1818–1828.
88. Bjorck T, Dahlen SE. Evidence indicating that leukotrienes C4, D4 and E4 are major mediators of contraction induced by anti-IgE in human bronchi. Agents Actions 1989; 26:87–89.
89. Bjorck T, Gustafsson LE, Dahlen SE. Isolated bronchi from asthmatics are hyperresponsive to adenosine, which apparently acts indirectly by liberation of leukotrienes and histamine. Am Rev Respir Dis 1992; 145:1087–1091.

2

Airway Hyperresponsiveness
Induction by T Cells

ERWIN W. GELFAND

National Jewish Center for
Immunology and Respiratory Medicine
Denver, Colorado

GARY L. LARSEN

National Jewish Center for
Immunology and Respiratory Medicine
and University of Colorado School of
Medicine
Denver, Colorado

I. Introduction

A fundamental feature of asthma is abnormal airway function such that the airways are more likely to become obstructed after exposure to a variety of stimuli. Extensive investigations have been conducted in both human and animal models of airway disease to define the mechanisms responsible for this abnormal state. This chapter will concentrate on studies that have addressed the potential of T cells to alter the function of airways by making them hyperresponsive, and the stimuli known to produce hyperresponsiveness. These pathways may be prime targets for studies addressing the genetic basis of asthma.

II. Airway Responsiveness

A heightened airway responsiveness (hyperresponsiveness) to a variety of stimuli is considered a hallmark of asthma. A basic knowledge of airway responsiveness in terms of definition and methods of assessment is important in understanding current concepts of asthma pathogenesis. This subject is dealt with initially since it has bearing on the discussion which follows.

A. Airway Responsiveness in Subjects with Asthma

Airway responsiveness is commonly defined as the ease with which airways narrow in response to various nonallergic and nonsensitizing stimuli [1,2]. In a clinical setting, the stimuli used to assess responsiveness most commonly include inhaled pharmacologic agents (histamine, methacholine) as well as natural physical stimuli (exercise, exposure to cold air). In the case of the commonly used methacholine challenge, the level of responsiveness is defined by assessing lung function before and after inhalation of increasing concentrations of methacholine. The more responsive the airways, the lower the amount of methacholine needed to decrease lung function. In this way, a provocative concentration (PC) of drug can be defined that causes a set decrease in lung function. Usually, this is a 20% decrease in FEV_1, and the responsiveness is reported as a PC_{20} in milligrams per milliliter of agonist. While even normal subjects may develop airway obstruction when inhaling these pharmacologic agents [3,4], subjects with asthma usually respond to much lower concentrations of agonist [5,6]. Thus, the airways of these individuals are hyperresponsive to these stimuli.

Within a group of asthmatic subjects, the level of airway responsiveness has been reported to correlate with the severity of asthma symptoms (wheeze, cough, chest tightness) as well as medication requirements in both adults [1,5] and children [6,7]. Thus, the most hyperresponsive asthmatics would be expected to have the most severe disease. While there can be great variability in responsiveness seen within groups of patients classified by disease severity [8], this general relationship has helped focus investigations on factors that can induce hyperresponsiveness.

The level of airway responsiveness is not static in either normal individuals or those with asthma, but may increase or decrease in response to various stimuli [9]. In general, stimuli that increase responsiveness and make asthma worse are found in our environment and have the ability to produce airway inflammation [10]. These stimuli include common viral respiratory infections [11–13], allergens [14,15], occupational agents [16,17], and air pollutants [18,19] including cigarette smoke [20–22]. From both clinical and mechanistic standpoints, the most intensely studied stimuli have been aeroallergens. Exposure of atopic individuals to allergens can lead to significant increases in airway responsiveness that persist for days, weeks, or months [14,15]. This heightened responsiveness is seen not only after exposure to allergen within the laboratory [14], but also as a consequence of natural exposure to the offending agent [15]. While the clinical consequences of an increase in responsiveness may be insignificant in normal individuals, this increase may lead to instability in subjects with asthma. In this respect, Cockcroft [23] proposed that a cycle can develop in which continuous or repeated exposure to allergen in sensitized individuals insidiously leads to increased airway responsiveness and more severe disease in that subsequent exposure to allergen and nonallergic stimuli more easily lead to airway obstruction. Clinical investigations in adults with asthma have documented that allergen exposure leads to an inflammatory reaction within the airways that is associated with obstruction and increased responsiveness (reviewed in Ref. 24).

B. Airway Responsiveness in Animal Models of Airway Disease

Several models of reversible airway obstruction have been developed in an attempt to better define the pathogenesis of disease processes that produce airway obstruction and hyperresponsiveness [25]. While no one model completely mimics asthma as found in humans, investigators have been able to study factors that lead to an increase in airway responsiveness in several species of animals. For reasons that will be discussed in more detail later, many of these models have been allergen-driven [26,27]. When larger species of animals have been employed for these studies, the methods of assessing airway responsiveness have been similar to those employed in humans. Thus, increasing concentrations of an agonist such as histamine [26] have been inhaled until a set decrease in airway function is achieved. In this way, a provocative concentration of drug can be defined. When smaller species of animals such as mice have been employed, responsiveness of the airways has been defined not only by inhalation challenges, but with other methods that are technically easier to employ. For example, increasing concentrations of methacholine have been administered intravenously to define the concentration of drug needed to produce a specific change in lung mechanics in mice. In this way, the effects of allergen sensitization on an index of airway responsiveness can be defined in this small species [28]. In addition, tracheas from normal and allergen-sensitized mice have been subjected to electrical field stimulation to cause the release of neurotransmitters (including acetylcholine) from neural tissue [29]. As reviewed in more detail later, repeated allergen exposure in certain stains of mice leads to an increased airway responsiveness to nerve stimulation in that the frequency of electrical field stimulation needed to produce 50% of the maximal contractile response (ES_{50}) decreases significantly. This alteration in airway function appears to be due to enhanced release of acetylcholine from nerves [30].

C. The Potential of T Cells to Induce Airway Responsiveness

The inflammatory nature of asthma in terms of the pathologic findings within airways has been appreciated for some time [31–34]. Various types of inflammatory cells are overrepresented within these airways, including eosinophils [35] and mast cells [36]. Initially, the studies were directed primarily at these types of cells in terms of how they might produce the abnormalities associated with and recognized clinically as asthma [37]. Recently, lymphocytes and associated IgE produc-

tion have attracted more attention in terms of investigations of asthma pathogenesis.

III. Induction of IgE Synthesis by T Cells

T lymphocytes play two essential roles in the induction of IgE synthesis. First,
they provide essential growth factors such as interleukin-4 (IL-4) and IL-13. In the
absence of these growth factors, IgE production is virtually eliminated. The signal
provided by IL-4 induces germline transcription of the Cε gene [38]. The second
signal is transmitted through direct physical interaction between T and B cells
which, in combination with IL-4, triggers the induction of functional ε-gene
transcription and IgE synthesis [39]. The requirement for T–B physical contact
can be substituted by monoclonal antibodies directed to the B-cell surface antigen
CD40 [40]. When both anti-CD40 antibody and IL-4 are added together to B cells,
large amounts of IgE are synthesized in vitro. The natural ligand for CD40 (gp39,
CD40 ligand) is a 33-kDa type II membrane glycoprotein expressed on the surface
of activated T-helper cells. In vivo, this interaction between CD40 ligand on
activated T cells with B-cell CD40 is essential for IL-4-dependent IgE synthesis [41].

A. Modulation of the Inflammatory Response and IgE
Synthesis by T-Cell Cytokines

Although IL-4 is the major cytokine known to cause isotype switching to IgE
synthesis, other cytokines can modulate IL-4-induced IgE synthesis. IL-5, a non-
isotype-specific B-cell growth factor and IL-6, a non-isotype-specific late B-cell
differentiation factor, both upregulate IgE synthesis induced by IL-4. In contrast,
interferon-γ inhibits IL-4-induced IgE synthesis [42]. IL-12 also is an effective
T-cell-derived factor which can inhibit IgE synthesis, at least in part through
triggering the secretion of interferon-γ [43].

The role of T cells in the regulation and expression of allergic and asthmatic
responses goes beyond the ability to simply provide "help" for IgE synthesis. A
number of T-cell-derived cytokines play major roles in determining the nature of
the airway inflammatory response in asthma. IL-5, IL-3, and granulocyte macrophage colony-stimulating factor (GM-CSF) enhance eosinophil differentiation
[44,45], maturation [46,47], endothelial adherence [48], activation [49], and degranulation [50]. IL-5 primes eosinophils for chemotaxis [51], and IL-3 and GM-
CSF may also lead to eosinophil accumulation [52–54]. The proinflammatory
cytokine TNF-α has multiple actions on neutrophils and eosinophils, and upregulates adhesion molecules on endothelium [55,56]. RANTES also leads to eosinophil accumulation [57]. IL-4 and IL-3 also serve as mast cell growth factors [58,
59]. IL-8 is an important chemoattractant for T cells and neutrophils [60].

This complex interaction between different cytokines and the inflammatory response has been used to support the concept of two major CD4$^+$ T-helper (T$_H$) cell subsets. The T$_{H1}$ subset of proinflammatory cytokines secrete IL-1, IL-2, IFN-γ, IL-6, and TNF-α. In contrast, the T$_{H2}$ subset supports IgE synthesis by producing IL-4, IL-5, IL-10, and TGF-β. IL-13, IL-3, and GM-CSF are produced by both subsets. The mechanisms which regulate the differentiation of resting T cells into T$_{H1}$ versus T$_{H2}$ cells is being actively investigated. The actual cytokine environment in which the cell is activated may play a major role in this differentiative step.

B. IgE and Airway Hyperresponsiveness

As presented below, many studies of airway hyperresponsiveness and T cells in both human and animal models have focused on allergen-induced changes in airways function. There are several reasons for this. Based on epidemiologic information, the hypothesis has been advanced that asthma may almost always be related to some type of IgE-related reaction, regardless of patient age. In this respect, Burrows and co-workers [61] showed that the prevalence of asthma in a population was closely related to the serum IgE level. Sears et al. [62] also found in children without histories of asthma or atopic disease that there was a significant correlation between serum IgE and the proportion with airway hyperresponsiveness. Thus, the presence of serum IgE has been associated with both the prevalence of asthma and the proportion of a group of children with airway hyperresponsiveness to methacholine. While these observations suggest that T cells might exert their effects in terms of airway hyperresponsiveness via control of IgE production, it is also likely that T cells exert their effects via non-IgE-dependent mechanisms through production and release of proinflammatory cytokines as reviewed above.

IV. Lymphocytes and Airway Responsiveness in Humans

In subjects with asthma, while many inflammatory cells may participate in disease pathogenesis, work to date suggests important roles for mast cells, eosinophils, and T cells [63–66]. In this section, clinical studies indicating that T cells are able to induce airway hyperresponsiveness are reviewed. In these studies, the number and types of T cells within the airways have been assessed after use of one of two procedures to obtain the cells: bronchoalveolar lavage with analysis of the cells obtained from the fluid, or endobronchial biopsy with analysis of the cells within the tissue. While many studies employing lavage and biopsy of subjects with asthma have been performed, preference is given to those in which T cells have been correlated with measures of airway responsiveness.

A. Studies Involving Bronchoalveolar Lavage

One of the first studies to analyze lymphocytes obtained by bronchoalveolar lavage from the airways of subjects with asthma was performed by Gonzalez et al. [67]. The focus of this work was to define the potential contribution of CD4+ and CD8+ lymphocytes to allergen-induced early and late asthmatic responses. The investigators found that after allergen bronchoprovocation, there was a decrease in CD4+ T cells and an increase in CD8+ cells in BAL from subjects that had only an immediate asthmatic response after allergen challenge. This pattern was not seen in subjects who also developed a late asthmatic response, suggesting that mobilization of a certain type of T cell into the lung might be associated with prevention of this late-phase reaction. While the investigators did not assess airway responsiveness, this study was among the first to suggest that lymphocytes within the airways might modulate airway function.

Subsequent studies employing lavage have attempted to correlate activated T cells with the level of airway responsiveness. In this respect, Walker et al. [68] assessed T-cell activation and eosinophils within bronchoalveolar lavage in 17 subjects with asthma and compared the results to similar investigations in normal controls. Compared to normal individuals, BAL from asthmatics contained significantly increased numbers of both CD4+ and CD8+ T cells, with these cells expressing elevated levels of T cell activation markers (interleukin-2 receptor [CD25], HLA-DR, and very late activation antigen-1 [VLA-1]). A close correlation was found between the numbers of lavage CD4+/CD25+ T cells and the number of eosinophils. In addition, the numbers of activated T cells and eosinophils were both related to the severity of asthma as assessed by impairment of FEV_1 and the level of responsiveness of the airways to methacholine. The results were interpreted by the investigators to suggest that recruitment and activation of lymphocytes and eosinophils are fundamental to the pathogenesis of asthma.

Recent work by Robinson et al [69] has confirmed and extended the study cited above. In this study, both bronchial washings and bronchoalveolar lavage fluid were obtained from 29 atopic asthmatic patients and 13 normal volunteers. T-cell phenotypes and activation status were defined by flow cytometry. CD4+ T cells from the asthmatics were activated when compared to controls as demonstrated by co-expression of CD25 on the cells. In both normals and asthmatics, the CD4+ T cells were of the memory phenotype (CD45RO). Within the group with asthma, there was a significant association between CD4+/CD25+ lymphocytes and asthma symptom scores, airway responsiveness to methacholine, and baseline FEV_1. The percentage of eosinophils within lavage fluid correlated with the asthma symptom score, while significant relationships were also found between the percentage of epithelial cells in BAL and both the FEV_1 and airway responsiveness. The authors suggested that selective activation of memory CD4+ T cells contributes to the eosinophil accumulation, airway responsiveness, and symptoms seen in the asthmatic population.

B. Studies Employing Biopsies from Airways

Studies utilizing biopsy material from airways of asthmatics have also been able to address the relationship between the presence of activated lymphocytes in tissue and measures of airway responsiveness. This was first reported by Azzawi et al. [63], who studied atopic asthmatic subjects as well as atopic nonasthmatic controls and normal healthy controls. Biopsies from both central and subsegmental bronchi were obtained at the time of fiberoptic bronchoscopy. The investigators found that there was a significant increase in the number of CD25$^+$ T cells in the more central airways in the asthmatics versus both other groups. Eosinophil numbers were greatly increased in the asthmatic subjects at both levels of the airways. Hyperresponsive subjects (asthmatics, some atopic nonasthmatics) had a significantly higher percentage of CD25$^+$ cells in central airways and of cells positive for a marker for eosinophil cationic protein (EG2) at both levels of airway. In a subsequent study with a similar design [70], these investigators also found that the ratio of EG2$^+$ cells to cells positive for a panleukocyte marker (CD45) correlated with the provocative concentration of methacholine causing a 20% drop in FEV$_1$. As with the lavage studies noted above, the conclusion of these studies was that recruitment and "activation" of lymphocytes and eosinophils are important in asthma pathogenesis.

While the work quoted in the above paragraphs has dealt primarily with atopic asthmatics, one recent study suggests that similar pathogenic processes in terms of T cells may be operative in both the atopic and nonatopic (intrinsic) asthmatic. Bentley et al. [35] used immunohistochemistry and a panel of monoclonal antibodies to compare T-lymphocyte, eosinophil, macrophage, and neutrophil infiltration in bronchial biopsy specimens from allergic and nonallergic asthmatics as well as normal controls. The group of intrinsic asthmatics had an intense mononuclear cell infiltrate with a significant increase in total leukocytes as well as CD4$^+$ and CD68$^+$ cells (macrophages) compared to both the normal controls and the extrinsic asthmatics. The numbers of CD25$^+$ and EG2$^+$ cells were both significantly elevated in the two groups of asthmatics compared to normal subjects. When airways responsiveness to methacholine was plotted versus the numbers of EG2$^+$ cells in the airways of the groups with asthma, a significant correlation was observed. These observations suggest that T-lymphocyte activation and eosinophil infiltration are common features in both intrinsic and extrinsic asthma.

V. T Lymphocytes and Airway Responsiveness in Animal Models

Although animal models may share only some of the features of human asthma, we have learned a great deal from these models, especially linking T cells, IgE production, and altered airway responsiveness. A role for T lymphocytes has been established in those species where reagents are available for identifying, isolating, and transferring T cells in animals exposed to antigen by inhalation.

A. Rats

In Brown-Norway rats actively sensitized to ovalbumin (OVA), a marked increase in airway responsiveness to inhaled acetylcholine after OVA exposure was induced in association with an increase in eosinophil and lymphocyte counts in bronchoalveolar lavage fluid [71]. Despite treatment with either dexamethasone or cyclosporin A, there was little effect on the induction of airway hyperresponsiveness, although eosinophil and lymphocyte influx were inhibited. The authors concluded that specific inhibition of T-lymphocyte activation in this species of rat was not sufficient to inhibit the induction of airway hyperresponsiveness despite suppressing allergen-induced eosinophilia in BAL fluid. In a similar approach to antigen-induced, IgE-mediated allergic airway inflammation, the presence of inflammatory cells in the airways did not always cause airway hyperresponsiveness [72].

In both IgE high- and low-responder rats, repeated exposure to antigen may indeed lead to the development of tolerance, with a progressive reduction in the allergic response of adult animals to the sensitizing antigen [73]. This contrasts with the consequences of allergen exposure during the neonatal period, where increased allergic sensitization may prevail. The development of antigen-specific immunological tolerance, especially of the IgE isotype, was transferable to naive syngeneic animals by $CD8^+$ splenic T cells that lacked α or β chains of the T-cell receptor (TCR) [74]. Kinetic studies on T-cell reactivity in aerosol-exposed rats demonstrated biphasic $CD4^+$ T_{H2}-like responses which were terminated coincident with IgE antibody production and at the same time that MHC class 1-restricted, OVA-specific, interferon-γ-producing $CD8^+$ T cells first appeared [75]. These phenomena were best demonstrated in animals expressing a low IgE responder phenotype, but were observed in high-responder rats as well.

Alveolar macrophages may play an important role in balancing immune responses in the lung in response to aerosolized antigen. In presensitized, aerosol-challenged animals, depletion of alveolar macrophages is associated with increases in local T-cell memory-dependent plasma cell responses and the accumulation of activated T cells in the lung [76,77]. A major function of alveolar macrophages would therefore be the dampening of secondary immune responses to inhaled antigens. In contrast, alveolar macrophages are known to release IL-1β, which, when instilled in the tracheas of Brown-Norway rats, induced inflammatory changes characterized by increases in neutrophil counts in BAL fluid and increased airway responsiveness to bradykinin [78].

The infiltration of inflammatory cells, including T cells, into tissues from the vascular space is facilitated by a series of adhesion molecules. Recently, leukocyte-endothelial adhesion pathways have been shown to be important in the development of airway hyperresponsiveness. One pathway involves the very late antigen-4 (VLA-4), which binds to the vascular cell adhesion molecule-1 (VCAM-1) on endothelial cells [79]. VLA-4, a member of the β-integrin family, is highly expressed on lymphocytes. Blocking of VLA-4 in Brown-Norway rats sensitized to OVA was associated with markedly reduced early- and late-phase responses. The number and composition of cells in the airways were unaffected by the antibody treatment.

B. Mice

A number of studies have been carried out in mice where knowledge of the immune system and availability of important reagents have provided new insight into the role of T cells in the development of airway hyperreactivity. In one model, mice were sensitized to picryl chloride via the skin and subsequently challenged intranasally [80,81]. Between 24 and 48 h after challenge, peribronchial and perivascular accumulation of macrophages and lymphocytes was noted. This was accompanied by an increase in pulmonary resistance and hyperreactivity of isolated trachea preparations to carbachol; dynamic compliance was unchanged. The response was antigen-specific and T-cell-dependent, since athymic (nude) mice developed no hyperreactivity. This hyperreactivity could be transferred by T cells from sensitized mice. These data support the conclusion that T cells which are involved in the delayed-type hypersensitivity response to picryl chloride can induce airway hyperreactivity. The role of the inflammatory infiltrate in the development of airway hyperresponsiveness was less clear.

A/J mice develop airway hyperreactivity in response to intravenously administered methacholine, and markedly increased numbers of pulmonary inflammatory cells following intraperitoneal sensitization and intratracheal challenge with sheep red blood cells [82]. Eosinophils were a prominent part of the inflammatory infiltrate. In-vivo depletion of CD4$^+$ T cells using an anti-CD4 monoclonal antibody prevented the development of both airway hyperreactivity and the infiltration of eosinophils, leading to the conclusion that altered airway responsiveness in this model was dependent on CD4$^+$ T lymphocytes and that eosinophils were the effectors of this response.

Similar results were obtained in BALB/c mice immunized to OVA intraperitoneally and challenged with aerosolized OVA [83,84]. Eosinophils began to infiltrate the trachea of these animals approximately 9 h after challenge and persisted for 48 h. In-vivo depletion of CD4$^+$ T cells by antibody decreased the infiltration of eosinophils. In contrast, depletion of CD8$^+$ T cells had no significant effect on OVA-induced eosinophil infiltration in the trachea. Pretreatment with anti-IL-5 antibody also decreased OVA-induced infiltration of eosinophils, suggesting that IL-5 mediates this eosinophil recruitment. Intraperitonel administration of recombinant interferon-γ (IFN-γ) prevented antigen-induced eosinophil recruitment by inhibiting CD4+ T-cell infiltration.

We have developed a model in the mouse where sensitization is achieved by repeated exposure to antigen exclusively through the airways and in the absence of adjuvant. Sensitization in this way resulted in a predominant IgE response, immediate cutaneous hypersensitivity, and an enlargement of the local or peribronchial lymph nodes (PBLN). Two different methods confirmed that sensitization in this way led to an alteration in airway responsiveness (AR). The first approach detected changes in airway conductance in vivo by body plethysmography after intravenous challenge with increasing concentrations of methacholine [28]. Sensitized mice exhibited heightened bronchoconstrictive responses compared to nonsensitized mice. The second method monitored AR in vitro [29]. Tracheal smooth muscle preparations were exposed to electrical field stimulation at constant voltage with increasing frequencies. The ES_{50} values (the frequency of electrical field stimulation resulting in half-maximal contraction of airway smooth muscle) were calculated from the electrical frequency dose–response curve. In sensitized mice a significantly lower ES_{50} was seen compared to values in nonsensitized animals.

The increase in AR to electrical field stimulation may have resulted from increased release of acetycholine from airway parasympathetic nerve endings [30]. In antigen-sensitized animals, a significant increase in acetylcholine release was demonstrated, although the dose–response to acetylcholine of isolated tracheal segments was comparable to that of nonsensitized animals. The results suggested that repeated airway exposure to allergen is associated with the development of an IgE responsive state and altered neural control of airways with increased release of acetylcholine from neural terminals. This increase in release of acetycholine was associated as well with loss of function of the M2 muscarinic autoreceptor in tracheas from immune animals.

Passive transfer of cells from the peribronchial lymph nodes (PBLN) of OVA-sensitized animals was capable of transferring this increase in AR, provided that the naive recipients were exposed to a single OVA inhalation 48 h prior to assessment [29]. In parallel to the increase in AR, the capacity to produce IgE and develop immediate cutaneous reactivity was also noted [85]. Similar results were obtained using inhalation and sensitization to ragweed [85,86]. These data indicated that the local lymphoid tissue at the site of sensitization could transfer responsiveness to the allergens. Further, it demonstrated that despite the development of IgE (or IgG1)-mediated responses, the development of altered airway function was dependent on challenge with the specific allergen via the airways. This was confirmed in a different approach where, to elicit strong IgE antibody production, mice were sensitized to OVA through the skin [87]. Animals sensitized in this way and that demonstrated equivalent serum IgE antibody responses and cutaneous reactivity to OVA nevertheless failed to demonstrate increased AR to electrical field stimulation in the absence of at least a single airway challenge.

Examination of the T cells in the enlarged PBLN of BALB/c mice sensitized to OVA revealed significant expansion of the Vβ8.1/8.2 population, and to a lesser extent, Vβ2$^+$ and Vβ14$^+$ cells [88]. When assayed for their ability to help OVA-primed B cells to produce immunoglobulin, it appeared that only Vβ8.1/8.2$^+$ T cells (from PBLN or spleen) could support IgE production. In contrast, Vβ2$^+$ cells from sensitized animals not only failed to help IgE production, they inhibited IgE production when co-cultured with Vβ8.1/8.2$^+$ cells. Transfer of Vβ8.1/8.2$^+$ T cells from sensitized animals into naive recipients passively transferred the capacity to develop allergen-specific IgE, immediate cutaneous reactivity and, following a single inhalation challenge, increased AR [89]. Co-transfer of Vβ2$^+$ T cells from sensitized (but not nonsensitized) mice prevented these responses. It appears that T cells bearing different Vβ elements are differentially involved in the in-vitro and in-vivo regulation of IgE production. Preliminary studies relate some of these differences to the cytokine profile exhibited by sensitized cells: Vβ8$^+$ T cells secrete increased amounts of IL-4. Moreover, these studies support a link between IgE and altered airway responsiveness.

Additional support for the association between IgE and increased AR comes from studies in a second strain of mice [29]. SJL/J mice, sensitized in the identical manner, do not develop IgE (they are poor producers of IL-4), but mount an IgG response (IgG2a, IgG2b, and IgG3). In the absence of IgE, they do not develop immediate cutaneous reactivity, nor is airway function altered. It is of interest that SJL/J mice are deficient in Vβ8$^+$ T cells.

The Vβ specific activity of the T cells in this model requires explanation. It is unlikely that intrathymic differentiation directs thymocytes bearing different T-cell receptors or different Vβ elements along different pathways. One possibility is that the association between receptor structure and T-cell function may relate to antigen specificity and antigen presentation. T cells bearing Vβ8 respond well to OVA. These T cells recognize a major antigenic peptide, OVA 323-339, in association with IA^d [90]; the peptide recognized by Vβ2$^+$ T cells is not known and, conceivably, these cells would encounter antigen on a different antigen-presenting cell (APC), other than the APC interacting with the OVA-specific Vβ8$^+$ T cells. Thus different APCs may drive T cells along different maturational pathways, possibly with different patterns of interleukin production.

When we examined the T-cell response to sensitization by OVA peptide 232-339, we saw similar levels of IgE antibody production, immediate skin test responses, and increased AR, as observed following sensitization to native OVA [91]. However, whereas native OVA resulted in expansion of both Vβ8.1$^+$ and Vβ8.2$^+$ T cells, the peptide led to the selective expansion of Vβ8.1$^+$ T cells. There was no expansion of Vβ2$^+$ T cells in response to sensitization with this peptide.

We also examined the response to sensitization to a different allergen, ragweed (RW) [86]. Following exposure to RW via the airway, IgE and IgG1 anti-

RW antibodies were detected, immediate skin test responses were elicited, and increased AR was observed in tracheal smooth muscle preparations exposed to electrical field stimulation. Histologic examination of the airways and lung revealed the presence of an inflammatory infiltrate in the mucosa and submucosa of the airways. Analysis of the frequency of Vβ-expressing T-cell subsets indicted that sensitization to RW stimulated the expansion of Vβ8.1$^+$, Vβ8.2$^+$ and Vβ13$^+$ T cells in PBLN and Vβ8.1$^+$, Vβ8.2$^+$, Vβ8.3$^+$, Vβ9$^+$, and Vβ14$^+$ T cells in the spleen. Co-culture of these subsets of T cells with RW-primed B cells showed that in the presence of RW, Vβ8.2 (and to a lesser degree Vβ9$^+$) T cells stimulated IgE and IgG1 production, whereas Vβ14$^+$ T cells stimulated IgG2a, and Vβ8.1$^+$, Vβ8.2$^+$, and Vβ9$^+$ T cells triggered IgG3 production. Further, transfer of Vβ8.2 T cells from sensitized mice stimulated the full spectrum of immediate hypersensitivity responses in naive recipients. These data provide additional documentation for the pivotal role of specific Vβ-expressing T-cell subsets in both the stimulation of IgE and IgG1 production as well as in the development of altered AR.

As discussed above for the rat, tolerance to IgE production following repeated antigen exposure can be induced by CD8$^+$ T cells [92]. Sensitization in BALB/c mice via repeated exposure to inhaled OVA resulted in an increase in CD8$^+$ T cells in the spleens of these animals. Transfer of CD8$^+$ T cells from the spleens of sensitized animals to sensitized recipients reduced serum IgE anti-OVA responses, decreased the immediate cutaneous response to intradermal antigen challenge, and normalized AR. A high percentage of these CD8$^+$ T cells were positive for IFN-γ, implying that this cytokine may be a relevant mediator of the functions of CD8$^+$ T cells in this model of allergen-induced sensitization.

Following a different protocol, parenteral challenge with OVA plus aluminum hydroxide adjuvant in several murine strains also resulted in the development of primary IgE responses. Repeated exposure to aerosolized OVA following sensitization reduces the capacity of these mice to generate IgE responses. This "IgE-selective tolerance" could be induced by CD8$^+$ T cells which released high levels of IFN-γ and have been characterized as γδ$^+$ T cells [93].

In light of the ability of IFN-γ to modulate IgE responses, the effectiveness of targeting IFN-γ therapy was demonstrated in our model of allergen-induced sensitization via the airways [94]. Previous studies emphasized the ability of parenteral IFN-γ to inhibit in-vitro and in-vivo IgE production [42,95]. At least in clinical usage, parenteral IFN-γ has had only limited success. When mice sensitized to OVA via the airways were given IFN-γ intraperitoneally (25,000 U/day) for 3 days prior to and on each of the 10 days of the sensitization protocol, total serum IgE levels were reduced by 50% but there was little effect on the development of the immediate hypersensitivity responses and altered AR. In contrast, when IFN-γ was given by nebulization, there were dramatic reductions in specific IgE and IgG1 antibody levels, reduced cutaneous reactivity, and normalization of

AR. These data demonstrate that the route of IFN-γ administration is a critical factor if we are to modulate this T-cell-dependent, immediate allergic response to sensitization via the airways.

C. Other Species of Animals

Guinea Pigs

Guinea pigs have served as excellent models of allergen-induced early and late-phase airways obstruction, but the relative paucity of immunologic reagents has limited these studies. The kinetics and phenotype of T lymphocytes infiltrating the airways of guinea pigs undergoing late-phase asthmatic reactions were studied following sensitization and challenge with OVA via the airways [96]. Induction of hypersensitivity was associated with an increase in mucosal cell numbers which consisted primarily of CD8+ T cells. Following allergen challenge, eosinophil numbers increased, and the T-cell accumulation consisted largely of CD3+/CD8- cells. Early on, eosinophil numbers correlated with CD8+ T cells, whereas at later times the correlation was with CD3+/CD8- cells. In guinea pigs sensitized to OVA, eosinophil accumulation and airway hyperreactivity were prevented by anti-IL-5 antibody treatment [97]. Preincubation of guinea pig eosinophils with antibody to the α4 subunit of the very late activation antigen-4 (VLA-4), which binds to vascular adhesion molecule-1 (VCAM-1), inhibits their accumulation in inflammatory sites. Airway hyperreactivity induced by OVA inhalation and triggered by methacholine is accompanied by increased numbers of eosinophils in the airways and CD4+ and CD8+ T cells in the bronchial wall. Treatment of sensitized guinea pigs with anti-VLA-4 antibody abrogated antigen-induced airway hyperreactivity to methacholine and the cellular infiltration [98].

Primates

There are a few studies on the role of T cells in primates sensitized to antigen and that subsequently develop heightened AR. In one model utilizing Ascaris-sensitized cynomolgus monkeys, inhalation of Ascaris was associated with increased responsiveness to inhaled methacholine and eosinophil infiltration of the airways [99]. Treatment with monoclonal antibody to ICAM-1 attenuated both airway eosinophilia and hyperresponsiveness. This group also examined the role of endothelial leukocyte adhesion molecule-1 (ELAM-1) in the development of acute airway inflammation and late-phase airway obstruction in this model of Ascaris-sensitized monkeys [100]. They demonstrated that a single inhaled exposure to antigen rapidly upregulated expression of ELAM-1 on vascular endothelium that correlated with neutrophil influx into the lungs and the onset of late-phase airway obstruction. Pretreatment with a monoclonal antibody to ICAM-1 had no effect on the influx of neutrophils. In contrast, treatment with an antibody to ELAM-1 blocked both the influx of neutrophils and the late-phase airway obstruction.

VI. Summary and Conclusions

A fundamental feature of asthma is abnormal airway function, such that the airway are hyperresponsive to a variety of stimuli. Clinical studies have associated heightened airway responsiveness with activated T lymphocytes and eosinophils within the airways as assessed by bronchoalveolar lavage and endobronchial biopsy. More mechanistic studies using several species of animals, including inbred strains of mice with passive transfer of murine T cells, has provided insight into how these cells might change airway function. While these observations suggest that T cells might exert their effect in terms of enhancing airway responsiveness via control of IgE production, it is also likely that T cells exert additional effects via non-IgE-dependent mechanisms through production and release of proinflammatory cytokines. Additional clinical studies as well as work with animal models of airway disease will further define the properties of T cells that allow them to influence the functioning of airways within mammalian species.

Acknowledgments

This work was supported in part by National Institutes of Health grant HL-36577.

References

1. Hargreave FE, Dolovich J, O'Byrne PM, Ramsdale EH, Daniel EE. The origin of airway hyperresponsiveness. J Allergy Clin Immunol 1986; 78:825–832.
2. Colasurdo GN, Larsen GL. Airway hyperresponsiveness. In: Busse W, Holgate S, eds. Asthma and Rhinitis. Boston: Blackwell, 1994:1044–1056.
3. Hopp RJ, Bewtra A, Nair NM, Townley RG. The effect of age on methacholine response. J Allergy Clin Immunol 1985; 76:609–613.
4. Tepper RS. Airway reactivity in infants: a positive response to methacholine and metaproterenol. J Appl Physiol 1987; 62:1155–1159.
5. Juniper EF, Frith PA, Hargreave FE. Airway responsiveness to histamine and methacholine: relationship to minimum treatment to control symptoms of asthma. Thorax 1981; 36:575–579.
6. Murray AB, Ferguson AC, Morrison B. Airway responsiveness to histamine as a test for overall severity of asthma in children. J Allergy Clin Immunol 1981; 68: 119–124.

7. Avital A, Noviski N, Bar-Yishay E, Springer C, Levy M, Godfrey S. Nonspecific bronchial reactivity in asthmatic children depends on severity but not on age. Am Rev Respir Dis 1991; 144:36–38.

8. Amaro-Galvez R, McLaughlin FJ, Levison H, Rashed N, Galdes-Sebaldt M, Zimmerman B. Grading severity and treatment requirements to control symptoms in asthmatic children and their relationship with airway hyperreactivity to methacholine. Ann Allergy 1987; 59:298–302.

9. Larsen GL. Asthma in children. N Engl J Med 1992; 326:1540–1545.

10. Wilson MC, Irvin CG, Larsen GL. Inflammation and asthma. Semin Respir Med 1987; 8:279–286.

11. Empey DW, Laitenen LA, Jacobs L, Gold WM, Nadel JA. Mechanisms of bronchial hyperreactivity in normal subjects after upper respiratory tract infection. Am Rev Respir Dis 1976; 113:131–139.

12. Hall WJ, Hall CB, Speers DM. Respiratory syncytial virus infection in adults. Clinical, virologic, and serial pulmonary function studies. Ann Intern Med 1978; 88: 203–205.

13. Lemanske RF Jr, Dick EC, Swenson CA, Vrtis RF, Busse WW. Rhinovirus upper respiratory infection increases airway hyperreactivity and late asthmatic reactions. J Clin Invest 1989; 83:1–10.

14. Cartier A, Thomson NC, Frith PA, Roberts R, Hargreave FE. Allergen-induced increase in bronchial responsiveness to histamine: relationship to the late asthmatic response and change in airway caliber. J Allergy Clin Immunol 1982; 70:170–177.

15. Boulet LP, Cartier A, Thomson NC, Roberts RS, Dolovich J, Hargreave FE. Asthma and increases in nonallergic bronchial responsiveness from seasonal pollen exposure. J Allergy Clin Immunol 1983; 71:399–406.

16. Lam S, Wong R, Yeung M. Nonspecific bronchial reactivity in occupational asthma. J Allergy Clin Immunol 1979; 63:28–34.

17. Chan-Yeung M. Occupational asthma. Chest 1990; 98:148S–161S.

18. Orehek J, Massari JP, Gayrard P, Grimaud C, Charpin J. Effect of short-term, low-level nitrogen dioxide exposure on bronchial sensitivity of asthmatic patients. J Clin Invest 1976; 57:301–307.

19. Seltzer J, Bigby BG, Stulbarg M, et al. O_3-induced change in bronchial reactivity to methacholine and airway inflammation in humans. J Appl Physiol 1986; 60:1321–1326.

20. Martinez FD, Antognoni G, Macri F, et al. Parental smoking enhances bronchial responsiveness in nine-year-old children. Am Rev Respir Dis 1988; 138:518–523.

21. Young S, Le Souëf PN, Geelhoed GC, Stick SM, Turner KJ, Landau LI. The influence of a family history of asthma and parental smoking on airway responsiveness in early infancy. N Engl J Med 1991; 324:1168–1173.

22. Menon P, Rando RJ, Stankus RP, Salvaggio JE, Lehrer SB. Passive cigarette smoke-challenge studies: increase in bronchial hyperreactivity. J Allergy Clin Immunol 1992; 89:560–566.

23. Cockcroft DW. Mechanism of perennial allergic asthma. Lancet 1983; 2:253–256.

24. O'Bryne PM, Dolovich J, Hargreave FE. Late asthmatic responses. Am Rev Respir Dis 1987; 136:740–751.

25. Larsen GL. Experimental models of reversible airway obstruction. In: Crystal RG, West JB, Barnes PJ, Cherniack NS, Weibel ER, eds. The Lung: Scientific Foundations. New York: Raven Press, 1991:953–965.

26. Marsh WR, Irvin CG, Murphy KR, Behrens BL, Larsen GL. Increases in airways reactivity to histamine and inflammatory cells in bronchoalveolar lavage following the late asthmatic response in an animal model. Am Rev Respir Dis 1985; 131: 875–879.

27. Murphy KR, Wilson MC, Irvin CG, et al. The requirement for polymorphonuclear leukocytes in the late asthmatic response and heightened airways reactivity in an animal model. Am Rev Respir Dis 1986; 134:62–68.

28. Renz H, Smith HR, Henson JE, Ray BS, Irvin CG, Gelfand EW. Aerosolized antigen exposure without adjuvant causes increased IgE production and increased airways responsiveness in the mouse. J Allergy Clin Immunol 1992; 89:1127–1138.

29. Larsen GL, Renz H, Loader JE, Bradley KL, Gelfand EW. Airway response to electrical field stimulation in sensitized inbred mice: passive transfer of increased responsiveness with peribronchial lymph nodes. J Clin Invest 1992; 89:747–752.

30. Larsen GL, Fame TM, Renz H, et al. Increased acetylcholine release in tracheas from allergen-exposed IgE-immune mice. Am J Physiol 1994; 266 (Lung Cell Mol Physiol 10): L263–L270.

31. Dunnill MS. The pathology of asthma, with special reference to changes in the bronchial mucosa. J Clin Pathol 1960; 13:27–33.

32. Dunnill MS, Massarella GR, Anderson JA. A comparison of the quantitative anatomy of the bronchi in normal subjects, in status asthmaticus, in chronic bronchitis, and in emphysema. Thorax 1969; 24:176–179.

33. Richards W, Patrick JR. Death from asthma in children. Am J Dis Child 1965; 110: 4–23.

34. Cutz E, Levison H, Cooper DM. Ultrastructure of airways in children with asthma. Histopathology 1978; 2:407–421.

35. Bentley AM, Menz G, Storz CHR, et al. Identification of T lymphocytes, macrophages, and activated eosinophils in the bronchial mucosa in intrinsic asthma. Relationship to symptoms and bronchial responsiveness. Am Rev Respir Dis 1992; 146:500–506.

36. Gibson PG, Allen CJ, Yang JP, et al. Intraepithelial mast cells in allergic and nonallergic asthma. Assessment using bronchial brushings. Am Rev Respir Dis 1993; 148:80–86.

37. Djukanović R, Roche WR, Wilson JW, et al. Mucosal inflammation in asthma. Am Rev Respir Dis 1990; 142:434–457.

38. Shapira SK, Jabara HH, Thienes CF, et al. Deletional switch recombination occurs in IL-4 induced isotype switching to IgE expression by human B cells. Proc Natl Acad Sci USA 1991; 88:7528–7532.

39. Vercelli D, Jabara HH, Arai K-I, Geha RS. Induction of human IgE synthesis requires interleukin 4 and T/B cell interactions involving the T cell receptor/CD3 complex and MHC class II antigens. J Exp Med 1989; 169:1295–1307.

40. Shapira SK, Vercelli D, Jabara HH, Fu SM, Geha RS. Molecular analysis of the induction of immunoglobulin ε synthesis in human B cells by interleukin 4 and engagement of CD40 antigen. J Exp Med 1992; 175:289–292.

41. Spriggs MK, Fanslow WC, Armitage RJ, Belmont J. The biology of the human ligand for CD40. J Clin Invest 1993; 13:373–380.

42. Pene J, Rousset F, Briere F, et al. IgE production by normal human lymphocytes is induced by interleukin 4 and suppressed by interferons γ and α and prostaglandin ε. Proc Natl Acad Sci USA 1988; 85:6880–6884.

43. Kiniwa M, Gately M, Gubler U, Chizzonite R, Fargeas C, Delespesse G. Recombinant interleukin-12 suppresses the synthesis of immunoglobulin ε by interleukin-4 stimulated human lymphocytes. J Clin Invest 1992; 90:262–266.

44. Campbell HD, Tucker WQJ, Hort Y, et al. Molecular cloning, nucleotide sequence, and expression of the gene encoding human eosinophil differentiation factor (interleukin 5). Proc Natl Acad Sci USA 1987; 84:6629–6633.

45. Jabara HH, Ackerman SJ, Vercelli D, et al. Induction of interleukin-4-dependent IgE synthesis and interleukin-5-dependent eosinophil differentiation by supernatants of a human helper T-cell clone. J Clin Immunol 1988; 8:437–446.

46. Saito H, Hatake K, Dvorak AM, et al. Selective differentiation and proliferation of haematopoietic cells induced by recombinant human interleukins. Proc Natl Acad Sci USA 1988; 85:2288–2292.

47. Sonoda Y, Arai N, Ogawa M. Humoral regulation of eosinophilopoiesis *in vitro*: analysis of the targets of interleukin 3, granulocyte/macrophage colony-stimulating factor (GM-CSF), and interleukin-5. Leukemia 1989; 3:14–18.

48. Walsh GM, Hartnell A, Wardlaw AJ, Kurihara K, Sanderson CJ, Kay AB. IL-5 enhances the *in vitro* adhesion of human eosinophils, but not neutrophils, in a leukocyte integrin (CD11/18)-dependent manner. Immunology 1990; 71:258–265.

49. Lopez AF, Sanderson CJ, Gamble JR, Campbell HD, Young JG, Vadas MA. Recombinant human interleukin 5 is a selective activator of human eosinophil function. J Exp Med 1988; 167:219–224.

50. Fujisawa T, Abu-Ghazaleh R, Kita H, Sanderson CJ, Gleich GJ. Regulatory effect of cytokines on eosinophil degranulation. J Immunol 1990; 144:642–646.

51. Sehmi R, Wardlaw AJ, Cromwell O, Kurihara K, Waltmann P, Kay AB. Interleukin-5 selectively enhances the chemotactic response of eosinophils obtained from normal but not eosinophilic subjects. Blood 1992; 79:2952–2959.

52. Warringa RAJ, Koenderman L, Kok PTM, Krekniet J, Bruijnzeel PLB. Modulation and induction of eosinophil chemotaxis by granulocyte-macrophage colony- stimulating factor and interleukin-2. Blood 1991; 77:2694–2700.

53. Rothenberg ME, Owen WF, Silberstein DS, et al. Human eosinophils have prolonged survival, enhanced functional properties, and become hypodense when exposed to human interleukin 3. J Clin Invest 1988; 81:1986–1992.

54. Owen WF Jr, Rothenberg ME, Silberstein DS, et al. Regulation of human eosinophil viability, density, and function by granulocyte/macrophage colony-stimulating factor in the presence of 3T3 fibroblasts. J Exp Med 1987; 166:129–141.

55. Pober JS, Gimbrone MA, Lapierre LA, et al. Overlapping patterns of activation of human eondothelial cells by interleukin 1, tumor necrosis factor, and immune interferon. J Immunol 1986; 137:1893–1896.

56. Springer TA. Adhesion receptors of the immune system. Nature 1990; 346:425–434.

57. Kameyoshi Y, Dorschner A, Mallet AI, Christophers E, Schroder J-M. Cytokine RANTES released from thrombin-stimulated platelets is a potent attractant for human eosinophils. J Exp Med 1992; 176:587–592.

58. Ihle JN, Keller J, Oroszalan S, et al. Biologic properties of homogeneous interleukin 3. Demonstration of WEHI-3 growth factor activity, mast cell growth factor activity, P cell-stimulating factor activity, and histamine-producing cell-stimulating factor activity. J Immunol 1983; 131:282–287.

59. Hamaguchi Y, Kanakura Y, Fujita J, et al. Interleukin 4 as an essential factor for *in vitro* clonal growth of murine connective tissue-type mast cells. J Exp Med 1987; 165:268–273.

60. Leonard EJ, Skeel A, Yoshimura T, Noer K, Kutvirt S, van Epps K. Leukocyte specificity and binding of human neutrophil attractant/activation protein 1. J Immunol 1990; 144:1323–1330.

61. Burrows B, Martinez FD, Halonen M, Barbee RA, Cline MG. Association of asthma with serum IgE levels and skin-test reactivity to allergens. N Engl J Med 1989; 320:271–277.

62. Sears MR, Burrows B, Flannery EM, Herbison GP, Hewitt CJ, Holdaway MD. Relation between airway responsiveness and serum IgE in children with asthma and in apparently normal children. N Engl J Med 1991; 325:1067–1071.

63. Azzawi M, Bradley B, Jeffery PK, et al. Identification of activated T lymphocytes and eosinophils in bronchial biopsies in stable atopic asthma. Am Rev Respir Dis 1990; 142:1407–1413.

64. Beasley R, Roche WR, Roberts JA, Holgate ST. Cellular events in the bronchi in mild asthma and after bronchial provocation. Am Rev Respir Dis 1989; 139:806–817.

65. Wardlaw AJ, Dunnette S, Gleich GJ, Collins JV, Kay AB. Eosinophils and mast cells in bronchoalveolar lavage in subjects with mild asthma. Relationship to bronchial hyperreactivity. Am Rev Respir Dis 1988; 137:62–69.

66. Laitinen LA, Laitinen A, Haahtela T. Airway mucosal inflammation even in patients with newly diagnosed asthma. Am Rev Respir Dis 1993; 147:697–704.

67. Gonzalez MC, Diaz P, Galleguillos FR, Ancic P, Cromwell O, Kay AB. Allergen-induced recruitment of bronchoalveolar helper (OKT4) and suppressor (OKT8) T-cells in asthma. Relative increases in OKT8 cells in single early responders compared with those in late-phase responders. Am Rev Respir Dis 1987; 136:600–604.

68. Walker C, Kaegi MK, Braun P, Blaser K. Activated T cells and eosinophilia in bronchoalveolar lavages from subjects with asthma correlated with disease severity. J Allergy Clin Immunol 1991; 88:935–942.

69. Robinson DS, Bentley AM, Hartnell A, Kay AB, Durham SR. Activated memory T helper cells in bronchoalveolar lavage fluid from patients with atopic asthma:

relation to asthma symptoms, lung function, and bronchial responsiveness. Thorax 1993; 48:26–32.

70. Bradley BL, Azzawi M, Jacobson M, et al. Eosinophils, T-lymphocytes, mast cells, neutrophils, and macrophages in bronchial biopsy specimens from atopic subjects with asthma: comparison with biopsy specimens from atopic subjects without asthma and normal control subjects and relationship to bronchial hyperresponsiveness. J Allergy Clin Immunol 1991; 88:661–674.

71. Elwood W, Lötvall JO, Barnes PJ, Chung KF. Effect of dexamethasone and cyclosporin A on allergen-induced airway hyperresponsiveness and inflammatory cell responses in sensitized Brown-Norway rats. Am Rev Respir Dis 1992; 145:1289–1294.

72. Kips JC, Cuvelier CA, Pauwels RA. Effect of acute and chronic antigen inhalation on airway morphology and responsiveness in actively sensitized rats. Am Rev Respir Dis 1992; 145:1306–1310.

73. Sedgwick JD, Holt PG. Suppression of IgE responses in inbred rats by repeated respiratory tract exposure to antigen: responder phenotype influences isotype specificity of induced tolerance. Eur J Immunol 1984; 14:893–897.

74. McMenamin C, Oliver J, Girn B, et al. Regulation of T-cell sensitization at epithelial surfaces in the respiratory tract: suppression of IgE responses to inhaled antigens by CD3$^+$ TcR α^-/β^- lymphocytes (putative γ/δ T cells). Immunology 1991; 74:234–239.

75. McMenamin C, Holt PG. The natural immune response to inhaled soluble protein antigens involves major histocompatibility complex (MHC)-class I-restricted CD4$^+$ T cell-dependent immune deviation resulting in selective suppression of IgE production. J Exp Med 1993; 178:889–899.

76. Thepen T, McMenamin C, Oliver J, Kraal G, Holt PG. Regulation of immune response to inhaled antigen by alveolar macrophages: differential effect of *in vivo* alveolar macrophage elimination on the induction of tolerance vs. immunity. Eur J Immunol 1991; 21:2845–2850.

77. Thepen T, McMenamin C, Girn B, Kraal G, Holt PG. Regulation of IgE production in presensitized animals: *in vivo* elimination of alveolar macrophages preferentially increases IgE responses to inhaled allergen. Clin Exp Allergy 1992; 22:1107–1114.

78. Tsukagoshi H, Sakamoto T, Xu W, Barnes PJ, Chung KF. Effect of interleukin-1β on airway hyperresponsiveness and inflammation in sensitized and non-sensitized Brown-Norway rats. J Allergy Clin Immunol 1994; 93:464–469.

79. Rabb HA, Olivenstien R, Issekutz TB, Renzi PM, Martin JG. The role of the leukocyte adhesion molecules VLA-4, LFA-1, and Mac-1 in allergic airway response in the rat. Am J Respir Crit Care Med 1994; 149:1186–1191.

80. Garssen J, Nijkamp FP, van der VLiet H, van Loveren H. T cell mediated induction of airway hyperreactivity in mice. Am Rev Respir Dis 1991; 144:931–938.

81. Enander I, Ulfgnen AK, Nygnen H, et al. Regulation of the delayed hypersensitivity reaction in the lung reflected as mononuclear, mast cell and mucous cell appearance after T helper cell depletion and adoptive transfer Int Arch Allergy Appl Immunol 1987; 82:361–363.

82. Gavett SH, Chen X, Finkelman F, Wills-Karp M. Depletion of murine CD4+ T lymphocytes prevents antigen-induced airway hyperreactivity and pulmonary eosinophilia. Am J Respir Crit Care Med 1994; 10:587–893.

83. Nakajima H, Iwamoto I, Tomoe S, et al. CD4+ T-lymphocytes and interleukin-5 mediate antigen-induced eosinophil infiltration into the mouse trachea. Am Rev Respir Dis 1992; 146:374–377.

84. Iwamoto I, Nakajima H, Endo H, Yoshida S. Interferon γ regulates antigen-induced eosinophil recruitment into the mouse airways by inhibiting the infiltration of CD4+ T cells. J Exp Med 1993; 177:573–576.

85. Saloga J, Renz H, Lack G, et al. Development and transfer of immediate cutaneous hypersensitivity in mice exposed to aerosolized antigen. J Clin Invest 1992; 91:133–140.

86. Renz H, Saloga J, Bradley KL, et al. Specific Vβ T-cell subsets mediate the immediate hypersensitivity response to ragweed allergen. J Immunol 1993c; 151:1907–1917.

87. Saloga J, Renz H, Larsen GL, Gelfand EW. Increased airways responsiveness in mice depends on local challenge with antigen. Am J Respir Crit Care Med 1994; 149:65–70.

88. Renz H, Bradley KL, Marrack P, Gelfand EW. T cells expressing variable elements of T-cell receptor β8 and β2 chain regulate murine IgE production. Proc Natl Acad Sci USA 1992; 89:6438–6442.

89. Renz H, Bradley K, Saloga J, Loader J, Larsen GL, Gelfand EW. T cells expressing specific Vβ elements regulate IgE production and airways responsiveness *in vivo*. J Exp Med 1993; 177:1175–1180.

90. Shimonkevitz R, Colon S, Kappler JW, Marrack P, Grey HM. Antigen recognition by H-2 restricted T cells. II A tryptic ovalbumin peptide that substitutes for processed antigen. J Immunol 1984; 133:2067–2074.

91. Renz H, Bradley K, Larsen GL, McCall C, Gelfand EW. Comparison of the allergenicity of ovalbumin and ovalbumin peptide 323-339. Differential expansion of Vβ-expressing T-cell populations. J Immunol 1993; 151:7206–7213.

92. Renz H, Lack G, Saloga J, et al. Inhibition of IgE production and normalization of airways responsiveness by sensitized CD8 T cells in a mouse model of allergen-induced sensitization. J Immunol 1994; 152:351–360.

93. McMenamin C, Pimm C, McKersey M, Holt PG. Regulation of IgE responses to inhaled antigen in mice by antigen specific γδ T cells. Science 1994; 265:1869–1871.

94. Lack G, Renz H, Saloga J, et al. Nebulized but not parenteral IFN-γ decreases IgE production and normalizes airways function in a murine model of allergen sensitization. J Immunol 1994; 152:2546–2554.

95. Finkelman FD, Katona IM, Mosmann TR, Coffman RL. IFN-γ regulates the isotypes of Ig secreted during *in vivo* humoral immune responses. J Immunol 1988; 140:1022–1029.

96. Frew AF, Mobel R, Azzawi M, et al. T lymphocytes and eosinophils in allergen-induced late-phase asthmatic reactions in the guinea pig. Am Rev Respir Dis 1990; 141:407–413.

97. Mauser PJ, Pitman A, Witt A, et al. Inhibitory effect of the TRFK-5 anti-IL-5 antibody in a guinea pig model of asthma. Am Rev Respir Dis 1993; 148:1623–1627.

98. Pretolani M, Ruffie C, Lapa e Silva JR, Joseph D, Lobb RR, Vorgaftig BB. Antibody to very late activation antigen 4 prevents antigen-induced bronchial hyperreactivity and cellular infiltration in the guinea pig airways. J Exp Med 1994; 180:795–805.

99. Wegner CD, Gundel RH, Reilly P, Haynes N, Letts LG, Rothlein R. Intercellular adhesion molecule-1 (ICAM-1) in the pathogenesis of asthma. Science 1990; 247: 451–459.

100. Gundel RH, Wegner CD, Torcellini CA, et al. Endothelial leukocyte adhesion molecule-1 mediates antigen-induced acute airway inflammation and late-phase airway obstruction in monkeys. J Clin Invest 1991; 88:1407–1411.

3

Role of T Cells in Virus-Induced Asthma

JAMES E. GERN and WILLIAM W. BUSSE

University of Wisconsin Medical School
Madison, Wisconsin

I. Introduction

Respiratory viruses are common causes of asthma exacerbations. As such, viral infections may be one of several environmental factors which, in concert with genetic factors, are responsible for the development of asthma. Surveys utilizing virus culture or increases in virus-specific antibody titers estimated that between a quarter and a half of wheezing episodes in children were associated with a viral upper respiratory infection (URI) [1–3]. Using a much more sensitive polymerase chain reaction assay, Johnston and colleagues found that 78% of wheezing children tested positive for a picornavirus (most likely rhinovirus), compared to 12% of age-matched controls [4]. Respiratory syncytial virus (RSV), parainfluenza virus (PIV), and influenza A infections are also frequently associated with increased asthma symptoms [1]. In adults with asthma, Nicholson and colleagues used similar techniques to demonstrate that 44% of severe and 54% of less severe episodes of wheezing were associated with rhinovirus infection [5]. Moreover, virus-induced asthma may be severe: 42% of hospitalizations for asthma in children are associated with URI [6], and these episodes may be fatal. Finally, there are data to suggest that infection with some respiratory viruses during infancy may increase the subsequent incidence of wheezing, especially in children from atopic families [7].

Despite a strong clinical relationship between viral URIs and the development of asthma symptoms, mechanisms for lower airway abnormalities are just beginning to be recognized. Virus infection can directly disrupt lower airway physiology through toxic effects on airway epithelial cells or neural elements [1], but there is now increasing evidence that viruses may indirectly worsen airway function in asthma by inducing immune responses that augment preexisting airway inflammation. For example, subjects with either naturally acquired colds or those infected experimentally with respiratory viruses transiently develop heightened bronchial responsiveness [8–12] and an increased likelihood of developing a late allergic response to inhaled antigen [8]. Since the T cell is an essential element in immune responses to respiratory viruses, and has also been implicated in the pathogenesis of asthma, virus/T-cell interactions may be of primary importance in the pathogenesis of virus-induced asthma symptoms. In this chapter we discuss the respiratory viruses associated with asthma and corresponding host defense mechanisms, and review in detail what is known of specific T-cell/virus interactions. With these concepts in mind, the mechanisms by which virus-induced T-cell responses may play a role in the pathogenesis of asthma will be developed.

II. Respiratory Viruses Associated with Asthma

There are relatively few viruses that are particularly likely to cause lower airway wheezing and asthma exacerbations. In young children, RSV, PIV, and rhinovirus (RV) produce wheezing frequently, while RV, coronavirus, and influenza are most commonly implicated in older children and adults [1,2,5]. Greater knowledge of the protein functions, structure, and replicative cycles of these viruses (Table 1) has led to an improved understanding of virus-specific cellular immune responses, and may lead to new approaches to treat virus-induced asthma as well.

A. Rhinovirus

Human RVs are a group of 101 serologically defined picornaviruses that are the most frequent cause of the common cold [13]. The cell receptor for 90% of RV strains is ICAM-1 [14–16], and the so-called minor-group RV strains bind to the low-density lipoprotein receptor [17]. The ICAM-1 binding sites are located within "canyons" on the surface of the virion that are small enough to prevent the binding of antibody [13,18]. Neutralizing antibodies bind around this cleft, and may sterically inhibit viral attachment or uncoating. Once attached to a susceptible cell, the virus is endocytosed and its positive sense RNA-genome released [19]. This is followed by a rapid shutdown of the host messenger RNA and protein

Table 1 Viral Pathogens Commonly Associated with Increased Asthma Symptoms

Virus (genus)	Family	Genome	Cellular receptor	Major T-cell epitopes	Neutralizing antibody targets	Host cells that support viral replication	Species affected	Comments
RV	Picornaviridae	ssRNA (+strand)	1. ICAM-1 2. LDL receptor	VP1 surface proteins	VP4 surface proteins	Epi	Human, monkey	101 serotypes
RSV	Paramyxoviridae	ssRNA (−strand)	Sialic acid	Proteins G and F, nucleoprotein	Proteins G and F	Epi, lymph, mono	Human, many mammals	Syncytia formation
Influenza	Orthomyxoviridae	Segmented ssRNA (−strand)	Sialic acid	Core and surface proteins	NA, HA	Epi, lymph, mono	Human, mouse	Antigenic variation
Parainfluenza	Paramyxoviridae	ssRNA (−strand)	Sialic acid	Unknown	HN, fusion protein (F)	Epi, host cell must cleave F protein	Human, monkey, rodents, birds	
Coronavirus	Coronaviridae	Polyadenylated ssRNA (+strand)	Unknown	Unknown	E2	Epi	Human, many mammals, birds	2 serotypes, high antigenic variation

synthesis, and then escalation of host synthesis of viral RNA and proteins [20,21]. Infectious virions are released following cell lysis. RV replicates inside some, but not all, cells that have surface ICAM-1. Ciliated and nonciliated epithelial cells permit RV replication in vitro [22], while blood monocytes and airway macrophages that also express ICAM-1 on their surface do not [23]. Whether other airway cells that express ICAM-1, such as B lymphocytes, activated T lymphocytes, or eosinophils, are also susceptible to RV infection or activation is unknown.

B. RSV

RSV is a paramyxovirus consisting of single-stranded RNA with a lipoprotein envelope [24]. There are two subgroups of RSV that may circulate through a community simultaneously [25]. Immunogenic surface proteins include protein G and a fusion protein (F), and neutralizing antibodies are specific for one of these two antigens [26]. Protein G is an attachment protein that binds to sialic acid, which is present on the surface of many mammalian cells [27]. The fusion protein is required for the virus to gain entry into the cell, and may participate in syncytia formation. The ssRNA is of negative polarity, which requires that positive-strand mRNA be synthesized initially, from which viral proteins are translated. Viral replication occurs in the cytoplasm, and results either in cell lysis or the formation of syncytia, which are multinucleated cells formed by the fusion of adjacent cells.

C. Influenza A

Influenza is an orthomyxovirus with a segmented single-stranded RNA genome. The influenza capsule contains two major antigens for neutralizing antibodies: hemagglutinin (HA), which is an attachment protein that binds to sialic acid residues [28], and neuraminidase (NA), which participates in viral budding and inhibits self-aggregation [29]. Influenza viruses are classified as type A, B, or C according to variations in their nucleoprotein and matrix proteins. Antigenic determinants of influenza A and/or B surface proteins change from one year to the next through two mechanisms [30]. Small changes in surface protein epitopes are thought to be the result of two or more point mutations in the HA or NA genes. Larger antigenic "shifts" occur less often, perhaps once per decade, and may be due to either genetic reassortment or the reactivation of a previous dormant serotype. The key to influenza's genetic reassortment is the segmented genome, which contains 10 genes on eight separate pieces of single-stranded RNA. When two different strains of influenza A infect the same host, a reshuffling of the genetic material can occur, leading to the production of a unique virus strain with a mixture of genetic segments from each parent strain. Influenza A can infect many species of mammals and birds, and additional genetic variation can arise from the cross-species mixing of viral stains. Influenza replicates in a variety of cells in vitro, including epithelial cells, monocytes, and lymphocytes [31], and replication is facilitated by cleavage with trypsin [32]. Influenza RNA replication is similar to that of RSV, except that viral replication requires the participation of elements in the host cell nucleus [33]. Replication occurs throughout the respiratory tract, and viral titers correlate with disease severity [34].

D. Parainfluenza Virus

Parainfluenza viruses are in the same family as respiratory syncytial virus and share some properties with RSV, such as the negative-strand RNA genome and the ability to form multinucleated syncytial cells [27]. Sendai virus is a closely related rodent paramyxovirus that provides an excellent animal model for the study of PIV infection. Like influenza, PIV has both hemagglutination and neuraminidase activity, but these activities are contained on a single protein, dubbed HN. Neutralizing antibodies bind to either the HN or fusion (F) proteins [35], but reinfection in the presence of moderate levels of neutralizing antibody may occur. PIV infects epithelial cells of the upper and lower respiratory tract in infants, but infection in older children and adults is presumed to be limited to the upper airway.

E. Coronavirus

Coronaviruses are large enveloped viruses that have a unique plus-stranded RNA genome that resembles mRNA in having a capped polyadenosine tail [36]. Coronaviruses are second only to rhinoviruses as a cause of the common cold, and some types may also cause acute enteritis. Human and animal coronaviruses have been classified into four groups, based on antigenic differences in envelope glycoproteins, but only two serotypes of human coronaviruses have been defined [37]. Neutralizing antibodies are generally specific for the E2 attachment protein, which binds to a host cell receptor of uncertain identity. Although the range of host cells in vivo has not yet been determined, it is interesting that some cell lines may support coronavirus infection for a prolonged period of time without any apparent cytotoxicity [38]. Infection may also lead to cell lysis or syncytia formation [39]. As is the case with orthomyxoviruses and paramyxoviruses, proteolytic cleavage of coronaviruses may potentiate virulence, probably by activating the E2 protein [36]. Host-cell protease activity may therefore be an important determinant of infectivity.

F. Common Features of Viruses Associated with Asthma

Several similarities exist among the viruses discussed above. First, all are single-stranded RNA viruses that produce large numbers of progeny within a very short time. Although this is obviously advantageous for the preservation of the viral genome, it also provides a very potent immunologic stimulus. By the time that specific T-cell-mediated antiviral responses have been mobilized, there may be a large viral antigen load to deal with, increasing the chances that normal airway tissues will become damaged through a "bystander effect."

In addition, several of these families of viruses have the ability to cause repeated infections. Rhinoviruses, coronaviruses, and influenza viruses accomplish this by shifting antigenic determinants, while RSV and PIV cause reinfection despite moderately high neutralizing antibody titers. The effects of repeated infection with antigenically similar proteins is not known, but could be a potent inflammatory stimulus. In the following section we examine the host responses to common respiratory viruses.

III. Host Antiviral Immune Defenses

Host antiviral defenses generally are directed either toward preventing viral attachment to the targeted cell or interrupting viral replication at an early stage by rapidly identifying and then destroying virus-infected cells before complete virions have been synthesized. These defenses may be either nonspecific or specific for a particular virus, with the latter being dependent on T-cell participation.

A. Nonspecific Antiviral Defenses

The respiratory mucous layer represents a significant barrier that viruses must penetrate in order to attach to their primary target, the airway epithelial cell. Particles entrapped in this viscous layer are shuttled to the gastrointestinal tract by a current generated by beating cilia. In addition to serving as a barrier, respiratory mucous contains a number of nonspecific antiviral factors, such as proteolytic enzymes [40] that may destroy or inhibit viral attachment proteins.

Respiratory mucous also contains cells with nonspecific antiviral effects. Greater than 90% of the cells in lower airway secretions from normal subjects are macrophages, while epithelial cells are the predominant cell in nasal secretions [41]. The cellular makeup of respiratory mucous may change dramatically during inflammation induced by either infectious or allergic stimuli. After viral infection, neutrophils are among the first cells recruited to the respiratory epithelium and mucus [42]. Although both neutrophils and macrophages may nonspecifically phagocytose viral particles, this activity is more effective when viruses are bound by antibody [43], and is further enhanced by complement activation. Activated neutrophils produce a number of virucidal substances including superoxide [44], myeloperoxidase [45], and defensins [46].

In addition to respiratory mucous and phagocytes, NK cells may be an important source of natural immunity to viral infection. The phenotypic classification of NK cells is confusing, since they were initially defined by an activity: the lysis of either tumor cells or virus-infected cells in a non-MHC-restricted manner and without immunological priming [47]. This distinguishes the cell with NK activity from CD8$^+$ cytotoxic T cells that lyse virus-infected cells only after the viral peptides have been presented bound to MHC class I molecules. It is clear that there are several distinct cell types that share NK cell activity, including $\gamma\delta$ and some $\alpha\beta$ T cells; and non-T cells that express CD2, CD16 (high-affinity IgG receptor), and CD56 (function unknown) on their surface [47]. NK cells may be able to nonspecifically lyse virus-infected cells by recognizing stress proteins such as adhesion molecules on the cell surface. After binding to the target cell, the NK cell degranulates in a directed fashion, releasing perforin [48] and other substances that result in cell death. These findings suggest that NK cells may play a role in controlling virus-infected cells before more specific CD8$^+$ T cells can be generated, but so far there is little direct evidence of their role in respiratory infections.

B. Specific Antiviral Immune Responses

The T cell is key to both specific antibody formation and MHC-restricted cytotoxicity, adaptive immune responses that are the most effective antiviral defense mechanisms. During a primary infection, viral antigens are captured in the airway lining or mucous layer by antigen presenting cells (APC) such as the dendritic cell [49] or the airway macrophage. These cells move to the tonsils or regional lymph nodes, where antigen presentation occurs [50], APC possess proteolytic enzymes which cut viral proteins into small peptides. These peptides then bind to MHC class I or II molecules in the cytoplasm and are transported to the surface of the cell, where they may be presented to "naive" T cells, which have not previously been exposed to antigen. Viral peptides bound to MHC class I and class II molecules stimulate CD8$^+$ and CD4$^+$ T cells, respectively. Optimal antigen presentation and T-cell stimulation requires the participation of other cell surface molecules such as CD2/CD28 and ICAM-1/LFA-1 [51,52]. These molecules assist in cell-to-cell adhesion, and in some cases also are capable of transducing signals to the T-cell nucleus. Once the T cell has been stimulated by a viral antigen, changes in the surface adhesion molecules occur that may direct the cell to leave the lymph node and enter the peripheral circulation. Expression of the lymph node homing receptor LECAM-1 (recognized by the antibody MEL-14) is reduced, while other adhesion molecules, e.g., LFA-1 and VLA-4, are upregulated [53]. The circulating T cells then bind to the inflamed area of the respiratory tract due to a local increase in expression of other complementary adhesion molecules such as ICAM-1 and VCAM-1. Once in the mucosa, the cells are exposed to high levels of viral antigen, which may drive further differentiation into either cytolytic or memory lymphocytes. The majority of T cells that track into the airway are CD8$^+$ cells, and in mouse models of influenza or Sendai virus infection, peak influx occurs 1 week after inoculation [54,55]. Limiting dilution studies demonstrate that the number of virus-specific cells in the respiratory mucosa also peaks 7 days after inoculation, but it is apparent that other lymphocytes that are not specific for viral proteins are also drawn into the airway [50,54].

Following primary infection, memory cells that are specific for respiratory viruses are distributed throughout the mucosal surfaces and the spleen. Reinfection produces a rapid and pronounced lymphocytic response, leading to an influx of both CD4+ and CD8+ cells into the respiratory tract [56]. Blood and splenic lymphocyte numbers decrease during this same time period, and in the mouse, return to normal by 1–2 weeks.

Activated CD4+ T cells may have several distinct antiviral activities. First, T-cell "help" is required to produce antibody capable of neutralizing viruses. Respiratory mucus contains large amounts of immunoglobulin, mostly of the IgA and IgG isotypes. Antibodies may provide the host with immunity toward infection with specific viruses by binding to viral coat proteins that are essential for either virus attachment or uncoating. Antibody would therefore be expected to be most effective in interrupting the extracellular portion of the virus life cycle. Recent data have also suggested that IgA may also be able to bind to intracellular viral proteins as well, since IgA must be transported through epithelial cells in its journey from the lymphocyte to the respiratory secretions [57]. Activated CD4+ T cells provide the signals that enable the B cell to switch from virus-specific IgM production to IgG and IgA, isotypes that confer antiviral immunity, and may aid in virus killing as well. In addition, CD4+ T cells are needed for affinity maturation, small modifications in antibody structure that increase antibody-binding avidity.

T-cell-derived cytokines such as IFN-γ, TGF-β, and IL-2 may have antiviral activities beyond their effects on antibody synthesis [58]. IFN-γ and TGF-β may inhibit viral replication directly [59,60], and both IFN-γ and IL-2 potentiate the antiviral functions of other cell types such as NK cells and CD8+ T cells. IFN-γ and IL-4 increase the expression of specific arrays of adhesion molecules [61–63], which recruit additional inflammatory cells into the airway during viral infection and also determine what type of cells are attracted. Surprisingly, despite the multiple antiviral properties of IFN-γ, transgenic mice lacking a functional IFN-γ gene mount effective cell-mediated and humoral immune responses after inoculation with influenza [64]. Finally, the cytokine milieu may direct the differentiation of naive T cells into either Th1 or Th2 helper T cells [65]. Cells exposed to antigen in the presence of IL-4 may be more likely to develop into Th2 cells that secrete cytokines associated with allergic inflammation, such as IL-4 and IL-5. On the other hand, naive cells that are activated by antigen in the presence of IL-12 are likely to develop into Th1 cells, which may inhibit allergic responses and potentiate antiviral cell-mediated responses.

Once cells are infected with virus, T-cell-mediated cytotoxicity is the most effective means of eradicating infection. CD8+ T cells "recognize" viral peptides bound to MHC class I molecules on the surface of infected cells. Activated cytotoxic T cells may kill infected cells via several pathways, including directed secretion of perforin, induction of apoptosis, and the secretion of cytokines such as IFN-γ that directly inhibit viral replication. Cytotoxic T cells are capable of recognizing and destroying infected cells rapidly, before virus replication has occurred. Mice or humans lacking functional CD8+ cells are impaired in their ability to eradicate viral infections, underscoring the importance of cytotoxic T cells in this regard [50,66].

IV. T-Cell Responses to Specific Respiratory Viruses

Rhinovirus, RSV, and influenza A are the viruses most closely identified with asthma exacerbations, and current information pertaining to T-cell responses to these viruses are reviewed in the following sections.

A. T-Cell Response to Rhinovirus

Several studies have focused on the cellular response to RV infection in humans, but animal studies are hampered by the fact that RV does not bind to rodent ICAM-1 [67]. Acute RV illnesses are characterized by increased numbers of neutrophils and lymphocytes in nasal secretions 3–4 days following inoculation [42,68]. Levandowski reported that peripheral blood lymphopenia paralleled lymphocyte migration into nasal secretions following inoculation with RV25 [69]. Symptom scores correlated with the decline in peripheral blood CD4+ but not CD8+ cells [69]. In contrast, Skoner and colleagues did not find an acute decrease in peripheral blood lymphocytes after experimentally infecting subjects with a different serotype (RV39) [70]. In both studies, peripheral blood lymphocyte numbers increased between 4 and 7 days after inoculation. The increase in circulating T cells coincides with resolution of symptoms, and lymphocyte counts remain elevated for at least 2 weeks. Moreover, Hsia et al. found evidence that peripheral blood lymphocytes from RV experimentally infected humans were activated, as they generated more IL-2 and interferon-γ (IFNγ) ex vivo and had enhanced antigen-induced blastogenesis [71]. Mononuclear cells incubated with RV in vitro produce interferon activity as measured in a plaque-forming assay, although the response is strain-dependent [72]. Blastogenic responses to RV are increased for up to 6 weeks after inoculation, and are serotype-specific in humans [73]. In contrast, studies of T cells generated from RV-vaccinated mice have indicated that RV T-cell epitopes are located on regions of surface proteins that are highly conserved among different RV serotypes [74].

In addition to activating RV-specific T cells as evidenced by enhanced blastogenesis, RV can also nonspecifically activate T cells. When ^{35}S-labeled RV16 is incubated with monocytes and T cells purified from peripheral blood, RV binds mainly to monocytes, and this binding is ICAM-1-dependent. In unseparated cells, the binding of RV to monocytes is followed by increased T-cell expression of CD69, an early activation marker [75]. These findings suggest that T cells that are not virus-specific may still be activated during viral infection, increasing the potential for airway inflammation. This mechanism may be especially relevant in asthma due to the increased numbers of T cells in the airway.

B. T-Cell Response to RSV

T-cell proliferative responses to inactivated RSV or RSV antigens are increased between 7 days and 1 month after the onset of symptoms [76,77]. Cytotoxic T cells can be demonstrated in the peripheral blood of adults who had presumably had a past RSV infection [78]. In infants with acute RSV infections, cytotoxic T cells were most often recovered from the peripheral blood during the first 2 weeks after onset of symptoms [79]. Cytotoxic T-cell responses are directed at the nucleoprotein or fusion protein in both in the human and the mouse [78,80]. The fusion protein may be a particularly important antigen, as it stimulates both CD4+ and CD8+ T-cell responses, and immunogenic epitopes on the F protein have been mapped [81]. The G protein, which is a primary target of neutralizing antibodies, primarily stimulates CD4+ T cells [78,82]. Immunosuppressed individuals may develop particularly severe RSV infections, or shed virus for prolonged periods of time [83].

C. T-Cell Response to Influenza

Peripheral blood lymphocyte counts fall between 2 and 6 days after inoculation with influenza [84]. Influenza-specific T-cell proliferative responses in peripheral blood then increase and fall to baseline levels 28 days after inoculation [85]. During this time period, influenza-specific cytotoxic T cells can also be detected [86], which may react to several different strains of influenza A [30]. As is the case with other viral infections, cytolytic T cells are important in clearing influenza-infected cells [66]. Transgenic mice that lack β_2 microglobulin have an impaired ability to clear influenza virus infection, but can clear mild infections [87]. The specificity of CD4+ T cells parallels the relative proportions of proteins within a virion, and includes both core and surface proteins [88]. These CD4+ T cells are crucial for the generation of influenza-specific antibody, and it has been shown that CD4+ T cells may also participate in the clearance of virus-infected cells by directing the synthesis of anti-HA antibody [89]. CD4+ cells probably play a lesser role in cytotoxic T-cell responses. For example, mice that are treated with an anti-CD4 monoclonal antibody and then infected with influenza are able to produce adequate numbers of virus-specific cytotoxic T cells to clear virus from the lung [54].

  Hennet and colleagues used bronchoalveolar lavage to determine the kinetics of cytokine production in mice that were inoculated with a lethal dose of influenza [90]. IL-1, IL-6, GM-CSF, and TNFα were detected within 1 day of inoculation, followed closely by IFN-γ, which may have been secreted by T cells or NK cells. Neither IL-2 nor IL-4, which are T-cell-derived cytokines, were detected during the 6-day experiment. The authors suggested that either the T cells were not activated by a primary infection within the time frame of the experiment, or the cytokines were produced in low concentrations or at an alternative site.

V. Virus Strategies for Evading Adaptive Immune Responses

Many viral pathogens have evolved mechanisms to dodge antiviral immune responses, or even to use components of the immune response to their own advantage [91–93]. The viruses associated with asthma have likewise adapted to the environment in the respiratory tract using a variety of strategies. First, since virus-specific antibody provides immunity by preventing viral attachment, several viruses have evolved mechanisms to avoid humoral immunity. For example, it is usual for many strains of RV to "circulate" through any given community at one time, thus increasing the chances of infecting hosts without serotype-specific neutralizing antibody. In contrast, influenza evades neutralizing antibodies through an extremely high rate of antigenic evolution, characterized by periodic major (antigenic shift) and minor (antigenic drift) changes in HA and NA antigenic epitopes. Although antibody to HA or NA confers immunity to infection and immunologic memory is prolonged, influenza A is able to dodge adaptive immune responses by varying the antigenic determinants of its surface proteins from year to year. Finally, the formation of syncytia by RSV, PIV, and coronavirus could allow these viruses to spread from cell to cell without being exposed to extracellular immune effectors such as antibody.

RSV is a poor immunogen, and infants in particular have an impaired capacity to form neutralizing antibody. While high levels of passively acquired maternal anti-RSV antibody are protective, reinfection is common despite the presence of neutralizing antibody [94]. Several factors may contribute to reduced immunogenicity. First, RSV infects immune cells and may directly suppress their function. RSV can replicate in macrophages [95], and RSV antigens can be detected in circulating monocytes during acute infection [96]. Second, RSV is a poor interferon inducer relative to other respiratory viruses [72,97]. Since interferon has direct antiviral properties, increases cell-mediated immune responses, and may participate in antibody synthesis as well, the relatively low induction of interferon may facilitate RSV infection. Finally, Roberts and colleagues have measured production of net IL-1 inhibitor activity by RSV-infected monocytes [98]. Given the wide range of immune functions attributed to IL-1, virus-mediated inhibition of this cytokine could reduce the effectiveness of several antiviral immune responses. For example, IL-1 and other acute-phase cytokines increase the expression of adhesion molecules such as ICAM-1 in the airway, and this may aid in the recruitment of inflammatory cells to the site of infection. Unlike other respiratory pathogens, such as influenza A, RSV does not increase ICAM-1 expression on monocytes, and RSV inhibits the clustering of infected mononuclear cells [99]. IL-1 also serves as a cofactor for lymphocyte proliferation by inducing HLA-DR and the high-affinity IL-2 receptor. During RSV infection, these responses are blunted, and mitogen-driven lymphocyte proliferation is inhibited [100]. Preincubation with live RSV in vitro also inhibits proliferation in response to inactivated RSV or RSV proteins [100,101]. Since IL-1 also participates in other immune responses, such as antibody production, it is anticipated that RSV might have other immunosuppressive properties as well. Thus, RSV-driven production of IL-1 inhibitor may decrease virus-specific T-cell responses that are necessary to kill virus-infected cells.

Like RSV, influenza virus infects lymphocytes and monocytes and can adversely affect immune cell function. Peripheral blood leukocyte counts are typically depressed during the acute phase of infection [84]. Mononuclear cells infected in vitro have decreased proliferation in response to both antigen and mitogen, and infected individuals have both decreased delayed-type hypersensitivity skin tests and lymphocyte blastogenic responses [102,103]. It is interesting that monocytes must be present for influenza to infect lymphocytes in vitro [31]. In addition to inhibiting lymphocyte responses, influenza infection has been associated with other immune abnormalities, including decreased phagocyte chemotaxis and bacteriocidal capacity [30]. Clinical immunosuppression due to influenza virus infection is evident as bacterial infections, especially with *S. Pneumoniae* or *N. Meningitidis*, are frequent complications.

RV infections often precede bacterial upper airway infections such as otitis media [104,105]. Since ICAM-1 and its natural ligand LFA-1 participate in several cellular immune processes such as cell recruitment, antigen presentation, and B-cell activation [51,106–109], it is possible that RV could disrupt local immunity through via binding to ICAM-1. We have preliminary data that RV inhibits antigen-specific T-cell proliferation, but does not inhibit mitogen, IL-2, or alloantigen-induced T-cell proliferation [110]. These findings suggest that RV interferes with antigen presentation and is not directly toxic to lymphocytes. If such events also occur in the airway, the specific anti-RV immune responses could be delayed, increasing the probability of successful RV replication. In addition, suppression of local airway immunity might increase the probability of secondary infectious complications.

In summary, respiratory viruses have evolved unique strategies to avoid immune detection by antibody. RV, RSV, and influenza all have developed rapid replicative cycles, which generally yield a new generation of virions before the host is able to mobilize virus-specific (and highly effective) immune responses such as virus-specific antibody or cytotoxic T cells. In addition, RSV, influenza A, and RV all have means of specifically delaying cell-mediated responses, either by infecting monocytes and lymphocytes, producing cytokine inhibitors, or interacting with key immune cell proteins such as ICAM-1. It is possible that some or all of these same interactions may be relevant in the pathogenesis of virus-induced asthma symptoms.

VI. T-Cell/Virus Interactions and Asthma

As discussed previously, interactions between respiratory viruses and T cells are complex. Virus infection induces the rapid expansion of virus-specific T cells; this response could change airway physiology as cytokines are produced, virus-infected cells are lysed by cytotoxic T cells, and virus-specific antibodies bind to their targets. It is also clear that viruses may influence the function of T cells in the airway that are not virus-specific. Such changes may be accomplished by direct infection of T cells or accessory cells, or by stimulating other airway cells to secrete mediators, cytokines, or cytokine inhibitors that in turn may alter the function of allergen-specific T cells. Several of these virus/T-cell interactions have the potential to contribute to asthmatic allergic inflammation. Ongoing studies are beginning to accumulate to lend support to these hypotheses.

A. Enhanced T-Cell Recruitment

To define virus effects on inflammatory cell recruitment directly, Fraenkel et al. experimentally infected normal and allergic subjects with RV [111]. No changes in histology were detected within the nasal mucosal biopsies during infection. No changes in histology were detected within the nasal mucosal biopsies during infection. Bronchial biopsies, in contrast, had increased numbers of CD3, CD4, and CD8[+] lymphocytes in normal and asthma subjects during the cold. Calhoun et al. also studied the effect of RV16 on cell recruitment in experimentally infected allergic rhinitis subjects, and then studied the recruitment of inflammatory cells into the lower airway after either antigen or saline segmental lung challenge [112]. RV infection caused a significant increase in the antigen-induced influx of total inflammatory cells and eosinophils 48 h after antigen challenge. In nonallergic subjects, there was no effect of RV16 on cell recruitment into lower airway secretions. These studies indicate that viral infections may increase the recruitment of T cells and eosinophils into the airway. Furthermore, cell recruitment is enhanced only in allergic subjects, which may account for the differences in clinical consequences of viral URI in allergic or asthma patients versus normal subjects. Virus infection probably promotes increased T-cell recruitment by inducing cytokine secretion from airway cells. For example, macrophages and monocytes stimulated in vitro with RV, RSV, or influenza A produce acute-phase cytokines such as IL-1β, TNFα, and interferon-α [98,113,114]. RV and influenza also stimulate interferon production [72,97,115,116], and there are preliminary data that virus infection stimulates IL-8 secretion by epithelial cells and perhaps other cell types as well [117–119]. IL-1β, TNFα, and IFN-γ are strong inducers of adhesion molecule expression on endothelial cells, which would in turn promote recruitment of inflammatory cells into the airway. In addition, IL-8 is a potent T-cell chemotactic agent, active at picomolar concentrations [120].

Influenza virus may also recruit leukocytes to the lung in a novel fashion. Colden-Stanfield and colleagues found that influenza infection of human umbilical vein endothelial cells (HUVEC) increased 28-fold the adhesion of HL-60 cells, a neutrophil cell line [121]. This increased adherence was abolished either by anti-HA antibody, or by treating the HL-60 cells with neuraminidase. These findings suggest that sialic acid residues on the leukocytes were binding to HA expressed on the surface of virus-infected HUVEC, providing an example of an adhesion molecule of viral origin.

In the mouse, there is evidence that the majority of T cells recruited to the lower airway in response to virus infection are not virus-specific T cells (supra vide). Presumably, any lymphocyte with the right combination of adhesion receptors could attach to endothelial cells in the respiratory tract and migrate into the airway mucosa or mucus layer. The net result of this "bystander" effect may be to attract more allergen-specific cells into the airway, as well as providing a mechanism by which viral infections could enhance allergen-induced responses. Although there is currently no direct evidence to support this hypothesis, the end result would be an increase in asthma symptoms.

B. Do Virus-Specific T Cells Promote Lower Airway Obstruction?

Virus-Specific T-Cell Proliferation and Asthma Symptoms

T cells control the adaptive immune responses to both viruses and allergens, but there are little data regarding the participation of virus-specific T cells in the pathogenesis of asthma exacerbation. Welliver et al. prospectively studied RSV-specific T-cell proliferative responses in 39 infected infants. Proliferative responses were higher both acutely and between 20 and 60 days after infection in the group of children with wheezing (either bronchiolitis or asthma) [122]. The question as to whether virus-specific T-cell proliferation correlates with lower airway dysfunction has yet to be settled, as two other studies were unable to confirm the correlation between disease manifestations and RSV-specific lymphocyte proliferation [76,77].

Lower Airway Pathology Related to CD8+ Cells

Animal studies indicate that virus-specific cytotoxic cells have the potential to cause lung injury. Cannon et al. irradiated mice, and then treated groups of mice with either intranasal RSV, intravenous RSV-specific T cells, or both [123]. Five days after the treatment, 4 out of 5 mice given both T cells and virus died, compared to none in the other groups (Fig. 1). Viral culture and histological examination of lung tissue revealed that infected mice that were given RSV-specific T cells were able to eliminate the virus but had increased infiltration of neutrophils and pulmonary hemorrhage. Similarly, transferring virus-primed CD4+ or CD8+ T cells may enhance lung inflammation in mice that are subsequently infected with influenza [124], and certain influenza-specific CD4+ clones may have similar effects [125]. These findings confirm that cytotoxic T cells are necessary to kill virus-infected cells, but also suggest that virus-specific T cells may also damage surrounding lung tissue after antigen exposure. If such events also occur in human airways, increased asthma symptoms may follow.

Enhancement of Inflammatory Cell Function by Virus-Specific T Cells

Another possibility is that T cells stimulated by viral peptides augment the inflammatory functions of inflammatory cells that are present in the asthmatic, but not the normal airway. For instance, several investigators have demonstrated that respiratory viruses increase basophil histamine release in vitro [72,126–128]. Ida et al. showed that human leucocytes infected with interferon-inducing respiratory viruses produced a soluble factor to enhance histamine release [126]. Interferon produced similar effects, implying a possible role in causation. Chonmaitree found that RSV, RV, and influenza A were each able to enhance anti-IgE-induced histamine release from human leukocytes [72]. In this study, however, histamine

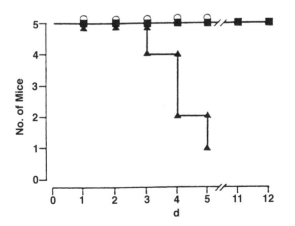

Figure 1   Survival of γ-irradiated BALB/c mice after RSV infection and/or transfer of an RSV-specific cytotoxic T cell clone at day 0. Treatments were: (○) RSV inoculation; (■) 8 × 10⁶ RSV-specific T cells; (▲) RSV inoculation + 8 × 10⁶ RSV-specific T cells. RSV-infected mice were killed on day 5 for lung RSV assays.

release was observed even when virus-induced interferon was not detectable. In a follow-up study, supernates from peripheral blood leukocytes stimulated with influenza A or RSV were found to induce histamine release from fresh mononuclear cells [129]. The soluble histamine-releasing factor was not identified as any known cytokine. Huftel et al. found that T-cell depletion abrogates the ability of influenza A to release histamine from leukocytes, and suggested that T cells may be the source of the histamine release-enhancing factor(s) [130]. Candidates for this T-cell-derived histamine releasing factor include members of the intercrine/chemocrine family of cytokines, including RANTES and MCIP, which have potent histamine-releasing activity and are also strong eosinophil chemotactic agents. Finally, Calhoun and colleagues experimentally infected allergic rhinitis subjects with RV16, and then performed segmental allergen challenge before, during, and after RV infection [131]. RV infection alone had little effect on airway histamine levels, but RV infection significantly increased BAL histamine in response to allergen challenge. These findings indicate that several respiratory viruses can enhance leukocyte histamine release, possibly by stimulating T-cell cytokine production. Since enhanced basophil histamine release correlates with airway reactivity [132], it is possible that this effect may be a relevant mechanism by which viral infections increase asthma symptoms.

Production of Virus-Specific IgE

The generation of virus-specific IgE would provide an obvious link between the immune response to virus and enhancement of allergic inflammation. In this case, inflammatory cells bearing IgE receptors could be "sensitized" by binding virus-specific IgE. Cross-linking of IgE molecules by virus would then trigger mast cell activation and release of inflammatory mediators such as histamine, leukotrienes, and cytokines, leading to typical asthmatic inflammation. Welliver and colleagues detected RSV-specific IgE bound to epithelial cells in the secretions of children with bronchiolitis [133]. Using double immunofluorescent staining, cell-bound IgE was found in 70–80% of nasopharyngeal washings, and virtually all of the IgE-positive cells also stained positive for RSV antigen. In a second study, RSV-specific IgE was detected with ELISA in the nasal secretions of 79 children with documented RSV infection [134]. Higher levels of virus-specific IgE were associated with wheezing versus nonwheezing illnesses, hypoxia, and greater histamine levels in nasal secretions. Bui and colleagues reported a similar association between RSV-specific IgE antibodies in the serum and the presence of wheezing illnesses [135]. Parainfluenza virus-specific IgE may play a similar role in virus-induced wheezing [136–138]. It has since been suggested that infants who develop high levels of RSV-specific IgE after primary infection may be more likely to experience recurrent wheezing 4 years after the initial viral infection [136]. In addition, several studies have documented the presence of mast cell mediators such as histamine and leukotrienes in secretions during RSV and parainfluenza infections [133,134,139]. Together, these observations imply that virus-specific IgE may participate in the pathogenesis of virus-induced wheezing in infancy, and may predispose the patient or recurrent episodes of wheezing. Whether IgE antibodies play a role in virus-induced wheezing in the older asthmatic has not yet been established.

Effects of Virus Infection on Th1 Versus Th2 Lymphocytes

Lymphocytes may be classified into Th1 or Th2 subgroups on the basis of the cytokines that they generate upon activation [140]. Lymphocytes that are stimulated by viral antigens have usually been found to produce IL-2 and IFN-γ, and are thus Th1-like. This cytokine profile, however, is not usually associated with asthma pathogenesis. In contrast, studies that have examined lymphokine production in allergic or asthmatic airways have found an increase in Th2-like cytokines such as IL-5 [141–143], and reported no increase in IFN-γ [141].

How, then, might Th1 responses induced by viral infections increase allergic or asthmatic inflammation? One possible explanation is that viruses may not elicit a pure Th1 response. For example, we know from the studies of Welliver [133, 134,144] and Bui [135] that virus-specific IgE is associated with wheezing in RSV and parainfluenza-infected infants. IgE synthesis requires the presence of either IL-4 [145] or IL-13 [146], which are both synthesized by Th2 lymphocytes. This is indirect evidence that RSV and parainfluenza virus infection induce the synthesis of at least some Th2 cytokines. Alwan et al. tested this possibility by vaccinating mice with recombinant vaccinia viruses (rVV) that expressed individual RSV protein [82,147]. Mice vaccinated with rVV-protein G developed pulmonary eosinophilia upon infection with RSV [147]. Furthermore, analysis of protein G-specific T cells from vaccinated mice yielded a Th2 cytokine profile, with large amounts of IL-4 and IL-5 bioactivity [82]. Passive transfer of these cells into mice that are then inoculated with RSV causes intense pulmonary eosinophilia and potentiates RSV-mediated pulmonary pathology [148]. In contrast, fusion protein-specific T cells consisted of a mixture of CD8+ and Th1-type CD4+ cells, and had little effect on pulmonary pathology [82,148]. This has not yet been verified in humans, but suggests that certain RSV proteins stimulate Th2 cells that increase airway inflammation and lead to increased morbidity.

A second possibility is that Th1 cytokines may upregulate the inflammatory functions of effector cells in virus-induced asthma; there is some in-vitro data to support this hypothesis. Valerius et al. incubated peripheral blood eosinophils from healthy donors with different cytokines and measured effects on eosinophil survival and function [149]. In these in-vitro experiments, recombinant IFN-γ potentiated both eosinophil survival and antibody-dependent cytotoxicity, suggesting that Th1 cytokines may also contribute to asthmatic inflammation.

C. Nonspecific Enhancement of T-Cell Inflammatory Function by Respiratory Viruses

Cytokine Production

In addition to effects on virus-specific T cells, respiratory viruses induce cytokine secretion from a variety of other cells in vitro, including macrophages [23,98, 113,114], monocytes [114], fibroblasts [150,151], and epithelial cells [117,119, 151]. These data suggest that virus-induced cytokines may enhance the effects of airway T cells, and it is possible that these cytokines either directly or indirectly contribute to asthma pathogenesis. For example, both IL-1 and TNF, which are induced by several respiratory viruses, enhance lymphocyte IL-2 receptor expression and antigen-driven T-cell proliferation [152,153]. IL-6, which may be induced from epithelium and fibroblasts by several viruses, synergizes with IL-1 in promoting T-cell proliferation [154]. Rhinovirus stimulates peripheral blood monocytes to produce IFN-α [155], which may increase the expression of the early activation marker CD69 on T cells and NK cells [156].

Data regarding in-vivo cytokine production in the airways of virus-infected humans are also beginning to appear. For instance, Balfour-Lynn et al. reported that TNF-α levels were increased in the upper airway secretions of wheezing infants infected with RSV [157]. Calhoun and colleagues experimentally infected with type 16 RV subjects with allergic rhinitis, performed segmental allergen challenge, and then measured cytokines in lower airway secretions. RV infection increased the amounts of both TNF-α and IFN-γ secreted into the lower airway in response to allergen challenge [158]. These models of virus-induced asthma suggest that virus infection may modify allergen-specific T cell responses in the lower airway, but these findings will need to be validated by additional studies examining the effects of virus infection on lower-airway T cells in subjects with asthma.

Viral Superantigens

Several viruses contain proteins that act as superantigens [159,160], which activate T cells by binding to specific Vβ regions to T-cell receptors [161]. Whereas the frequency of virus-specific cells in the airway might be 1 in 1000, superantigens may activate 5–30% of T cells, depending on the frequency of the relevant Vβ regions [161]. If respiratory viruses also contain superantigens, they could activate lymphocytes involved in asthma pathogenesis, potentially increasing both airway inflammation and asthma symptoms.

VII. Summary

Viral respiratory infections are a major cause of asthma exacerbations and provide unique insight into pathogenic mechanisms of this disease. There is increasing evidence that the increased severity of airway disease in allergic and asthmatic individuals with colds is due to unique interactions between the immune response to RV and preexisting airway inflammation. Characterization of T-cell antiviral responses, in both normal and allergic subjects, will provide valuable new information toward defining the mechanisms of wheezing with colds.

References

1. Cypcar D, Busse WW. Role of viral infections in asthma. Immunol Allergy Clin N Am 1993; 13:745–766.

2. Pattemore PK, Johnston SL, Bardin PG, Viruses as precipitants of asthma symptoms. I. Epidemiology. Clin Exp Allergy 1992; 22:325–336.

3. Duff AL, Pomeranz ES, Gelber LE, et al. Risk factors for acute wheezing in infants in infants and children: viruses, passive smoke, and IgE antibodies to inhalant allergens. Pediatrics 1993; 92:535–540.

4. Johnston SL, Pattemore PK, Sanderson G, et al. Community study of role of viral infections in exacerbations of asthma in 9- 11-year-old children. Br Med J 1995; 310:1225–1229.

5. Nicholson KG, Kent J, Ireland DC. Respiratory viruses and exacerbations of asthma in adults. Br Med J 1993; 307:982–986.

6. Mcintosh K, Ellis EF, Hoffman LS, Lybass TG, Eller JJ, Fulginiti VA. The association of viral and bacterial respiratory infection with exacerbations of wheezing in young asthmatic children. J Pediatr 1973; 82:578–590.

7. Morgan WJ, Martinez FD. Risk factors for developing wheezing and asthma in childhood. Pediatr Clin N Am 1992; 39:1185–1203.

8. Lemanske RF Jr, Dick EC, Swenson CA, Vrtis RF, Busse WW. Rhinovirus upper respiratory infection increases airway hyperreactivity and late asthmatic reactions. J Clin Invest 1989; 83:1–10.

9. Picken JJ, Niewoehner DE, Chester EH. Prolonged effects of viral infections of the upper respiratory tract upon small airways. Am J Med 1972; 52:738.

10. Blair HT, Greenberg SB, Stevens PM, Bilunos PA, Couch RB. Effects of rhinovirus infection on pulmonary function of healthy human volunteers. Am Rev Respir Dis 1976; 114:95–102.

11. Empey DW, Laitinen LA, Jacobs L, Gold WM, Nadel JA. Mechanisms of bronchial hyperreactivity in normal subjects after upper respiratory tract infection. Am Rev Respir Dis 1976; 113:131–139.

12. Cheung D, Dick EC, Timmers MC, De Klerk EPA, Spaan WJM, Sterk PJ. Rhinovirus inhalation causes prolonged excessive airway narrowing to methacholine in asthmatic subjects *in vivo*. Am J Respir Crit Care Med 1994; 149(suppl):A47(abstr).

13. Dick EC, Inhorn SL. Rhinoviruses. In: Feigin RD, Cherry JD, eds. Textbook of Pediatric Infectious Diseases, 3rd ed. Philadelphia: W.B. Saunders, 1992; 1507–1532.

14. Staunton DE, Merluzzi VJ, Rothlein R, Barton R, Marlin SC, Springer TA. A cell adhesion molecule, ICAM-1, is the major surface receptor for rhinoviruses. Cell 1989; 56:849–853.

15. Tomassini JE, Graham D, DeWitt CE, Lineberger DW, Rodkey JA, Colonno RJ. cDNA cloning reveals that the major group rhinovirus receptor on HeLa cells is intercellular adhesion molecule 1. Proc Natl Acad Sci USA 1989; 86:4907–4911.

16. Greve JM, Davis G, Meyer AM, et al. The major human rhinovirus receptor is ICAM-1. Cell 1989; 56:839–847.

17. Hofer F, Gruenberger M, Kowalski H, et al. Members of the low density lipoprotein receptor family mediate cell entry of a minor-group common cold virus. Proc Natl Acad Sci USA 1994; 91:1839–1842.

18. Johnston SL, Bardin PG, Pattemore PK. Viruses as precipitants of asthma symptoms. III. Rhinoviruses: molecular biology and prospects for future intervention. Clin Exp Allergy 1993; 23:237–246.

19. Rueckert RR. Picornaviridae and their replication. In: Fields BN, Knipe DM, Chanock RM, et al., Virology, 2nd ed. New York: Raven Press, 1990:507–546.

20. Etchison D. Human rhinovirus 14 infection of HeLa cells results in the proteolytic cleavage of the p220 cap binding complex subunit and inactivates globin mRNA translation *in vitro*. J Virol 1985; 54:634–638.

21. Lucas-Lenard JM. Inhibition of cellular protein synthesis after infection. In: Perez-Bercoff R, ed. The Molecular Biology of Picornaviruses. New York: Cambridge University Press, 1979:73–99.

22. deArruda E, Mifflia TE, Gwaltney JMJ, Winther B, Haydin FG. Localization of rhinovirus replication *in vitro* with *in situ* hybridization. J Med Virol 1991; 54:634–638.

23. Gern JE, Galagan DM, Dick EC. Rhinovirus enters but does not replicate inside monocytes and airway macrophages. J Immunol 1996; 156:621–627.

24. Mcintosh K, Chanock RM. Respiratory syncytial viruses. In: Fields BN, Knipe DM, Chanock RM, et al., Virology, 2nd ed. New York: Raven Press, 1990:1045–1074.

25. Hendry RM, Talis AL, Godfrey E, Anderson LJ, Fernie BF, Mcintosh K. Concurrent circulation of antigenically distinct strains of respiratory syncytial virus during community outbreaks. J Infect Dis 1986; 153:291–297.

26. Walsh EE, Hall CB, Briselli M, Brandriss MW, Schlesinger JJ. Immunization with glycoprotein subunits of respiratory syncytial virus to protect cotton rats against viral infection. J Infect Dis 1987; 155:1198–1204.

27. Kingsbury DW. Paramyxoviridae and their replication. In: Fields BN, Knipe DM, Chanock RM, et al., Virology, 2nd ed. New York: Raven Press, 1990:945–962.

28. Wiley DC, Skehel JJ. The structure and function of the hemagglutinin membrane glycoprotein of influenza virus. Annu Rev Biochem 1987; 56:365–394.

29. Colman PM, Ward CW. Structure and diversity of influenza virus neuraminidase. Curr Topics Microbiol Immunol 1985; 11:177–255.

30. Murphy BR, Webster RG. Orthomyxoviruses. In: Fields BN, Knipe DM, Chanock RM, et al., Virology, 2nd ed. New York: Raven Press, 1990:1091–1152.

31. Mock DJ, Domurat F, Roberts NJ, Walsh EE, Licht MR, Keng P. Macrophages are required for influenza virus infection of human lymphocytes. J Clin Invest 1987; 79:620–624.

32. Klenk HD, Rott R, Orlich M, Blodorn J. Activation of influenza A viruses by trypsin treatment. Virology 1975; 68:426–439.

33. Kingsbury DW. Orthomyxoviridae and their replication. In: Fields BN, Knipe DM, Chanock RM, et al., Virology, 2nd ed. New York: Raven Press, 1990:1075–1089.

34. Murphy BR, Chalhub EG, Nusinoff SR, Kasel J, Chanock RM. Temperature-sensitive mutants of influenza virus. III. Further characterization of the ts-1[E] influenza A recombinant (H3N2) virus in man. J Infect Dis 1973; 128:479–487.

35. Spriggs MK, Murphy BR, Prince GA, Olmsted RA, Collins PL, Expression of the F and HN glycoproteins of human parainfluenza virus type 3 recombinant vaccinia viruses: contribution of the individual proteins to host immunity. J Virol 1987; 67: 3416–3423.

36. Holmes KV. Coronaviridae and their replication. In: Fields BN, Knipe DM, Chanock RM, et al., Virology, 2nd ed. New York: Raven Press, 1990:841–856.

37. Dick EC, Inhorn SL. Coronaviruses. In: Feigin RD, Cherry JD, eds. Textbook of Pediatric Infectious Diseases, 3rd ed. Philadelphia: W. B. Saunders, 1992; 1498–1506.

38. Chaloner-Larsson G, Johnson-Lussenburg CM. Establishment and maintenance of a persistent infection of L132 cells by human coronavirus strain 229E. Arch Virol 1981; 69:117–129.

39. Bruckova M, Mcintosh K, Kapikian AZ, Chanock RM. The adaptation of two human coronavirus strains (OC38 and OC43) to growth in cell monolayers. Proc Soc Exp Biol Med 1970; 135:431–435.

40. Kaliner MA. Human nasal host defense and sinusitis. J Allergy Clin Immunol 1992; 90:424–430.

41. Bascom R, Pipkorn U, Lichtenstein LM, Naclerio RM. The influx of inflammatory cells into nasal washings during the late response to antigen challenge. Am Rev Respir Dis 1988; 138:406–412.

42. Levandowski RA, Weaver CW, Jackson GG. Nasel secretion leukocyte populations determined by flow cytometry during acute rhinovirus infection. J Med Virol 1988; 25:423–432.

43. Tamura M, Webster RG, Ennis FA. Antibodies to HA and NA augment uptake of influenza A viruses into cells via Fc receptor entry. Virology 1991; 182:211–219.

44. Busse WW, Vrtis RF, Steiner R, Dick EC. In vitro incubation with influenza virus primes human polymorphonuclear leukocyte generation of superoxide. Am J Respir Cell Mol Biol 1991; 4:347–354.

45. Yamamoto K, Miyoshi-Koshio T, Utsuke Y, Mizuno S, Suzuki K. Virucidal activity and viral protein modification by myeloperoxidase: a candidate for defense factor of human polymorphonuclear leukocytes against influenza virus infection. J Infect Dis 1991; 164:8–14.

46. Lehrer RI, Lichtenstein AK, Ganz T. Defensins: antimicrobial and cytotoxic properties of mammalian cells. Annu Rev Immunol 1993; 11:105–128.

47. Podack ER. Killer and natural killer cells: function of non-major histocompatibility complex-restricted killer cells. In: Lachmann PJ, Peters DK, Rosen FS, Walport MJ, eds. Clinical Aspects of Immunology, 5th ed. Boston: Blackwell Scientific Publications, 1993:619–633.

48. Krahenbuhl O, Tschopp J. Perforin-induced pore formation. Immunol. Today 1991; 12:399–403.

49. Knight SC, Macatonia SE, Roberts MS, Harvey JJ, Patterson S. Dendritic cells and antigen presentation. In: Thomas DB, ed. Viruses and the Cellular Immune Response. New York: Marcell Dekker, 1993:49–74.

50. Doherty PC, Allen W, Eichelberger M. Roles of $\alpha\beta$ and gamma-delta T cell subsets in viral immunity. Annu Rev Immunol 1992; 10:123–151.

51. Tohma S, Hirohata S, Lipsky PE. The role of CD11a/CD18-CD54 interactions in human T cell-dependent B cell activation. J Immunol 1991; 146:492–499.

52. Teunissen MBM, Rongen HAH, Bos JD. Function of adhesion molecules, lymphocyte function associated antigen-3, and intercellular adhesion molecule-1 on human epidermal Langerhans cells in antigen-specific T cell activation. J Immunol 1994; 152:3400–3409.

53. Andersson EC, Christensen JP, Marker O, Thomsen AR. Changes in cell adhesion molecule expression on T cells associated with systemic virus infection. J Immunol 1994; 152:1237–1245.

54. Allan W, Tabi Z, Cleary A, Doherty PC. Cellular events in the lymph node and lung of mice with influenza. J Immunol 1990; 144:3980–3986.

55. Doherty PC. Probes, protocols, and paradigms in the analysis of cell-mediated immunity in virus infections. In: Thomas DB, ed. Viruses and the Cellular Immune Response. New York: Marcell Dekker, 1993:1–13.

56. Kimpen JLL, Ogra PL. T cell redistribution kinetics after secondary infection of BALB/c mice with respiratory syncytial virus. Clin Exp Immunol 1993; 91:78–82.

57. Mazenec MB, Nedrud JG, Kaetzel CS, Lamm ME. A three-tiered view of the role of IgA in mucosal defense. Immunol Today 1993; 14:430–435.

58. Ramsay AJ, Ruby J, Ramshaw IA. A case for cytokines as effector molecules in the resolution of virus infection. Immunol Today 1993; 14:155–157.

59. Mestan J, Digel W, Mittnacht S, et al. Antiviral effects of recombinant tumor necrosis factor *in vitro*. Nature 1986; 323:816.

60. Gastl G, Huber C. The biology of interferon actions. Blut 1988; 56:193–199.

61. Schleimer RP, Sterbinsky SA, Kaiser J, et al. IL-4 induces adherence of human eosinophils and basophils but not neutrophils to endothelium. Association with expression of VCAM-1. J Immunol 1992; 148:1086–1092.

62. Dustin ML, Rothlein R, Bhan AK, Dinarello CA, Springer TA. Induction by IL 1 and interferon-gamma: tissue distribution, biochemistry, and function of a natural adherence molecule (ICAM-1). J Immunol 1986; 137:245–254.

63. Renkonen R, Mattila P, Majuri ML, Paavonen T, Silvennoinen O. IL-4 decreases IFN-gamma-induced endothelial ICAM-1 expression by a transcriptional mechanism. Scand J Immunol 1992; 35:525–530.

64. Graham MB, Dalton DK, Giltinan D, Braciale VL, Stewart TA, Braciale TJ. Response to influenza infection in mice with a targeted disruption in the interferon gamma gene. J Exp Med 1993; 178:1725–1732.

65. Romagnani S. Th1 and Th2 subsets of CD4+ T lymphocytes. Sci Am Sci Med 1994; May/June:68–77.

66. Fishaut M, Tubergen D, Mcintosh K. Cellular response to respiratory viruses with particular reference to children with disorders of cell-mediated immunity. J Pediatr 1980; 96:179–186.

67. Hastings GZ, Francis MJ, Rowlands DJ, Chain BM. Antigen processing and presentation of human rhinovirus to CD4 T cells is facilitated by binding to cellular receptors for virus. Eur J Immunol 1993; 23:1340–1345.

68. Turner RB. The role of neutrophils in the pathogenesis of rhinovirus infections. Pediatr Infect Dis J 1990; 9:832–835.

69. Levandowski RA, Ou DW, Jackson GG. Acute-phase decrease of T lymphocyte subsets in rhinovirus infection. J Infect Dis 1986; 153:743–748.

70. Skoner DP, Whiteside TL, Wilson JW, Doyle WJ, Herberman RB, Fireman P. Effect of rhinovirus 39 infection on cellular immune parameters in allergic and nonallergic subjects. J Allergy Clin Immunol 1993; 92:732–743.

71. Hsia J, Goldstein AL, Simon GL, Sztein M, Hayden FG. Peripheral blood mononuclear cell interleukin-2 and interferon-gamma production, cytotoxicity, and antigen-stimulated blastogenesis during experimental rhinovirus infection. J Infect Dis 1990; 162:591–597.

72. Chonmaitree T, Lett-Brown MA, Tsong Y, Goldman AS, Baron S. Role of interferon in leukocyte histamine release caused by common respiratory viruses. J Infect Dis 1988; 157:127–132.

73. Levandowski RA, Pachucki CT, Rubenis M. Specific mononuclear cell response to rhinovirus. J Infect Dis 1983; 148:1125.

74. Hastings GZ, Francis MJ, Rowlands DJ, Chain BM. Epitope analysis of the T cell response to a complex antigen: proliferative responses to human rhinovirus capsids. Eur J Immunol 1993; 23:2300–2305.

75. Vrtis RF, Dick EC, Brener KM, Busse WW. Rhinovirus 16 (RV16) activation of human peripheral blood mononuclear cells (PBMC) requires ICAM-1. J Allergy Clin Immunol 1994; 93:198(abstr).

76. Scott R, Pullan CR, Scott M, McQuillin J. Cell-mediated immunity in respiratory syncytial virus disease. J Med Virol 1984; 13:105–114.

77. Cranage MP, Gardner PS. Systemic cell-mediated and antibody responses in infants with respiratory syncytial virus infections. J Med Virol 1980; 5:161–170.

78. Bangham CRM, McMichael AJ. Specific human cytotoxic T cells recognize B-cell lines persistently infected with respiratory syncytial virus. Proc Natl Acad Sci USA 1986; 83:9183–9187.

79. Isaacs D, Bangham CRM, McMichael AJ. Cell-mediated cytotoxic response to respiratory syncytial virus in infants with bronchiolitis. Lancet 1987; ii: 769–771.

80. Bangham CRM, Openshaw PJM, Ball LA, King AMQ, Wertz GW, Askonas BA. Human and murine cytotoxic T cells specific to respiratory syncytial virus recognize the viral nucleoprotein (N), but not the major glycoprotein (G), expressed by vaccinia virus recombinants. J Immunol 1986; 137:3973–3977.

81. Levely ME, Bannow CA, Smith CW, Nicholas JA. Immunodominant T-cell epitope on the F protein of respiratory syncytial virus recognized by human lymphocytes. J Virol 1991; 65:3789–3796.

82. Alwan WH, Record FM, Openshaw PJM. Phenotypic and functional characterization of T cell lines specific for individual respiratory syncytial virus proteins. J Immunol 1993; 150:5211–5218.

83. Hall CB, Powell KR, MacDonald NE, et al. Respiratory syncytial virus infection in children with compromised immune function. N Engl J Med 1986; 315:77–81.

84. Douglas RGJ, Alford RH, Cate TR, Couch RB. The leukocyte response during viral respiratory illness in man. Annu Intern Med 1966; 64:521–530.

85. Dolin R, Murphy BR, Caplan EA. Lymphocyte blastogenic responses to influenza virus antigens after influenza infection and vaccination in humans. Infect Immun 1978; 19:867–874.

86. Ennis FA, Rook AH, Qu YH, et al. HLA restricted virus-specific cytotoxic T-lymphocyte responses to live and inactivated influenza vaccines. Lancet 1981; 2:887–891.

87. Bender BS, Croghan T, Zhang L, Small PA Jr. Transgenic mice lacking class I major histocompatibility complex-restricted T cells have delayed viral clearance and increased mortality after influenza virus challenge. J Exp Med 1992; 175:1143–1145.

88. Caton AJ, Gerhard W. The diversity of the CD4$^+$ T cell response in influenza. Sem Immunol 1992; 4:85–90.

89. Scherle PA, Palladino G, Gerhard W. Mice can recover from pulmonary influenza virus infection in the absence of class I-restricted cytotoxic T cells. J Immunol 1992; 148:212–217.

90. Hennet T, Ziltener HJ, Frei K, Peterhans E. A kinetic study of immune mediators in the lungs of mice infected with influenza-A virus. J Immunol 1992; 149:932–939.

91. Marrack P, Kappler J. Subversion of the immune system by pathogens. Cell 1994; 76:323–332.

92. Openshaw PJM, Odonnell DR. Asthma and the common cold—can viruses imitate worms. Thorax 1994; 49:101–103.

93. Gooding LR. Viral proteins that counteract host immune defenses. Cell 1992; 71: 5–7.

94. Salkind AR, Roberts NJ. Recent observations regarding the pathogenesis of recurrent respiratory syncytial virus infections—implications for vaccine development. Vaccine 1992; 10:519–523.

95. Panuska JR, Hertz MI, Taraf H, Villani A, Cirino NM. Respiratory syncytial virus infection of alveolar macrophages in adult transplant patients. Am Rev Respir Dis 1992; 145:934–939.

96. Domurat F, Roberts NJ, Walsh EE, Dagan R. Respiratory syncytial virus infection of human mononuclear leukocytes *in vitro* and *in vivo*. J Infect Dis 1985; 152:895–901.

97. Hall CB, Douglas RB, Simons RL, Geiman JM. Interferon production in children with respiratory syncytial, influenza and parainfluenza virus infections. J Pediatr 1978; 93:28–32.

98. Roberts NJ, Prill AH, Mann TN. Interleukin 1 and interleukin 1 inhibitor production by human macrophages exposed to influenza virus or respiratory syncytial virus. J Exp Med 1986; 163:511–519.

99. Salkind AR, Nichols JE, Roberts NJ. Suppressed expression of ICAM-1 and LFA-1 and abrogation of leukocyte collaboration after exposure of human mononuclear leukocytes to respiratory syncytial virus in vitro. J Clin Invest 1991; 88:505–511.

100. Salkind AR, McCarthy DO, Nichols JE, Donnelly SC, Walsh EE, Roberts NJ. Interleukin-1-inhibitor activity induced by respiratory syncytial virus: abrogation of

virus-specific and alternate human lymphocyte proliferative responses. J Infect Dis 1991; 163:71–77.

101. Preston FM, Beier PL, Pope JH. Infectious respiratory syncytial virus (RSV) effectively inhibits the proliferative T-cell response to inactivated RSV in vitro. J Infect Dis 1992; 165:819–825.

102. Roberts NJ, Nichols JE. Regulation of lymphocyte proliferation after influenza virus infection of human mononuclear leukocytes. J Med Virol 1989; 27:179–187.

103. Reed WP, Olds JW, Kisch AL. Decreased skin-test reactivity associated with influenza. J Infect Dis 1972; 125:398–402.

104. Arola M, Ruuskanen O, Ziegler T, et al. Clinical role of respiratory virus infection in acute otitis media. Pediatrics 1990; 86:848–855.

105. Sung BS, Chonmaitree T, Broemeling LD, et al. Association of rhinovirus infection with poor bacteriologic outcome of bacterial-viral otitis media. Clin Infect Dis 1993; 17:38–42.

106. Wegner CD, Gundel RH, Reilly P, Haynes N, Letts LG, Rothlein R. Intercellular adhesion molecule-1 (ICAM-1) in the pathogenesis of asthma. Science 1990; 247: 456–459.

107. Smith CW, Marlin SD, Rothlein R, Toman C, Anderson DC. Cooperative interactions of LFA-1 and Mac-1 with Intercellular Adhesion Molecule-1 in facilitating adherence and transendothelial migration of human neutrophils in vitro. J Clin Invest 1989; 83:2008–2017.

108. Van Seventer GA, Shimizu Y, Horgan KL, Luce F, Webb D, Shaw S. Remote T cell co-stimulation via LFA-1/ICAM-1 and CD2/LFA-3: demonstration with immobilized ligand/mAb and implication in monocyte-mediated co-stimulation. Eur J Immunol 1991; 21:1711–1718.

109. Sligh JE, Ballantyne CM, Rich SS, et al. Inflammatory and immune responses are impaired in mice deficient in intercellular adhesion molecule-1. Proc Natl Acad Sci USA 1993; 90:8529–8533.

110. Joseph BE, Murray SE, Gern JE. Rhinovirus selectively inhibits antigen-specific T cell proliferation. J Allergy Clin Immunol 1994; 93:203(abstr).

111. Fraenkel DJ, Bardin PG, Johnston SL, Wilson S, Sanderson G, Holgate ST. Nasal biopsies in human rhinovirus 16 infection: an immunohistochemical study. Am Rev Respir Dis 1992; 147:460(abstr).

112. Calhoun WJ, Reed HE, Stevens CA, Busse WW. Experimental rhinovirus 16 infection potentiates airway inflammation only in allergic subjects. Am Rev Respir Dis 1991; 143:A47.

113. Becker S, Quay J, Soukup J. Cytokine (tumor necrosis factor, IL-6, and IL-8) production by respiratory syncytial virus-infected human alveolar macrophages. J Immunol 1991; 147:4307–4312.

114. Gern JE, Galagan DM, Dick EC, Busse WW. Rhinovirus stimulates monocytes and airway macrophages to produce IL-1β and TNFα protein and mRNA. Am J Respir Crit Care Med 1994; 149:A357(abstr).

115. Vrtis RF, Dick EC, Busse WW. Rhinovirus 16 (RV16) causes lymphocyte generation of interferon-gamma. J Allergy Clin Immunol 1993; 91:262(abstr).

116. Roberts NJ, Hiscott J, Signs DJ. The limited role of the human interferon system response to respiratory syncytial virus challenge—analysis and comparison to influenza virus challenge. Microb Pathog 1992; 12:409–414.

117. Subauste MC, Jacoby DB, Proud D. Rhinovirus infection of a human bronchial epithelial cell line (BEAS-2B) induces cytokine release. Am J Respir Crit Care Med 1994; 149(suppl):A985.

118. Teran LM, Johnston SL, Shute JK, Church MK, Holgate ST. Increased levels of interleukin-8 in the nasal aspirates of children with virus-associated asthma. J Allergy Clin Immunol 1994; 93:272(abstr).

119. Becker S, Koren HS, Henke DC. Interleukin-8 expression in normal nasal epithelium and its modulation by infection with respiratory syncytial virus and cytokines tumor necrosis factor, interleukin-1 and interleukin-6. Am J Respir Cell Mol Biol 1993; 8:20–27.

120. Matsushima K, Oppenheim JJ. Interleukin 8 and MCAF: novel inflammatory cytokines inducible by IL-1 and TNF. Cytokine 1989; 1:2–13.

121. Colden-Stanfield M, Ratcliffe D, Cramer EB, Gallin EK. Characterization of influenza virus-induced leukocyte adherence to human umbilical vein endothelial cell monolayers. J Immunol 1993; 151:310–321.

122. Welliver RC, Kaul A, Ogra PL. Cell-mediated immune response to respiratory syncytial virus infection: relationship to the development of reactive airway disease. J Pediatr 1979; 94:370–375.

123. Cannon MJ, Openshaw PJM, Askonas BA. Cytotoxic T cells clear virus but augment lung pathology in mice infected with respiratory syncytial virus. J Exp Med 1988; 168:1163–1168.

124. Ada GL, Jones PD. The immune response to influenza infection. Curr Topics Microbiol Immunol 1986; 128:1–54.

125. Taylor PM, Esquivel F, Askonas BA. Murine CD4+ T cell clones vary in function in vitro and in influenza infection in vivo. Int Immunol 1990; 2:323–328.

126. Ida S, Hooks JJ, Siraganian RP, Notkens AL. Enhancement of IgE-mediated histamine release from human basophils by viruses: role of interferon. J Exp Med 1977; 145:892–896.

127. Busse WW, Swenson CA, Borden EC, Treuhauft MW, Dick EC. The effect of influenza A virus on leukocyte histamine release. J Allergy Clin Immunol 1983; 71:382–388.

128. Graziano FM, Tilton R, Hirth T, et al. The effect of parainfluenza 3 infection upon guinea pig basophil and lung mast cell histamine release. Am Rev Respir Dis 1989; 139:715–720.

129. Chonmaitree T, Lett-Brown MA, Grant JA. Respiratory viruses induce production of histamine-releasing factor by mononuclear leukocytes: a possible role in the mechanism of virus-induced asthma. J Infect Dis 1991; 164:592–594.

130. Huftel MA, Swensen CA, Borcherding WR, et al. The effect of T-cell depletion on enhanced basophil histamine release after *in vitro* incubation with live influenza-A virus. Am J Respir Cell Mol Biol 1992; 7:434–440.

131. Calhoun WJ, Dick EC, Schwartz LB, Swenson CA, Vrtis RF, Busse WW. Rhino-

virus (RV) 16 respiratory infection enhances airway histamine release to antigen. J Allergy Clin Immunol 1992; 89:230(abstr).

132. Gaddy JN, Busse WW. Enhanced IgE-dependent basophil histamine release and airway reactivity in asthma. Am Rev Respir Dis 1986; 134:969–974.

133. Welliver RC, Kaul TN, Ogra PL. The appearance of cell-bound IgE in respiratory-tract epithelium after respiratory-syncytial-virus infection. N Engl J Med 1980; 303:1198–1202.

134. Welliver RC, Wong DT, Sun M, Middleton EJ, Vaughan RS, Ogra PL. The development of respiratory syncytial virus-specific IgE and the release of histamine in nasopharyngeal secretions after infection. N Engl J Med 1981; 305:841–846.

135. Bui RHD, Molinaro GA, Kettering JD, Heiner DC, Imagawa DT, St Geme JW. Virus-specific IgE and IgG4 antibodies in serum of children infected with respiratory syncytial virus. J Pediatr 1987; 110:87–90.

136. Welliver RC, Wong DT, Rijnaldo D, Ogra PL. Predictive value of respiratory syncytial virus-specific IgE responses for recurrent wheezing following bronchiolitis. J Pediatr 1986; 109:776–780.

137. Loughlin GM, Taussig LM. Pulmonary function in children with a history of laryngotracheobronchitis. J Pediatr 1979; 94:365–369.

138. Gurwitz D, Corey M, Levison H. Pulmonary function and bronchial reactivity in children after croup. Am Rev Respir Dis 1980; 122:95–99.

139. Volvovitz B, Welliver RC, De Castro G, Krystofik DA, Ogra PL. The release of leukotrienes in the respiratory tract during infection with respiratory syncytial virus: role in obstructive airway disease. Pediatr Res 1988; 24:504–507.

140. Mossman TR, Coffman RL. T_{H1} and T_{H2} cells: different patterns of lymphokine secretion lead to different functional properties. Annu Rev Immunol 1989; 7:145–173.

141. Robinson DS, Hamid Q, Ying S, et al. Predominant T_{H2}-like bronchoalveolar T-lymphocyte population in atopic asthma. N Engl J Med 1992; 326:298–304.

142. Walker C, Bode E, Boer L, Hansel TT, Blaser K, Virchow J Jr. Allergic and nonallergic asthmatics have distinct patterns of T-cell activation and cytokine production in peripheral blood and bronchoalveolar lavage. Am Rev Respir Dis 1992; 146:109–115.

143. Hamid Q, Azzawi M, Ying S, et al. Expression of mRNA for Interleukin-5 in mucosal bronchial biopsies from asthma. J Clin Invest 1991; 87:1541–1546.

144. Welliver RC, Wong DT, Middleton EJ, Sun M, McCarthy N, Ogra PL. Role of parainfluenza virus-specific IgE in pathogenesis of croup and wheezing subsequent to infection. J Pediatr 1982; 101:889–896.

145. Vercelli D, Geha RS. Regulation of IgE synthesis in humans. J Clin Invest 1989; 9:75–81.

146. Punnonen J, Aversa G, Cocks BG, et al. Interleukin 13 induces interleukin 4-independent IgG4 and IgE synthesis and CD23 expression by human B cells. Proc Natl Acad Sci USA 1993; 90:3730–3734.

147. Openshaw PJM, Clarke SL, Record FM. Pulmonary eosinophilic response to respiratory syncytial virus infection in mice sensitised to the major surface glycoprotein G. Int Immunol 1992; 4:493.

148. Alwan WH, Kozlowska WJ, Openshaw PJ. Distinct types of lung disease caused by functional subsets of antiviral T cells. J Exp Med 1994; 179:81–89.

149. Valerius T, Repp R, Kalden JR, Platzer E. Effects of IFN on human eosinophils in comparison with other cytokines. J Immunol 1990; 145:2950–2958.

150. Zhu Z, Einarsson O, Landry M, Zheng T, Elias JA. Human rhinovirus 14 induction of cytokine production by human lung fibroblasts. Am J Respir Crit Care Med 1994; 149(suppl):A47(abstr).

151. Einarsson O, Panuska J, Zhu Z, Landry M, Elias J. Respiratory syncytial virus stimulation of interleukin-11 production by airway epithelial cells and lung fibroblasts. Am J Respir Crit Care Med 1994; 149(suppl):A47(abstr).

152. Yokota S, Geppert TD, Lipsky PE. Enhancement of antigen and mitogen-induced human T lymphocyte proliferation by TNF. J Immunol 1988; 140:531–536.

153. Dinarello CA, Cannon JG, Mier JW, et al. Multiple biological activities of human recombinant interleukin 1. J Clin Invest 1986; 77:1734–1739.

154. Elias JA, Trinchieri G, Beck J, et al. Synergistic interaction of IL-6 and IL-1 mediated the thymocyte stimulating activity produced by recombinant IL-1 in stimulated human fibroblasts. J Immunol 1989; 142:509–514.

155. Levandowski RA, Horohov DW. Rhinovirus induces natural killer-like cytotoxic cells and interferon alpha in mononuclear leukocytes. J Med Virol 1991; 35: 116–120.

156. Gerosa F, Tommasi M, Carra G, Gandini G, Tridente G, Benati C. Different sensitivity to interleukin 4 of interleukin 2- and interferon alpha-induced CD69 antigen expression in human resting NK cells and CD3+, CD4−, CD8− lymphocytes. Cell Immunol 1992; 141:342–351.

157. Balfourlynn IM, Valman HB, Wellings R, Webster ADB, Taylor GW, Silverman M. Tumour necrosis factor-alpha and leukotriene E_4 production in wheezy infants. Clin Exp Allergy 1994; 24:121–126.

158. Calhoun WJ, Murphy K, Jarjour NN, Dick EC, Stevens CA, Busse WW. Modulation of airspace interferon-gamma and tumor necrosis factor-α production following experimental rhinovirus 16 infection. Am Rev Respir Dis 1992; 145(suppl):A37(abstr).

159. Ignatowicz L, Kappler JW, Marrack P, Scherer MT. Identification of two V beta 7-specific viral superantigens. J Immunol 1994; 152:65–71.

160. Lafon M. Rabies virus superantigen. Res Immunol 1993; 144:209–213.

161. Drake CG, Kotzin BL. Superantigens: biology, immunology, and potential role in disease. J Clin Immunol 1992; 12:149–162.

4

G-Protein-Coupled Receptor Signaling in the Lung

STUART A. GREEN and STEPHEN B. LIGGETT

University of Cincinnati College of Medicine
Cincinnati, Ohio

I. Introduction

G-protein-coupled receptors (GPCRs) represent a diverse and highly significant superfamily of receptor proteins. These receptors are localized to the cell surface and, once activated, transduce their signals via membrane-associated guanine nucleotide-binding proteins (G proteins). To date, several hundred GPCRs have been identified by pharmacological and/or molecular cloning techniques. That so many different physiologic signaling events are accomplished via this same basic mechanism suggests that the process is highly efficient. Indeed, as will be discussed, signaling by GPCRs provides for remarkable amplification, whereby significant changes in cellular function are illicited by signals such as single photons, odors, and subnanomolar concentrations of agonists. In addition, it is clear that while the general scheme of signal transduction is the same within the superfamily, structural diversity has evolved which has provided for plasticity at virtually every step in the process, including expression, ligand binding, G-protein coupling, and regulation. A number of GPCRs are expressed in the lung, although the functional relevance of some of these receptors to lung physiology is not always evident. In some cases, molecular cloning has confirmed the existence of receptor species predicted by classical pharmacology. Such receptors play well-

67

recognized roles in the maintenance of lung physiology under resting conditions, as well as mediating compensatory events during pathophysiological conditions, and serve as targets for pharmacologic therapy. In other cases, new receptors have been identified for which a physiological function has not yet been firmly identified.

This chapter discusses GPCRs in the lung relevant to asthma, with an emphasis on the molecular basis of signal transduction and the potential aspects of the process where genetic variation may play a role in asthma. Before discussing individual receptors in the lung, it is useful to begin with an overview of GPCR structure, function, and regulation. In the discussion to follow, adrenergic and muscarinic receptors, which have been intensely studied in this regard, will serve as paradigms for GPCR signal transduction. This is particularly useful in reference to asthma, since both receptor families subserve significant roles in pulmonary physiology.

II. Structure of G-Protein-Coupled Receptors and Functional Correlates to Signal Transduction

A. Membrane Topology

GPCRs are membrane-delimited proteins that may undergo a variety of post-translational modifications, including N-linked glycosylation, palmitoylation, formation of disulfide bonds, and receptor phosphorylation [1,2]. Each of these receptors consists of seven hydrophobic regions which are believed to adopt alpha-helical conformations and to serve as transmembrane spanning domains (TMDs). Based on homologies with bacteriorhodopsin and bovine rhodopsin, as well as studies utilizing proteolytic digestion, epitope mapping, and site-directed mutagenesis, it is now well established that GPCRs orient themselves in the cell membrane such that the amino-terminal group is extracellular, the carboxy-terminal group is intracellular, and the transmembrane spanning domains are linked by three extracellular and three or four intracellular loops, depending on the presence of a palmitoylated cysteine residue within the proximal carboxy terminal tail (Fig. 1). In most cases, the transmembrane spanning domains serve as the ligand-binding site, while the intracellular connecting loops serve as coupling and regulatory domains.

B. Signal Transduction

The sine quo non of GPCRs is their common usage of G proteins in signal transduction. Signal transduction (Fig. 2) begins with binding of an agonist to the receptor, followed by adoption of an "activated" conformation of the receptor, which then binds to a specific G protein. It should be noted that this scenario is probably too simplistic, in that several GPCRs have been demonstrated in vitro to couple to G proteins in the absence of ligand [3]. Such receptor behavior is better

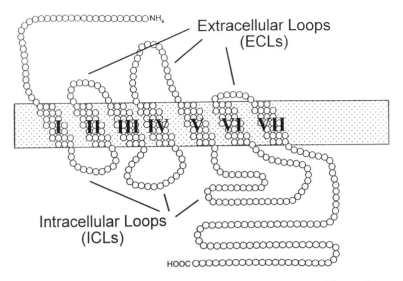

Figure 1 Schematic representation of putative membrane topology of G-protein-coupled receptors. Characteristic hydrophobic transmembrane spanning domains are indicated as I–VII. Also depicted are the extracellular amino-terminal tail, intracellular carboxy-terminal tail, and various intra- and extracellular loops.

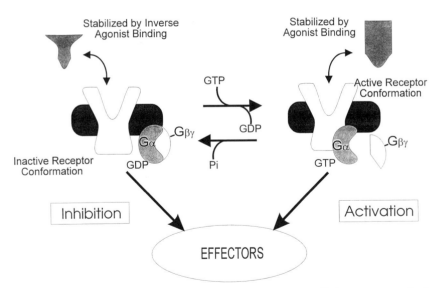

Figure 2 Signal transduction by G-protein-coupled receptors. Receptors may exist in either activated (right) or inactivated (left) conformations. Activated receptor conformations may be stabilized by agonist binding, and are accompanied by binding of G proteins and subsequent modulation of effector activity. Conversely, inactivated receptor conformations may be stabilized by inverse agonist binding. Receptor activation is also accompanied by dissociation of G proteins to G_α and $G_{\beta\gamma}$ subunits, either of which may interact with various effector moieties. See text for further discussion.

explained by a "two-state" equilibrium between activated and inactivated receptors, which may be influenced by the presence or absence of ligands. In such a scenario, ligands that promoted stabilization of the activated receptor conformation would serve as agonists, those that do not affect the activated/inactivated equilibrium would be neutral antagonists, and those that promoted the inactivated conformation serve as inverse agonists (sometimes referred to as negative antagonists). Activated receptors (such as those that occur following the binding of an agonist) adopt conformations which favor binding of the receptor to a G protein; in the case of agonist-promoted activation, this results in formation of the "ternary complex." This is accompanied by exchange of GTP for GDP bound to the G protein and subsequently by separation of G protein into G_α and $G_{\beta\gamma}$ subunits. These G_α and $G_{\beta\gamma}$ subunits activate or inactivate various effectors such as adenylyl cyclase, phospholipase C, and ion channels. Coupling to effectors by G_α subunits is accompanied by hydrolysis of G_α-bound GTP to GDP, which results in reassociation of G_α and $G_{\beta\gamma}$ and completes the receptor-activated portion of the cycle.

It is now known that within the well-recognized G proteins such as G_T (transducin), G_s, G_i, $G_q/_{11}$, G_o and G_z, that there are a number of isoforms of the α, β, and γ subunits. For example, at least three different $G_{i\alpha}$ isoforms are known, and a number of β-subunit isoforms and γ-subunit isoforms have been identified. Some progress has been made in identifying specific roles for these subunit isoforms, suggesting another degree of complexity in the signal transduction process.

C. Structural Determinants of Receptor Coupling

As stated above, signal transduction via GPCRs begins with binding of agonist to the receptor. Agonists (and antagonists) bind to their respective receptors by means of specific interactions with amino acids located within the transmembrane spanning domains. The best studied of these is that of the binding of catecholamines to the β_2AR. Using site-directed mutagenesis of recombinantly expressed β_2AR, Strader and colleagues demonstrated that two serine residues within the fifth transmembrane spanning domain (Ser204 and Ser207), as well as Asp113 within the third transmembrane domain, form key hydrogen bonds with the catechol hydroxyl and amino groups of epinephrine, respectively [4,5]. Muscarinic receptors (mAchRs) do not contain analogous serine residues within TMD5, but do contain an analogous aspartate residue within TMD3. This reflects the fact that the endogenous agonist for mAchRs, acetylcholine, does not contain a catechol moiety but does have an amino group. Interestingly, in both the m_1AchR and β_2AR, substitution of Asp113 with Asn impairs binding of receptor antagonists [6,7]; in the β_2AR, substitution with Gln confers partial agonist activity from some traditional antagonists [6]. Mutagenesis studies performed in the rat m_3AchR have revealed several threonine and tyrosine residues within TMDs III,

V, VI, and VII as critical for high-affinity acetylcholine binding, somewhat analogous to the serine residues described for the β_2AR above.

Agonist-bound receptors adopt (or become stabilized in) conformations which favor physical binding of the receptor to G protein with subsequent activation. The binding of agonist appears primarily to alter the conformation of the second and third intracellular loops of GPCRs which subserve these functions. The structures of these intracellular domains thus dictate which G proteins are bound/activated by a given receptor. Interestingly, recent studies with receptors that can couple to two G proteins have suggested that synthetic agonists can bind within the TMDs in such a way as to favor conformational changes that provide for coupling of the receptor to one, versus another, G protein [8,9]. Within the third intracellular loop, the proximal and distal portions appear to be critically important in the coupling process [6,10–15]. The conformation of these regions appear to be modulated by other domains within the loop. For example, β_1AR and β_2AR have highly conserved amino and carboxy portions of the third intracellular loop, but display different efficacies for coupling to G_s ($\beta_2AR > \beta_1AR$) [16,17]. The intervening sequences in the third intracellular loops are highly dissimilar. In particular, the β_1AR contains a proline-rich region within this domain. Although the tertiary structure of this proline-rich region is not known, it is likely that such a region would have significant conformational influence on the adjacent G-protein-coupling domains. In fact, deletion of this proline-rich intervening sequence of the β_1AR locus results in a significant improvement in β_1AR/Gs coupling, while substitution of the β_1AR sequence into the β_2AR attenuates G_s coupling [18]. For the muscarinic receptors, coupling specificity for the various G proteins is also localized within the intracellular domains. Chimeric mAchR receptors have taken advantage of the differences in mAchR/G protein-coupling specificity to study these interactions more precisely from a molecular standpoint. Using this approach, Wess and colleagues [13,19] and others [20] have shown that the first 16–21 amino acids of ICL3, and probably the distal portion of ICL3 as well, determine to a large degree the specificity of receptor/G-protein coupling.

D. Regulation of Signal Transduction

A number of GPCR-mediated signal transduction events are dynamically regulated; that is, there are equilibria between activating events, such as coupling of receptor to G protein, and events which tend toward inactivation. With regard to the latter, many GPCRs display a characteristic reduction in signal transduction intensity following prolonged exposure to agonists, a phenomenon termed desensitization or tachyphylaxis [21]. Several molecular mechanisms responsible for desensitization appear to be common among GPCRs. The three dominant mechanisms are phosphorylation of the receptors by various kinases, internalization (sequestration) of the receptor away from the cell surface, and downregulation of receptor number.

Phosphorylation of activated receptors occurs via at least two mechanisms by agonist-independent protein kinases such as PKA and PKC, and by agonist-dependent kinases termed G-protein-coupled receptor kinases or GRKs [2,21]. Phosphorylation of the β_2AR by PKA at consensus sites within the third intracellular loop and possibly the proximal carboxy-terminal tail occurs rapidly after activation of adenylyl cyclase and results in uncoupling of β_2AR from G_s. Phosphorylation by GRKs such as GRK2 (also referred to as βAR kinase or βARK) also occurs rapidly after receptor activation and results in receptor G-protein uncoupling. GRKs differ from agonist-independent kinases, however, in that (1) they do not require downstream second messengers such as cAMP, (2) receptor occupancy by agonist is required, and (3) the sites which serve as substrates for phosphorylation are distinct from those utilized by PKA and PKC. Since GRKs require receptor occupancy, desensitization via GRK-mediated phosphorylation is referred to as homologous. Desensitization via PKA or PKC may be either homologous (as occurs when the receptor itself initiates kinase activation) or heterologous (as occurs when a different receptor activates a kinase, which then phosphorylates the first receptor in an "innocent bystander" scenario). Heterologous desensitization may prove to be a significant mechanism of receptor cross-talk in the lung as well as other tissues and organs.

Knowing the molecular determinants of phosphorylation in a given receptor may provide the opportunity to enhance or block desensitization of that receptor. For example, identification of β_2AR-specific sequences that serve as substrates for GRKs such as GRK2 (βARK) could lead to the development of specific GRK2 inhibitors that might prolong β-agonist-mediated bronchial smooth muscle relaxation. Several studies have identified carboxy-terminal tail serines and threonines of the β_2AR as the likely site of GRK-mediated phosphorylation [22–24]. Mutated receptors in which these residues were substituted by alanines and glycines displayed a partial loss of agonist-promoted desensitization in transfected cells [22,23]. Substitution of serines within the PKA consensus sequences (RRSS) in the third intracellular loop and the cytoplasmic tail also results in receptors with depressed desensitization. The specificity of these mutations as representing phosphorylation sites was supported by whole-cell ^{32}P-labeling experiments performed under agonist exposure conditions similar to those described for the functional desensitization studies; the level of phosphorylation exhibited by each receptor was proportional to the level of functional desensitization observed [22]. Of note, while both kinases appeared to be functionally active at high (i.e., micromolar) concentrations of agonist, only the PKA sites appeared to be involved in desensitization at low (i.e., nanomolar) concentrations of agonist, a finding that was also observed in the phosphorylation studies. Thus, it appears that these kinases (PKA and GRKs) have evolved to respond to different agonist-exposure scenarios: PKA is principally active at low agonist exposure levels, such as those that might be observed due to circulating catecholamines, while higher agonist exposure levels (such as might be found in the lung after administration of inhaled β-agonist bronchodilators) activate the more receptor-specific GRK class of kinases as well as PKA. The precise serines or threonines phosphorylated in β_2AR by βARK are not known. Recent work by our group using site-directed mutagenesis of the α_{2A}AR has shown that all four serines in the EESSSS sequence of the third intracellular loop are phosphorylated by βARK during agonist-promoted desensitization of this receptor [25]. Similar motifs are present in the cytoplasmic tail of the β_2AR and probably represent the GRK phosphorylation sites.

At present, it is still not clear whether all GRKs utilize the same or similar sequences for binding and phosphorylation. This may become increasingly important, as it is also unclear which GRKs are expressed in various lung tissues. To date, GRKs 2, 3, 5, and 6 have been detected by Northern analysis in RNA prepared from whole-lung extracts [26–29], but more precise localization studies such as in-situ hybridization have not been reported in the lung. Thus, knowledge of GRK-specific recognition sequences, along with identification of cell type-specific expression of individual GRKs, may lead to tissue-specific pharmacological intervention in GPRC regulation events.

Phosphorylation of GPCRs by GRKs such as GRK2 involve a series of protein interactions which have only recently become evident (reviewed in Ref. 30). Phosphorylation by GRK2 requires G-protein βγ subunits, and can be inhibited by factors that deplenish the intracellular pool of such βγ subunits. This requirement of βγ subunits represents yet another level in the complexity of GPRC-mediated signal transduction, in that events mediated both by Gα subunits (such as cAMP-promoted activation of PKA) and by βγ subunits facilatory to GRK phosphorylation tend to uncouple the transduction pathways. I should also be noted that phosphorylation alone is not sufficient for β_2AR to become uncoupled to G_s. The interdiction of another protein, termed βarrestin, is required for functional desensitization. βarrestin is thought to specifically bind to regions of receptors phosphorylated by GRKs.

In contrast to the relatively defined structural domains for receptor phosphorylation, less is known about the requirements for receptor sequestration (internalization of receptor away from the cell surface) and downregulation (actual loss of receptor density) following agonist exposure. A prerequisite for sequestration is binding of agonist to the receptor. However, for the β_2AR, neither coupling to G protein nor activation of second-messenger pathways appear to be required. Mutagenesis studies of the β_2AR have identified a domain within the carboxy-terminal tail (NPXXY, which was first described in the LDL receptor [31]) that appears to be required for sequestration to occur [32,33]. Even so, other receptors that contain this motif, such as the β_1AR, β_3AR, and α_{2c}AR, do not undergo significant agonist-promoted sequestration. This suggests that the NPXXY motifs may be required, but are not sufficient, for sequestration to occur. Although receptor phosphorylation is also agonist-promoted and occurs within the intracellular domains of the receptor, the relationship between phosphorylation and sequestration is not clear. In the β_2AR, receptor phosphorylation does not appear to be required for sequestration, since mutated β_2AR lacking phosphorylation sites (described above) sequester normally. In contrast, mutation of phosphorylation sites within the m1AchR appears to ablate sequestration [34]. Other domains that are removed from the intracellular regions but nevertheless affect their conformation have also been shown to play a role in this process. For example, we have shown that a single point mutation within the fourth transmembrane spanning domain of the β_2AR, resulting in the substitution if Ile for Thr at codon 164 (a naturally occurring variant of the human β_2AR), results in significant attenuation of agonist-promoted sequestration [35]. The role of sequestration in the desensitization process may be threefold. Clearly, loss of surface receptors in a cell where there are few spare receptors can result in a loss of responsiveness. Since sequestration occurs during the time period after rapid phosphorylation but before downregulation, the process may be a mechanism for desensitization during this intermediate time period. In addition, recent studies have suggested that dephosphorylation of receptors may occur at the level of the internalized receptor. Finally, some of the receptors in the sequestered pool may eventually undergo degradation leading to a net loss of cellular receptor (downregulation). A pharmacologic method of blocking agonist-promoted sequestration could conceivably blunt or enhance desensitization. The latter effect may prove to be an effective means of desensitizing "unwanted" signal transduction pathways.

Downregulation of GPCRs occurs following prolonged (generally hours) exposure to agonists. This process differs from sequestration in that total receptor density (not just cell-surface expression) is decreased. In addition, whereas sequestration requires agonist occupancy of the receptor, downregulation may occur in the absence of agonist and may even occur following exposure to cAMP analogues, clearly indicating that sequestration and downregulation are independent phenomena. Nevertheless, it is possible that downregulation may at least partly reflect degradation of sequestered receptors, a possibility that is now being investigated [36,37]. Downregulation may occur due to changes in receptor synthesis rates (at either transcriptional, translational, and/or posttranslational steps) or in receptor degradation. Genetic determinants of downregulation are thus not confined to the coding regions of the gene. For example, Malbon and colleagues have identified a 35-kDa protein that binds to a short region (AUUUA) within the 3′ untranslated region of the β_2AR mRNA; this protein is upregulated by agonist exposure, and binding to the above pentamer is accompanied by destabilization of mRNA transcripts [38]. Receptor phosphorylation appears to be required, since mutated β_2AR lacking PKA phosphorylation sites fail to exhibit wild-type phosphorylation and downregulation following exposure to the membrane-permeable cAMP analog dibutyryl cAMP [39]. Notably, the decline in mRNA levels was not affected by this mutation, further supporting the notion of multiple pathways for downregulation to occur. Within the receptor protein itself, the structural determinants of GPCR downregulation also appear to be multiple and complex, located within both intra- and extracellular domains of the receptors. For example, mutation of Tyr350 and Tyr354 in the carboxy terminus of the β_2AR to alanines ablates agonist-promoted downregulation; however, substitution of either residue alone does not [40,41]. Two amino acids within the extracellular amino terminus (Arg16 and Gln27) are polymorphic in the β_2AR in the human population, resulting in Gly16 and Glu27, respectively [42]. When studied in recombinant cells and in primary cultures of human airway smooth muscle cells, these polymorphic variants exhibit markedly different downregulation phenotypes [43,44]. Specifically, cells expressing the Gly16 β_2AR undergo enhanced agonist-promoted downregulation, whereas cells expressing the Glu27 variant are resistant to such downregulation, compared to "wild-type" β_2AR. The implications of β_2AR polymorphisms to asthma [45–47] are discussed further elsewhere in this volume.

III. Diseases Caused by Mutations of GPCR Signal Transduction Components

Studies such as those discussed above have contributed substantially to our understanding of the relationship between receptor structure and function. Such studies have also revealed that small mutations can have significant effects on receptor function. Over the past few years, a number of diseases have been found to be due to mutations in genes which encode for components of G-protein signaling pathways [48–50]. These include those in which the receptor structure/ or the G-protein structure have been altered. Examples of such mutations are illustrated in Fig. 3.

At the receptor level, several types of mutations have been described. In X-linked nephrogenic diabetes insipitus, a number of different mutations have been found in the gene encoding for the V2 vasopressin receptor [51–53]. These include those that result in frame shifts, premature terminations, or altered amino acid residues in the TMDs and the third intracellular loop. These result in either a loss of expression of the intact receptor or expression of a receptor that fails to bind ligand or to activate G_s. Other diseases due to mutations in GPCRs leading to inactive receptors include those that cause familial glucocorticoid resistance (ACTH receptor) [54,55], familial hypercalciuric hypercalcemia (calcium-sensing receptor) [56], neonatal severe hyperparathyroidism (calcium-sensing receptor [56]), and retinitis pigmentosa (rhodopsin [57,58]). Although a human correlate has not yet been described, the dwarf *little* phenotype in mice has been found to be due to a point mutation in the growth hormone-releasing hormone

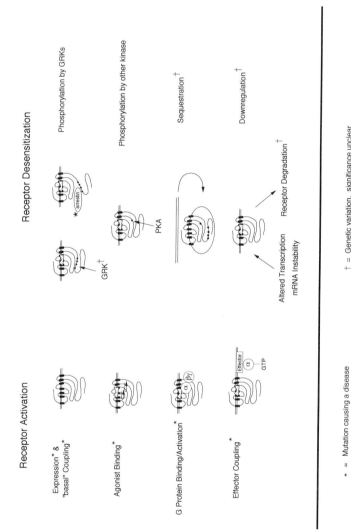

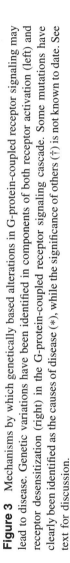

Figure 3 Mechanisms by which genetically based alterations in G-protein-coupled receptor signaling may lead to disease. Genetic variations have been identified in components of both receptor activation (left) and receptor desensitization (right) in the G-protein-coupled receptor signaling cascade. Some mutations have clearly been identified as the causes of disease (*), while the significance of others (†) is not known to date. See text for discussion.

receptor [59]. Also, mutations in the melanocyte-stimulatory hormone receptor result in mice with hypo- or hyperpigmentation, depending on whether the mutation results in an inactive or an overactive receptor [60]. Three human diseases are known to be caused by mutations that result in persistent activation of GPCRs. In familial male precocious puberty, a mutation in the luteinizing hormone (LH) receptor in the testis resulting in a receptor that is constitutively activated [61]. In some hyperfunctioning adenomas which result in hyperthyroidism, a mutation of the thyroid-stimulatory hormone (TSH) receptor also results in constitutive activation [62]. Both the LH and TSH receptors are coupled to G_s, and thus a persistent, and agonist-independent, increase in intracellular cAMP is noted. Finally, in one form of autosomal retinitis pigmentosa, mutations in rhodopsin result in constitutive activation [63].

Some diseases have been found which appear to be due to mutations in G proteins rather than the receptors. In the majority of patients with Albright's hereditary osteodystrophy, membrane $G_{s\alpha}$ activity is reduced. A number of different mutations in the $G_{s\alpha}$ gene have been described in these patients, including those that cause a disruption of mRNA synthesis and protein expression, and those that cause mutations which depress receptor–G_s coupling [49]. In acromegaly, the pituitary tumors have been shown to have somatic mutations in the $G_{s\alpha}$ gene resulting in decreased intrinsic GTPase activity, and thus more prolonged time in the active conformation [64]. The effect is an increase in cAMP and growth-hormone secretion from these cells. Somatic mutations in $G_{s\alpha}$ have also been reported in the McCune-Albright syndrome [65]. Studies of several other tumors have suggested that they may be due to mutations in $G_{i\alpha}$. Human diseases caused by mutations in other portions of the activation pathway have not been reported. Within the desensitization pathways, a recent study reports genetic variation in the structure of GRK4, although its relevance to function or disease is not known [66]. As is discussed further elsewhere in this volume, polymorphisms of the β_2AR in the amino terminus alter agonist-promoted downregulation and appear to act as disease modifiers in asthma. Another polymorphism of the β_2AR, in the fourth transmembrane spanning domain, depresses agonist-promoting sequestration.

IV. G-Protein-Coupled Receptors Relevant to Lung Physiology

Table 1 lists the cloned GPCRs that are known to be expressed in the lung and for which a role in asthma physiology has been proposed. Two classes of these, the muscarinic acetylcholine receptors (mAchRs) and the β-adrenergic receptors (βARs), have been extensively studied at both the pharmacological and molecular levels, and clearly play a significant role in lung function. Two others, the histamine and PAF receptors, have also been studied pharmacologically; molecu-

Table 1 Pulmonary G Protein-Coupled Receptors with Potential Physiological Roles in Asthma

Class	Receptor	Localization[a]	Actions	Agonists	G proteins	References
Adrenergic	β_1AR	alv epi, glands	??	norepinephrine	Gs	21, 74, 75, 77
	β_2AR	SM, alv epi, glands, AW epi, endo	↑ relaxation, ↓ inflammatory mediators, ↑ clearance secretions	epinephrine	Gs	
Muscarinic	m_1AchR	ganglia, glands, alv epi	?↑ secretion, ?↑ contraction	acetylcholine	Gq	67, 69–71
	m_2AchR	ganglia, SM	↓ contraction	acetylcholine	Gi	
	m_3AchR	SM, glands, epi, endo	↑ contraction, ↑ secretion	acetylcholine	Gq	
Histamine	H_1	SM, epi	↑ contraction, ↑ secretions	histamine	Gq/11	85–88
	H_3	SM	↓ contraction	histamine	Gi/Go	
PAF	PAF receptor	epi, macs, mast, inflamm. cells	multiple	PAF	Gi/Go ?Gs	89–94
Neuropeptide	VIP	SM, glands, arteries	↑ contraction, ↑ secretion	VIP	Gs	95, 96, 98–101
	B_2	SM, ?endo, ?epi	↑ contraction, vascular leakage	bradykinin	Gq, ?Gi	
Tachykinin	NK-1	SM	↑ contraction	substance P	Gq/11	102
	NK-2	SM	↑ contraction	neurolinin A	?Gq/11	
	NK-3	SM	↑ contraction	neurokinin B	?	
Interleukin	IL-8R(A+B)	epi, macs	↑ neutrophil chemotaxis, ↑ inflammatory mediators	IL-8	G_i, $G_{14/16}$	103–107

[a]Abbreviations: alv, alveolar; AW, airway; epi, epithelium; endo, endothelium; macs, macrophages; mast, mast cells; SM, smooth muscle.

lar studies of these receptors are now emerging. Several others, including the neuropeptide, tachykinin, and interleukin-8 (IL-8) receptors, are probably involved in asthma pathogenesis, although the data for these are still somewhat formulative. It should be emphasized that by no means is this list exhaustive, and current and future research will undoubtedly add new receptors (such as those for the leukotrienes) to this scheme.

A. Muscarinic Acetylcholine Receptors

Muscarinic acetylcholine receptors (mAchRs) modulate airways caliber through direct effects on airway smooth muscle (m_2AchR, m_3AchR) and perhaps via indirect effects on other tissues such as alveolar epithelium (m_1AchR) (reviewed in Ref. 67). (A fourth mAchR subtype, the m_4AchR, has been described in rodent lung [68] but not human, while the m_5AchR has not been reported in the lung of any species.) These receptors couple to different signal transduction pathways by virtue of their different G-protein specificities: the m_2AchR receptor couples to G_i (and thus inhibition of adenylyl cyclase), while the m_1AchR and m_3AchR receptor couple to G_q and the inositol phosphate second-messenger pathway. The m_3AchR receptor appears to be the principle mediator of smooth muscle contraction in the lung, although the m_1AchR and m_2AchR may also modulate smooth muscle tone via their effects on neurotransmission. Structurally, the mAchRs are distinguished by significant homology within the transmembrane spanning and ligand-binding domains, and significant sequence divergence within the large third intracellular loops [69].

The physiology of mAchRs in lung is complex and is incompletely understood [67]. Activation of postsynaptic m_3AchR on airway smooth muscle results in contraction via activation of phospholipase C and mobilization of intracellular calcium. This pathway may be attenuated by activation of presynaptic m_2AchR located on postganglionic nerves. In addition, some studies have suggested that activation of m_2AchR located on airways smooth muscle may mediate airways contraction via inhibition of adenylyl cyclase activity and subsequent decreases in intracellular levels of cAMP [70,71]. m_1AchRs located within parasympathetic ganglia are also believed to augment contractile parasympathetic signal transduction initiated by nicotinic transmission. At present, there are no definite examples of mAchR dysfunction that result in abnormalities in airway smooth muscle tone, although it has been suggested that a defect in prejunctional m_2AchR function may contribute to the increased bronchial hyperresponsiveness observed in some asthmatics [72,73]. Confirmation of these studies will depend on the development of subtype-selective agonists and antagonists for clinical use.

B. β-Adrenergic Receptors

Although there is extensive species-dependent differences in subtype distribution in the lung, in humans both β_1AR and β_2AR have been detected, with the β_2AR being predominate [74,75]. Like the mAchRs, β_2ARs have also been identified on human airway smooth muscle [75]. Agonists for these receptors (such as epinephrine, albuterol, and the newer, long-acting agents formoterol and salmeterol) mediate smooth muscle relaxation via coupling to G_s, activation of adenylyl cyclase, increases in intracellular cAMP, and activation of PKA. Activation of PKA may result in smooth muscle relaxation by one of several mechanisms, including inhibition of myosin light-chain phosphorylation, reduction in intracellular Ca^{2+} concentration by way of augmented Ca^{2+}/Na^+ exchange, and perhaps most importantly by activation of membrane K^+ channels. Activation of K^+ channels may also occur via direct coupling of $G_{s\alpha}$ to the channel. Interestingly, in cardiac tissues this mechanism may also lead to direct activation of voltage-gated Ca^{2+} channels [76]; if this also occurs in airway smooth muscle, it would be predicted to offset somewhat the relaxant effects of βAR stimulation.

βAR may also modify airways function through other mechanisms in addition to direct effects on airway smooth muscle (reviewed in Ref. 77). For example, β-agonists may inhibit cholinergic-mediated contraction via $β_2AR$ located on prejunctional nerves. β-Agonists also inhibit release of histamine from mast cells, thromboxane release from eosinophils, and possibly other mediators from neutrophils, lymphocytes, and macrophages. Other proposed β-agonist-mediated effects include increased ciliary beat frequency and alterations in vascular permeability. Most, if not all, of these effects are believed to be due to the $β_2AR$. While the $β_1AR$ has been detected in airways nerve ganglia, the majority of $β_1AR$ are in fact localized within the alveolar walls [74]. This is puzzling, since $β_1ARs$, by virtue of their increased affinity for norepinephrine, are believed to function only postjunctionally at sympathetic nerve junctions, of which there are none in the distal airways in humans.

There are perhaps four potential mechanisms for $β_2AR$-related dysfunction in asthma that have been proposed based on experimental evidence. As introduced earlier, the human $β_2AR$ is known to exist in at least six polymorphic forms based on point mutations at four loci within the coding region of the gene [42]. Two of these loci (codons 16 and 27 within the extracellular amino terminus of the receptor) exhibit markedly altered downregulation and desensitization phenotypes depending on the amino acids expressed, when studied in vitro [43,44]. In particular, cells containing Gly16 $β_2AR$ undergo enhanced agonist-promoted receptor downregulation, whereas cells expressing the Glu27 $β_2AR$ polymorphism are strongly resistant to such downregulation and desensitization. Recently, three groups have reported studies of human airway physiologic measurements based on $β_2AR$ genotype [78–80]. These studies, which in each case have supported the paradigm of genetically mediated $β_2AR$ dysfunction in airways pathophysiology, are discussed in detail elsewhere in this volume.

Second, a number of reports have investigated the role of anti-$β_2AR$ antibodies in individuals with asthma [81]. Some studies have revealed the apparent presence of antibodies in about the same percentage of normal subjects and those with asthma. With the cloning of the human β_2AR and development of antisera in animals, a recent study has suggested that anti-β_2AR antibodies are more prevalent in asthmatics [81]. Some of these antibodies, which are primarily of the IgM and IgG subtypes, exhibit effects on receptor expression and function when studied in recombinant cells. It thus appears plausible that, at least in some individuals, the presence of such antibodies may attenuate normal β_2AR function.

Third, several studies have suggested that various cytokines may modulate β_2AR-mediated signal transduction in lung cells. For example, Kelsen and colleagues observed that in cultured BEAS-2B human airway epithelial cells, treatment with recombinant IL-1β resulted in a two- to fourfold increase in βAR density, but a significant decrease in receptor-dependent and -independent formation of cAMP. These results were not observed following treatment with vehicle or with IL-2, suggesting that they were cytokine-specific [82]. Both TNF-α and IL-1 have been shown to attenuate isoproterenol-induced relaxation of precontracted guinea pig airways [83]. A similar attenuation in β-agonist-promoted signal transduction has also been observed following TGF-β1 treatment of cultured human tracheal smooth muscle cells [84]. Thus, during a disease such as asthma, where inflammation plays a prominent role, cytokine-mediated dysfunction of β_2AR may develop. The molecular basis of such dysfunction is not known.

Finally, several studies have suggested that β_2AR dysfunction may result from prior exposure to β-agonists, most likely reflecting the activation of molecular desensitization pathway as described above. To begin to assess this at the molecular level, we have recently determined whether administration of standard doses of inhaled β-agonist in humans causes desensitization of lung cell β_2AR [51]. Normal subjects underwent bronchoscopy with harvesting of bronchial epithelial cells and alveolar macrophages. β_2AR expression and function were assessed in vitro with both cell types. Subjects were then administered inhaled metaproterenol (10 mg) every 4 h for six consecutive doses. After such treatment, bronchoscopy with cell harvesting from the contralateral lung was then carried out as before and receptor expression and function determined. β_2AR expression decreased ~65% in both bronchial epithelial cells and alveolar macrophages after the in-vivo metaproterenol exposure. Receptor function was also depressed in both cell types. For alveolar macrophage β_2AR, an ~85% desensitization was observed. This was accompanied by a ~35% desensitization of the PGE$_2$ responses, but no change in the forskolin response. In bronchial epithelial cells, in-vivo exposure to inhaled metaproterenol induced a desensitization of the β_2AR which was not as profound, amounting to ~50% desensitization. No decrements in forskolin stimulated levels were noted, and PGE$_2$ responses were not depressed. Taken together, these results indicate that, at the cellular level, administration of β-agonists in conventional doses does result in desensitization of macrophage and epithelial β_2AR.

C. Other Receptors

Besides muscarinic and adrenergic receptors, other GPCRs appear by physiologic studies to play a significant role in lung function, but their molecular biology is less clear (Table 1). Histamine has long been recognized as a nonspecific constrictor of bronchial smooth muscle, as well as an activator of the inflammatory cascade acting at mast cells. Histamine H_1 receptors have been isolated from human lung cDNA libraries [85,86], but the cellular localization within the lung is not known. In cultured human airway epithelial cells, exposure to histamine results in activation of inositol phosphate turnover through the pertussis toxin (PTX)-insensitive G protein G_q [87]. Physiologic studies in isolated guinea pig trachea have also suggested the presence of an H_3 receptor that is coupled to smooth muscle relaxation, possibly via a PTX-sensitive G_i/G_o pathway; this pathway appears to be activated at low concentrations of histamine, whereas the H_1-mediated effects become predominate at higher agonist concentrations [88]. At present, there is no evidence for an H_2 receptor in human lung.

Platelet-activating factor (PAF) is a lipid mediator which is released from inflammatory cells and is believed to play a significant role in antigen-induced bronchial hyperresponsiveness (reviewed in Ref 89). The PAF receptor gene has been cloned from guinea pig lung [90] and human leukocytes [91], and in the human encodes a protein with the characteristic seven transmembrane spanning domains, which lacks sites for N-linked glycosylation. PAF receptors appear to be able to couple to different G proteins in a cell-dependent manner. In recombinant RBL-2H3 rat basophils expressing the human PAF receptor, Ca^{2+} mobilization induced by PAF is not blocked by PTX, but is inhibited by guanine nucleotide analogs, suggesting a role for a PTX-insensitive G protein [92]. Binding of PAF to recombinant Chinese hamster ovary cells expressing the guinea pig receptor is accompanied by activation of MAP kinase, production of inositol phosphates, and inhibition of adenylyl cyclase; however, these effects are differentially modulated by PTX, suggesting both PTX-sensitive and -insensitive pathways [93]. In guinea pig alveolar macrophages, PAF-mediated signaling appears to be partially modulated by both G_i and G_s [94]. Part of the difficulty in sorting out PAF-mediated signal transduction events may lie in the multiple inflammatory pathways that are activated along with PAF release. These include not only chemoattraction and activation of inflammatory cells, but also increases in vascular permeability, augmentation of smooth muscle contraction, and increases in bronchial hyperresponsiveness. Each of these responses is cell-type specific and thus may represent a unique signal transduction pathway.

Table 1 also lists receptors for neuropeptides such as vasointestinal peptide and bradykinin, tachykinins such as substance P, and interleukin-8 (IL-8). Vaso-intestinal peptide (VIP) binds to a 54-kDa receptor protein in rat lung, and is coupled to the G_s/adenylyl cyclase pathway [95]. VIP receptors have been localized in humans to airway smooth muscle, as well as submucosal glands and both pulmonary and bronchial arteries [96]. One report has indicated a loss of VIP receptor immunostaining in the lungs of asthmatics [97]. VIP administered by either inhaled or intravenous route results in relaxation of bronchial smooth muscle, perhaps by the same sequence of postreceptor event as occurs with the G_s-coupled β_2AR [98]. Bradykinin receptors located on canine smooth muscle are coupled to inositol phosphate turnover, most likely via either G_i and/or G_q [99]. Radioligand-binding studies have determined that the bradykinin receptor present in human lung membranes is of the B_2 subtype [100]. The guinea pig lung receptor is also of the B_2 subtype, and has been demonstrated to mediate increased microvascular leakage and bronchoconstriction following exposure to inhaled bradykinin [101]. Receptors for tachykinins such as substance P, neurokinin A, and neurokinin B have been localized to airway smooth muscle in several species, including human [102]. Substance P receptors (NK-1) and most likely neurokinin A receptors (NK-2) couple to G_q/11 and phosphoinositol turnover. Substance P and neurokinin A stimulate smooth muscle contraction, increases in mucus secretion, and increased vascular permeability. In addition, these compounds have in-vitro inflammatory effects such as promoting mast cell degranulation, although the clinical significance of this is uncertain [102]. Each of these effects may contribute to increased obstruction to airway flow.

Activation of the inflammatory cascade associated with bronchial asthma is also dependent at least in part on the activity of chemoattractant cytokines such as IL-8. IL-8 mRNA expression is upregulated in rabbit alveolar macrophages [103] and cultured human airway epithelial cells [104] following inflammatory stimuli. Two human neutrophil IL-8 receptors have been cloned [105,106], which have been designed IL-8RA and IL-8RB, respectively. Both of these are typical G-protein-coupled receptors. Interestingly, it appears that different regions of IL-8 are important for ligand receptor interactions between the two receptors (reviewed in Ref. 107). IL-8-promoted signal transduction appears to be mediated by both G_i and $G_{14/16}$ and subsequent phospholipase C activation, although the relative contribution of each receptor to these pathways has not been fully elucidated [107].

V. Summary

Recent evidence continues to implicate G-protein-coupled receptors as key mediators of lung function, and as potential sites of dysfunction in pathophysiological states such as bronchial asthma. Molecular approaches to elucidating the structural and functional domains of these receptors have vastly improved our understanding of signal transduction events that follow binding of ligands to receptor. As more receptors are identified by molecular cloning techniques, application of these data will further enhance this knowledge base. A number of human diseases are now known to be caused by mutations in genes encoding for various components in the signaling cascade. Given the importance of this signaling in lung function, the potential for genetically based GPCR dysfunction in asthma needs to be continued to be explored.

Acknowledgments

We gratefully acknowledge the assistance of Katie Gouge in the preparation of this manuscript.

References

1. Liggett SB, Raymond JR. Pharmacology and molecular biology of adrenergic receptors. In: Bouloux PM, ed. Catecholamines. Baillier's Clinical Endocrinology and Metabolism, 7th ed. London: W. B. Saunders, 1993:279–306.
2. Liggett SB. Molecular basis of G-protein coupled receptor signalling. In: Crystal R, West JB, Weibel ER, Barnes PJ, eds. The Lung: Scientific Foundations. New York: Raven Press, 1995 (in press).
3. Samama P, Cotecchia S, Costa T, Lefkowitz RJ. A mutation-induced activated state of the β_2-adrenergic receptor. J Biol Chem 1993; 268:4625–4636.
4. Strader CD, Candelore MR, Hill WS, Sigal IS, Dixon RAF. Identification of two serine residues involved in agonist activation of the β-adrenergic receptor. J Biol Chem 1989; 264:13572–13578.
5. Strader CD, Sigal IS, Candelore MR, Rands E, Hill WS, Dixon RAF. Conserved aspartic acid residues 79 and 113 of the β-adrenergic receptor have different roles in receptor function. J Biol Chem 1988; 263:10267–10271.
6. Strader CD, Candelore MR, Hill WS, Dixon RAF, Sigal IS. A single amino acid substitution in the β-adrenergic receptor promotes partial agonist activity from antagonists. J Biol Chem 1989; 264:16470–16477.
7. Fraser CM, Wang CD, Robinson DA, Gocayne JD, Venter C. Site-directed mutagenesis of M_1 muscarinic acetylcholine receptors: conserved aspartic acids play important roles in receptor function. Mol Pharmacol 1989; 36:840–847.
8. Eason MG, Kurose H, Holt BD, Raymond JR, Liggett SB. Simultaneous coupling of α_2-adrenergic receptors to two G-proteins with opposing effects: subtype-selective coupling of α_2C10, α_2C4 and α_2C2 adrenergic receptors to G_i and G_s. J Biol Chem 1992; 267:15795–15801.
9. Eason MG, Jacinto MT, Liggett SB. Contribution of ligand structure to activation of α_2AR subtype coupling to G_s. Mol Pharmacol 1994; 45:696–702.

10. Cheung AH, Huang RC, Graziano MP, Strader CD. Specific activation of Gs by synthetic peptides corresponding to an intracellular loop of the β-adrenergic receptor. FEBS Lett 1991; 279:277–280.

11. O'Dowd BF, Hnatowich M, Regan JW, Leader WM, Caron MG, Lefkowitz RJ. Site-directed mutagenesis of the cytoplasmic domains of the human β$_2$-adrenergic receptor. J Biol Chem 1988; 263:15985–15992.

12. Okamoto T, Murayama Y, Hayashi Y, Inagaki M, Ogata E, Nishimoto I. Identification of a G$_s$ activator region that is autoregulated via protein kinase A-dependent phosphorylation. Cell 1991; 67:723–730.

13. Wess J, Brann MR, Bonner TI. Identification of a small intracellular region of the muscarinic M$_3$ receptor as a determinant of selective coupling to PI turnover. FEBS Lett 1989; 258:133–136.

14. Cotecchia S, Ostrowski J, Kjelsberg MA, Caron MG, Lefkowitz RJ. Discrete amino acid sequences of the α$_1$-adrenergic receptor determine the selectivity of coupling to phosphatidylinositol hydrolysis. J Biol Chem 1992; 267:1633–1639.

15. Malek D, Munch G, Palm D. Two sites in the third inner loop of the dopamine D$_2$ receptor are involved in functional G protein-mediated coupling to adenylate cyclase. FEBS Lett 1993; 325:215–219.

16. Green S, Holt B, Liggett SB. β$_1$- and β$_2$-adrenergic receptors display subtype specific coupling to G$_s$. Mol Pharmacol 1992; 41:889–893.

17. Levy FO, Zhu X, Kaumann AJ, Birnbaumer L. Efficiency of β$_1$-adrenergic receptors is lower than that of β$_2$-adrenergic receptors. Proc Natl Acad Sci USA 1993; 90: 10798–10802.

18. Green S, Liggett SB. A proline-rich region of the third intracellular loop imparts phenotypic β$_1$- versus β$_2$-adrenergic receptor coupling and sequestration. J Biol Chem 1994; 269:26215–26219.

19. Wess J, Bonner TI, Dorje F, Brann MR. Delineation of muscarinic receptor domains conferring selectivity of coupling to guanine nucleotide-binding proteins and second messengers. Mol Pharmacol 1990; 38:577–523.

20. Lechleiter J, Hellmiss R, Duerson K, et al. Distinct sequence elements control the specificity of G protein activation by muscarinic acetylcholine receptor subtypes. EMBO J 1990; 9:4381–4390.

21. Liggett SB, Lefkowitz RJ. Adrenergic receptor-coupled adenylyl cyclase systems: regulation of receptor function by phosphorylation, sequestration and downregulation. In: Sibley D, Houslay M, eds. Regulation of cellular signal transduction pathways by desensitization and amplification. London: John Wiley, 1993:71–97.

22. Hausdorff WP, Bouvier M, O'Dowd BF, Irons GP, Caron MG, Lefkowitz RJ. Phosphorylation sites on two domains of the β$_2$-adrenergic receptor are involved in distinct pathways of receptor desensitization. J Biol Chem 1989; 264:12657–12665.

23. Liggett SB, Bouvier M, Hausdorff WP, O'Dowd B, Caron MG, Lefkowitz RJ. Altered patterns of agonist-stimulated cAMP accumulation in cells expressing mutant β$_2$-adrenergic receptors lacking phosphorylation sites. Mol Pharmacol 1989; 36:641–646.

24. Onorato JJ, Palczewski K, Regan JW, Caron MG, Lefkowitz RJ, Benovic JL. The

role of acidic amino acids in peptide substrates of the β-adrenergic receptor kinase and rhodopsin kinase. Biochemistry 1991; 30:5118–5125.

25. Eason MG, Moreira SP, Liggett SB. Four consecutive serines in the third intracellular loop are the sites for βARK-mediated phosphorylation and desensitization of the α_{2A}-adrenergic receptor. J Biol Chem 1995; 270:4681–4688.

26. Benovic JL, Deblasi A, Stone WC, Caron MG, Lefkowitz RJ. β-adrenergic receptor kinase: primary structure delineates a multigene family. Science 1989; 246:235–240.

27. Benovic JL, Onorato JJ, Arriza JL, et al. Cloning, expression and chromosomal localization of β-adrenergic receptor kinase 2. J Biol Chem 1991; 266:14939–14946.

28. Kunapuli P, Benovic JL. Cloning and expression of GRK5: a member of the G protein-coupled receptor kinase family. Proc Natl Acad Sci USA 1993; 90:5588–5592.

29. Benovic JL, Gomez J. Molecular cloning and expression of GRK6. J Biol Chem 1993; 268:19521–19527.

30. Lefkowitz RJ. G protein-coupled receptor kinases. Cell 1993; 74:409–412.

31. Chen Wen-Ji, Goldstein JL, Brown MS. NPXY, a sequence often found in cytoplasmic tails, is required for coated pit-mediated internalization of the low density lipoprotein receptor. J Biol Chem 1990; 265:3116–3123.

32. Hausdorff WP, Campbell PT, Ostrowski, Yu SS, Caron MG, Lefkowitz RJ. A small region of the β-adrenergic receptor is selectively involved in its rapid regulation. Proc Natl Acad Sci USA 1991; 88:2979–2983.

33. Barak LS, Tiberi M, Freedman NJ, Kwatua MM, Lefkowitz RJ,Caron MG. A highly conserved tyrosine residue in G-protein-coupled receptors is required for agonist-mediated β_2-adrenergic receptor sequestration. JBL 1994; 269:2790–2795.

34. Lameh J, Philip M, Sharma YK, Moro O, Ramachandran J, Sadee W. Hm1 muscarinic cholinergic receptor internalization requires a domain in the third cytoplasmic loop. J Biol Chem 1992; 267:13406–13412.

35. Green SA, Cole G, Jacinto M, Innis M, Liggett SB. A polymorphism of the human β_2-adrenergic receptor within the fourth transmembrane domain alters ligand binding and functional properties of the receptor. J Biol Chem 1993; 268:23116–23121.

36. von Zastrow M, Kobilka BK. Ligand-regulated internalization and recycling of human β_2-adrenergic receptors between the plasma membrane and endosomes containing transferring receptors. J Biol Chem 1992; 267:3530–3538.

37. von Zastrow M, Kobilka BK. Antagonist-dependent and independent steps in the mechanism of adrenergic receptor internalization. J Biol Chem 1994; 269:18448–18452.

38. Huang L, Tholanikunnel BG, Vakalopoulou E, Malbon CC. The M_r 35,000 β-adrenergic receptor mRNA-binding protein induced by agonists requires both an AUUUA pentamer and U-rich domains for RNA recognition. J Biol Chem 1993; 268:26769–26775.

39. Bouvier M, Collins S, O'Dowd BF, et al. Two distinct pathways for cAMP-mediated down-regulation of the β_2-adrenergic receptor. J Biol Chem 1989; 264:16786–16792.

40. Valiquette M, Bonin H, Hnatowich M, Caron MG, Lefkowitz RJ, Bouvier M. Involvement of tyrosine residues located in the carboxyl tail of the human β_2-adren-

ergic receptor in agonist-induced down-regulation of the receptor. Proc Natl Acad Sci USA 1990; 87:5089–5093.

41. Valiquette M, Bonin H, Bouvier M. Mutation of tyrosine-350 impairs the coupling of the β_2-adrenergic receptor to the stimulatory guanine nucleotide binding protein without interfering with receptor down-regulation. Biochemistry 1993; 32:4979–4985.

42. Reihsaus E, Innis M, MacIntyre N, Liggett SB. Mutations in the gene rn coding for the β_2-adrenergic receptor in normal and asthmatic subjects. Am J Respir Cell Mol Biol 1993; 8:334–339.

43. Green S, Turki J, Innis M, Liggett SB. Amino-terminal polymorphisms of the human β_2-adrenergic receptor impart distinct agonist-promoted regulatory properties. Biochemistry 1994; 33:9414–9419.

44. Green SA, Turki J, Bejarano P, Hall IP, Liggett SB. Influence of β_2-adrenergic receptor genotypes on signal transduction in human airway smooth muscle cells. Am J Respir Cell Mol Biol 1995; 13:25–33.

45. Liggett SB. Functional properties of human β_2-adrenergic receptor polymorphisms. News in Physiologic Sciences 1995; 10:265–273.

46. Liggett SB. Genetics of β_2-adrenergic receptor variants in asthma. Clin Exp Allergy 1995; 25:89–94.

47. Green SA, Turki J, Hall IP, Liggett SB. Implications of genetic variability of human β_2-adrenergic receptor structure. Pulmonary Pharmacol 1985; 8:1–11.

48. Raymond JR. Hereditary and acquired defects in signaling through the hormone-receptor-G protein complex. Am J Physiol 1994; 266:F163–F174.

49. Spiegel AM, Weinstein LS, Shenker A. Abnormalities in G protein-coupled signal transduction pathways in human disease. J Clin Invest 1993; 92:1119–1125.

50. Clapham DE. Mutations in G protein-linked receptors: novel insights on disease. Cell 1993; 75:1237–1239.

51. Turki J, Green SA, Newman KB, Meyers MA, Liggett SB. Human lung cell β_2-adrenergic receptors desensitize in response to *in vivo* administered β-agonist. Am J Physiol: Lung Cell Mol Physiol 1995; L709–L714.

52. Merendino JJ, Spiegel AM, Crawford JD, O'Carroll AM, Brownstein MJ, Lolait SJ. Brief report: a mutation in the vasopressin V2-receptor gene in a kindred with X-linked nephrogenic diabetes insipidus. N Engl J Med 1993; 328:1538–1541.

53. Holtzman EJ, Harris HW, Kolakowski LF, Guay-Woodford LM, Botelho B, Ausiello DA. Brief report: a molecular defect in the vasopressin V2-receptor gene causing nephrogenic diabetes insipidus. N Engl J Med 1993; 328:1534–1537.

54. Clark AJ, McLoughlin L, Grossman A. Familial glucocorticoid deficiency associated with point mutation in the adrenocorticotropin receptor. Lancet 1993; 341:461–462.

55. Weber A, Kapas S, Hinson J, Grant DB, Grossman A, Clark AJ. Functional characterization of the cloned human ACTH receptor: impaired responsiveness of a mutant receptor in familial glucocorticoid deficiency. Biochem Biophys Res Commun 1993; 197:172–178.

56. Pollak MR, Brown EM, Chou YW, et al. Mutations in the human Ca2+-sensing receptor gene cause familial hypocalciuric hypercalcemia and neonatal severe hyperparathyroidism. Cell 1995; 75:1297–1303.

57. Dryja TP, McGee TL, Lauri BA, et al. Mutations within the rhodopsin gene in

patients with autosomal dominant retinitis pigmentosa. N Engl J Med 1990; 323: 1302–1307.

58. Sung CH, Davenport CM, Hennessey JC, et al. Rhodopsin mutations in autosomal dominant retinitis pigmentosa. Proc Natl Acad Sci USA 1991; 88:6481–6485.

59. Lin S, Lin CR, Gukovsky I, Lusis AJ, Sawchenko PE, Rosenfeld MG. Molecular basis of the little mouse phenotype and implications for cell type-specific growth. Nature 1993; 364:208–213.

60. Robbins LS, Nadeau JH, Johnson KR, et al. Pigmentation phenotypes of variant extension locus alleles result from point mutations that alter MSH receptor function. Cell 1993; 72:827–834.

61. Shenker A, Laue L, Kosugi S, Merendino JJ, Minegishi T, Cutler GB. A constitutively activating mutation of the luteinizing hormone receptor in familial male precocious puberty. Nature 1993; 14:652–654.

62. Parma J, Duprez L, Van Sande J, et al. Somatic mutations in the thyrotropin receptor gene cause hyperfunctioning thyroid adenomas. Nature 1993; 365:649–651.

63. Robinson PR, Cohen GB, Zhukovsky EA, Oprian DD. Constitutively active mutants of rhodopsin. Neuron 1992; 9:725.

64. Landis CA, Masters SB, Spada A, Pace AM, Bourne HR, Vallar L. GTPase inhibiting mutations activate the alpha chain of Gs and stimulate adenylyl cyclase in human pituitary tumours. Nature 1989; 340:692–696.

65. Weinstein LS, Shenker A, Gejman PV, Merino MJ, Friedman E, Spiegel AM. Activating mutations of the stimulatory G protein in the McCune-Albright syndrome. N Engl J Med 1991; 325:1688–1695.

66. Sallese M, Lombardi MS, De Blasi A. Two isoforms of G protein-coupled receptor kinase 4 identified by molecular cloning. Biochem Biophys Res Commun 1994; 199:848–854.

67. Barnes PJ. Muscarinic receptor subtypes in airways. Life Sci 1993; 52:521–527.

68. Mak JC, Haddad EB, Buckley NJ, Barnes PJ. Visualization of muscarinic m4 mRNA and m4 receptor subtype in rabbit lung. Life Sci 1993; 53:1501–1508.

69. Wess J. Molecular basis of muscarinic acetylcholine receptor function. Trends Pharmacol Sci 1993; 14:308–313.

70. Lefort J, Pretolani M, Desquand S, Vargaftig BB. Muscarinic receptor subtypes coupled to generation of different second messengers in isolated tracheal smooth muscle cells. Br J Pharmacol 1991; 104:613–618.

71. Fernandes LB, Fryer AD, Hirshman CA. M2 muscarinic receptors inhibit isoproterenol-induced relaxation of canine airway smooth muscle. J Pharmacol Exp Ther 1992; 262:119–126.

72. Ayala LE, Ahmed T. Is there a loss of a protective muscarinic receptor mechanism in asthma? Chest 1989; 96:1285–1291.

73. Ind PW, Dixon CMS, Fuller RW, Barnes PJ. Anticholinergic blockade of beta-blocker induced bronchoconstriction. Am Rev Respir Dis 1989; 139:1390–1394.

74. Carstairs JR, Nimmo AJ, Barnes PJ. Autoradiographic visualization of β-adreno-receptor subtypes in human lung. Am Rev Respir Dis 1985; 132:541–547.

75. Hamid QA, Mak JC, Sheppard MN, Corrin B, Venter JC, Barnes PJ. Localization of beta-2 adrenoceptor messenger RNA in human and rat lung using in situ hybridization: correlation with receptor autoradiography. Eur J Pharmacol 1991; 206:133–138.

76. Yatani A, Brown AM. Rapid β-adrenergic modulation of cardiac calcium currents by a fast G-protein pathway. Science 1989; 245:71–74.

77. Nijkamp FP, Engels F, Henricks PAJ, Van Oosterhout AJM. Mechanisms of β-adrenergic receptor regulation in lungs and its implications for physiological responses. Physiol Rev 1992; 72:323–367.

78. Hall IP, Wheatley A, Wilding P, Liggett SB. Association of the Glu27 β_2-adrenoceptor polymorphism with lower airway reactivity in asthmatic subjects. Lancet 1995; 345:1213–1214.

79. Turki J, Pak J, Green S, Martin R, Liggett SB. Genetic polymorphisms of the β_2-adrenergic receptor in nocturnal and non-nocturnal asthma: evidence that Gly16 correlates with the nocturnal phenotype. J Clin Invest 1995; 95:1635–1641.

80. Holroyd KJ, Levitt RC, Dragwa C, et al. Evidence for β_2-adrenergic receptor (ADRB2) polymorphism at amino acid 16 as a risk factor for bronchial hyperresponsiveness (BHR). Am J Respir Crit Care Med 1995; 151:A673 (abstr).

81. Turki J, Liggett SB. Receptor-specific functional properties of β_2-adrenergic receptor autoantibodies in asthma. Am J Respir Cell Mol Biol 1995; 12:531–539.

82. Anakwe O, Zhou S, Benovic J, Aksoy M, Kelsen SG. Interleukins impair β-adrenergic receptor adenylate cyclase (βAR-AC) system function in human airway epithelial cells. Chest 1995; 107:138S–139S.

83. Willis-Karp M, Uchida Y, Lee JY, Jinot J, Hirata A, Hirata F. Organ culture with proinflammatory cytokines reproduces impairment of the β-adrenoceptor-mediated relaxation in tracheas of a guinea pig antigen model. Am J Respir Cell Mol Biol 1993; 8:153–159.

84. Nogami M, Romberger DJ, Renneard SI, Toews ML. TGF-β_1 modulates β-adrenergic receptor number and function in cultured human tracheal smooth muscle cells. Am J Physiol 1994; 266:L187–L191.

85. Moguilevsky N, Varsalona F, Noyer M, et al. Stable expression of human H1-histamine-receptor cDNA in Chinese hamster ovary cells. Pharmacologic characterization of the protein, tissue distribution of the messenger RNA and chromosomal localization of the gene. Eur J Biochem 1994; 224:489–495.

86. De Backer MD, Gommeven W, Moereels H, et al. Genomic cloning, heterologous expression and pharmacologic characterization of a human histamine H1 receptor. Biochem Biophys Res Commun 1993; 197:1601–1608.

87. Li H, Choe NH, Wright DT, Adler KB. Histamine provokes turnover of inositol phospholipids in guinea pig and human airway epithelial cells via an H1-receptor/G protein-dependent mechanism. Am J Respir Cell Mol Biol 1995; 12:416–424.

88. Cardell LO, Edvinsson L. Characterization of the histamine receptors in the guinea-pig lung: evidence for relaxant H3 receptors in the trachea. Br J Pharmacol 1994; 111:445–454.

89. Barnes PJ. Platelet activating factor and asthma. Ann NY Acad Sci 1991; 629:193–204.

90. Honda Z, Nakamura M, Miki I, et al. Cloning by functional expression of platelet-activating factor receptor from guinea-pig lung. Nature 1991; 349:342–346.

91. Kunz D, Gerard NP, Gerard C. The human leukocyte platelet-activating receptor. cDNA cloning, cell surface expression, and construction of a novel epitope-bearing analog. J Biol Chem 1992; 267:9101–9106.

92. Ali H, Richardson RM, Tomhave ED, Dubose RA, Haribabu B, Snyderman R.

Regulation of stably transfected platelet activating factor receptor in RBL-2H3 cells. Role of multiple G proteins and receptor phorphorylation. J Biol Chem 1994; 269: 24557–24563.

93. Honda Z, Takano T, Gotoh Y, Nishida E, Ito K, Shimizu T. Transfected platelet-activating factor receptor activates mitogen-activated (MAP) kinase and MAP kinase in Chinese hamster ovary cells. J Biol Chem 1994; 269:2307–2315.

94. Levistre R, Masliah J, Beveziat G. Stimulating and inhibiting guanine-nucleotide-binding regulatory protein involvement in stimulation of arachdonic-acid release by N-formyl-methinyl-leucyl-phenylalanine and platelet-activating factor from guinea pig alveolar macrophages. Eur J Biochem 1993; 213:295–303.

95. Kermode JC, Deluca AW, Zilberman A, Valliere J, Shreeve SM. Evidence for the formation of a functional complex between vasoactive intestinal peptide, its receptor and G_s in lung membranes. J Biol Chem 1992; 267:3382–3388.

96. Carstairs JR, Barnes PJ. Visualization of vasoactive intestinal peptide receptors in human and guinea pig lung. J Pharmacol Exp Ther 1986; 239:249–255.

97. Ollerenshaw S, Jarvis D, Woolcock A, Sullivan C, Scheibner T. Absence of immunoreactive vasoactive intestinal polypeptide in tissue from the lungs of patients with asthma. N Engl J Med 1989; 19:1244–1248.

98. Suid SI. Vasoactive intestinal polypeptide (VIP) in asthma. Ann NY Acad Sci 1991; 629:305–318.

99. Yang CM, Hsia HC, Luo SF, Hsieh JT, Ong R. The effect of cyclic AMP elevating agents on bradykinin and carbachol-induced signal transduction in canine cultured trachea smooth muscles cells. Br J Pharmacol 1994; 112:781–788.

100. Trifilieff A, Lach E, Dument P, Gies JP. Bradykinin binding sites in healthy and carcinomatous human lung. Br J Pharmacol 1994; 111:1228–1232.

101. Sakamoto T, Sun J, Barnes PJ, Chung KF. Effect of bradykinin receptor antagonist, HOE 140, against bradykinin- and vagal stimulation-induced airway responses in the guinea-pig. Eur J Pharmacol 1994; 251:137–421.

102. Barnes PJ. Sensory nerves, neuropeptides, and asthma. Ann NY Acad Sci 1991; 629: 359–370.

103. D'Angio CT, Sinkin RA, LoMonaco MB, Finklestein JN. Interleukin-8 and monocyte chemoattractant protein-1 mRNAs in oxygen-injured rabbit lung. Am J Physiol 1995; 268:L826–L831.

104. Kwon OJ, Au BT, Collins PD, et al. Tumor necrosis factor-induced interleukin-8 expression in cultured human airway epithelial cells. Am J Physiol 1994; 267:L398–L405.

105. Holmes WE, Lee J, Kuang W, Rice GC, Wood WI. Structure and functional expression of a human interleukin-8 receptor. Science 1991; 253:1278–1280.

106. Murphy PM, Tiffany HL. Cloning of a complementary DNA encoding a functional human interleukin-8 receptor. Science 1991; 253:1280–1283.

107. Ben-Baruch A, Michiel DF, Oppenheim JJ. Signals and receptors involved in recruitment of inflammatory cells. J Biol Chem 1995; 270:11703–11706.

5

Regulation of Smooth Muscle Contractility

RICHARD J. PAUL
University of Cincinnati College of Medicine
Cincinnati, Ohio

PRIMAL DE LANEROLLE
College of Medicine
University of Illinois at Chicago
Chicago, Illinois

I. Introduction

Mechanical activity in muscle is ultimately the result of actin–myosin filament interaction. This interaction is associated with enhanced ATP hydrolysis, which provides the immediate source of chemical energy for mechanical activity. Thus the mechanisms controlling actin–myosin interaction are key to understanding regulation of smooth muscle contraction/relaxation.

A common feature (though logically not necessary or sufficient) of activation of smooth muscle is an increase in intracellular calcium. Thus regulation of $[Ca^{2+}]_i$ is an important aspect of our understanding of regulation of smooth muscle contractility. An understanding of the mechanisms for transduction of the Ca^{2+} signal into activation of actin–myosin interaction form a second major component needed to understand how contractility is regulated. Finally, mechanisms that modulate the Ca^{2+} sensitivity of the smooth muscle response have recently been shown to be of considerable importance to smooth muscle physiology. By this is meant that for a given $[Ca^{2+}]_i$, the level of activation of actin–myosin interaction, or the number or activated cross-bridges, can be modulated. Moreover, the kinetics of this interaction, or cross-bridge cycle rate, can also be modulated independent of $[Ca^{2+}]_i$. This is the focus of much research activity, and it offers the potential for new therapeutic approaches. This review uses this logical framework, i.e., (1) regulation of $[Ca^{2+}]_i$, (2) Ca^{2+} signal transduction, and (3) modulation of Ca^{2+} sensitivity, to approach the multifaceted nature of regulation of smooth muscle contractility.

II. Regulation of $[Ca^{2+}]_i$

Regulation of intracellular calcium in smooth muscle has much in common with other cell types, particular skeletal and cardiac muscle. This literature has been extensively reviewed [1] and will be treated only briefly here. Our emphasis is on those aspects unique to smooth muscle. $[Ca^{2+}]_i$ is a balance of Ca^{2+} input and lowering mechanisms. Ca^{2+} input is multifaceted, with influx, exchangers, and release from internal storage systems playing major roles. Plasmalemma ion channels include voltage-dependent Ca^{2+} channels and nonselective ligand-gated channels. The latter are part of the mechanisms underlying "pharmacomechanical coupling," in which activation is independent of membrane potential [2]. This also includes agonist-mediated release of Ca^{2+} from intracellular storage sites in the sarcoplasmic reticulum (SR). SR release mechanisms include those involving the inositol 1,4,5-triphosphate (IP_3) receptor, which are activated by a cascade involving G-protein activation of phospholipase A and concomitant production of IP_3 and diacylglycerol (DAG). In addition, ryanodine receptors, Ca^{2+} release channels that play a major role in striated muscle, are found in smooth muscle. These channels can be activated by Ca^{2+} itself [3] and can integrate Ca^{2+} influx with internal organelle Ca^{2+} release.

Ca^{2+} extrusion and uptake rely on the plasmalemma and SR Ca^{2+} ATPases, about which much is known [4]. Of interest to smooth muscle activation is evidence for a restricted cytoplasmic region between the inner plasmalemmal surface and the peripheral SR. This "superficial buffer barrier" delays Ca^{2+} entry and may account for data suggesting that the SR may contribute to Ca^{2+} extrusion from the cell [5]. The latter is supported by evidence which indicates that inhibition of the SR Ca^{2+} pump results in a higher steady-state $[Ca^{2+}]_i$. Since one would anticipate that the SR storage capacity is finite, lower steady-state $[Ca^{2+}]_i$ with a competent SR imply a route for Ca^{2+} extrusion from the SR to the extracellular space. A hypothetical subsarcolemmal space is postulated to permit higher Ca^{2+} concentrations than the bulk cytosol, favoring the plasmalemmal Ca^{2+} pump and allowing gradients energetically suitable for Ca^{2+} extrusion by the Na–Ca exchange mechanisms. In addition to a possible role in Ca^{2+} extrusion, the SR has also been postulated to play a direct role in Ca^{2+} entry. Based on studies with SR Ca^{2+} pump inhibitors, Putney and Bird [6] suggest that the state of depletion of intracellular stores regulates Ca^{2+} influx. The relation of this "capacitative Ca^{2+} entry" to the postulated subsarcolemmal restricted space is not known. A distinct subsarcolemmal compartment has also been postulated from metabolic studies which suggest that the energy requirements of this region are supported by a membrane-associated glycolytic cascade [7]. This hypothesis has been recently supported by data which show that Ca^{2+} homeostasis and normal excitation–contraction coupling in smooth muscle are dependent on the presence of glucose, independent of cellular ATP content [8]. An understanding of the function of this subcellular domain will likely be central to our understanding of the regulation of $[Ca^{2+}]_i$.

As may be anticipated, there are many sites for modulation of the channels, pumps, and exchangers responsible for regulation of $[Ca^{2+}]_i$ [1]. Of recent interest is the role played by phospholamban, a protein associated with the SR Ca^{2+} pump. This protein inhibits the SR Ca^{2+} pump, and inhibition is relieved by phosphorylation. This protein plays a major role in β-adrenergic effects on cardiac muscle [9] and has been implicated in cGMP-mediated effects in vascular smooth muscle [10]. Using a recently developed mouse model in which the phospholamban gene has been ablated [11], the steady-state dose (KCl, phenylephrine) isometric force relations for the aorta without phospholamban were shifted significantly to the right compared to aorta from wild-type mice [12]. Lower $[Ca^{2+}]_i$ for any given Ca^{2+} influx due to a more active SR Ca^{2+} pump in the absence of phospholamban is postulated to account for this observation. These data support a role for the SR in steady-state regulation of $[Ca^{2+}]_i$ and suggest that phospholamban modulation of the SR Ca^{2+} pump may play a significant role in regulation of smooth muscle $[Ca^{2+}]_i$.

III. Ca^{2+} Signal Transduction

A. Biochemical Studies

Our understanding of the major differences in regulation of actin–myosin interaction in smooth muscle from that of striated muscle evolved from biochemical studies on isolated actomyosin ATPase. The addition of purified actin to myosin purified from striated muscle leads to a marked increase in the myosin ATPase activity. The thin-filament proteins tropomyosin and troponin inhibit this activation. The Ca^{2+} transduction mechanism involves the binding of Ca^{2+} to a subunit of troponin (TnC), which leads to a change in the position of tropomyosin on actin, removing its inhibition of actin–myosin interaction. In contrast, the Mg-ATPase of purified smooth muscle myosin is not activated by actin. Rather than removal of an inhibiting factor, smooth muscle myosin requires an activator. There is no troponin complex in smooth muscle, and early evidence suggested a thick-filament-based regulatory mechanism [13]. The search for the activating factor was advanced when it was found that phosphorylation of the 20-kDa light chain (LC_{20}) stimulated the actin-activated Mg-ATPase activity of smooth muscle myosin [14]. The Ca^{2+} sensitivity was resolved by Hartshorne and colleagues [15,16], who demonstrated that the myosin-regulatory light-chain kinase (MLCK), an enzyme that specifically catalyzes the phosphorylation of LC_{20}, requires the Ca^{2+}-binding protein calmodulin for its activity. This schema for regulation of smooth muscle contractility is depicted in Fig. 1. An increase in $[Ca^{2+}]_i$ results in binding of Ca^{2+} to calmodulin. The Ca^{2+}/calmodulin complex then binds to and activates myosin-regulatory light-chain kinase. The activated enzyme phosphorylates LC_{20}, transforming myosin into a form that can interact with actin and hydrolyze ATP. Unlike striated muscle, in which relaxation simply reverses the activation process, i.e., decreasing $[Ca^{2+}]_i$ leads to dissociation of Ca^{2+} from TnC and subsequent inhibition of actin–myosin interaction by tropomyosin, relaxation in smooth muscle requires a second element. While decreasing $[Ca^{2+}]_i$ inactivates MLCK, dephosphorylation of LC_{20} requires a phosphatase. Regulation of this phosphatase is an active area of research (see below).

The paradigm based on these biochemical data is that Ca^{2+} regulates smooth muscle contraction by regulating myosin light-chain kinase activity, which, in turn, controls actin–myosin interaction. This hypothesis has been the source of much research activity over the past decade. As with most central dogmas, there is substantial supportive evidence and an equally impressive number of exceptions.

B. Evidence from Permeabilized Smooth Muscle

There is strong evidence that phosphorylation/dephosphorylation regulates the actin-activated Mg ATPase of purified smooth muscle myosin [17]. Studies using permeabilized or "skinned" smooth muscle have also provided convincing data implicating myosin phosphorylation/dephosphorylation as a major site for regulation of actin–myosin interaction and contractility. Various degrees of membrane permeability can be achieved, permitting experimental control over a number of major conditions including Ca^{2+} and ATP concentrations and specific components of the phosphorylation/dephosphorylation cascade. In these preparations, isometric force is dependent on the $[Ca^{2+}]$ and, more specifically, the Ca^{2+} sensitivity of isometric force [18–20] and velocity of shortening increase with the concentration of calmodulin in the bathing medium. Calmodulin antagonists [21] and a specific calmodulin-binding peptide [22] can completely inhibit isometric force in the presence of Ca^{2+}, indicating an absolute dependence of contractility on calmodulin.

The use of ATPγS, a substrate for MLCK but only a poor substrate for phosphatase [23], with permeabilized fibers further supports a primary role for this pathway. Incubation of skinned fibers with ATPγS in the presence of Ca^{2+} leads to virtually irreversible thiophosphorylation of myosin LC_{20}. After thiophosphorylation, contractility in skinned fibers is independent of Ca^{2+} or calmodulin and requires only ATP to support the actin–myosin interaction [24]. Interestingly,

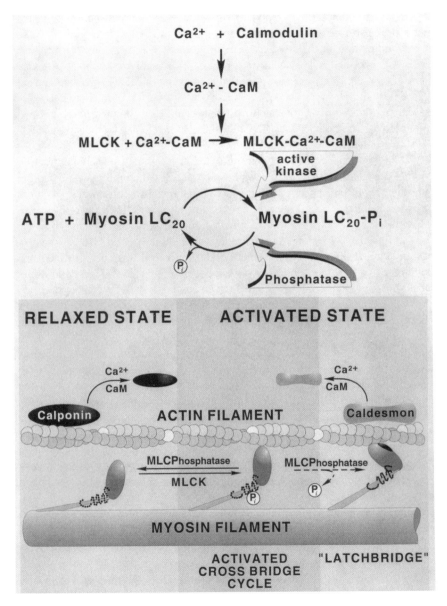

Figure 1 Major pathways for regulation of smooth muscle contractility. Myosin LC_{20} phosphorylation/dephosphorylation by myosin regulatory light-chain kinase (MLCK) and phosphatase (MLCP) is the major pathway for activation/relaxation. The thin-filament proteins, calponin and caldesmon, are also postulated to modulate contractility. Dephosphorylation of an attached myosin molecule may also lead to a slower detachment rate, leading to the so-called latch state. (See text for details.)

activation of skinned fibers requires Mg^{2+}, but after thiophosphorylation, isometric force in skinned fiber can be maintained in the absence Mg^{2+} [25,26]. These studies indicate that Mg-ATP is required for activation and further implicate the involvement of a kinase in the process. The involvement of MLCK was advanced by the discovery that proteolytic cleavage of MLCK produced a fragment that could phosphorylate LC_{20} independent of Ca^{2+}/calmodulin [27]. When the constitutively active, truncated MLCK was added to skinned fibers in Ca^{2+}-free solution, a contraction was elicited which was mechanically indistinguishable from that induced by Ca^{2+} [24,28].

The significance of LC_{20} phosphorylation to smooth muscle contractility was also approached in terms of the phosphatase. Based on the central paradigm, enhancement of phosphatase activity should inactivate smooth muscle. Addition of a phosphatase-enriched fraction from bovine aorta was first shown to enhance relaxation in skinned fibers [29]. A purified bovine aortic phosphatase produced parallel reductions in isometric force, shortening velocity and LC_{20} phosphorylation in skinned fibers [30,31]. Similarly, Haeberle et al. [32] demonstrated that both force and LC_{20} phosphorylation were decreased in a dose-dependent fashion by addition of the catalytic subunit of phosphatase 1. The importance of a phosphatase in regulation has also been demonstrated through the use of various phosphatase inhibitors, such as okadaic acid, calyculin b, or microcystin. Consistent with regulation by LC_{20} phosphorylation/dephosphorylation, all of these phosphatase inhibitors are associated with activation in skinned fibers. Phosphatase inhibition also increases both force and LC_{20} phosphorylation in intact smooth muscle, as shown in Fig. 2. Until recently, phosphatase activity was not thought to be regulated, but studies of the regulation of phosphatase activity as a modulator of smooth-muscle Ca^{2+} sensitivity is an area of intense research activity [33]. This will be discussed further in the section on modulation of Ca^{2+} sensitivity.

The studies on skinned fibers strongly supports the hypothesis that myosin phosphorylation/dephosphorylation is necessary and, in fact, likely to be sufficient for regulation of actin–myosin interaction in permeabilized smooth muscle. Generalizations to intact smooth muscle, however, must be made cautiously, as the permeabilization procedures may themselves alter the signal transduction process.

C. Intact Smooth Muscle

Pressure injection of the constitutively active MLCK into single smooth muscle cells elicits a contraction [34], despite low $[Ca^{2+}]_i$. This suggests that other Ca^{2+}-dependent pathways, whether inhibitory or stimulatory, do not regulate—that is, activate—smooth muscle actin–myosin interaction. These data do not rule out the existence of other mechanisms that may modulate this interaction. This and the data from skinned fiber studies suggest that LC_{20} phosphorylation/dephosphory-

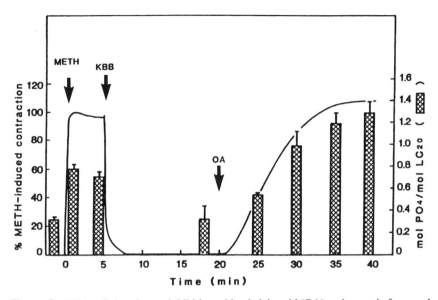

Figure 2   Effect of phosphatase inhibition with odadaic acid (OA) on isometric force and LC_{20} phosphorylation in lamb tracheal smooth muscle. Fibers were first contracted by applying 1 μM methacholine (METH) for 5 min followed by 50 μM OA for 15 min after washing out the methacholine with Krebs-bicarbonate buffer (KBB). The fibers were frozen at various times and LC_{20} phosphorylation was quantitated. The solid line represents the isometric force generated by a representative fiber. Each bar represents mean $\pm$ SE ($n =$ 5–10) for the phosphorylation measurements. Adapted from Obara et al. (1989).

lation is the major activator of actin–myosin interaction. If LC_{20} phosphorylation is central to regulation of actin–myosin interaction in living smooth muscle, there should be precise relationships between (1) the time courses of phosphorylation and force production, (2) the extent of LC_{20} phosphorylation and the steady-state level of force generated, and (3) the time courses of dephosphorylation and relaxation. These relationships have been studied extensively for airways (tracheal) smooth muscle, as shown in Fig. 3 and Table 1. There is a fair amount of variability in the literature, likely due to different techniques and the difficulty of making LC_{20} phosphorylation measurements in living tissue. However, in general, LC_{20} phosphorylation precedes force generation [35–37], and LC_{20} dephosphorylation precedes relaxation [38,39]. This is also true for other smooth muscle types, with similar studies on vascular [40–44], uterine [45–48], and intestinal smooth muscle [49]. As the database grows, there are exceptions to the association of force with LC_{20}-P_i [50]. If there is a consensus, most smooth muscle researchers would agree that LC_{20} phosphorylation is required to initiate contraction and

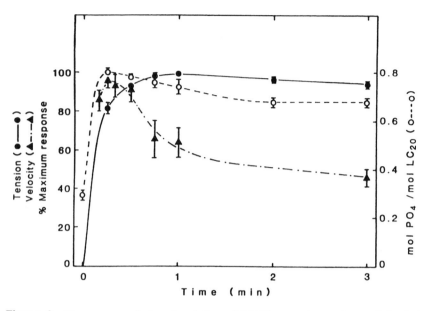

Figure 3 Time course of phosphorylation of 20-kDa myosin regulatory light-chain (LC_{20}), unloaded shortening velocity (V_{us}) and isometric force. Lamb tracheal smooth muscle fibers were stimulated with 10^{-6} M methacholine. Force (●) and LC_{20} phosphorylation (○) were measured in the same fibers; V_{us} (▲) was measured in a separate set of fibers. From Obara and de Lanerolle (1989).

dephosphorylation required for relaxation. However, the relationship between LC_{20}-P_i and steady-state force and the existence of other mechanisms for modulation of both force and shortening velocity remain controversial.

The observations that underlie this controversy are shown in Fig. 3. With constant stimulation, isometric force (an index of the number of activated cross-bridges) increases monotonically to a sustained maximum value. In contrast, LC_{20}-P_i in most smooth muscles achieves a maximum shortly after initiation of the stimulation, then decreases to a steady-state value. There is a wide range of reported values in terms of the ratio of the peak to steady-state value and the extent to which the steady-state values exceeds the initial baseline (Table 1). This is due partly to the temporal resolution with respect to determination of when the maximum value occurs and in terms of sensitivity of the assay to discriminate changes from baseline. The shape of the LC_{20}-P_i transient also varies with stimulus and tissue type; for example, in hog carotid artery the peak may be between 30% and 40% and steady state about 25%, which differ significantly from the

Table 1 Summary of LC_{20} Phosphorylation and Velocity Data from Studies on Tracheal Smooth Muscle[a]

Ref.	Agonist and dose	Resting	LC_{20} phosphorylation (mol PO_4/mol LC_{20}) Peak (30–60 s)	Maintained (>3 min)
114	10^{-6} M Carb	0.13	0.75	0.27
76	10^{-6} M Carb	0.10*	0.80*	0.11
40	10^{-5} M Carb	0.12	0.46 (100%)	0.20* (49%)
Mean ± SE		0.12 ± 0.01	0.67 ± 0.11	0.19 ± 0.05
30	10^{-4} M Meth	0.25	0.45	0.55
28	10^{-4} M Meth	0.29	0.62	0.49
39	10^{-6} M Carb	0.14	0.68 (100%)	0.46 (21%)
21	10^{-5} M Carb	0.13	0.66	0.47
62	10^{-7} M Carb	0.09		0.42
88	10^{-6} M Meth	0.29	0.80 (100%)	0.68 (46%)
124	10^{-7} M Carb	0.09*	0.70	0.60*
75	3×10^{-7} M Meth	0.12	0.40 (100%)	0.44 (27%)
LC_{20} PO_4 Mean ± SE		0.18 ± 0.03	0.62 ± 0.05	0.51 ± 0.03
Velocity Mean ± SE			100%	36 ± 8%

[a]In all the studies summarized, tracheal muscles were stimulated with a muscarinic agonist and myosin phosphylation was measured at or near its peak value and after it had stabilized (3–120 min). In some cases, phosphorylation values had to be extrapolated from the figures, and these are identified with asterisks. Velocity (parentheses underneath phosphorylation data) are expressed on the basis of the peak velocity value as being 100%. Data shown on top are from studies performed before 1985; with the exception of Refs. 28 and 30, the data on bottom are from studies performed since 1985. Carb, carbachol; Meth, methacholine. Adapted from P. de Lanerolle and R.J. Paul, Am. J. Physiol. 261: L1-L14, 1991.

values for tracheal muscle shown in Table 1. However, the key question raised is how LC_{20}-P_i, which decreases with the duration of stimulation, can regulate the number of activated cross-bridges, which presumably remain constant as evidenced by the maintained isometric force.

Another key mechanical observation, highlighted by Murphy and colleagues [42], was that the shortening velocity (an index of the rate of cross-bridge cycling) reaches a maximum value shortly after initiation of the stimulus but then declines to a steady-state value some two- to threefold lower (Fig. 3). Based on correlations between shortening velocity and LC_{20}-P_i, they proposed that LC_{20}-P_i

regulates cross-bridge cycle rate and hence shortening speed and postulated that dephosphorylated, slowly cycling cross-bridges, termed "latchbridges," underlie force maintenance [42].

This hypothesis is appealing for a number of reasons. First, a number of studies indicate that $[Ca^{2+}]_i$ after stimulation shows a transient behavior parallel to that of LC_{20}-P_i [51–53], consistent with Ca^{2+} regulation of MLCK. Second, smooth muscles maintain force very efficiently. Energy utilization is high during force generation but then decreases (two- to fourfold) during tension maintenance [54]. The hypothesis that LC_{20}-P_i regulates cycle rate could also provide a mechanistic basis for the special energetic characteristics of smooth muscle. Since these initial studies, a number of supportive correlations [51] as well as exceptions [50] have been reported.

At present, there is no clear consensus as to the relations among LC_{20}-P_i, steady-state isometric force, and velocity in living smooth muscle. Smooth muscle can be activated in the absence of LC_{20}-P_i by Mg^{2+} [55], Mn^{2+} [56], polylysine [57,58], and preincubation with vanadate [59], as shown in studies using permeabilized tissues. Oxidation of some protein may be involved, and at least some of the characteristics of these contractures are similar to those elicited by LC_{20}-P_i. Moreover, the force elicited by these agonists is generally not additive but rather complementary to that elicited by LC_{20}-P_i; i.e., maximum phosphorylation of LC_{20} by exposure to these agents does not further increase force. This suggests that the activation pathway for some of these agents may parallel that of LC_{20}-P_i, but the site of oxidation and the mechanism(s) remain to be elucidated.

Given the significance of smooth muscle regulation to diseases such as asthma, the mechanisms here are subject to intense research activity. In one school of thought, LC_{20}-P_i is proposed to be essential for initiating contraction, but other Ca^{2+}-dependent mechanisms are postulated to be involved during force maintenance [60]. This received early impetus from studies which suggested that LC_{20}-P_i decreased to near baseline levels during sustained contractions, but isometric force retained Ca^{2+}-sensitivity. This led to a search for additional mechanisms regulating dephosphorylated "latchbridges." However, in most recent studies, LC_{20}-P_i is reported to be significantly elevated above the resting level in the steady state after stimulation (Table 1). There are a number of thin-filament-associated proteins that have been proposed as smooth muscle regulatory proteins, including leitonin [61], caldesmon [62], and calponin [63]. The strongest evidence is at the biochemical level [64], indicating that all these proteins bind to the thin filament and inhibit the actin-activated ATPase of myosin. Regulation is conferred by Ca^{2+}-dependent phosphorylation, and/or binding by Ca^{2+}/calmodulin, which weakens the binding of these proteins to actin. It should be noted, however, that there are some reports indicating that these proteins can bind to myosin [65] and enhance its ATPase in the absence of actin. As both calponin and caldesmon bind to actin, competitive interactions between these proteins may also be important to their proposed inhibitory functions [66].

There is considerable biochemical evidence supporting thin-filament-based modulatory mechanisms. However, at the physiological level, the evidence for a functional role of thin-filament proteins is yet controversial. A relatively new model system, the so-called motility assays, bridges between biochemical studies, which assess the effects of thin-filament-associated proteins on myosin ATPase, and studies on more structured permeabilized smooth muscle. These studies measure filament velocity of either myosin-coated beads on actin cables or that of actin filaments on myosin-coated nitrocellulose plates. The results are mixed in terms of the function of caldesmon and calponin. Sellers and colleagues [67] reported that increasing caldesmon concentration inhibited actin filament velocity in a graded manner, whereas calponin inhibited actin sliding in a more "all-or-none" fashion. Similar findings for caldesmon were reported by Okagaki et al. [68]. On the other hand, Haeberle and colleagues [69] reported that caldesmon had no effect on filament velocity when its monomeric form was preserved by DTT. They proposed that caldesmon has a "tethering" effect, facilitating actin filament interaction with the myosin-coated surface. Haeberle also reported [70] that calponin increased actin binding to myosin while decreasing filament velocity twofold, suggesting that calponin inhibits the rate of dissociation of actin from myosin.

There is less evidence for thin-filament regulation in the more intact muscle models, but studies in this area are gaining in momentum. Partially this is due to the early expectations of a regulator paralleling the skeletal troponin/tropomyosin, which is an on–off regulator of skeletal actin–myosin interaction at the thin-filament level. The studies with ATPγS or the Ca^{2+}-independent MLCK indicating that activation by LC_{20}-P_i can occur in the absence of Ca^{2+} indicate that a Ca^{2+}-dependent inhibitor of actin–myosin interaction in smooth muscle is unlikely. On the other hand, thin-filament proteins which modulate the cross-bridge cycle rate remain attractive candidates for the slowing of velocity with duration of stimulation. Recently, caldesmon (CaD) and proteolytic fragments of CaD were reported to inhibit force in permeabilized gizzard smooth muscle [71,72], though similar studies in taenia coli were negative (Paul, unpublished observations). A peptide inhibitor of the binding of CaD to actin was reported to increase isometric force, presumably by competing with endogenous CaD in studies of permeabilized single cells of ferret aorta and portal vein [73]. Calponin added to permeabilized smooth muscle has also been reported to inhibit isometric force [74]. Using fibers activated by thiophosphorylation with ATPγS, addition of calponin in the absence of Ca^{2+} was found to have a more pronounced inhibitory effect on shortening velocity than isometric force [75]. In both these latter studies, phosphorylated calponin was not effective, suggesting a potential path for regulation involving protein kinase C. Phosphorylation of CaD by MAP kinase [76], potentially activated by a tyrosine kinase [77], provides another interesting scenario for regulation of smooth muscle and integration with an important pathway for regulation of smooth muscle proliferation.

Studies on the role of LC_{20}-P_i and its relation to the proposed thin-filament modulatory proteins remains enigmatic. There is considerable controversy as to the extent and distribution of the thin-filament proteins. Both calponin and caldesmon are reported to co-localize with the contractile apparatus and cytoskeleton of smooth muscle cells [78,79]. However, the extent of actin filaments containing CaD is only 35–45% of the total thin filaments in vascular smooth and slightly less in visceral muscle based on selective extraction [80]. Others report significantly lower values for aorta and higher for visceral smooth muscle [81]. It is not clear whether the thin filaments containing the modulatory proteins lie in distinct domains, but the stoichiometry poses a problem to theories of regulation in that there appears to be a significant number of thin filaments that would not contain the proposed modulatory proteins.

A second area of considerable controversy arising from studies on intact smooth muscle concerns the in-vivo evidence for phosphorylation of the modulatory proteins. It appears that while Ca^{2+}/calmodulin can reverse the inhibition of ATPase in vitro, the concentrations required are not consistent with in-vivo modulation. Thus phosphorylation of the thin filament proteins appears to be the more likely avenue for regulation. However, efforts to correlate phosphorylation of the thin-filament proteins with altered contractility in vivo have been mixed. There are data favoring phosphorylation [50,82–84], and equally strong data suggesting it is not [85–87]. The type of stimulation, the tissue type, and the time course of phorphorylation are all factors to be considered in interpretation of these data. In sum, the evidence for some form of modulation of smooth muscle contractility at the level of the thin filament continues to grow, but unequivocal evidence for its functional role in vivo remains elusive.

A second school of thought, pioneered by Murphy and colleagues, postulates that the slowing of shortening velocity and energy utilization with the duration of stimulation in intact smooth muscle can be explained by LC_{20}-P_i alone, without invoking any other regulatory mechanism. Their "latch" theory involves one critical assumption which postulates that when a phosphorylated cross-bridge is dephosphorylated while attached to actin, the rate constant for dissociation of this complex, termed latchbridge, is decreased. Using a four-state model and computer simulation, the time course of isometric force development and the biphasic time course of LC_{20}-P_i could be readily predicted by this model [88]. Incorporating this concept with previous models permitted shortening velocity to be included [89] and also explained the decrease in velocity with duration of stimulation as well as the apparent correlation of shortening velocity with LC_{20}-P_i.

This model was challenged on energetic grounds [90]. Using the original four-state model, it was shown that the curvilinear relation between ATP utilization and isometric force predicted by the model appeared to conflict with the linear behavior reported for smooth muscle [91]. Moreover, the predicted energy utilization associated with myosin phosphorylation/dephosphorylation by the model, 87% in the original four-state model [88,89] and 50% in the coupled version [92], exceeded the values of approximately 20% based on experimental data in living tissue [54]. This curvilinearity was suggested to be compatible with experimental data, giving the limited range of LC_{20}-P_i, associated with physiological levels of stimulation [92]. In addition, new energetics experiments [93] supported earlier data [94] indicating that at high levels of stimulation and LC_{20}-P_i, the relation between ATP utilization and force was nonlinear. However, in recent studies, ATP utilization at long muscle lengths, where force was significantly reduced, was used to assess the energy utilization not associated with actin–myosin interaction [95]. In these studies on intact hog carotid artery, suprabasal energy utilization at long muscle lengths was reduced to approximately 25% of that at the optimal length for force generation. These data support the conclusions from some [96,97] but not all [98] studies on permeabilized smooth muscles indicating that myosin phosphorylation/dephosphorylation is only a moderate determinant of total energy utilization during contraction. For completeness, it should be noted that four-state models invoking cooperative activation of nonphosphorylated cross-bridges [98] or simply a large detachment rate constant for activated cross-bridges [90] can also simulate smooth muscle behavior. Whether these current energetic data can be included in a simple four-state model remains to be determined. In sum, models of regulation based only on LC_{20}-P_i are attractive because of their simplicity. They are not incompatible with additional modulation at the thin filament level, and it remains likely that some combination of these theories may be necessary to completely explain the behavior of intact smooth muscle.

IV. Modulation of Smooth Muscle Ca^{2+} Sensitivity

Perhaps the area of most intense current activity involves an understanding of the mechanisms which underlie the modulation of smooth muscle Ca^{2+} sensitivity. Development of therapeutic approaches to smooth muscle-related diseases has focused largely on interventions at the level of altering $[Ca^{2+}]_i$. However, recent studies have indicated that modulation of the response of smooth muscle at a constant $[Ca^{2+}]_i$ may be equally important to regulation of smooth muscle contractility. Early studies by Morgan and Morgan [52], using aequorin light production as an index of $[Ca^{2+}]_i$, demonstrated that the relation between $[Ca^{2+}]_i$ and force was dependent on the mode of stimulation. Agonist-based stimulation was associated with a higher level of force per given $[Ca^{2+}]_i$ than that associated with KCl depolarization, which has since been verified in a number of studies [2]. In addition, there is also evidence that the relations between LC_{20}-P_i and isometric force can also be varied [71]. There is experimental evidence to support four separate or interactive mechanisms that can affect the responsiveness of a smooth muscle to a given level of $[Ca^{2+}]_i$. Although the involvement of any of these mechanisms in modulating smooth muscle contractility remains controversial, the evidence in support of each of them, and their shortcomings, are described below.

One mechanism involves the modulation of MLCK activity by covalent modification. Since MLCK is activated by the binding of the Ca^{2+}-calmodulin complex [15], covalent modifications that decrease the affinity of MLCK for the Ca^{2+}-calmodulin complex result in a decreases in MLCK activity, LC_{20}-P_i, and force. MLCK is known to be phosphorylated by cyclic AMP-dependent protein kinase (cAPK) [99–101] and the type II multifunctional Ca^{2+}-calmodulin-dependent kinase (CaMKII) [102,103]. Modulation of MLCK activity by phosphorylation by cAPK is particularly relevant to the study of airway smooth muscle because agents that increase intracellular cyclic AMP levels result in myosin dephosphorylation and relaxation of tracheal smooth muscle [38,104]. Moreover, pretreating tracheal smooth muscles with isoproterenol attenuates both the rates of myosin light-chain phosphorylation and force generation by lamb tracheal smooth muscle [105], as shown in Fig. 4. Lastly, the airway hyperreactivity associated with asthma has been suggested to be related to a lack of responsiveness to elevation in cyclic AMP level [106–108].

In-vitro studies have demonstrated that MLCK is phosphorylated at two sites, termed sites A and B, by cAPK. Phosphorylation of both sites decreases the affinity (K_{Cam}) of MLCK for Ca^{2+}/calmodulin [100,101]. Thus, at any submaximal $[Ca^{2+}]_i$, fewer phosphorylated MLCK molecules will be activated by the available Ca^{2+}/calmodulin complexes than unphosphorylated MLCK molecules. This, in turn, can theoretically result in a lower level of LC_{20}-P_i and less force generation by a smooth muscle. One approach for testing this hypothesis has been to label the ATP in smooth muscles with ^{32}P, stimulate the smooth muscles with various contracting and relaxing agents, immunoprecipitate MLCK, and analyze the level of MLCK phosphorylation. This type of experiment has demonstrated 1 mol PO_4/mol MLCK in resting muscle and that this increases to 2 mol PO_4/mol MLCK following forskolin treatment [104]. These changes in MLCK phosphorylation were shown to be specific to an increase in intracellular cyclic AMP levels, because methacholine or methacholine followed by atropine, which do not increase cyclic AMP levels, did not result in an increase in MLCK phosphorylation [104].

Although the data described above support the idea that stoichiometric increases in MLCK phosphorylation could be involved in cyclic AMP-mediated relaxation of smooth muscle, two additional pieces of information are needed to fully evaluate the importance of this mechanism. First, it is essential to correlate an increase in MLCK phosphorylation with a decrease in MLCK activity following treatment with agents that increase cyclic AMP levels. This is a difficult experiment to execute, because it requires either inhibiting all other protein kinases without affecting MLCK activity and phosphorylation levels while performing the activity assay or purifying MLCK from small pieces of tissue and assaying activity in isolation. Second, it is important to establish the MLCK sites that are phosphorylated. MLCK can be phosphorylated by protein kinase C (PKC) [109] and CaMKII [102,103], and one study has suggested that up to six MLCK sites are phosphorylated following stimulation with various agents [110]. Sorting through all of these phosphorylation sites and performing reliable activity assays represents a difficult task that is required to truly understand the importance of MLCK phosphorylation in cyclic AMP-mediated relaxation of airway muscle.

MLCK phosphorylation by CaMKII has also been suggested to affect Ca^{2+} sensitivity and smooth muscle contractility [111]. Initial biochemical studies showing that MLCK phosphorylation by CaMKII results in a decrease in the affinity of MLCK for the Ca^{2+}/calmodulin complex [102,103] have been followed by experiments demonstrating MLCK phosphorylation in contracting smooth muscles [111]. Since the phosphorylation of MLCK could be abolished by agents that inhibit CaMKII, it was concluded that this enzyme was catalyzing the phosphorylation of MLCK in contracting muscles. However, the calcium concentration required for half-maximal phosphorylation of myosin light chains and MLCK were 250 and 500 nM, respectively. This means that a higher $[Ca^{2+}]_i$ concentration is required to affect the phosphorylation of MLCK, which is inconsistent with the notion that this is an important modulatory reaction for two reasons. First, the higher calcium concentration is a reflection of the activation kinetics of CaMKII and suggests that the activation of this enzyme and the resulting phosphorylation of MLCK occur after phosphorylation of myosin light chains. Second, there should be sufficient Ca^{2+}/calmodulin complexes within the cell at the higher $[Ca^{2+}]_i$ to overcome the effects of phosphorylating MLCK. These two points make it difficult to visualize how MLCK phosphorylation by CaMKII is involved in modulating smooth muscle contractility, and additional experiments are needed to fully understand the role of MLCK phosphorylation, by either cAPK or CaMKII, in affecting Ca^{2+} sensitivity and the contractile properties of smooth muscle.

A second mechanism for affecting Ca^{2+} involves the direct manipulation of ATP hydrolysis by the phosphorylated myosin. MLC_{20} is phosphorylated on Ser 19 and Thr 18 by MLCK [112]. Phosphorylation of Ser 19 appears to be the critical element in activating smooth muscle and nonmuscle myosins. MLC_{20} is also phosphorylated by PKC, but on Ser 1, Ser 2, and Thr 8 [112,113]. Phosphorylation by PKC, alone, has no effect on ATP hydrolysis by smooth muscle and nonmuscle myosins, whereas phosphorylation by PKC of myosin previously phosphorylated by MLCK attenuates the rate of ATP hydrolysis [114]. That is, myosin phosphorylated by both PKC and MLCK has a lower rate of ATP hydro-

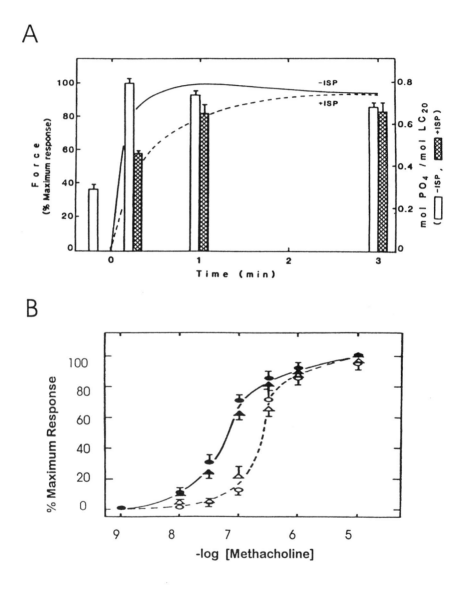

lysis than myosin phosphorylated by MLCK, alone [114]. These in-vitro results suggested that multiple-site phosphorylation by two separate protein kinases with different activation kinetics could affect ATP hydrolysis by myosin and the contractility. This hypothesis is supported by the observation that the addition of phorbol esters, which activate PKC, results in a slow, sustained smooth muscle contraction [115–117]. However, analysis of the MLC_{20} phosphorylation sites have not demonstrated the phosphorylation of the relevant sites following phorbol ester treatment [118–121]. These data have questioned the role of myosin phosphorylation by PKC in affecting the contractile properties of smooth muscle.

A third possibility is that modulating phosphatase activity affects the Ca^{2+} sensitivity of smooth muscles. The extent and rate of LC_{20}-P_i at any time during smooth muscle contraction or relaxation reflects the balance between MLCK and MLC_{20} phosphatase activities [122]. Mechanisms that shift this balance by inhibiting MLC_{20} phosphatases will increase the rate or extent of LC_{20}-P_i, at any given level of $[Ca^{2+}]_i$, and, hence, the contractile properties of the muscle. There are many phosphates that have been shown to dephosphorylate phosphorylated MLC_{20} [123], but little is known about the mechanisms that regulate these enzymes.

Nevertheless, it has been suggested that G-protein-coupled inhibition of myosin phosphatases may play a role in Ca^{2+} sensitization of smooth muscles [2]. This was based on the observation that addition of GTPγS to smooth muscle fibers permeabilized with staphylococcal alpha toxin increases force and LC_{20}-Pi_i, at constant myolasmic Ca^{2+} [124], and inhibits MLC_{20} phosphatase activity in smooth muscles [125]. Although the G-protein involved has not been identified,

---

Figure 4   (A) Effects of isoproterenol (ISP) pretreatment on LC_{20} phosphorylation and contractile properties of lamb tracheal smooth muscle. Fibers were stimulated with 10^{-6} M methacholine. Broken line represents force produced by fibers preincubated with 10^{-6} M isoproterenol for 5 min; solid line represents force produced by control fibers (mean ± SE, $n = 5$–7). Open and cross-hatched bars indicate LC_{20} phosphorylation in control fibers and ISP-treated fibers, respectively. LC_{20} phosphorylation values in the two groups are significantly different (i.e., $P \leq 0.05$) only at 15 s ($P \leq 0.001$) after addition of methacholine as determined by a Student's t test. (B) Effect of isoproterenol on methacholine dose–response relationships for isometric force and LC_{20} phosphorylation. Fibers were frozen at 3 min after methacholine stimulation and the level of LC_{20} phosphorylation was determined. Force was expressed as percent maximal active tension. Data from control fibers (●, ▲) and fibers preincubated with 10^{-6} M M ISP (○, △) for 5 min, were analyzed separately. ●, Tension in control fibers; ○, tension in ISP-treated fibers; ▲, LC_{20} phosphorylation in control fibers; △, LC_{20} phosphorylation in ISP-treated fibers. Adapted from Obara and de Lanerolle (1989).

the observation that AlF_4^- can also sensitize permeabilized smooth muscles suggest that heterotrimeric G proteins may be involved in this process [126]. The Ca^{2+}-sensitizing effects of GTPγS may involve arachidonic acid metabolism. Addition of arachidonic acid to smooth muscles permeabilized with staphylococcal alpha toxin at constant, submaximal Ca^{2+} increases LC_{20}-P_i and contracts the muscle [127]. In addition, the same investigators have shown that arachidonic acid also inhibits the activity of a multisubunit phosphatase by dissociating the subunits of this enzyme [127]. Since G proteins, by definition, are activated by the binding GTP, the observed effects of GTPγS in permeabilized smooth muscles are consistent with a mechanism that involves G-protein-coupled activation of phospholipase A_2, an increase in intracellular arachidonic acid, the inhibition of MLC_{20} phosphatase(s) by the arachidonic acid, an increase in LC_{20}-P_i due to a shift in the MLCK/phosphatase activity ratio, and an increase in force in the absence of changes in $[Ca^{2+}]_i$. This mechanism could also be involved when smooth muscles are stimulated by any agent that activates G proteins, such as α_1-adrenergic receptor agonists [128].

The fourth putative mechanism involves thin-filament proteins. Much of the impetus for the interest in thin-filament regulatory mechanisms has come from studies on calponin and caldesmon. Calponin is a smooth muscle-specific protein that has a molecular weight of 34,000. It is a highly abundant protein that co-localizes with tropomyosin and actin in smooth muscle cells [129]. Calponin binds actin, tropomyosin, and Ca^{2+}-calmodulin. Calponin is phosphorylated by PKC and CaMKII, and the unphosphorylated, but not the phosphorylated form, inhibits actomyosin ATPase activity in vitro [63]. Caldesmon is expressed in both smooth muscle and nonmuscle cells. The smooth muscle form of caldesmon is an elongated protein of 87 kDa. It is also located on actin filaments, and the carboxy terminal contains a binding site for actin, tropomyosin, and Ca^{2+}-calmodulin. Purified caldesmon inhibits the actin-activated ATPase activity of smooth muscle myosin and the movement of actin filaments in an in-vitro motility assay [67]. Caldesmon is phosphorylated by PKC, and phosphorylation by PKC decreases the ability of caldesmon to inhibit ATP hydrolysis by actin and myosin [130]. The Ca^{2+}-calmodulin-binding characteristics and the inhibition of actomyosin ATPase activity by calponin and calmodulin have stimulated great interest in the involvement of these proteins in smooth muscle contractility. The evidence for and against direct modulation of the actin–myosin interaction in smooth muscle cells by these proteins has been described above. What follows describes the possible indirect involvement of these proteins in modulating smooth muscle contractility.

Experiments on smooth muscle fibers or single cells with permeabilized membranes have shown that certain agents, such as GTPγS [124] and phenylephrine [128], induced a contraction at constant myoplasmic $[Ca^{2+}]$. Subsequent experiments correlated phenylephrine-induced force generation, at constant

$[Ca^{2+}]$, with the translocation of the specific, calcium-independent, epsilon iso-form of PKC [131]. The ϵ-PKC could then have downstream effects by one of two pathways. One pathway involves the phosphorylation of calponin. Phosphoryla-tion of calponin would relieve the inhibitory effects of this protein on ATP hydrolysis by actin and myosin, thereby resulting in an increase in force without a change in $[Ca^{2+}]_i$ or LC_{20}-P_i. The second pathway involves the activation of the ras pathway by ϵ-PKC and the subsequent phosphorylation of caldesmon by the mitogen-activated protein kinase (MAP kinase) [76]. Immunofluorescence and digital imaging microscopy on isolated smooth muscle cells have suggested that prolonged phenylephrine treatment results in the eventual redistribution of MAP kinase to the vicinity of the contractile filaments, and that this redistribution can be blocked by PKC inhibitors [131]. Although these data are suggestive, consider-able experimental data are needed to conclude that either pathway is actively involved in modulating smooth muscle contractility.

V. Summary

Our understanding of the regulation of smooth muscle contractility has advanced considerably in the past two decades. Control of intracellular $[Ca^{2+}]_i$ is a key element in which the smooth muscle cell shares many common features with excitable cells and its skeletal muscle counterparts. However, the transduction of the Ca^{2+} signal at the contractile filament level is now known to be dramatically different. The major transduction system in smooth muscle involves the thick filaments, rather than the thin-filament linked, troponin/tropomyosin system of skeletal muscle. Phosphorylation of the myosin regulatory light chain by a $Ca^{2+}/$ calmodulin-dependent kinase is a central step in the activation process. Since this step involves covalent modification, it is slower than the simple binding/unbinding of Ca^{2+} to troponin C in the skeletal muscle contraction/relaxation cycle. However, it affords additional sites for control of smooth muscle contractility, in particular at the level of the phosphatase required in deactivation. Although much is known, the exact role of myosin LC_{20} phosphorylation/dephosphorylation is yet a subject of considerable controversy. LC_{20}-P_i likely is involved not only in the regulation of the number of activated cross-bridges, but also in the regulation of the cross-bridge cycle and hence contractile velocity and energetics. Moreover, the regula-tion of myosin LC_{20}-P_i also provides an avenue for modulation of contractility at constant $[Ca^{2+}]_i$. The modulation of contractile response for a given $[Ca^{2+}]_i$ is an area of considerable interest to the understanding of the regulation of smooth muscle contractility as well as to potential therapeutic approaches. Of particular interest in this regard is the role of potential thin-filament proteins, such as caldesmon and calponin, in the modulation of Ca^{2+} sensitivity, again an area of considerable controversy. Thus, while having made significant advances over the past decades, our understanding of the regulation of smooth muscle contractility remains an existing area for future studies.

References

1. Sperelakis N, Ohya Y. Electrophysiology of vascular smooth muscle. In: Sperelakis N, ed. Physiology and Pathophysiology of the Heart, 3rd ed. Boston: Kluwer, 1995: 859–894.

2. Somlyo AP, Somlyo AV. Signal transduction and regulation in smooth muscle. Nature 1994; 372:231–236.

3. Iino M. Calcium-induced calcium release mechanism in guinea pig taenia caeci. J Gen Physiol 1989; 94:363–383.

4. Wuytack F, Raeymakers L, De Smedt H, et al. Ca(2+)-transport ATPases and their regulation in muscle and brain. Ann NY Acad Sci 1991; 671:82–91.

5. Chen Q, van Breemen C. The superficial buffer barrier in venous smooth muscle: sarcoplasmic reticulum refilling and unloading. Br J Pharmacol 1993; 109(2): 336–343.

6. Putney JW Jr, Bird GS. The signal for capacitative calcium entry. Cell 1993; 75(2): 199–201.

7. Ishida Y, Riesinger I, Walliman T, Paul RJ. Compartmentation of ATP synthesis and utilization in smooth muscle: roles of aerobic glycolysis and creatine kinase. In Saks V, Ventura-Clapier R, eds. Cellular Energetics: Role of Coupled Creatine Kinases. Mol Cell Biochem 1994; 133/134:39–50.

8. Zhang C, Paul RJ. Excitation-contraction coupling and relaxation in porcine carotid arteries are specifically dependent on glucose. Am J Physiol 1994; 267:H1996–H2004.

9. Edes I, Kranias EG. Regulation of cardiac sarcoplasmic reticulum function by phospholamban. Membrane Biochem 1989; 7:175–192.

10. Lincoln TM, Cornwell TL. Towards an understanding of the mechanism of action of cyclic AOMP and cyclic GMP in smooth muscle relaxation. Blood Vessels 1991; 28:129–137.

11. Luo W, Grupp IL, Harrer J, et al. Targeted ablation of the phospholamban gene is associated with markedly enhanced myocardial contractility and loss of B-agonist stimulation. Circ Res 1994; 75:401–409.

12. Lalli J, Luo W, Kranias EG, Paul RJ. Decreased vascular sensitivity in aorta from transgenic phospholamban deficient mice. Circulation 1994; 90(4):I356.

13. Bremel RD. Myosin linked calcium regulation in vertebrate smooth muscle. Nature 1974; 252:405–407.

14. Sobieszek A. Vertebrate smooth muscle myosin. Enzymatic and structural properties. In: Stephens NL, ed. The Biochemistry of Smooth Muscle. Baltimore, MD: University Park Press, 1977:413–443.

15. Dabrowska RD, Aromatorio DK, Sherry JMF, Hartshorne DJ. Composition of the myosin light chain kinase from chicken gizzard. Biochem Biophys Res Commun 1977; 78:1263–1272.

16. Dabrowska R, Sherry JMF, Aromatorio DK, Hartshorne DJ. Modulator protein as a component of myosin light chain kinase from chicken gizzard. Biochemistry 1978; 17:253–258.

17. Sellers JR, Pato MD, Adelstein RS. Reversible phosphorylation of smooth muscle myosin, heavy meromyosin, and platelet myosin. J Biol Chem 1981; 256:13137–13142.

18. Cassidy PS, Kerrick WGL, Hoar PE, Malencik DA. Exogenous calmodulin increases Ca^{2+} sensitivity of isometric tension activation and myosin phosphorylation in skinned smooth muscle. Pfluegers Arch 1980; 387:115–120.

19. Rüegg JC, Paul RJ. Vascular smooth muscle. Calmodulin and cyclic AMP-dependent protein kinase alter calcium sensitivity in porcine carotid skinned fibers. Circ Res 1982; 50:394–399.

20. Sparrow MP, Pfitzer G, Gaglemann M, Rüegg JC. Effect of calmodulin, Ca^{2+}, and cAMP protein kinase on skinned tracheal smooth muscle. Am J Physiol 1984; 246: C308–C314.

21. Cassidy PS, Hoar PE, Kerrick WGL. Inhibition of Ca^{2+}-activated tension and myosin light chain phosphorylation in skinned smooth muscle strips by the phenothiazines. Pfluegers Arch 1989; 414:282–285.

22. Rüegg JC, Zeugner C, Strauss JD, et al. A calmodulin-binding peptide relaxes skinned muscle from guinea-pig taenia coli. Pfluegers Arch 1989; 414:282–285.

23. Sherry JMF, Gorecka A, Aksoy MO, Dabrowska R, Hartshorne DJ. Roles of calcium and phosphorylation in the regulation of the activity of gizzard myosin. Biochemistry 1978; 17:4411–4418.

24. Walsh MP, Bridenbaugh R, Hartshorne DJ, Kerrick WGL. Phosphorylation-dependent activated tension in skinned gizzard muscle fibers in the absence of Ca^{2+}. J Biol Chem 1982; 257:5987–5990.

25. Arner A, Hellstrand P. Effects of calcium and substrate on force-velocity relation and energy turnover in skinned smooth muscle of the guinea pig. J Physiol 1985; 360: 347–365.

26. Paul RJ, Rüegg JC. Role of magnesium in activation of smooth muscle. Am J Physiol 1988; 255 (Cell Physiol 24):C465–C472.

27. Walsh MP, Dabrowska R, Hinkins S, Hartshorne DJ. Calcium-independent myosin light chain kinase of smooth muscle. Preparation by limited chymotryptic digestion of the calcium ion dependent enzyme, purification and characterization. Biochemistry 1982; 21:1919–1925.

28. Mrwa W, Guth K, Ruegg JC, et al. Mechanical and biochemical characterization of the contraction elicited by a calcium-independent myosin light chain kinase in chemically skinned smooth muscle. Exp Basel 1985; 41:1002–1005.

29. Rüegg JC, DiSalvo J, Paul RJ. Soluble relaxation factor from vascular smooth muscle: a myosin light chain phosphatase. Biochem Biophys Res Commun 1982; 106:1126–1133.

30. Bialojan C, Rüegg JC, DiSalvo J. Phosphatase-mediated modulation of actin-myosin interaction in bovine aortic actomyosin and skinned porcine carotid artery. Proc Soc Exp Biol Med 1985; 178:36–45.

31. Bialojan C, Merkel L, Rüegg JC, Gifford D, DiSalvo J. Prolonged relaxation of

detergent-skinned smooth muscle involves decreased endogenous phosphatase activity. Soc Exp Biol Med 1985; 178:648–652.

32. Haeberle JR, Hathaway DR, De Paoli-Roach AA. Dephosphorylation of myosin by the catalytic subunit of a type-1 phosphatase produces relaxation of a chemically skinned uterine smooth muscle. J Biol Chem 1985; 260:9965–9968.

33. Kitazawa T, Kobayashi S, Horiuti KE, Somlyo A, Somlyo A. Role of the phosphatidylinositol cascade G-protein and modulation of the contractile response to Ca^{2+}. J Biol Chem 1989; 264:5339–5342.

34. Itoh T, Ikebe M, Kargacin GJ, Hartshorne DJ, Kemp BE, Fay FS. Effects of modulators of myosin light-chain kinase activity in single smooth muscle cells. Nature 1989; 338:164–167.

35. de Lanerolle P, Stull JT. Myosin phosphorylation during contraction and relaxation of tracheal smooth muscle. J Biol Chem 1980; 255:9993–10,000.

36. de Lanerolle P, Condit JR, Tanenbaum M, Adelstein RS. Myosin phosphorylation, agonist concentration and contraction of tracheal smooth muscle. Nature 1982; 298: 871–872.

37. Merkel L, Gerthoffer WG, Torphy TJ. Dissociation between myosin phosphorylation and shortening velocity in canine trachea. Am J Physiol 1990; 258:C524–C532.

38. de Lanerolle P. cAMP, myosin dephosphorylation, and isometric relaxation of airway smooth muscle. J Appl Physiol 1988; 64:705–709.

39. Gerthoffer WT. Calcium dependence of myosin phosphorylation and airway smooth muscle contraction and relaxation. Am J Physiol 1986; 250 (Cell Physiol 19):C597–C604.

40. Aksoy MO, Murphy RA, Kamm KE. Role of Ca^{2+} and myosin light chain phosphorylation in regulation of smooth muscle. Am J Physiol 1982; 242 (Cell Physiol 11): C109–C116.

41. Aksoy MO, Mras S, Kamm KE, Murphy RA. Ca^{2+}, cAMP, and changes in myosin phosphorylation during contraction of smooth muscle. Am J Physiol 1983; 245 (Cell Physiol 14):C255–C270.

42. Dillon PG, Aksoy MO, Driska SP, Murphy RA. Myosin phosphorylation and the cross-bridge cycle in arterial smooth muscle. Science 1981; 211:495–497.

43. Ledvora RF, Barany K, VanderMeulen DL, Barron JT, Barany M. Stretch-induced phosphorylation of the 20,000 dalton light chain of myosin in arterial smooth muscle. J Biol Chem 1983; 258:14080–14083.

44. Rembold CM, Murphy RA. Myoplasmic calcium, myosin phosphorylation, and regulation of the crossbridge cycle in swine arterial smooth muscle. Circ Res 1986; 58:803–815.

45. Csabina S, Barany M, Barany K. Stretch-induced myosin light chain phosphorylation in rat uterus. Arch Biochem Biophys 1986; 249:374–381.

46. Haeberle JR, Hott JW, Hathaway DR. Regulation of isometric force and isotonic shortening velocity by phosphorylation of the 20,000 dalton myosin light chain of rat uterine smooth muscle. Pfluegers Arch 1985; 403:215–219.

47. Janis RA, Barany K, Barany M, Sarmiento JG. Association between myosin light

chain phosphorylation and contraction of rat uterine smooth muscle. Mol Physiol 1981; 1:3–11.

48. Nishikori K, Weisbrodt NW, Sherwood OD, Sanborn BM. Effects of relaxin on rat uterine myosin light chain kinase activity and myosin light chain phosphorylation. J Biol Chem 1983; 258:2468–2474.

49. Butler TM, Siegman MJ, Mooers SU. Chemical energy usage during shortening and work production in mammalian smooth muscle. Am J Physiol 1983; 244 (Cell Physiol 13):C234–C242.

50. Gerthoffer WT. Regulation of the contractile element of airway smooth muscle. Physiology 1991; 261:L15–L28.

51. Rembold CM, Murphy RA. Histamine concentration and Ca^{2+} mobilization in arterial smooth muscle. J Muscle Res Cell Motil 1993; 14:325–333.

52. Morgan JP, Morgan KG. Stimulus-specific patterns of intracellular calcium levels in smooth muscle of ferret portal vein. J Physiol 1989; 256 (Cell Physiol):C96–C100.

53. Bradley AB, Morgan KG. Alterations in cytoplasmic calcium sensitivity during porcine coronary artery contractions as detected by aequorin. Physiology 1987; 385: 437–448.

54. Paul RJ. Smooth muscle: mechanochemical energy conversion, relations between metabolism and contractility. In: Johnson LR, et al., eds. Physiology of the Gastrointestinal Tract, Vol. 1, 2nd ed. New York: Raven Press, 1987:483–506.

55. Barsotti R, Ikebe M, Hartshorne DJ. Effects of Ca^{2+}, Mg^{2+} and myosin phosphorylation on skinned smooth muscle fibers. Am J Physiol 1987; 252(5 pt. 1):C543–C554.

56. Kerrick WGL, Hoar PE. Mn^{2+} activates skinned smooth muscle cells in the absence of smooth muscle myosin. J Biol Chem 1985; 260:13146–13153.

57. Szymanski PT, Strauss JD, Doerman GE, DiSalvo J, Paul RJ. Polylysine stimulates smooth muscle actomyosin ATPase activity and contraction in skinned fibers in the absence of light chain phosphorylation. Am J Physiol 1992; 262:C1446–1455.

58. Szymanski PI, Doermann GE, Ferguson DG, Paul RJ. Polylysine activates smooth muscle myosin ATPase via induction of a 10S-6S transition. Am J Physiol 1993; 265:C379–C386.

59. Lalli J, Obara K, Paul RJ. Vanadate oxidation elicits a contracture in skinned guinea pig taenia coli independent of myosin light chain (LC_{20}) phosphorylation. Biophys J 1994; 66:A410.

60. Marston S, Pritchard K, Redwood C, Taggart M. Ca^{2+}-regulation of the thin filament: biochemical mechanisms and physiological role. Biochem Soc Trans 1988; 16:494–497.

61. Ebashi S, Mikawa T, Hirata M, Toyo-Oka T, Nonomura Y. Regulatory proteins of smooth muscle. In: Casteels R, Godfraind T, Ruegg JC, eds. Excitation-Contraction Coupling in Smooth Muscle. Amsterdam: Elsevier/North-Holland, 1977:325–334.

62. Sobue K, Muramoto Y, Fujita M, Kakiuchi S. Purification of a calmodulin-binding protein from chicken gizzard that interacts with F-actin. Proc Natl Acad Sci USA 1981; 78:5652–5655.

63. Winder SJ, Walsh MP. Smooth muscle calponin. J Biol Chem 1990; 265:10148–10155.

64. Lehman W. Calponin and the composition of smooth muscle thin filaments. J Muscle Res Cell Motil 1991; 12:221–224.
65. Szymanski PJ, Tao T. Interaction between calponin and smooth muscle myosin. FEBS Lett 1993; 334(3):379–382.
66. Makuch R, Birukov K, Shirinsky V, Dabrowska R. Functional interrelationship between calponin and caldesmon. J Biochem 1991; 280(pt 1):33–38.
67. Shirinsky VP, Biryukov KG, Hettasch JM, Sellers JR. Inhibition of the relative movement of actin and myosin by caldesmon and calponin. J Biol Chem 1992; 267(22):15886–15892.
68. Okagaki T, Higashi-Fujime S, Ishikawa R, Takano-Ohmuro H, Kohama K. In vitro movement of actin filaments on gizzard smooth muscle myosin: requirement of phosphorylation of myosin light chain and effects of tropomyosin and caldesmon. J Biochem 1991; 109(6):858–866.
69. Haeberle JR, Trybus KM, Hemric ME, Warshaw DM. The effects of smooth muscle caldesmon on actin filament motility. J Biol Chem 1992; 267(32):23001–23006.
70. Haeberle JR. Calponin decreases the rate of cross-bridge cycling and increases maximum force production by smooth muscle myosin in an in vitro motility assay. J Biol Chem 1994; 269(17):12424–12431.
71. Pfitzer G, Zeugner C, Troschka M, Chalovich JM. Caldesmon and a 20-kDa actin-binding fragment of caldesmon inhibit tension development in skinned gizzard muscle fiber bundles. Proc Natl Acad Sci USA 1993; 90(13):5904–5908.
72. Pfitzer G, Fischer W, Chalovich JM. Phosphorylation-contraction coupling in smooth muscle: role of caldesmon. Adv Exp Med Biol 1993; 332:195–202.
73. Katsuyama H, Wang CL, Morgan KG. Regulation of vascular smooth muscle tone by caldesmon. J Biol Chem 1992; 267(21):14555–14558.
74. Itoh T, Suzuki S, Suzuki A, Nakamura F, Naka M, Tamaka T. Effects of exogenously applied calponin on Ca^{2+}-regulated force in skinned smooth muscle of the rabbit mesenteric artery. Eur J Physiol 1994; 427:301–308.
75. Obara K, Szymanski PJ, Tao T, Paul RJ. Calponin inhibits shortening velocity and isometric force in skinned taenia coli smooth muscle. J Biophys 1995; 68:A75.
76. Adam LP, Hathaway DR. Identification of mitogen-activated protein kinase phosphorylation sequences in mammalian h-Caldesmon. FEBS Lett 1993; 322(1):56–60.
77. DiSalvo J, Steusloff A, Semenchuk L, Satoh S, Kolquist K, Pfitzer G. Tryosine kinase inhibitors suppress agonist-induced contraction in smooth muscle. Biochem Biophys Res Commun 1993; 968–974.
78. Takeuchi K, Takahashi K, Abe M, et al. Co-localization of immunoreactive forms of calponin with actin cytoskeleton in platelets, fibroblasts and vascular smooth muscle. J Biochem 1991; 109(2):311–316.
79. North AJ, Gimona M, Cross RA, Small JV. Calponin is localized in both the contractile apparatus and the cytoskeleton of smooth muscle cells. J Cell Sci 1994; 107(3):437–444.
80. Lehman W, Denault D, Marston S. The caldesmon content of vertebrate smooth muscle. Biochim Biophys Acta 1993; 1203(1):53–59.
81. Haeberle JR, Hathaway DR, Smith CL. Caldesmon content of mammalian smooth

muscles. Comment in: J Muscle Res Cell Motil 1992:13(5):582–585. J Muscle Res Cell Motil 1992:13(1):81–89.

82. Winder SJ, Allen BG, Fraser ED, Kang HM, Kargacin GJ, Walsh MP. Calponin phosphorylation in vitro and in intact muscle. J Biochem 1993; 296(pt 3):827–836.

83. Adam LP, Milio L, Brengle B, Hathaway DR. Myosin light chain and caldesmon phosphorylation in arterial muscle stimulated with endothelin-1. J Mol Cell Cardiol 1990; 22(9):1017–1023.

84. Abe Y, Kasuya Y, Kudo M, et al. Endothelin-1-induced phosphorylation of the 20-kDa myosin light chain and caldesmon in porcine coronary artery smooth muscle. Jpn J Pharmacol 1991; 57(3):431–435.

85. Gimona M, Sparrow MP, Strasser P, Herzog M, Small JV. Calponin and SM 22 isoforms in avian and mammalian smooth muscle. Absence of phosphorylation in vivo. Eur J Biochem 1992; 205(3):1067–1075.

86. Barany M, Rokolya A, Barany K. Absence of calponin phosphorylation in contracting or resting arterial smooth muscle. FEBS Lett 1991; 279(1):65–68.

87. Barany M, Barany K. Calponin phosphorylation does not accompany contraction of various smooth muscles. Biochim Biophys Acta 1993; 1179(2):229–233.

88. Hai C-M, Murphy RA. Cross-bridge phosphorylation and regulation of latch state in smooth muscle. Am J Physiol 1988; 254:C99–106.

89. Hai C-M, Murphy RA. Regulation of shortening velocity by cross-bridge phosphorylation in smooth muscle. Am Physiol 1988; 255:C86–94.

90. Paul RJ. Smooth muscle energetics and theories of cross-bridge regulation. Am J Physiol 1990; 258:C369–375.

91. Paul RJ. The chemical energetics of vascular smooth muscle. Intermediary metabolism and its relation to contractility. In: Bohr DF, Somlyo AP, Sparks HV, eds. Handbook of Physiology, Section on Circulation II. American Physiology Society 1980:201–235.

92. Hai C-M, Murphy RA. Adenosine 5′-triphosphate consumption by smooth muscle as predicted by the coupled four-state cross-bridge model. Biophysical 1992; 61:530–541.

93. Wingard CJ, Paul RJ, Murphy RA. Dependence of ATP consumption on cross-bridge phosphorylation in swine carotid smooth muscle. J Physiol 1994; 111–117.

94. Krisanda JM, Paul RJ. Energetics of isometric contraction in porcine carotid artery. Am J Physiol 1984; 246:C510–C519.

95. Wingard CJ, Browne AK, Paul RJ, Murphy RA. The ATP cost of covalent regulation in swine carotid artery. J Biophys 1995; 68:A168.

96. Kenney RE, Hoar PE, Kerrick WG. The relationship between ATPase activity, isometric force, and myosin light-chain phosphorylation and thiophosphorylation is skinned smooth muscle fiber bundles from chicken gizzard. J Biol Chem 1990; 265 (15):8642–8649.

97. Paul RJ, Wendt IR, Walker JS, Gibbs CL. Smooth muscle energetics: testing theories of crossbridge regulation. In: Sperelakis N, Woods JD, eds. Frontiers in Smooth Muscle Research. New York: A. R. Liss, 1990:29–38.

98. Butler TM, Narayan SR, Mooers SU, Siegman MJ. Rapid turnover of myosin light

chain phosphate during cross-bridge cycling in smooth muscle. Am Physiol 1994; 267(4 pt 1):C1160–1166.

99.   Adelstein RS, Conti MA, Hathaway DR, Klee CB. Phosphorylation of smooth muscle myosin light chain kinase by the catalytic subunit of adenosine $3':5'$-monophosphate-dependent protein kinase. J Biol Chem 1978; 253:8347–8350.

100.   Conti MA, Adelstein RS. The relationship between calmodulin binding and phosphorylation of smooth muscle myosin kinase by the catalytic subunit of $3':5'$ cAMP-dependent protein kinase. J Biol Chem 1981; 256:3178–3181.

101.   Nishikawa M, de Lanerolle P, Lincoln TM, Adelstein RS. Phosphorylation of mammalian myosin light chain kinases by the catalytic subunit of cyclic AMP-dependent protein kinase and by cyclic GMP-dependent protein kinase. J Biol Chem 1984; 259:8429–8436.

102.   Hashimoto Y, Soderling TR. Phosphorylation of smooth muscle myosin light chain kinase by Ca^{2+}/calmodulin-dependent protein kinase II: comparative study of the phosphorylation sites. Arch Biochem Biophys 1990; 278:41–45.

103.   Ikebe M, Reardon S. Phosphorylation of smooth myosin light chain kinase by smooth muscle Ca^{2+}/calmodulin-dependent multifunctional protein kinase. J Biol Chem 1990; 265:8975–8978.

104.   de Lanerolle P, Nishikawa M, Yost DA, Adelstein RS. Increased phosphorylation of myosin light chain kinase after an increase in cyclic AMP in intact smooth muscle. Science 1984; 223:1415–1417.

105.   Obara K, de Lanerolle P. Isoproterenol attenuates myosin phosphorylation and contraction of tracheal muscle. J Appl Physiol 1989; 66:2017–2022.

106.   Gold WM. The role of cyclic nucleotides in airway smooth muscle. In: Nadel JA, ed. Physiology and Pharmacology of the Airways. New York: Marcel Dekker, 1980:123.

107.   Rinard GA, Jensen A, Puckett M. Hydrocortisone and isoproterenol effects on trachealis, cAMP and relaxation. J Appl Physiol 1983; 55:1609–1613.

108.   Szentivanyi A. The β-adrenergic theory of the atopic abnormality in bronchial asthma. J Allergy 1968; 42:203–232.

109.   Nishikawa M, Shirakawa S, Adelstein RS. Phosphorylation of smooth muscle myosin light chain kinase by protein kinase C. J Biol Chem 1985; 260:8978–8983.

110.   Stull JT, Hsu LC, Tansey MG, Kamm KE. Myosin light chain kinase phosphorylation in tracheal smooth muscle. J Biol Chem 1990; 265:16683–16690.

111.   Tansey MG, Luby-Phelps K, Kamm KE, Stull JT. Ca^{2+}-dependent phosphorylation of myosin light chain kinase decreases the Ca^{2+} sensitivity of light chain phosphorylation within smooth muscle cells. J Biol Chem 1994; 269:9912–9920.

112.   Bengur AR, Robinson EA, Appella E, Sellers JR. Sequence of the sites phosphorylated by protein kinase C in the smooth muscle myosin light chain. J Biol Chem 1987; 262:7613–7617.

113.   Ikebe M, Hartshorne DJ, Elzinga M. Phosphorylation of the 20,000-dalton light chain of smooth muscle myosin by the calcium-activated, phospholipid-dependent protein kinase. J Biol Chem 1987; 262:9569–9573.

114.   Nishikawa M, Hikada H, Adelstein RS. Phosphorylation of smooth muscle heavy meromyosin by calcium-activated phospholipid-dependent protein kinase. J Biol Chem 1983; 258:14069–14072.

115. Chatterjee M, Tejada M. Phorbol ester-induced contraction in chemically skinned vascular smooth muscle. Am J Physiol 1986; 251 (Cell Physiol 20):C356–C361.

116. Jiang MJ, Morgan KG. Intracellular calcium levels in phorbol ester-induced contractions of vascular muscle. Am J Physiol 1987; 253 (Heart Circ Physiol 22):H1365–H1371.

117. Singer HA, Baker KM. Calcium dependence of phorbol 12,13-dibutyrate-induced force and myosin light chain phosphorylation in arterial smooth muscle. J Pharmacol Exp Ther 1987; 243:814–821.

118. Colburn JC, Michnoff CH, Hsu LC, Slaughter CA, Kamm KE, Stull JT. Sites phosphorylated in myosin light chain in contracting smooth muscle. J Biol Chem 1988; 263:19166–19173.

119. Kamm KE, Hsu LC, Kubota Y, Stull JT. Phosphorylation of smooth muscle myosin heavy and light chains. J Biol Chem 1989; 264:21223–21229.

120. Singer HA, Oren JW, Benscoter HA. Myosin light chain phosphorylation in ^{32}P-labeled rabbit aorta stimulated by phorbol 12,13-dibutyrate and phenylephrine. J Biol Chem 1989; 264:21215–21222.

121. Sutton TA, Haeberle JR. Phosphorylation by protein kinase C of the 20,000-dalton light chain of myosin in intact and chemically skinned vascular smooth muscle. J Biol Chem 1990; 265:2749–2754.

122. de Lanerolle P, Paul RJ. Myosin phosphorylation/dephosphorylation and the regulation of airway smooth muscle contractility. Am J Physiol 1991; 261 (Lung Cell Mol Physiol 5):L1–L14.

123. Cai S, Nowak G, de Lanerolle P. Myosin dephosphorylation as mechanism of relaxation of airway smooth muscle, In: Raeburn D, Giembycz, MA, eds. Airway Smooth Muscle: Biochemical Control of Contraction and Relaxation. Basel: Birkhauser Verlag, 1994:223–251.

124. Kitazawa T, Kobayashi S, Horiuti K, Somlyo AV, Somlyo AP. Receptor-coupled, permeabilized smooth muscle. J Biol Chem 1989; 264:5339–5342.

125. Kitazawa T, Masuo M, Somlyo AP. G protein-mediated inhibition of myosin light-chain phosphatase in vascular smooth muscle. PNAS 1991; 88(20):9307–9310.

126. Kawase T, Van Breemen C. Aluminum fluoride induces a reversible Ca^{2+} sensitization in α-toxin permeabilized vascular smooth muscle. Eur Pharm 1992; 214:39–44.

127. Gong MC, Fugslang M, Alessi D, et al. Arachidonic acid inhibits myosin light chain phosphatase and sensitizes smooth muscle to calcium. Biol Chem 1992; 21492–21498.

128. Collins EM, Walsh MP, Morgan KG. Contraction of singular vascular smooth muscle cells by phenylephrine at constant $[Ca^{2+}]$. Am Physiol 1992; 262:H754–H762.

129. Winder SJ, Walsh MP. Calponin: thin filament-linked regulation of smooth muscle contraction. Cell Signaling 1993; 5:677–686.

130. Vorotnikok AV, Gusev NB, Hua S, Collins JH, Redwood CS, Marston SB. Phosphorylation of aorta caldesmon by endogenous proteolytic fragments of kinase C. J Muscle Res Cell Motil 1995; 15:37–48.

131. Khalil RA, Morgan KG. PKC-mediated redistribution of mitogen-activated protein kinase during smooth muscle cell activation. Am Physiol 1993; 265:C406–C411.

6

Macrophages and Antigen Presentation

WILLIAM J. CALHOUN

University of Pittsburgh
Pittsburgh, Pennsylvania

I. Introduction

Macrophages are found in virtually every organ and tissue. In the lung, alveolar macrophages (AM), interstitial macrophages, and intravascular macrophages have been described. These cells subserve a variety of critical functions, including nonspecific host defense, immunologic induction to novel antigens and activation to recall antigens, and regulation of immune-inflammatory responses (reviewed in Ref. 1). An ever-expanding literature suggests that these cells may also contribute to the development and resolution of inflammation asthma. Moreover, by virtue of their ability to present antigen, macrophages are a principal pathway by which lymphocytes are alerted to foreign antigen (both novel and recall), and therefore are also poised to regulate this aspect of the immune response. This chapter reviews the relationships among macrophages, asthma, and antigen presentation in the regulation of immune-inflammatory responses within the context of critical pathways that may be genetically altered in the disease.

II. Overview of Macrophages

A. Origin and Fate

Alveolar macrophages are derived from bone marrow progenitor cells which traverse the circulation as blood monocytes, migrate to the pulmonary interstitium where they are recognized as interstitial macrophages [2], and cross the alveolar–capillary membrane to reside in the airspace. Studies of the effects of bone marrow transplantation on AM in both animals and humans have confirmed that the majority of these cells in the airspace in the resting state are recently (<100 days) derived from marrow cells (express donor genotype). However, human AM can and do proliferate [3], and this mechanism may contribute to maintaining the resident population of AM, particularly in inflamed lung. The degree to which this mechanism may contribute to macrophagic inflammation in asthma is unknown. These cells may migrate to regional lymph nodes, undergo apoptosis and phagocytosis in situ, or migrate to the mucociliary escalator to be carried to the pharynx (reviewed in Ref 4).

B. Phenotypic and Functional Characteristics of Lung Macrophages

Expression of Surface Antigens

AM express a variety of surface proteins which mediate immune-inflammatory functions. These include receptors for immunoglobins IgG (FcγR1/CD64, FcγR2/CD32, FcγR3/CD16), IgA, and IgE (FcϵR2/CD23), complement (CR1/CD35, CR3/CD11b-CD18), lipopolysaccharide/LPS-binding protein (CD14), transferrin (CD71), glucocorticoids, histamine, leukotrienes, lectins, and cytokines [5–8]. In addition, these cells express adhesion molecules (LFA-1/CD11a-CD18, ICAM-1/CD54) and proteins of major histocompatibility (MHC) class I and II necessary for cell–cell interactions and the process of antigen presentation. Many of these surface molecules are expressed constitutively, and are upregulated by activation. When activated, macrophages may also express receptor for IL-2 (Tac antigen/CD25) and show heightened expression of low-affinity IgE receptor (CD23).

Phagocytosis and Antigen Presentation

A principal function of AM is engulfment and clearance of senescent cells, foreign proteins, and invading microorganisms. In the latter two cases, AM can initiate an immune response by the process of antigen presentation (vide infra). Although AM can ingest particles not coated with immunoglobulin or complement, such opsonins markedly increase the efficiency of uptake (reviewed in Ref 1). The uptake of nonopsonized bacteria may be mediated by the CD18-chain surface molecules (CD11a-CD18/LFA-1, CD11b-CD18/CR3, and CD11c-CD18/p150,

95) as well as the LPS/LPS-binding protein receptor CD14 (reviewed in Ref. 9). Following ingestion, protein components may be partially degraded to oligopeptides, and expressed on the surface in the context of MHC class I or II antigens. These complexes can interact with the T-cell receptor (TCR) on T lymphocytes expressing CD8 or CD4 antigens, respectively, to initiate an immunologic response. This aspect of macrophage physiology is explored in more detail in a subsequent section. The role that T lymphocytes, particularly helper (CD4+) cells, play in asthma has received intense scrutiny over the past decade. In that T lymphocytes can respond only to antigen presented in the context of MHC class II antigens, and that AM are probably the principal APC in the lower respiratory tract, the potential for the coordination and regulation of inflammation in asthma by macrophages should not be overlooked.

Secretory Products of Alveolar Macrophages

Upon activation, alveolar macrophages secrete a broad panoply of products into either endosomic/lysosomic vacuoles or the extracellular space (Table 1). These can be broadly summarized as oxidants, antioxidants, lipid mediators, proteases and enzymes, antiproteases, and cytokines and growth factors. There is evidence that the specific effector response of the AM differs depending on both the nature

Table 1   Secretory Products of Macrophages[a]

Oxidants	*Antioxidants and antiproteases*
Superoxide anion	Glutathione
Hydrogen peroxide	α_1-Antitrypsin
Hydroxyl radical	α_2-Macroglobulin
Reactive nitrogen species [12, 125]	Tissue inhibitor of metalloproteinase
Lipid mediators	*Proteases and enzymes*
Prostaglandins/thromboxanes	Lysozyme
Leukotrienes	β-Glucuronidase
Platelet-activating factor	Acid hydrolases
Cytokines and growth factors	Angiotensin-converting enzyme
IL-1α, IL-1β, IL-1 receptor antagonist	Collagenase
IL-6	Elastase
Interferon-α, -β, -γ	Plasminogen activator
Macrophage inflammatory proteins 1 and 2 [126]	
TNF-α	
IL-8	
TGF-α, TGF-β	
Platelet-derived growth factor	

[a]Adapted with permission from Ref. 10.

of the stimulus and on the specific pathways of intracellular signal transduction [10]. Recent investigations have shown that macrophages transcribe and translate the inducible form of nitric oxide synthase, that induction by interferon-γ (IFN-γ) and lipopolysaccharide (LPS) is regulated by upstream (5′) sequences (consisting of cooperative binding sites for NF-κB, NF-IL6, and IFN-related promoters), and that the resulting production of nitric oxide is inhibitable by chemical inhibitors of nitric oxide synthase [11,12]. Moreover, in addition to its host defense functions and effects on vascular tone, nitric oxide may have autocrine effects on monocyte mobility [13]. An intriguing, expanding, yet mechanistically incomplete literature suggests that nitric oxide could be involved in the pathogenesis of asthma, particularly with respect to vasodilation and capillary leak [14,15].

C. Macrophage Heterogeneity

Existing data confirm that AM are heterogeneous, and that subpopulations of both tissue and AM have distinct functional, mediator, and inflammogen profiles. AM can be fractionated by buoyant density, and functional characteristics of these subpopulations can then be defined. Higher-density cells appear to have enhanced chemotactic motility [16], cytokine release [17], superoxide production [18], and exhibit other functional differences [19]. In contrast, lower-density cells secrete plasminogen activator and inhibit the release of superoxide anion by unfractionated macrophages [19,20]. Therefore, higher-density cells appear to have greater potential for promoting inflammation. Another useful distinction is that FcR (immunoglobulin receptor)-positive cells more prominently secrete prostaglandin E_2 (PGE_2) and tumor necrosis factor-α (TNF-α), and participate in nonspecific responses, whereas FcR-negative cells present antigen more efficiently and participate in initiating antigen-specific immune responses [1]. However, the evaluation of subpopulations of AM in asthma remains in its infancy. The accumulated body of knowledge about macrophage subpopulations in asthma is relatively small, and information regarding this topic is incorporated into the corresponding functional sections.

III. Macrophages in Asthma

Alveolar macrophages are the most prevalent cells in the airways of normal subjects, symptomatic, or asymptomatic asthmatics. Although eosinophils are clearly quite characteristic of asthma, and their presence and activation status correlate with its severity [21–23], the critical processes which control eosinophil influx and activation are not known. It has been proposed that AM subserve this regulatory role in asthma [24,25]. This section reviews the extensive literature that has developed over the last decade, which collectively supports the concept that macrophages, particularly alveolar macrophages, are important participants in the generation, maintenance, and resolution of airway inflammation in asthma and allergic diseases (reviewed in Refs. 24, 26, and 27). Collectively, the existing literature suggests that macrophages may play a pivotal role in asthma and allergic disease by directing the recruitment and activation of inflammatory cells, by generating factors which directly promote bronchospasm and tissue injury, and by production and release of cytokines which modulate and control the airway inflammatory response.

A. Rational for Investigating Alveolar Macrophages in Asthma

The evidence that alveolar macrophages contribute to airway inflammation in asthma can be grouped in four broad areas. First, AMs are the most numerous cell of both the conducting airways and the distal airspace in health, in quiescent asthma, and in clinically active asthma. Following antigen challenge of allergic volunteers, the numerical increase in AM exceeds that of eosinophils, neutrophils, or other cells. Although these data do not prove a link between AM and asthmatic inflammation, additional data suggest that specific recruitment of AM to the airway occurs during the development of allergic inflammation, which could argue for a pathogenic role. Hence, AM are in the correct anatomic compartment to influence the physiology of the airway. Second, AM bear low-affinity surface receptors for IgE (FcεRII, CD23) and can be activated for proinflammatory functions by binding of antigen to IgE linked to those receptors. In this way, the development of antigen-specific IgE responses which predispose to mast cell degranulation upon antigen exposure also may provide a pathway by which AM are activated. Third is the capability of AM to produce a broad range of mediators, cytokines, and inflammogens which are plausibly or experimentally linked to asthma and allergic responses. Lastly, AM from asthmatics and other allergic subjects are functionally and phenotypically distinct from normal macrophages, and from AM in other pulmonary diseases.

B. Aspects of AM Physiology and Function Relevant to Asthma

Prevalence of AM in the Airspace

Alveolar macrophages are the most prevalent cell in the human airspace, both in normal subjects [28], and in asthmatics [29,30]. In addition to their principal location in the alveoli and distal airspaces, they are also quite numerous in the *conducting* airway [31]. These conducting-airway macrophages may comprise as much as 25% of all airspace macrophages. Thus, the number and state of functional activation of these cells would be expected to play a major role in the regulation of inflammation in the airway, and thereby to influence airway physiology. Macrophages are both resident in and recruited to the airspace in asthma. Following antigen challenge, the increase in AM numerically exceeds that of eosinophils, neutrophils, or lymphocytes [30,32–34]. This observation holds even following segmental airway antigen challenge and the attendant intense eosinophilic inflammation [18,32,33,35]; cf. Ref. 30. In fact, with the exception of studies using the intense stimulus of segmental antigen bronchoprovocation by ourselves and others, AM outnumber other airspace cells by a ratio of 4:1 or more [18]. Although macrophages logically must be present in the airspace in order to influence it, the mere presence of these cells do not necessarily implicate them in the pathogenesis of disease. Additional data link AM phenotypes and functions to the development of airway inflammation.

Antigen Activation of AM by IgE-Dependent Mechanisms

Alveolar macrophages and mononuclear cells express low-affinity receptors for IgE (FcεRII, CD23) [36]. The proportion of monocytes and macrophages expressing CD23 is increased in allergic patients (up to 80%) compared to normals (8–20%), and is further enhanced following airway antigen challenge [37–39]. Of interest, CD23 expression is also heightened in hypersensitivity pneumonitis (66% [40]), suggesting that enhanced CD23 expression by monocytic cells might be a marker for macrophage activation, or pathogenically linked to immunologically mediated pulmonary diseases. The expression of CD23 by defined subpopulations of AM in asthma has not, however, been critically investigated. Via these receptors, AM are activated by antigen to release eicosanoids [41–45], to transcribe and secrete cytokines (IL-1β and TNF-α) [39], to produce superoxide anion (SO), to release lysosomal enzymes [44,46], and to augment cytotoxicity [47]. Although many in-vitro studies have been conducted using IgE–anti-IgE complexes, AM bearing IgE can also be activated specifically and directly by antigens to which the host is allergic (i.e., IgE confers antigenic specificity) [48], suggesting that the in-vitro observations have relevance in vivo. Collectively, the observation of CD23 expression by monocytic cells (augmented in atopic states), the presence of increased circulating IgE levels in this situation, and the demonstration of AM activation by specific antigen in an IgE-CD23-dependent manner all strongly suggest that this pathway is important in regulation of airway inflammation in atopic asthma. Whether or not IgE differentially activates subpopulations of AM in asthma has not been critically evaluated. The degree to which IgE-dependent activation of AM participates in nonallergic asthma, exercise/hyperpnea-induced bronchospasm, or bronchial obstruction related to irritants or viruses also remains an open question. However, existing data suggest that AM activation does not occur in exercise asthma [49].

Mediator, Inflammogen, and Cytoregulatory Factor Release by Activated AM

Upon activation, alveolar macrophages and mononuclear cells release a plethora of compounds which have been implicated in or linked to asthma. A representative but not exhaustive list is found in Table 2. These factors can be broadly grouped as (1) chemotactic factors, (2) cytokines and other cell-activating factors, (3) target tissue (smooth muscle and mucous gland) activators, and (4) direct inflammogens. Obviously, a number of these factors have multiple activities, so the grouping is not exclusive. In this section, the data which directly link release of these factors by macrophage/monocytes to regulation of airway inflammation and asthma is reviewed.

Chemotactic Factors

No chemotactic factors which specifically and selectively recruit only eosinophils have yet been identified. However, there is little question that chemotactic factors do direct the migration of granulocytes and other inflammatory cells, which may be modulated by selective expression of addressins, selectins, integrin adhesion molecules, or other factors. Thus, chemotactic factor release by AM and other cells is likely important in the regulation of airway inflammation. Following activation, macrophages and monocytes release physiologically important amounts of leukotriene B_4 (LTB_4) [43,50], complement fragments [51,52], interleukin-8 (IL-8) [53], and a neutrophil chemotactin distinct from IL-8 [54], all of which can serve to recruit granulocytes. Leukotriene B_4 is a potent neutrophil and

Table 2 Mononuclear Phagocyte Products with a Putative Role in Asthma Syndromes[a]

Eicosanoids	
Leukotrienes B_4, C_4, D_4	
5-Hydroxyeicosatetraenoic acid	
PGE_2, $F_{2\alpha}$, D_2	
Thromboxanes	
Platelet-activating factor	Macrophage-derived mucus secretagogue
Cytokines	
IL-1, TNF-α	
Eosinophil-activating factors (GM-CSF [79])	
Endothelins [93]	Histamine-releasing factors
Superoxide anion	
β-Glucuronidase	Neutral proteases

[a]Adapted with permission and modifications from Ref. 26.

eosinophil chemotactin [55], and thereby could contribute to the intense neu-trophilic influx which occurs early after antigen challenge [32], as well as the later eosinophilic response [30,35]. In addition, activated AM produce platelet-activating factor (PAF), a chemotactin which may have some selectivity for eosinophils [55]. Recently, Corrigan et al. have demonstrated another protein neutrophil chemotactic factor in supernatants from monocytes obtained from patients with acute severe asthma [54]. Collectively, these data suggest that monocyte/macrophages are likely active participants in recruiting inflammatory cells to the airway in asthma.

Cell Activating Factors

As noted above, mononuclear cells transcribe and secrete the phlogistic cytokines IL-1β and TNF-α following stimulation of the low-affinity receptor for IgE (FcϵR2; CD23) by IgE immune complexes [39]; these factors are also released upon stimulation with environmental and occupational antigens [56,57]. Mono-cytes and macrophages also produce TNF-α, IL-6, GM-CSF, and other soluble factors which potentiate inflammatory responses [58–60]. Finally, human mono-cytes release IL-10 (cytokine synthesis-inhibiting factor), which may serve down-regulating functions, at least in part by autocrine suppression of TNF-α release [61,62]. A selected overview of this area will be reviewed. More complete dis-cussions have recently been published [58,63]. However, with respect to asthma, very little is known about the cytokine profiles of subpopulations of AM and their relationships to potentiation and resolution of asthmatic airway inflammation.

Interleukin-1 (IL-1), a pluripotent cytokine, plays a central role in control of inflammatory responses [64]. In the environment of the airway, AM are probably the most important source of IL-1. Interleukin-1 activates lymphocytes, induces mucus secretion [65], primes mast cells for enhanced mediator release, and may act directly as a histamine-releasing factor [66]. Spontaneous release of IL-1 by AM is about 10-fold greater in cells obtained from asthmatics compared to normal subjects, but lipopolysaccharide (LPS)-stimulated release is comparable. These data suggest that AM in asthma are activated in situ for release of IL-1. Of considerable interest, no differences between IL-1 release from allergic versus nonallergic asthmatic AM could be detected, suggesting that activation of AM for IL-1 secretion in asthma may be independent of allergic status [67]. This finding is consistent with the observation that bronchoalveolar lavage (BAL) fluids of nonallergic asthmatics have increased levels of IL-1β [60,68,69]. In patients with symptomatic asthma, BAL fluid concentrations of IL-1β are significantly greater than those of either normal subjects [68], or asymptomatic asthmatics [60]. Borish and colleagues have also investigated the concentration of IL-1β in BAL fluids, and its production by purified AM [69]. Nocturnal samples (4 a.m.) of BAL fluids from asthmatics contained significantly greater concentrations of IL-1β than normal controls. In addition, IL-1β mRNA transcripts were identified (exclusively in AM by in-situ hybridization) in purified AM populations, and mRNA expression could be blocked by oral prednisone (50 mg) given 11 h prior to BAL [69]. Production of an IL-1 inhibitor by AM and monocytes from asthmatics (distinct from prostaglandin E_2) has also been demonstrated [70]. This factor is released in response to either anti-IgE or specific antigen. Thus, AM in asthma secrete both IL-1 and its inhibitors. Increased IL-1 secretion, diminished inhibitor release, enhanced intracellular or extracellular processing, decreased expression of "decoy" receptors for IL-1, or some combination thereof might be expected to favor inflammation. Conversely, alterations of these factors in the opposite directions could lead to reduced inflammation. Understanding the balance and control of these processes should lead to greater insights into the regulation of inflammation in asthma.

Elias et al. have shown that human AM of high buoyant density have enhanced release of IL-1, suggesting that a shift toward high-density cells would favor IL-1-mediated inflammation [17]. Clearly, density increases do occur in allergic subjects following antigen challenge, but the suggestion that high-density AM produce more IL-1 in this specific setting has not been evaluated in human asthma. It is plausible to hypothesize that alterations of AM subpopulations represent a pathogenic mechanism of disordered regulation of inflammation in asthma, but that suggestion has not yet been critically tested.

Tumor necrosis factor-α (TNF-α) is principally a product of activation macrophages and monocytes [71], and promotes the secretion of IL-1, IL-6, and GM-CSF by mononuclear cells [72]. Moreover, it primes eosinophils for leukotriene release and potentiates expression of ICAM-1 on epithelial cells and thereby could plausibly potentiate eosinophil recruitment and activation in asthma (reviewed in Ref. 58). The recruitment of neutrophils in IgE-dependent allergic late-phase reactions has also been shown to be at least partially a consequence of TNF-α release [73]. TNF-α concentrations in BAL fluids are higher in symptomatic compared to asymptomatic asthmatics [60], and in allergic subjects compared to controls [74]. Recent data suggest that TNF-α may be necessary for a late-phase airway response to antigen. Gosset and colleagues performed BAL in allergic asthmatics 18 h following antigen challenge and found significantly increased AM production of TNF-α in those asthmatics with a late-phase response. Moreover, there was no overlap in TNF-α production between those with late-phase responses and those without: AM production of TNF-α in each of 5 subjects with a late response exceeded that of any of those subjects with only an immediate response. These data suggest that TNF-α could be a determinant of late inflammatory responses. TNF-α may also play a role in exacerbations of asthma related to viral infections. Infection of monocytes by respiratory syncytial virus in vitro leads to potentiated secretion of TNF-α [75], and concentrations are increased in BAL fluids following antigen challenge in relationship to experimental rhinovirus 16 infection in humans [76]. Taken in aggregate, current data support the concept that TNF-α is an important regulator of airway inflammatory responses, and may be centrally involved in asthma.

Granulocyte-macrophage colony-stimulation factor (GM-CSF) has eosinophil-activating and survival-enhancing properties, and is also a histamine-releasing factor for basophils [77]. Peripheral blood concentrations of GM-CSF in patients with acute asthma are significantly higher than normal, and all toward normal following corticosteroid therapy [78]. Alveolar macrophages from asthmatic but not normal subjects spontaneously release GM-CSF, which potentiates LTC_4 production by eosinophils [79]. These observations suggest that AM in asthma are activated to secrete GM-CSF in asthmatics, and therefore are poised to upregulate airway inflammation by eosinophils.

Notably, however, GM-CSF also has striking effects on monocytic cells which may be of more direct relevance to asthma and allergic disease. In macrophages grown in the presence of GM-CSF, expression of receptors for the downregulating cytokine TGF-β is markedly diminished compared to those exposed to CSF-1 [80], which would likely render the macrophages resistant to the "anti-inflammatory" effects of TGF-β. (TGF-β, and IL-4, synergize with IL-10 to downregulate macrophage function [81].) Moreover, GM-CSF-exposed macrophages are insensitive to PGE_2 with respect to suppression of TNF-α and nitric oxide release [82]. Thus, an effect of GM-CSF (prominently expressed during allergic reactions) on macrophages may be to permit them to remain immunologically and functionally activated, and thus possibly to contribute to the persistent inflammation which characterizes asthma.

Histamine-releasing factors (HRFs) are a diverse group of cytokines produced by a wide variety of cells (reviewed by Ref. 83). They serve to induce or augment the release of histamine from basophils and mast cells. Monocytes and macrophages are important sources of HRF [84]. The putative role of these factors in asthma has been recently reviewed [85]. Although the mechanisms by which HRF potentiate histamine release are not totally clear, several observations of mononuclear cell-derived HRF shed some light on this question. First, most investigators find that the effect of HRF is dependent on the presence of basophil-bound IgE; stripping IgE from the cells by brief treatment with lactic acid generally abrogates the potentiating effect of HRF on histamine release. Second, treatment of these "stripped" basophils with IgE-containing serum, generally obtained from asthmatics, restores HRF-induced histamine release [86–88]. Lastly, one group has suggested that a specific subtype of IgE ("IgE⁺") is responsible for mediating the effects of HRF [86]. Other investigators have not, however, observed this distinction [87].

Chonmaitree and colleagues have recently demonstrated that monocytes infected in vitro with either respiratory syncytial virus or influenza A produced increased histamine-releasing factor, and suggested that this mechanism might play a significant role in the exacerbation of asthma related to viral respiratory tract infections [89]. At least one type of HRF is produced spontaneously by mononuclear cells from asthmatics, and production is further augmented following in-vitro antigen challenge. Although the specific pathogenic roles of these factors has not been entirely defined, it is clear that both partially characterized species unrelated to known cytokines [90], and better-known cytokines released by AM (e.g., IL-1, GM-CSF) can both provoke and augment histamine release from sensitive basophils and mast cells via IgE-dependent mechanisms.

Smooth Muscle and Mucus Gland Activators

Leukotriene C_4 (LTC_4), a product of eosinophils, mast cells, and macrophages, is a potent smooth muscle constrictor. AM release LTC_4 in response to antigen in a time-, does-, and IgE-dependent manner [41,42]. Human monocytic cells also appear to release this mediator in response to IgE immune complexes [91]. Further, following local antigen challenge, prostaglandin D_2 (PGD_2, a bronchial smooth muscle spasmogen) is found at high concentration in the airway [92]. Although it is a mast cell product, PGD_2 can also be synthesized by AM [45]. In addition, human macrophages transcribe and secrete endothelins 1 and 3, which strongly regulate smooth muscle tone. Moreover, levels of endothelin 1 are sharply upregulated by either lipopolysaccharide or phorbol myristate acetate, suggesting that inflammogenic stimuli might promote the production of endothelin 1 in vivo [93].

AM also release products which potentiate mucus secretion, at least in vitro. Leukotriene B_4 (LTB_4) and a small-molecular-weight product of AM and monocytes are two of these meditors [94]. In addition, IL-1 (particularly IL-1β) has been shown to promote dose-dependent secretion of mucous glycoproteins [65]. Thus, AM not only can regulate the recruitment and activation of inflammatory cells, it also may contribute more directly to physiologic abnormalities by induction of mucus hypersecretion and alteration in smooth muscle tone.

Direct Inflammogens

AM release β-glucuronidase, neutral proteases, and other lysosomal enzymes following cross-linking of the IgE receptor [44,95]. These agents could plausibly amplify the inflammatory response, but their contribution to asthma has not yet been established. Superoxide (SO) anion, in contrast, bears a direct and convincing relationship to airway inflammation and physiology in asthma. One stimulus for the release of SO by human AM is cross-linking the IgE receptor [95]. Superoxide anion is an inflammogen, a bronchoconstrictor, and a cause of bronchial hyperresponsiveness, at least in cats and guinea pigs [96,97]. Several laboratories have demonstrated a relationship between SO release and human asthma. Spontaneous release of SO by BAL cells and purified AM is increased in asthmatics [30,98] and is further augmented following antigen challenge [18,30]. Further, in that high-density AM subpopulations exhibit increased release of SO (vide infra), the regulation of these subpopulations of AM is clearly an important factor to explore to understand SO-driven (and perhaps other inflammogen-related) airway inflammation in asthma.

Phenotypic and Functional Differences

AM from asthmatics are phenotypically and functionally distinct from normal. They spontaneously secrete IL-1 [67,69] and the eosinophil activator GM-CSF [79], and express mRNA for this cytokine [99]. Spontaneous release of reactive oxygen species by AM is increased in asthmatics and allergic subjects [30,98], and is further augmented following antigen challenge [30]. The buoyant density of AM from asymptomatic asthmatics is considerably less than that of healthy subjects [29], but may increase after antigen challenge [18]. Although the implications of altered density profiles of AM in asthma are not entirely clear, subpopulations of AM subserve different immune-effector functions in other inflammatory pulmonary diseases [19,100] and may do so in asthma. In animals, low-density AM serve to inhibit SO release by other macrophages [20]. If application to human asthma, this observation suggests that an increase in AM density would augment SO-driven inflammation in two ways: (1) by increasing the proportion of high-density cells which have enhanced SO release (vide infra), and (2) by reducing the suppressive effects of low-density AM.

Summary

Collectively, these data demonstrate that AM can be activated in asthma by IgE-dependent mechanisms to produce inflammogens, cytokines, and eicosanoids which promote and maintain airway inflammation. Their quantitative contribution to the inflammatory burden of the airway, their role in initiating or provoking the response (particularly in nonallergic asthma), the distribution of these factors among AM subpopulations, and the nature of putative interactions with structural and infiltrating cells are fruitful areas for future investigation.

IV. Macrophages and Antigen Presentation

A. General Concepts

Major Histocompatibility Complex (MHC) Restriction of Antigen Presentation

Recognition and elimination of foreign antigens are essential for host defense, and require the cooperation of macrophages, T and B lymphocytes, and granulocytes. As noted above, following IgE or nonspecific activation, AM can secrete factors which recruit and activate granulocytes. The immunospecificity of the response, however, relies on antigen recognition by T lymphocytes, which in turn is dependent on presentation of an antigenic determinant in the context of MHC antigens on the surface of an antigen-presenting cell (APC) such as a macrophage. This important concept, that T cells can only respond to antigen expressed in association with MHC proteins, underscores the critical role of AM in initiating and regulating immune-inflammatory responses in the lung, as AM are the most numerous APC in the airspace. Other cells known to subserve APC function include B lymphocytes and dendritic cells [101,102].

T-lymphocytes expressing the CD8 surface marker ($T_{s/c}$) recognize antigens presented with MHC class I molecules (human HLA-A, B, and C determinants). Conversely, CD4$^+$ T cells (T_H) recognize antigens in association with MHC molecules of class II (human HLA-DP, -DQ, and -DR determinants). Mature, circulating T lymphocytes express either CD4 or CD8 in essentially a mutually exclusive manner. Thus, T lymphocytes will respond in a dichotomous manner to antigen presented in the context of either class I or class II proteins. These molecular concepts underlie the long-observed MHC-restricted nature of antigen presentation [102,103].

Peptide Recognition by T-Cell Receptors

It is important to contrast antigen recognition by T lymphocytes via T-cell receptors (TCR) and that of immunoglobulins. The TCR recognize peptide fragments of 6–20 amino acid residues, and recognition appears to be principally of primary structure (amino acid sequence) [104]. These fragments may retain no conformational similarity to the native protein, and conceivably may be derived from an interior sequence not accessible from extramolecular sites, and therefore not available for antibody binding. The inability of T cells to distinguish native and denatured protein has long been recognized, and is a consequence of this extensive protein processing (reviewed in Ref. 105). In contrast, antibodies recognize foreign epitopes by their three-dimensional structure (primary, secondary, tertiary, and quaternary structures may all contribute to antigenic determinants).

The Major Histocompatibility Complex

The MHC in humans comprises some 4000 kilobases located on the short arm of chromosome 6. The MHC in humans is extremely polymorphic at both class I and class II loci. These polymorphisms underlie both the selectivity of peptide fragment binding to MHC proteins via polymorphism in the antigen-binding cleft (thereby dictating to which antigen-derived peptides a response can be mounted), and the specificity of association with the complementary TCR via polymorphism near the surface of the class I or II molecule which interacts with the TCR [106]. The MHC region encodes the three families of class I antigens (HLA-A, -B, and

-C), three families of class II antigens (-DR, -DP, and -DQ), the transporter associated with antigen processing (TAP) protein subunits 1 and 2 (which are also polymorphic), TNF-α and -β, and other immune-response genes [102,107].

Pathways for Antigen Processing and Presentation

Two major pathways for antigen processing have been described: endogenous and exogenous [102,103,108]. In general, exogenous proteins are ingested, denatured, unfolded, and subtotally digested in acidic endosomic vesicles to peptides of 15–20 residues, and subsequently expressed on the cell membrane in association with class II MHC molecules. Macrophages are thought to use this pathway predominantly. Endogenous proteins (self-antigens, viral proteins) synthesized in the rough endoplasmic reticulum or on free ribosomes are partially degraded and translocated by TAP transporter(s) to the Golgi, where the fragments associate with class I MHC molecules. This complex is then expressed on the cell surface (Fig. 1). However, exceptions to this general principle are described ([108]; reviewed in [109]). Thus, the process of antigen presentation is critically dependent on the temporal and spatial coordination of antigen ingestion or synthesis, subtotal proteolysis, specificity and activity of the TAP system, synthesis of MHC glycoproteins, associated of the peptide fragment and MHC molecules, and translocation of the assembly to the cell surface.

Class I MHC-Associated Antigen Presentation

Class I proteins are expressed on the surface of all nucleated cells. In functional configurations, they are composed of a heavy chain, β_2-microglobulin, and a bound (presented) peptide of 8–11 amino acid residues in length. Longer peptides may be bound to class I protein intracellularly, but those bound to class I molecules presented on the surface are overwhelmingly of lengths 8–11 residues [102]. Two α helices form a peptide-binding cleft in which six pockets (A–F) have been identified [110]. High-affinity binding of the peptide is facilitated by interaction of the amino terminus with the A pocket, the carboxyl terminus with the F pocket, and by hydrogen bonds between the heavy chain and the peptide bond groups of the bound peptide (reviewed in Ref. 102). Peptide binding affinity is highly dependent on length, with 8–11 residues typically associated with high-affinity binding. Beyond optimal length, binding may be dramatically reduced by addition of one or two residues. Moreover, different class I alleles differentially bind certain residues located at specific positions within the peptide (reviewed in Ref 106).

Class I heavy chains are associated with β_2-microglobulin in the endoplasmic reticulum (EF) [111]. Cytosolic proteins (including those of viral origin) are thought to be transported to the Golgi/ER by the heterodimeric protein TAP embedded in the membrane of the ER [112,113]. TAP expression and function is necessary for efficient processing of peptides destined for class I expression.

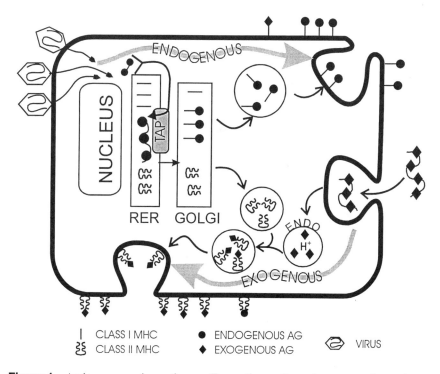

Figure 1 Antigen-processing pathways. Two pathways for antigen processing and presentation are depicted. In the endogenous pathway, cytosolic proteins (self-antigens, viral proteins, etc.) are partially degraded to peptides of 8–11 amino acids length, and are transported to the endoplasmic reticulum by TAP proteins, where association with MHC antigens of class I occurs. These complexes are then translocated to the cell surface, where they may interact with T lymphocytes expressing CD8 (suppressor/cytotoxic T cells). The exogenous pathway processes extracellular, usually foreign, protein. These molecules are ingested, and the phagosomic vesicle fuses with an acidic endosome. Acidic proteases subtotally digest the protein into peptides of 15–20 residues. MHC class II proteins are transported through the cytoplasm in transport vesicles which fuse with the acidic endosomes. Subsequently, association of the peptide and MHC class II protein occurs, and the complex is expressed on the cell surface. These complexes then interact with T cells expressing CD4 (helper/inflammatory) T cells.

Most endogenous protein is expressed with class I molecules, and most exogenous with class II proteins. A small fraction of endogenous peptide may associate with class II molecules, and some exogenous peptide may be expressed in association with class I MHC proteins.

Abbreviations: RER, rough endoplasmic reticulum; GOLGI, Golgi apparatus; TAP, transporter associated with antigen processing.

Adapted from Ref. 109 with permission.

Moreover, TAP is polymorphic, and different alleles exhibit specificity for residues of the carboxyl terminus of transported peptides. In this regard, Heemels and colleagues have recently shown that peptides with a hydrophobic carboxyterminal residue were transported by either cim[a] and cim[b] alleles, but peptides with histidine, lysine, or arginine were transported solely by cim[a] [107]. This observation outlines yet another layer of restriction of immune responses utilizing class I antigens: Only those peptide fragments transportable by the specific TAP allele can be associated intracellularly with MHC class I molecules.

Intracellular assembly, however, is not essential for surface expression of functional class I MHC molecules, as the heavy chain–β_2-microglobulin complex can associate with synthetic peptides added to the extracellular space [114]. Extending this concept, Kozlowski and colleagues recently demonstrated that processing of protein destined for association with class I molecules occurs in serum via at least two pathways: (1) the carboxydipeptidase angiotensin converting enzyme [ACE], and (2) a serum protease not inhibitable by captopril (a selective ACE inhibitor) [108]. These data suggest that the processing and presentation of peptide fragments for association with class I molecules is considerably more complex than is depicted in Fig. 1.

Class II MHC-Associated Antigen Presentation

Expression of class II MHC molecules is limited to APC: macrophages, B-lymphocytes, and dendritic cells of Langerhans. Functional class II MHC molecules are heterodimers of 31-kDa α and 28-kDa β chains, and are thought to present a peptide-binding cleft similar to that of class I molecules. However, the peptide length preference is probably somewhat longer (15–20 amino acids). The acidic and proteolytic environment of the endosomic compartment is essential for both processing and presentation of antigen to CD4[+] cells, as disruption of either acidification or proteolysis selectively blocks functional class II antigen presentation [106,115]. Upon fusion of transport vesicles containing the class II heterodimer with the acidic endosomes containing proteolysis products, peptide binds to the $\alpha\beta$ dimer and the complexes are transported to the cell surface [103,116]. Of note, peptides presented in association with class II antigens typically generate a broader range of responses than do those presented with class I molecules. This distinction has been attributed in part to the finite repertoire of peptides of <11 residues, which is smaller than that of the roughly 20-residue chain bound by class II molecules. Other explanations include tighter control of class I than class II TCR-linked responses [106]. In addition, detailed observations have shown that the primary amino acid sequence of a peptide determines the avidity of its binding to specific class II alleles; peptide presentation is therefore biased toward those combinations of fragments and class II alleles which associate rapidly and with high affinity. This interaction between antigenic fragments and products of the host genome is an important determinant of which particular peptide fragments are ultimately presented to CD4$^+$ T lymphocytes, and to which an immune response can be generated [116].

Gautam and colleagues have investigated the structural requirements for peptide presentation in association with MHC class II molecules. Using synthetic peptides in a model of experimental autoimmune encephalitis, a T-cell-mediated disease, they observed that specific amino acid residues were differentially responsible for TCR reactivity, and that position-specific residues which conferred maximal helper T-cell responses could be recognized in the context of a fragment as small as a hexapeptide [104]. Because viral and bacterial proteins might share short sequences with host proteins, and thus be able to induce autoreactive T-lymphocyte clones, this observation has obvious possible implications for both autoimmune disorders and infectious exacerbations of preexisting inflammatory diseases such as asthma.

Stimulation of macrophages with a variety of cytokines induces increased expression of class II molecules. Both GM-CSF and IFN-γ upregulate presentation of foreign protein (native bovine insulin) by macrophages. However, recent studies have shown that antigen presentation and expression of class II proteins are differentially regulated. In vitro, presentation was most markedly enhanced by GM-CSF, whereas expression of MHC class II antigens was increased more by IFN-γ. Forms of bovine insulin which require no proteolysis, in contrast, were presented with greater efficiency by IFN-γ-treated macrophages as a consequence of greater class II molecule expression. Inhibition of macrophage proteases, or blockade of endosome acidification, resulted in increased antigen presentation by IFN-γ-, but not GM-CSF-treated macrophages. These data suggested that the relatively weakly enhanced antigen presentation by macrophages treated with IFN-γ could have resulted from excessive degradation of antigenic peptides [117]. Thus, efficient presentation of antigen by macrophages is a carefully coordinated process of antigen ingestion, expression and activation of proteases and proton pumps, synthesis of MHC class II molecules and related proteins, and numerous other factors. Interruption of this highly regulated process in a selective and specific manner may prove to have useful therapeutic implications in immunologic diseases, perhaps including asthma.

Recent data have suggested that heat shock proteins (HSP) may also participate in the processing and presentation of antigen by APCs. These highly conserved proteins are induced by elevation in ambient temperature and other environmental insults. Murine and human APC express a member of the HSP70 family on their surfaces. This 72-kDa protein binds peptides and is immunologically cross-reactive between mouse and human cells. Human monocytes expressing the LPS/LPS-binding-protein receptor CD14 also constitutively express an antigenic determinant reactive with this HSP. Moreover, blocking this HSP determinant with a neutralizing monoclonal antibody markedly reduced the ability of the monocytes to present antigen [118].

It has been hypothesized that HSPs also serve to convey cytosolic peptides to the endoplasmic reticulum, at least for tumor- and viral-derived proteins released by cytolysis into the extracellular space [119]. Although the mechanisms involved have yet to be fully clarified, these observations suggest that members of the HSP family may participate in initial stages of binding, internalization, and processing of extracellular protein antigens.

B. Heterogeneity of Pulmonary Antigen-Presenting Cells

Havenith and colleagues have demonstrated that BAL mononuclear cells can be separated by autofluorescence into high-fluorescence and low-fluorescence populations. Moreover, the high-fluorescence cells had cytomorphology typical of AM, whereas the low-fluorescence cells were smaller and more monocytelike. In addition, high-fluorescence cells migrated to a lower buoyant density (<1.065 g/mL), whereas low-fluorescence cells exhibited greater density ($1.065–1.079$ g/mL). Thus, by morphologic, fluorimetric, and density criteria, airspace mononuclear cells could be separated into two populations. Of note, functional studies also demonstrated marked differences between these two populations. Stimulation of primed T lymphocytes by high- and low-fluorescence AM in the presence of specific antigen was performed in order to examine the capabilities of these macrophage subpopulations to present specific antigen. These studies demonstrated that the low-density, high-fluorescence fraction (AM-like cells) produced dose-dependent *inhibition* of antigen presentation, whereas the high-density, low-fluorescence fraction (monocytelike cells) produced dose-dependent *stimulation* of antigen presentation [120]. These observations confirm that subpopulations of AM differ markedly not just quantitatively, but qualitatively in their ability to present antigen and to initiate an immunologic response. It is reasonable to hypothesize, therefore, that alterations in resident AM subpopulations which occur as a consequence of viral infection, antigen exposure [18], or other cause might have a profound impact on the immunologic environment of the lung, and could qualitatively alter airway inflammation in asthma.

C. Possible Differential Effects of Macrophage Subsets on Antigen Presentation to T_{H1} and T_{H2} Lymphocytes

Controversy exists with respect to whether a particular type of APC preferentially presents antigen to a specific T_H subset. It has been suggested that macrophage antigen presentation preferentially induces T_{H1} subsets, and that B-cell presentation may favor T_{H2} activation [121] (reviewed in Refs. 122–124). However, superantigen presentation by B cells results in a preferential T_{H1} response, unless exogenous IL-4 is simultaneously present [123]. Thus, although the hypothesis is that the type of APC regulates the nature of the subsequent immunologic response, convincing data which unequivocally confirm this hypothesis are not yet available. Whether specific macrophage subpopulations activate preferentially a subset of T lymphocytes also remains unknown. Such putative regulation could occur at several levels. Differences in phagocytosis, endosomal acidification, proteolytic enzyme production, regulation of MHC class II molecules, regulation of cytokine production, L-arginine and nitric oxide metabolism, and release of other immunomodulatory substances all could be rationally implicated in generation of selective T_{H1} or T_{H2} responses [1]. Because prostaglandin E_2 (PGE_2) differentially blocks the production of cytokines by T_{H1} cells, the accumulation of macrophages with heightened PGE_2 secretion at the site of inflammation might be expected to be associated with heightened T_{H2} lymphocyte activation. Similarly, IFN-γ inhibits the proliferation of T_{H2} but not T_{H1} clones, but does not impair their ability to secrete cytokines (reviewed in Ref. 124). Thus, secretion or release of IFN-γ by macrophages would be expected to antagonize the development of a functional T_{H2} response.

V. Summary and Future Directions

Macrophages subserve both afferent- and efferent-arm functions in the immune system, and are the principal phagocytes in the lower respiratory tract in both healthy and asthmatic humans. They are poised to initiate and regulate immunologic and inflammatory responses in the airway by virtue of their anatomic locale, the variety of receptors by which activation can be achieved, the repertoire of secretory products elaborated following activation, and the obligate control they exert over MHC class II–CD4$^+$ lymphocyte interactions. The recent interest in the possible pathogenic role of T_{H2} lymphocytes in allergic asthma, coupled with the necessity of antigen presentation by immunologically capable APC including macrophages, makes a strong case for additional investigation into the participation of alveolar macrophages in the pathogenesis of asthma. Additional studies linking specific MHC alleles with airway hyperresponsiveness and/or asthma, in the presence and absence of atopy, will provide a foundation for understanding asthma at a genetic level. These observations may then permit detailed molecular studies to be conducted to examine the primary structure of allergenic peptides and the relationship of their structure to (1) the avidity of class II MHC protein binding, and (2) the preference for presentation of T_{H1} and T_{H2} lymphocytes. Because changes in macrophage populations are also observed in asthma, additional investigation of these subpopulations is also required to examine the possibility of differential effects on the immunologic and inflammatory responses characteristic of asthma.

Acknowledgments

This work was supported in part by a Career Investigator Grant from the American Lung Association and the American Lung Association of Western Pennsylvania.

References

1. Rutherford MS, Witseli A, Schook LB. Mechanisms generating functionally hetero-geneous macrophages: chaos revisited. J Leuk Biol 1993; 53:602–618.
2. Kobzik L, Godleski JJ, Barry BE, Brain JD. Isolation and antigenic identification of hamster lung interstitial macrophages. Am Rev Respir Dis 1988; 138:908–914.
3. Bitterman PB, Saltzman LE, Adelberg S, Ferrans VJ, Crystal RG. Alveolar macro-phage replication: one mechanism for the expansion of the mononuclear phagocyte population in the chronically inflamed lung. J Clin Invest 1984; 74:460–469.
4. Hocking WG, Golde DW. The pulmonary alveolar macrophage. N Engl J Med 1979; 301:580–887 & 639–645.
5. Stahl PD. The mannose receptor and other macrophage lectins. Curr Opin Immunol 1992; 4:49–52.
6. Gauldie J, Richards C, Lamontagne L. Fc receptors for IgA and other immunoglobu-lins on resident and activated alveolar macrophages. Mol Immunol 1983; 20:1029–1037.
7. Sibille Y, Reynolds HY. Macrophages and polymorphonuclear neutrophils in lung defense and injury. Am Rev Respir Dis 1990; 141:471–500.
8. Herscowitz HB. In defense of the lung: paradoxical role of the pulmonary alveolar macrophage. Ann Allergy 1985; 55:634–648.
9. Wright SD, Detmers PA. Receptor mediated phagocytosis. In: Crystal RG, West JB, eds. The Lung: Scientific Foundations. New York: Raven Press, 1991:539–551.
10. Crystal RG. Alveolar macrophages. In: Crystal RG, West JB, eds. The Lung: Scientific Foundations. New York: Raven Press, 1991:527–538.
11. Lowenstein CJ, Alley EW, Raval P, et al. Macrophage nitric oxide synthase gene: two upstream regions mediate induction by interferon-γ and lipopolysaccharide. Proc Natl Acad Sci USA 1993; 90:9730–9734.
12. Weisz A, Oguchi S, Cicatiello L, Esumi H. Dual mechanism for the control of inducible-type NO synthase gene expression in macrophages during activation by interferon-γ and bacterial lipopolysaccaride. J Biol Chem 1994; 269:8324–8333.
13. Belenky SN, Robbins RA, Rubinstein I. Nitric oxide synthase inhibitors attenuate human monocyte chemotaxis *in vitro*. J Leuk Biol 1993; 53:498–503.
14. Kharitonov SA, Yates D, Robbins RA, Logan-Sinclair R, Shinebourne EA, Barnes PJ. Increased nitric oxide in exhaled air of asthmatic patients. Lancet 1994; 343:133–135.
15. Persson MG, Zetterstrom O, Agrenius V, Ihre E, Gustafsson LE. Single-breath nitric oxide measurements in asthmatic patients and smokers. Lancet 1994; 343:146–147.
16. Brannen AL, Chandler DB. Alveolar macrophage subpopulations' responsiveness to chemotactic stimuli. Am J Pathol 1988; 132:161–166.

17. Elias JA, Schreiber AD, Gustilo K, et al. Differential IL-1 elaboration by unfrac-tionated and density fractionated human alveolar macrophages and blood monocytes: relationship to cell maturity. J Immunol 1985; 135:3198–3204.

18. Calhoun WJ, Reed HE, Moest DR, Stevens CA. Enhanced superoxide production by alveolar macrophages and airspace cells, airway inflammation, and alveolar macrophage density changes follow segmental antigen bronchoprovocation in allergic subjects. Am Rev Respir Dis 1992; 145:317–325.

19. Holian A, Dauber JH, Diamond MS, Danielle RP. Separation of bronchoalveolar cells from guinea pig on continuous gradients of Percoll: functional properties of fractionated lung macrophages. J Reticuloendothel Soc 1983; 33:157–164.

20. Zeidler RB, Flynn JA, Arnold JC, Conley NS. Subpopulation of alveolar macrophages inhibits superoxide anion production by macrophages. Inflammation 1987; 11:371–379.

21. Bousquet J, Chanez P, Lacoste JY, et al. Eosinophilic inflammation in asthma. N Engl J Med 1990; 323:1033–1039.

22. Walker C, Kaegi MK, Braun P, Blaser K. Activated T-cells and eosinophilia in bronchoalveolar lavages from subjects with asthma correlated with disease severity. J Allergy Clin Immunol 1991; 88:935–942.

23. Pretolani M, Ruffie C, Joseph D, et al. Role of eosinophil activation in the bronchial reactivity of allergic guinea pigs. Am J Respir Crit Care Med 1994; 149:1167–1174.

24. Fuller RW. The role of the alveolar macrophage in asthma. Respir Med 1989; 83: 177–178.

25. Lee TH, Lane SJ. The role of macrophages in the mechanisms of airway inflammation in asthma. Am Rev Respir Dis 1992; 145:S27–S30.

26. Rankin JA. The contribution of alveolar macrophages to hyperreactive airway disease. J Allergy Clin Immunol 1989; 83:722–729.

27. Calhoun WJ, Jarjour NN. Macrophages and macrophage diversity. In: Busse WW, Holgate ST, eds. Asthma and Rhinitis. Boston: Blackwell, 1995; 467–473.

28. The BAL Cooperative Study Group. Bronchoalveolar lavage constituents in healthy individuals, idiopathic pulmonary fibrosis, and selected comparison groups. Am Rev Respir Dis 1990; 141:S169–S202.

29. Chanez P, Bousquet J, Couret I, et al. Increased numbers of hypodense alveolar macrophages in patients with bronchial asthma. Am Rev Respir Dis 1991; 144: 923–930.

30. Calhoun WJ, Bush RK. Enhanced reactive oxygen species metabolism of airspace cells and airway inflammation following antigen challenge in human asthma. J Allergy Clin Immunol 1990; 86:306–313.

31. Eschenbacher WL, Gravelyn TR. A technique for isolated airway segment lavage. Chest 1987; 92:105–109.

32. Liu MC, Hubbard WC, Proud D, et al. Immediate and late inflammatory responses to ragweed antigen challenge of the peripheral airway in allergic asthmatics. Cellular, mediator, and permeability changes. Am Rev Respir Dis 1991; 144:51–58.

33. Calhoun WJ, Jarjour NN, Gleich GJ, Stevens CA, Busse WW. Increased airway inflammation with segmental *versus* aerosol antigen challenge. Am Rev Respir Dis 1993; 147:1465–1471.

34. Diaz P, Gonzalez MC, Galleguillos FR, et al. Leukocytes and mediators in bronchoalveolar lavage during allergen-induced late-phase asthmatic reactions. Am Rev Respir Dis 1989; 139:1383–1389.

35. Sedgwick J, Calhoun WJ, Gleich GJ, et al. Immediate and late airway response of allergic rhinitis patients to segmental antigen challenge: characterization of eosinophil and mast cell mediators. Am Rev Respir Dis 1991; 144:1274–1281.

36. Melewicz FM, Kline LE, Cohen AB, Spiegelberg HL. Characterization of Fc receptors for IgE on human alveolar macrophages. Clin Exp Immunol 1982; 49: 364–370.

37. Melewicz FM, Zeiger RS, Mellon MH, et al. Increased peripheral blood monocytes with Fc receptors for IgE in patients with severe allergic disorders. J Immunol 1981; 126:1592–1595.

38. Carroll MP, Curham SR, Walsh G, et al. Activation of neutrophils and monocytes after allergen- and histamine-induced bronchoconstriction. J Allergy Clin Immunol 1985; 75:290–296.

39. Borish L, Mascali JJ, Rosenwasser LJ. IgE-dependent cytokine production by human peripheral blood mononuclear phagocytes. J Immunol 1991; 146:63–67.

40. Pforte A, Breyer G, Prinz JC, et al. Expression of the Fc-receptor for IgE (FcεRII, CD23) on alveolar macrophages in extrinsic allergic alveolitis. J Exp Med 1990; 171:1163–1169.

41. Rankin JA, Hitchcock M, Merrill WW, Bach MB, Brashler JA, Askenase PW. IgE-dependent release of leukotriene C_4 from alveolar macrophages. Nature 1982; 297: 329–331.

42. Rankin JA, Hitchcock M, Merrill WW, et al. IgE immune complexes induced immediate and prolonged release of leukotriene C_4 (LTC_4) from rat alveolar macrophages. J Immunol 1984; 132:1993–1999.

43. Rankin JA. IgE immune complexes induce LTB_4 release from rat alveolar macrophages. Ann Inst Pasteur Immunol 1986; 137:364–367.

44. Fuller RW, Morris PK, Richmond R, et al. Immunoglobulin E-dependent stimulation of human alveolar macrophages: significance in type 1 hypersensitivity. Clin Exp Immunol 1986; 65:416–426.

45. MacDermott J, Kelsey CR, Waddell KA, et al. Synthesis of leukotriene B_4 and prostanoids by human alveolar macrophages: analysis by gas chromatography/mass spectroscopy. Prostaglandins 1984; 27:163–177.

46. Tonnel AB, Gosset PH, Joseph M, et al. Stimulation of alveolar macrophages in asthmatic patients after local provocation test. Lancet 1983; i:1406–1408.

47. Spiegelberg HL. Structure and function of Fc receptors for IgE on lymphocytes, monocytes, and macrophages. Adv Immunol 1984; 35:61–88.

48. Joseph M, Tonnel AB, Torpier G, et al. Involvement of immunoglobulin E in the secretory process of alveolar macrophages from asthmatic patients. J Clin Invest 1983; 71:221–230.

49. Jarjour NN, Calhoun WJ. Exercise-induced asthma is not associated with mast cell activation or airway inflammation. J Allergy Clin Immunol 1992; 89:60–68.

50. Martin TR, Raugi G, Merritt T, Henderson WR Jr. Relative contribution of leuko-

triene B_4 to the neutrophil chemotactic activity produced by the resident human alveolar macrophage. J Clin Invest 1987; 80:1114–1124.

51. Nathan CF. Secretory products of macrophages. J Clin Invest 1987; 79:319–326.

52. McPhaden AR, Hamilton AO, Lappin D, Whaley K. Synthesis and secretion of complement components by mononuclear phagocytes. In: Dean and Jessup, eds. Mononuclear Phagocytes: Physiology and Pathology. Boston: Elsevier, 1985: 139–159.

53. Van Damme J, Van Beeumen J, Opdenakker G, Billiau A. A novel, NH_2-terminal sequence-characterized human monokine possessing neutrophil chemotactic, skin-reactive, and granulocytosis promoting activity. J Exp Med 1988; 167:1364–1376.

54. Corrigan CJ, Collard P, Nagy L, Kay AB. Cultured peripheral blood mononuclear cells derived from patients with acute severe asthma ("status asthmaticus") spontaneously elaborate a neutrophil chemotactic activity distinct from interleukin-8. Am Rev Respir Dis 1991; 143:538–544.

55. Sigal CE, Valone FH, Holtzman MJ, Goetz EJ. Preferential human eosinophil chemotactic activity of platelet activating factor (PAF). Clin Exp Immunol 1987; 7:179–184.

56. Siracusa A, Vecchiarelli A, Brugnami G, Marabini A, Felicioni D, Severini C. Changes in interleukin-1 and tumor necrosis factor production by peripheral blood monocytes after specific bronchoprovocation test in occupational asthma. Am Rev Respir Dis 1992; 146:408–412.

57. Enk C, Mosbech H. Interleukin-1 production by monocytes from patients with allergic asthma after stimulation in vitro with lipopolysaccharide and *Dermatophagoides pteronyssinus* mite allergen. Int Arch Allergy Appl Immunol 1988; 85: 308–311.

58. Calhoun WJ, Kelley J. Cytokines in the respiratory tract. In: Chung F, Barnes P, eds., Pharmacology of the Respiratory Tract: Clinical and Experimental. New York: Marcel Decker, 1993:253–288.

59. Gosset P, Tsicopoulos A, Wallaert B, et al. Increased secretion of tumor necrosis factor α and interleukin-6 by alveolar macrophages consecutive to the development of the late asthmatic reaction. J Allergy Clin Immunol 1991; 88:561–571.

60. Broide DH, Lotz M, Cuomo AJ, Coburn DA, Federman EC, Wasserman SI. Cytokines in symptomatic airways. J Allergy Clin Immunol 1992; 89:958–967.

61. Malefyt RdW, Abrams J, Bennett B, Figdor CG, de Vries JE. Interleukin 10 inhibits cytokine synthesis by human monocytes: an autoregulatory role of IL-10 produced by monocytes. J Exp Med 1991; 174:1209–1220.

62. Muldoon SR, Hinton K, Calhoun WJ. Modulation of IL-1β and TNF-α by IL-10 in peripheral blood monocytes—evidence of down-regulation. Am J Respir Crit Care Med 1994; 149:A1099.

63. Kelley J. Cytokines of the lung. Am Rev Respir Dis 1990; 141:765–788.

64. Dinarello CA. Interleukin-1 and interleukin-1 antagonism. Blood 1991; 77:1627–1652.

65. Cohan VL, Scott AL, Dinarello CA, Prendergast RA. Interleukin-1 is a mucus secretagogue. Cellular Immunol 1991; 136:425–434.

66. Subramanian N, Bray MA. Interleukin-1 can provoke histamine release from mast cells. J Immunol 1987; 138:271–275.

67. Pujol J-L, Cosso B, Daures J-P, Clot J, Michel F-B, Goddard P. Interleukin-1 release by alveolar macrophages in asthmatic patients and healthy subjects. Int Arch Allergy Appl Immunol 1990; 91:207–210.

68. Mattoli S, Mattoso VL, Soloperto M, Allegra L, Fasoli A. Cellular and biochemical characteristics of bronchoalveolar lavage fluid in symptomatic nonallergic asthma. J Allergy Clin Immunol 1991; 87:794–802.

69. Borish L, Mascali JJ, Dishuck J, Beam WR, Martin RJ, Rosenwasser LJ. Detection of alveolar macrophage-derived IL-1β in asthma. J Immunol 1992; 149:3078–3082.

70. Gosset P, Lassale P, Tonnel AB, et al. Production of an interleukin-1 inhibitory factor by human alveolar macrophages from normals and allergic asthmatic patients. Am Rev Respir Dis 1988; 138:40–46.

71. Schollmeier K. Immunologic and pathophysiologic role of tumor necrosis factor. Am J Respir Cell Mol Biol 1990; 3:11–12.

72. Vilček J, Lee TH. Tumor necrosis factor. J Biol Chem 1991; 266:7313–7316.

73. Wershil BK, Wang Z-S, Gordon JR, Galli SJ. Recruitment of neutrophils during IgE-dependent cutaneous late phase reactions in the mouse is mast cell dependent. J Clin Invest 1991; 87:446–453.

74. Calhoun WJ, Murphy K, Stevens CA, Jarjour NN, Busse WW. Increased interferon-γ and tumor necrosis factor-α in bronchoalveolar lavage fluid after antigen challenge in allergic subjects. Am Rev Respir Dis 1992; 145:A638.

75. Panuska JR, Midulla F, Cirino NM, et al. Am J Physiol 1990; 259:L396–L402.

76. Calhoun WJ, Dick EC, Schwartz LB, Busse WW. A common cold virus, rhinovirus 16, potentiates airway inflammation in allergic subjects following segmental antigen bronchprovocation. J Clin Invest 1994; 94:2200–2208.

77. Haak-Frendsho M, Arai N, Arai K-I, et al. Human recombinant granulocyte macrophage colony stimulating factor and interleukin-3 cause basophil histamine release. J Clin Invest 1988; 82:17–19.

78. Brown PH, Crompton GK, Greening AP. Proinflammatory cytokines in acute asthma. Lancet 1991; 338:590–593.

79. Howell CF, Pujol JL, Crea AEG, et al. Identification of an alveolar macrophage-derived activity in bronchial asthma that enhances leukotriene C_4 generation by human eosinophils stimulated by ionophore A23187 as a granulocyte-macrophage colony stimulating factor. Am Rev Respir Dis 1989; 140:1340–1347.

80. Falk LA, Ruscetti FW. Modulation of TGF-β1 receptor expression by macrophage activating agents. In: Oppenheim JJ, Powanda MC, Kluger MJ, Dinarello CA, eds. Molecular and Cellular Biology of Cytokines. New York: Wiley-Liss, 1990: 179–183.

81. Oswald IP, Gazzineli RT, Sher A, James SL. IL-10 synergizes with IL-4 and transforming growth factor-β to inhibit macrophage cytotoxic activity. J Immunol 1992; 148:3578–3582.

82. Rutherford MS, Schook LB. Macrophage function in response to PGE_2, L-arginine deprivation, and activation by colony-stimulating factors is dependent on hematopoietic stimulus. J Leuk Biol 1993; 52:228–235.

83. Lichtenstein LM. Histamine releasing factors and IgE heterogeneity. J Allergy Clin Immunol 1988; 81:814–820.

84. Schulman ES, Liu MC, Proud D, MacGlashan DW Jr, Lichtenstein LW, Plaut M. Human lung macrophages induced histamine release from basophils and mast cells. Am Rev Respir Dis 1985; 131:230–235.

85. Alam R. Cytokines and bronchial hyperreactivity. Agents Actions Suppl 1990; 31:147–162.

86. MacDonald SM, Lichtenstein LM, Proud D, et al. Studies of IgE-dependent histamine releasing factors: heterogeneity of IgE. J Immunol 1987; 139:506–512.

87. Alam R, Forsythe PA, Rankin JA, Boyars MC, Lett-Brown MA, Grant JA. Sensitivity of basophils to histamine releasing factor(s) of various origins: dependency on allergic phenotype of the donor and surface-bound IgE. J Allergy Clin Immunol 1990; 86:73–81.

88. Liu MC, Proud D, Lichtenstein LM, et al. Human macrophage-derived histamine releasing activity is due to an IgE-dependent factor(s). J Immunol 1986; 136:2588–2595.

89. Chonmaitree T, Lett-Brown MA, Grant JA. Respiratory viruses induce production of histamine releasing factor by mononuclear leukocytes: a possible role in the mechanism of virus-induced asthma. J Infect Dis 1991; 164:592–594.

90. Baeza ML, Reddigan SR, Kornfeld D, et al. Relationship of one form of human histamine-releasing factor (HRF) to connective tissue activating peptide-III. J Clin Invest 1990; 85:1516–1521.

91. Ferreri NR, Howland WC, Spiegelberg H. Release of leukotriene C_4 and B_4 and prostaglandin E_2 from human monocytes stimulated with aggregated IgG, IgA and IgE. J Immunol 1986; 136:4188–4193.

92. Murray JJ, Tonnel AB, Brash AR, et al. Release of prostaglandin D_2 into human airways during acute allergen challenge. N Engl J Med 1986; 315:800–804.

93. Ehrenreich H, Anderson RW, Fox CH, et al. Endothelins, peptides with potent vasoactive properties, are produced by human macrophages. J Exp Med 1990; 172:1741–1748.

94. Marom Z, Shellhammer JH, Kaliner M. Human pulmonary macrophage-derived mucus secretagogue. J Exp Med 1984; 159:844–860.

95. Tonnel M, Tonnel AB, Capron A, Voisin C. Enzyme release and superoxide anion production by human alveolar macrophages stimulated with immunoglobulin E. Clin Exp Immunol 1980; 40:416–422.

96. Katsumata U, Miwa M, Icinose M, et al. Oxygen radicals produce airway constriction and hyperresponsiveness in anesthetized cats. Am Rev Respir Dis 1990; 141:1158–1161.

97. Fang ZX, Lai Y-L. Oxygen radicals in bronchoconstriction of guinea pigs elicited by isocapnic hyperpnea. J Appl Physiol 1993; 74:627–633.

98. Cluzel M, Damon M, Chanez P, et al. Enhanced alveolar cell luminol-dependent chemiluminescence in asthma. J Allergy Clin Immunol 1987; 80:195–201.

99. Broide DH, Firestein GS. Endobronchial allergen challenge in asthma. J Clin Invest 1991; 88:1048–1053.

100. Calhoun WJ, Salisbury SM. Heterogeneity in cell recovery and superoxide produc-

tion in buoyant density defined subpopulations of human alveolar macrophages from healthy volunteers and sarcoidosis patients. J Lab Clin Med 1989; 114:682–690.

101. Unanue ER, Allen PM. The basis for the immunoregulatory role of macrophages and other accessory cells. Science 1987; 236:551–557.

102. Urban RG, Chicz RM, Vignali DAA, Strominger JL. The dichotomy of peptide presentation by class I and class II MHC proteins. Chem Immunol 1993; 57: 197–234.

103. Unanue ER, Cerottini J-C. Antigen presentation. FASEB J 1989; 3:2496–2502.

104. Gautam AM, Lock CB, Smilek DE, Pearson CI, Steinman L, McDevitt HO. Minimum structural requirements for peptide presentation by major histocompatibility complex class II molecules: implications in induction of autoimmunity. Proc Natl Acad Sci USA 1994; 91:767–771.

105. Buus S, Sette A, Grey HM. The interaction between protein derived immunogenic peptides and Ia. Immunol Rev 1987; 98:115–141.

106. Yewdell JW, Bennink JR. Antigen processing: a critical factor in rational vaccine design. Sem Hematol 1993; 30:26–34.

107. Heemels MT, Schumacher TN, Wonigeit K, Ploegh HL. Peptide translocation by variants of the transporter associated with antigen processing. Science 1993; 262: 2059–2063.

108. Kozlowski S, Corr M, Shirai M, et al. Multiple pathways are involved in the extracellular processing of MHC class I restricted peptides. J Immunol 1993; 151: 4033–4044.

109. Hance AJ. Accessory-cell–lymphocyte interactions. In: Crystal RG, West JB, eds. The Lung: Scientific Foundations. New York: Raven Press, 1991:483–498.

110. Saper MA, Bjorkman PJ, Wiley DC. Refined structure of the human histocompatibility antigen HLA-A2 at 2.6 Å resolution. J Mol Biol 1991; 219:277–319.

111. Krangel MS, Orr HT, Strominger JL. Assembly and maturation of HLA-A and HLA-B antigens *in vivo.* Cell 1979; 34:979–991.

112. Monaco JJ, Cho S. Attaya M. Transport protein gene in the murine MHC: possible implications for antigen processing. Science 1990; 250:1723–1726.

113. Lapham CK, Bacik I, Yewdell JW, et al. Class I molecules retained in the endoplasmic reticulum bind antigenic peptides. J Exp Med 1993; 177:1633–1641.

114. Townsend A, Ohlen C, Bastin J, Ljunggren HG, Foster L, Karre K. Association of class I major histocompatibility heavy and light chains induced by viral peptides. Nature 1989; 340:443–448.

115. McCoy KL, Schwartz RH. The role of intracellular acidification in antigen processing. Immunol Rev 1988; 106:129–147.

116. Nelson CA, Harding CV, Unanue ER. Biochemical anatomy of antigen presentation. Cold Spring Harbor Symp Quant Biol 1992; 57:557–563.

117. Frosch S, Bonifas U, Reske-Kunz AB. The capacity of bone marrow derived macrophages to process bovine insulation is regulated by lymphokines. Int Immunol 1993; 5:1551–1558.

118. Manara GC, Sansoni P, Badiali-de Georgi L, et al. New insights suggesting a possible role of a heat shock protein 70-kD family related protein in antigen processing/presentation phenomenon in humans. Blood 1993; 82:2865–2871.

119. Srivastava PK, Udono H, Blachere NE, Li Z. Heat shock proteins transfer peptides during antigen processing and CTL priming. Immunogenetics 1994; 39:93–98.

120. Havenith CEG, Breedijk AJ, van Miert PPMC, et al. Separation of alveolar macrophages and dendritic cells via autofluorescence: phenotypical and functional characterization. J Leukocyte Biol 1993; 53:504–510.

121. Gajewski TF, Pinnas M, Wong T, Fitch FW. Murine Th1 and Th2 clones proliferate optimally in response to distance antigen presenting cell populations. J Immunol 1991; 196:1750–1758.

122. Paulnock DM. Macrophage activation by T-cells. Curr Opin Immunol 1992; 4:344–349.

123. Gollob KJ, Nagelkerken L, Coffman RL. Endogenous retroviral superantigen presentation by B-cells induces the development of type 1 CD4$^+$ T-helper lymphocytes. Eur J Immunol 1993; 23:2565–2571.

124. Gajewski TF, Schell SR, Nau G, Fitch FW. Regulation of T-cell activation: differences among T-cell subsets. Immunol Rev 1989; 111:79–110.

125. Isobe K-I, Nakashima I. Nitric oxide production from a macrophage cell line: interaction with autologous and allogenic lymphocytes. J Cell Biochem 1993; 53:198–205.

126. Sherry B, Horii Y, Manogue KR, Widmer U, Cerami A. Macrophage inflammatory proteins 1 and 2: an overview. Cytokines 1992; 4:117–130.

7

Genetic Control of T-Cell and T-Cell Cytokine Expression in Asthma

LANNY J. ROSENWASSER

National Jewish Center for Immunology and Respiratory Medicine
Denver, Colorado

I. Introduction

Asthma is a respiratory disease characterized by reversible airway obstruction caused primarily by irritation and inflammation within the airways. This inflammation and irritation is associated with the phenomena of bronchial hyperresponsiveness to recall challenge with various agonists or allergens to which a susceptible individual with asthma may be responsive [1]. Asthma is a life-long disease once it is contracted. There may be long periods of remission between exacerbations of the disease, and the disease may range between very mild episodic to chronic severe daily interference with airway function. For many people, the most significant trigger for this asthmatic syndrome are specific allergens proteins found in the indoor and outdoor environment that trigger a specific limb of the immune response associated with the production of the antibodies of the IgE isotype. This proclivity to associate asthma with isotype expression goes beyond even the specific selection of allergen reactivity with the IgE, since population studies have shown a link between total as well as specific IgE and skin test reactivity and asthma within populations [2–4]. Nonetheless, asthma is a relatively heterogeneous disease, and for that reason identification of a predominant or major set of genes responsible for the hereditary contribution to asthma may be quite difficult. That asthma is a complex genetic disease is without doubt, since previous studies have identified both familial clustering associated with the disease as well as twin studies that show a greater prevalence of disease in monozygotic as opposed to dizygotic twins [5,6]. This chapter reviews the contribution of T-cell-based immune responses to allergen as a model for studying potential branch points and candidate genes for genetic control of asthma. We present the rationale for examining the particular genetic control of T-cell-related cytokines in asthma's potential candidate genes, and we highlight some of the experimental results that we have recently generated looking at the promoter regions of the cluster of cytokine genes on human chromosome 5q.

II. Cellular Interactions in the Immune Response to Allergens in the Airway and Lungs of Asthmatics

When an allergen is inhaled, there are interactions between cells generated during an immune response that are involved in the sensitization, elicitation, and recall of allergen triggers for induction of asthmatic inflammation. With the development of fiber-optic bronchoscopy, bronchoalveolar lavage, and transbronchial biopsy, it has become clear that the pathogenesis of the inflammation seen in asthmatic airways rests heavily on the contribution of a series of cells to this particular inflammation, and in fact a case can be made that the Th2 subset of CD4$^+$ T lymphocytes is particularly involved in the recognition of allergen and the generation of a set of cytokines that are characteristically associated with asthmatic, allergic, and generalized airway inflammation. This section systematically reviews the interactions between subsets of inflammatory cells involved in airway responses and identifies potential branch points for genetic control of responses.

When an inhaled allergen first encounters the airway, a number of specific antigen presenting cells (APCs) are present within the airway that might first intercept the allergen, process it through cell biological mechanisms, and generate various enzymes and subcellular organelles such that fragments of the allergen are redisplayed on class II MHC and class I MHC molecules of airway lining cells. The major antigen-presenting cells within the airway include professional antigen presenters such as dendritic cells and bronchial macrophages; both of these cells are involved in specific presentation to T cells, and the role of airway dendritic cells in selectively activating T lymphocytes has been well established by various laboratories. The role of macrophages in this process in the airway is somewhat diminished by demonstration of some dampening of expression of accessory molecules beyond MHC on the airway macrophages as opposed to dendritic cells. Table 1 lists the major and minor APCs of the airways. Other cells within the airway, particularly antigen-specific B cells, endothelial cells, epithelial cells, smooth muscle cells, and even mast cells and eosinophils, can act under some

Table 1 APCs of the Airway

Major cells	Effector function
Macrophages	APC, cytokines, mediators
Dendritic cells	APC, cytokines, mediators
B cells	APC, Ig production, mediators
Minor cells	Effector function
Epithelial	APC, cytokines, mediators
Endothelial	APC, cytokines, mediators
Mast cells	Cytokines, mediators, specific responses (IgE)
Eosinophils	Cationic proteins, cytokines, mediators

Note: APC, antigen-presenting cells; Ig, immunoglobulin.

circumstances as antigen-presenting cells related to their exposure to factors such as cytokines and in particular interferon-γ and GM-CSF and IL-4 as cytokines that are capable of upregulating class II MHC expression on many of the resident and inflammatory cells found in the bronchi in asthma. Antigen presentation is a complex process, as alluded to earlier. Initially, an allergen is taken up into the cytosol by pinocytotic vesicles and merges with subcellular organelles and lysosomes to form secondary lysosomes. Within the secondary lysosomes, low pH and the presence of various kinds of proteases and transporters generate a small fragment of an allergen that can then bind in the antigen fragment-binding pocket within the three-dimensional structure of the HLA class II MHC molecules. Beyond this delivery of the first specific signal to the T cell by the antigen-presenting cell, other accessory functions can be subserved by the APC. These include expression of other membrane molecules including B7.1, B7.2 (CD80, CD86) interacting with CD28 and CTLA-4 on the T-lymphocyte membrane, ICAM-1, LFA-1 interactions on the APC T-cell membranes, and the interaction of VLA-4 and VCAM-1 between APCs and T lymphocytes. In addition to these adhesion molecule interactions, production of soluble factors including IL-1 and IL-6 as potential second signals for the IL-1 and IL-6 receptors on T cells may also constitute a secondary accessory signal for T-cell activation involved in antigen presentation. Obviously, all of these factors potentially are candidate genes for asthmatic involvement, since CD4 Th2-like T cells are so critically involved in allergic asthmatic reactions.

The major cell type with which antigen-presenting macrophages and dendritic cells interact in the airway is the CD4$^+$ subset of T cells [7,8]. Table 2 lists the major classes and subpopulations of T cells and notes their major functions. T lymphocytes are prominent among the various populations of airway cells, and their importance lies in their major role in the recognition of inhaled allergen proteins. The T lymphocytes arrive from bone marrow-derived precursors se-

Table 2 Classification of T Lymphocytes

CD2/CD3 mature T cells	Specificity	Function
CD8 TCRαβ	Class I MHC and peptide	Cytotoxicity Immunoregulation
CD4 (TH1) TCRαβ	Class II MHC and peptide (allergen)	Delayed-type hypersensitivity and host defense IL-2, IL-3, IFN-γ, lymphotoxin, GM-CSF
CD4 (TH2) TCRαβ	Class II MHC and peptide (allergen)	Antibody synthesis (IgE) IL-4, IL-5, IL-9, IL-10, IL-3, GM-CSF
CD4⁻, CD8⁻ TCRγδ	Unknown CD1, heat shock proteins	Epithelial defense

lected by thymic maturation through a complicated selection and deletion process that occurs during T-cell maturation. The T cells that emerge during this process populate peripheral lymphoid tissues, including lymph nodes within the bronchial alveolar wall. The majority of such cells display unique combinations of cell surface proteins. It is these proteins that differentiate and function within the mature T-cell compartment. Most mature T cells—in fact, the overwhelming majority of cells that have been selected through the thymus—express on the surface the protein markers CD2 and CD3 and CD3 must be co-expressed for specific T-cell receptors to be present. The specific T-cell receptors, namely, the alpha and beta proteins that are present on the cell surface membranes of T cells and that react with self class II MHC molecules or HLA-D molecules, are complex proteins that are developed through molecular recombination events. In fact, the association and recombination of various gene segments involved in specific recognition of the protein allergens depends on various receptors comprised of the various regions. For example, the T-cell-receptor alpha chain comprises a variable region, a joining region, and a constant region, whereas the beta chain is composed of a variable region, a diversity region, a joining region, and a constant region. These seven genetic segments make up the two proteins that are involved directly in recognizing inhaled foreign allergens in the airway. Once the CD3 population of T cells have differentiated into mature T cells, they can be further developed in terms of the ability of a particular subset of T cells to help B cells produce antibodies or to help macrophages and other accessory cells express delayed-type hypersensitivity. This so-called differentiation of the CD4 subpopulation of T cells into Th2⁺ cells versus Th1⁺ cells clearly delineates these different subpopulations. There has been much research on this subdivision in the past few years, which has shown that the Th1 subpopulation of CD4 T helper cells is the population of cells involved in the mediation of delayed-type hypersensitivity.

The cytokines made by these cells are effector molecules that contribute to host defense, and hence infection with an intercellular parasite leads to generation of a T-cell response that is characterized by the production of interferon-γ and lymphotoxin. IL-4, IL-5, and the T-cell cytokines involved in antibody switch and production, including IgE isotype switch, are more characteristic of the alpha–beta-bearing T-cell receptor-bearing cells of the Th2 subpopulation. This subpopulation of cells is quite prominent in responses to allergens in the airway, both in vitro and in vivo, and CD4$^+$ Th2 cells have enhanced capability for producing IL-4, IL-5, and other cytokines that are involved in the generation of allergic antibody responses and allergic inflammation. More important, activation of these cytokine genes of the Th2 type may be very important in the generation of underlying allergic asthmatic inflammation. Other T-cell subpopulations do not seem to play a primary role in asthma, such as the CD8$^+$ T cell subset that includes specific alpha–beta T-cell receptor-bearing cells restricted to class I targets and involved in CTL killing. Another subpopulation of CD8$^+$ T cells may have cytotoxic effects via natural killer activity, and these particular cells may be quite important. Other subpopulations of T cells include the T-cell receptor CD3$^+$ T cells that bear gamma–delta T-cell receptors. These cells are thought to play a role in epithelial defense, although the specificity of their ligands and the actual mechanism by which they are involved in host defense, let alone asthma, is as yet undefined.

Other cells that are of great importance in the airway include mast cells, eosinophils, and basophils. These cells are allergic effector cells. Mast cells are capable of binding specific allergens through the fact that the cells bear high-affinity Fc receptors for IgE. Bridging of IgE antibody molecules with the actual allergens and the IgE Fc receptors leads to activation of the mast cells, which then are triggered to release the contents of their granules as well as other stored mediators. The cross-linking event also induces a biochemical activation that leads to newly synthesized mediators such as leukotrienes and prostaglandins and PAF and may involve nuclear activation such that cytokine gene activation may be turned on in these mast cells that have been activated. Eosinophils are the major effector cells in the airway that play a significant role in inducing inflammation associated with responses to allergens. Eosinophils are derived from bone marrow precursors, and production of mature eosinophils is stimulated by the action of cytokines such as GM-CSF, IL-3, and IL-5. They also are involved in prolonging eosinophil survival in vivo and in vitro. IL-5 is another activator that has an effect on the ability of eosinophils to chemotax and move to a chemoattractant signal. The chemokines, including RANTES, also are very effective eosinophil chemotactic factors, as is a newly described substance known as EOTAXIN. These cells all play a major role with their capability of making various mediators, including enzymes, cationic proteins, leukotrienes, prostaglandins, and platelet-activating factor, and in generating the ongoing intense inflammation associated with asthmatic responses. Any of these mediators or any of the proteins that mark these cells specifically may be potential candidate genes for dysregulation in asthma.

III. Cytokines Involved in Asthmatic Response

Cytokines are relatively small-molecular-weight proteins, usually between 10 and 40 kDa in size, that have multiple pleotropic effects on multiple target tissues. The role of these cytokines in allergic responses has recently been recognized [9]. There are a particular set of cytokines involved in inducing allergic reactions, primarily by governing immune reactions to generate an IgE response and by the ability of various groups of cytokines to generate activated eosinophils, mast cells, and basophils at sites of allergic inflammation. There are five or six major cytokine families, including the interferons, growth and differentiative factors, tumor necrosis factors, colony-stimulating factors, histamine-releasing factors or chemokines, and the interleukins. These proteins all may cross-interact at various levels and at various targets, and the distinction between an interleukin and an interferon may be somewhat artificial. The significant cytokines that are involved in the generation of allergic responses are summarized in Tables 3 and 4. As noted previously, there is a differentiation of these cytokines into so-called Th1- and Th2-like cytokines for the T-cell cytokines that are generated in response to allergens and for the promulgation of allergen-specific responses. Of significant interest in the past few years has been the identification that the development of a Th2-type T-cell response occurs when allergen stimulates naive Th0-like cell in the presence of IL-4 [10]. Similarly, the development of the Th2 lineage of T-cell subsets involves allergen- or antigen-specific stimulation of a Th0 cell in the presence of the cytokine IL-12 [11]. The genetic control of these cytokines has

Table 3 Cytokine-Induced Airways and Allergic Inflammation

Function	Cytokine	Activity
IgE	IL-4, IL-13	IgE isotype switch
	IL-2, IL-5, IL-6	B-cell stimulation with IL-4
	IFN-γ	Inhibits IL-4
	IL-10	Inhibits IFN-γ
	IL-12	Induces IFN-γ
Eosinophilia	IL-3, IL-5, GM-CSF, IL-1,	Eosinophilopoietins and
	tumor necrosis factor (TNF)	activators
Mast cell, Basophil	IL-3, IL-4, IL-9, IL-10	Mast-cell growth factors
development and	hematopoietic stem cell factor	
activation	RANTES, CTAP-III, NKF-p23,	Histamine-releasing factors
	NAP-2, MCAF	

Table 4 Human CD4 T-Cell Subsets

TH1	TH2
IFN-γ	IL-4
LT (TNF-β)	IL-5
	IL-9
Both and TH0	
IL-3	
GM-CSF	
IL-2[a]	
IL-6[b]	
IL-10[b]	
IL-13	

[a]TH1 in mouse.
[b]TH2 in mouse.

become a focus of significant interest, since many of the genes that code for the cytokines have been found on the long arm of human chromosome 5 and linkage studies in various populations have suggested that indeed the area of chromosome 5q31-33 may be an area of intense locus control in asthma.

IV. Genetic Variation in Cytokine Genes

The genetic predisposition to asthma and atopy has been a difficult area for study for many years, likely because in this complex genetic disease, manifestations of the disease require alternative combinations of various sets of genes acting independently or synergistically to produce a complex phenotype such as the clinical syndrome of asthma. Furthermore, the possibility that different sets of genes may contribute differently in different populations also must be considered, as must the issues of the length and nature of environmental exposures, and selection of asthmatic and atopic phenotypes through the interaction of both these environmental and genetic factors. That a genetic component plays a role is without question, since multiple family studies as well as monozygotic and dizygotic twin studies demonstrate that anywhere between 30% and 60% of the contribution of the factors involved in the generation and expression of atopy and asthma may be due to genetic inheritance. Not only is atopy a potential marker for the inheritance of asthma, familial clustering of bronchial hyperresponsiveness is another marker that has been examined utilizing laboratory markers and physiology, and this has been assessed in families with atopy and asthma. Therefore this linkage to both atopy and bronchial hyperresponsiveness has been accomplished utilizing family studies, linkage analysis, and other means of examining the genetics of complex disease. We are entering an era where multiple attempts to identify familial and genetic susceptibility to complex disease may be examined by utilizing microsatellite markers through the entire genome, which may identify potential hotspots or hits within the genome that might identify candidate genes that might be in linkage dysequilibrium with marker hits. This approach has only been begun to be applied to familial studies with asthma, and within the next few years many studies may be forthcoming on this approach [12,13]. The standard approach utilizing candidate genes to identify likely candidates for contributions to the genetics of asthma and atopy has been the norm for the past few years while data have been developing. Table 5 lists different categories of potential candidate genes of atopy and allergy, all of which may be related potentially to the type of allergic and immunologic dysregulation demonstrated on pathologic and immunopathologic studies of asthma. As noted in Table 5, these factors may include

Table 5 Candidate Genes of Atopy and Asthma

	Examples
Recognition elements	TCR-α V/J/C
TCR genes	TCR-β V/D/J/C
HLA genes	HLA-DRα,β
	HLA-DPα,β
	HLA-DQα,β
Cytokines influencing allergic phenotype	
Eosinophil growth, activation, and apoptosis-inhibiting factors	IL-5, IL-3, GM-CSF, eotaxin, RANTES
Mast-cell growth factors	IL-3, IL-9, IL-10, nerve growth factor, TFG-β
Histamine-releasing factors	MCP-1, MCP-3, RANTES, HRF-p23
IgE isotype switch factors	IL-4, IL-13
Inhibition of IgE isotype switch	Interferon-γ, IL-12
Pro-inflammatory cytokines	IL-1α, IL-1β, TNF-α, IL-6
Anti-inflammatory cytokines	TGF-β, IL-10, IL-6
TH1/TH2-determining cytokines	IL-12/IL-4
Receptors	
IgE	FcϵR1 β chain, FcϵRII (CD23)
Cytokine gene receptors	IFN-γR β-chain, M-CSF, type II IL-1R
Adhesion molecules	VLA-4, VCAM-1, ICAM-1, LFA-1
Corticosteroid receptor	Grl-hsp90; NF-κB, I-κB
Neurogenic receptors	β_2-adrenergic, cholinergic receptors
Nuclear transcription factors	AP-1, NFIL-2a, Oct-1, STAT-1, NFAT, STAT-6, gaf

all of the genes involved in T-cell and NHC-linked recognition, cytokines that influence the allergic phenotype, receptors for various materials including adhesion molecules, steroid receptors, neurogenic receptors, and even nuclear transcription factors which may play a role in the expression of genes that influence other candidate genes. Besides these various candidate genes, the beginnings of identification of vesicular chromosomal linkage with asthma and atopy, particularly from the point of view of immune responsiveness, has been identified. Initial reports on the genetics of asthma linked some responses to human chromosome 6, and identified the association of HLA markers and possibly TNF by linkage to allergen reactivity in asthmatic populations [14]. A number of studies over the years have been published on this particular mechanism. More recently, information concerning potential associations of markers linked to chromosome 14 and presumably the alpha chain of the T-cell receptor in asthmatic, atopic populations has also been reported [15]. It has also been reported by a number of groups that a marker on chromosome 11q13 has been associated with asthma and atopic sensitivity, and while the initial reports of this linkage have not been well confirmed, some groups have confirmed this association and further identification of potential polymorphisms with the beta chain of the high-affinity IgE Fc receptor that might be associated with this particular marker and/or the functional association of atopy and asthma with this marker [16,17]. More recently, a number of groups have shown linkage to both atopy and bronchial hyperresponsiveness to a number of the genes present on human chromosome 5q31-33 [18–22]. Within this cluster are the genes for many of the Th2-like cytokines involved in IgE production and allergic inflammation, and two groups have identified different markers within this region as being linked in various populations to asthma and atopy. As mentioned previously, asthma and atopy may develop secondary to the transcriptional dysregulation of these T-lymphocyte-related cytokines. The same genes that code for cytokines and influence IgE production, bone marrow stimulation, and allergic inflammation may also be sites of genetic control for these kinds of responses. Our group has investigated the presence of potential polymorphisms within this gene cluster to identify markers which may link to transcriptional dysregulation in asthmatic kindreds. These polymorphisms were first identified in the 5′ promoter region of the genes within 5q31-33 via the technique of polymerase chain reaction (PCR), initiated single-stranded conformational polymorphisms (SSCP), and as heterodimers of PCR products [23,24]. Such polymorphisms may reflect either base exchanges which regulate gene transcription directly, or alternatively, they may be linked in other ways to gene dysregulation. Of the six cytokine genes assayed in this manner in the 5′ regions of these genes on chromosome 5, three SSCP were identified, one each in the IL-3, IL-9 and IL-4 5′ regions, and confirmed by heteroduplex analysis. These polymorphisms were then further evaluated via DNA sequencing, and the functionality of the IL-4 promoter polymorphism was studied in significant detail.

A. Approach

Families with and without asthma were drawn from the subject sample followed by the Asthma Risk Study which has been conducted at the National Jewish Center. Our study group consisted of 20 asthmatic families (more than four family members each, at least one of whom had asthma) and five control (nonasthmatic families). Control families are nuclear families in which no member has elevated IgE or a personal history of asthma or respiratory symptoms. The presence of asthma was documented by evaluation at the National Jewish Center through history, physical examination, and the presence of reversible airway disease upon pulmonary function testing. DNA was isolated from peripheral blood using a DNA extraction kit (BRL, Bethesda, MD). Whole blood was lysed, washed, and digested with proteinase K. After digestion, the solution was extracted two times with phenol:chloroform:isoamyl alcohol (25:24:1) and two to three times with chloroform alone. DNA was ethanol precipitated and resuspended at 0.5 μg/μL in water (via OD 260-nm absorption).

Single-stranded conformational polymorphisms (SSCP) was performed on the upstream promoter regions of five relevant chromosome five genes, IL-3, IL-4, IL-5, IL-9, and GM-CSF, according to standard techniques. Approximately 500–1000 nucleotide sequences were analyzed in fragments, each $\approx$250–325 nucleotides in length. Primer sequences were synthesized on an Applied Biosystems 381A DNA synthesizer (Foster City, CA). To perform the SSCP analyses, PCR was performed on genomic DNA (100 ng) in the presence of g33P-ATP, primers (40 pmol/μL) Taq polymerase dNTPs (1.25 mM each), and reaction buffer. After initial denaturation (5 min at 94°C), we performed 30 PCR cycles at 1 min each at 94°C, 60°C, and 72°C. PCR product (10 μL) was diluted in 50 μL of 0.1% SDS/10 mM EDTA, and 5.0 μL of this was mixed with 6.0 μL of formamide dye (95%). Samples were denatured (94°C for 3 min) and chilled rapidly to 4°C. The denatured DNA (2 μL) was loaded on a 4.5% nondenaturing acrylamide gel under four conditions: 4°C and 22°C, with and without 5% glycerol. Electrophoresis was performed with constant monitoring of temperature; to minimize heating during the electrophoresis, a fan was used to blow air against the glass plates. After electrophoresis, the gels were dried and autoradiography was performed.

To confirm any polymorphisms detected via SSCP and to detect any additional polymorphisms which might have been missed, analysis of DNA heteroduplexes was performed. Heteroduplexes were analyzed on DNA fragments generated using the primers described for SSCP. PCR was performed as described (without 33P-ATP). After the final thermal cycle was completed, the Taq polymerase was inactivated through the additional of EDTA. Samples were denatured (95°C for 3 min), and the reaction mixture was slowly cooled over 30 min to 37°C. PCR product with dye markers underwent acrylamide electrophoresis (MDE Gel, AT Biochem, Inc., Malvern, PA) at 20 V/cm. Leaving the gel adhered to one glass plate, the DNA was stained in 0.6X TBE containing ethidium bromide (1 μg/mL) for 15 min. The gels were destained and visualized via transillumination.

DNA was extracted from the acrylamide from each of the two wild-type and two polymorphic bands detected by SSCP. Both strands of the DNA were extracted and sequenced separately, for additional accuracy. This was accomplished by applying fluorescent markers to the acrylamide gel and overlaying the developed X-ray paper on the gel. The region containing the DNA was identified, excised, and the DNA electrophoretically extracted. The DNA was PCR amplified using the original primers used in the SSCP analysis and purified from agarose (Gene Clene, Bio 101, Inc., La Jolla, CA). DNA sequencing was performed on a commercial dsDNA cycle system (BRL) using Taq polymerase. Nested primers were synthesized and 33P end-labeled via T4 polynucleotide kinase (BRL). Reactions consisted of template DNA ($\approx$50 fmol), Taq DNA polymerase (2.5 U), sequencing buffer, and the appropriate termination mix. Initial denaturation (95°C, 30 s at 55°C, and 60 s at 70°C) was followed by 10 cycles of 30 s at 95°C and 60 s at 60°C. Reactions were denatured, loading on a sequencing acrylamide gel (Lone Ranger, AT Biochem), and electrophoresed at 60–65 W. Gels were dried and autoradiography performed.

B. Results

We have examined the DNA from families with and without asthma to explore the association of the potential for polymorphisms within the promoter region of six cytokine genes identified within the 5q gene cluster. We found polymorphisms in three of the six promoter regions, IL-3, IL-4, and IL-9. The PCR primers for the entire regions for all six cytokine genes are presented in Table 6. Table 7 identifies the position and frequency of promoter polymorphisms in the asthmatic kindreds. In Fig. 1 the IL-4 promoter polymorphism is illustrated, and by sequencing one can see that a C-to-T exchange at position −590 bp from the open reading frame of the IL-4 is associated with this polymorphism. In Fig. 1, what is of interest in the C-to-T exchange that occurs at position −590 bp up from the open reading frame in the 5′ region of the IL-4 gene is the fact that this particular exchange occurs at the confluence of two inverted palindromes. It should be noted that this particular sequence in this particular region of the IL-4 promoter has no consensus sequence for the binding site for any of the known transcription factors. Hence, either an unknown or a previously unrecognized binding sequence must exist for this particular area of the promoter to be transcriptionally active. The fact that it is at the confluence of two inverted palindromes speaks very highly to the likelihood of significant transcriptional regulation at this particular point. In fact, subsequent experiments just alluded to in the results and discussion, support the idea that this is a highly transcriptionally active site. In data not shown, the association of this promoter polymorphism with total serum IgE can be demon-

Table 6 PCR Primers for SSCP

Gene	Nucleotides[a]		Oligo sequence
IL-5	5′	−451−−427	TAAGACAGATTAATCTAGCCACAGT
	3′	−258−−278	GGGTTAATACATCATTGCCCC
	5′	−278−−258	GGGGCAATGATGTATTAACCC
	3′	25−1	AACTCAAATGCAGAAGCATCCTCAT
IL-9	5′	−523−−503	GCAACCTCAGTCTTACTATGC
	3′	−231−−253	GTTGAGTACTGAAATGCTGAAGG
	5′	−253−−231	CCTTCAGCATTTCAGTACTCAAC
	3′	24−1	AGGTAAGGACCATGGCCAGAAGCAT
IL-3	5′	−450−−425	GCCACCCACCAGGACCAAGCAGGGC
	3′	−188−−212	CCACAGACGTAATTATTCATCCATG
	5′	−212−−188	CATGGATGAATAATTACGTCTGTGG
	3′	25−1	GGAGCAGGACGGGCAGGCGGCTCAT
IL-4	5′	−1140−−1118	GGTGGGGCACTGACTAGGAGGGC
	3′	−826−−850	CTCAATGATCCTCCCACCTCAGCC
	5′	−844−−820	GGTGGGAGGATCATTGAGCTGGG
	3′	−535−−558	GGGGCTCCTTCTCTGCATAGAGGC
	5′	−555−−535	GCCTCTATGCAGAGAAGGAGCCCC
	3′	−229−−250	CCTGTGAAATCAGACCAATAGG
	5′	−250−−229	CCTATTGGTCTGATTTCACAGG
	3′	29−3	GGGGGAAGCAGTTGGGAGGTGAGACCC
IL-13	5′	−771−−751	CCTAGGCAGGCAACATAGTG
	3′	−471−−491	GCTATGGGAATTTGGGGAGT
	5′	−521−−501	TTTAAGAGACTGGTTCATCG
	3′	−220−−240	ACTTATTGAGAAGGGTCCAG
	5′	−271−−251	TAAACCCACCCAGATCTTGG
	3′	20−1	TGGTCAACAAAAGCGCCATG
GM-CSF	5′	−461−−437	GAGGAAGGCTGGAGTCAGAATGAGG
	3′	−295−−318	GGCTGCCCCCTCCCTCTGAGGGGC
	5′	−318−−295	GCCCCTCAGAGGGAGGGGGCAGCC
	3′	24−1	AGAGCAGCAGGCTCTGCAGCCACAT

[a]Position from open reading frame.

Table 7 Promoter Polymorphisms

Cytokine	Position	Polymorphism	5′ from ORF	Frequency
IL-4	5q31	C to T	−590	33/95
IL-3	5q31	T to C	−68	26/102
IL-9	5q31	A to C	−351	12/72

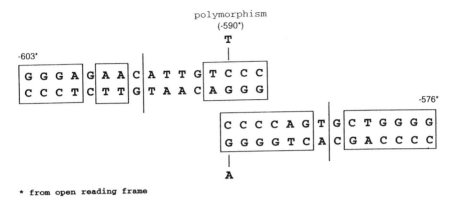

Figure 1   Adjacent palindrome sequences flank the IL-4 promoter polymorphism.

strated significantly in affected families that have this polymorphism such that those with the T or polymorphism structure have a significantly higher total serum IgE than those who have the C at position −590. This change is associated with functional changes as well in that transfection of promoters that have this C-to-T exchange identifies greater transfected luciferase activity with the T-polymorphism structure as opposed to the C wild-type structure. Furthermore, electromobility shift assays (EMSA) demonstrate that more nuclear transcription factors are bound to the promoter polymorphism sequence as opposed to the wild-type sequence, so the T in position −590 will bind more nuclear transcription factor than the C-position oligonucleotide in EMSA studies [20,21]. Further evaluation of the actual activity associated with this C-to-T exchange in terms of the nature of the transcription factor binding is under intense study [25]. The possibility that this C-to-T exchange −590 bp from the open reading frame is significant is suggested from our initial data. Additional subjects will need to be studied and correlations to clinical parameters sought in order to further assess the relevance of these polymorphisms to the development of asthma. These studies are currently underway. The fact that a disease can be manifested by promoter abnormalities as opposed to coding region abnormalities is also significant in these studies, and the identification of the extract transcriptional regulation and transcription factors that are involved in the cytokine gene regulation with this genetic polymorphism will be critical and are beginning to be defined. Further work to confirm the identification of this site as important in the genetics of asthma and atopy by linkage analysis will also be necessary. Nonetheless, the atopic asthmatic IL-4 and to a lesser extent IL-3 and IL-9 promoter polymorphisms are the beginning of the dissection of potential molecular mechanisms for linkage analysis and marker association in family studies with asthma. Overall, the likelihood that one set or even a closely linked set of interacting genes and coregulated genes is the primary genes involved in the regulation of asthma is not likely. It is more likely that sets of genes with totals of greater than 15 to 20 to 25 genes may be all dysregulated in asthma, with each set interacting in a unique way and contributing something to asthma in different populations that undergo different environmental stresses and exposures. The complex genetics of a syndrome such as asthma is somewhat daunting, since numerous molecular variants may also be possible in these circumstances. However, the identification of a large number of sets of genes that may be dysregulated in asthma needs to be approached in a direct and analytical way, so that assessment of risk and screening of populations at risk can be begun even if a particular gene that is identified may not contribute more than 5% or 8% of the genetic contribution to a disease such as asthma. The next 5 to 10 years in this area should be exciting and may provide significant insights into the heretofore unsuspected mechanisms involved in the clinical syndrome known as bronchial asthma.

Acknowledgments

I would like to recognize all of my co-workers who have worked on this particular project, in particular, Larry Borish, Dwight Klemm, Mary Klinnert, and Mark Leppert, who have collaborated in various parts of this project, and the excellent assistance of Hiroaki Inamura, Julie Dresback, and Jim Mascali in doing the various experiments alluded to in this chapter. This work was funded by U.S. Public Health Service grants AI35156 and HL36577.

References

1. Broide DH, Firestein GS. Endobronchial allergen challenge in asthma. Demonstration of cellular source of granulocyte macrophage colony-stimulating factor by in situ hybridization. J Clin Invest 1991; 88:1048–1053.
2. Burrows B, Martinez FD, Halonen M, Barbee RA, Cine MG. Association of asthma with serum IgE levels and skin-test reactivity to allergens. N Engl J Med 1989; 320: 271–277.
3. Burrows B, Sears MR, Flannery EM, Herbison GP, Holdaway MD. Relationship of bronchial responsiveness assessed by methacholine to serum IgE, lung function, symptoms, and diagnosis in 11-year-old New Zealand children. J Allergy Clin Immunol 1992; 90:376–385.
4. Burrows B, Sears MR, Flannery EM, Herbison GP, Holdaway MD. Relationship of bronchial responsiveness to allergy skin test reactivity, lung function, respiratory symptoms, and diagnosis in 13-year-old New Zealand children. J Allergy Clin Immunol 1995; 95:548–556.

5. Hopp RJ, Bewtra AK, Watt GD, Nair NM, Townley RG. Genetic analysis of allergic disease in twins. J Allergy Clin Immunol 1984; 73:265–270.

6. Hopp RJ, Townley RG, Biven R, Bewtra AK, Nair NM. The presence of airway reactivity before the development of asthma. Am Rev Respir Dis 1990; 141:2–8.

7. Robinson DS, Hamid Q, Ying S, et al. Predominant Th2-like bronchoalveolar T-lymphocyte population in atopic asthma. N Engl J Med 1992; 326:298–304.

8. Wierenga EA Snock M, DeGroot C, et al. Evidence for compartmentalization of functional subsets of CD4$^+$ T lymphocytes in atopic patients. J Immunol 1990; 144: 4651–4656.

9. Borish L, Rosenwasser LJ. Update on cytokines. J Allergy Clin Immunol. In press.

10. Seder RA, Paul WE, Davis MM, de St. Groth BF. The presence of interleukin 4 during in vitro priming determines the lymphokine-producing potential of CD4 T cells from T cell receptor transgenic mice. J Exp Med 1992; 176:1091–1098.

11. Manetti R, Parronchi GP, Giudizi MG, et al. Natural killer cell stimulatory factor (interleukin 12[IL-12]) induces T helper type 1 (Th1)-specific immune responses and inhibits the development of IL-4-producing Th cells. J Exp Med 1993; 177:1199–1204.

12. Collins FS. Positional cloning: let's not call it reverse anymore. Nature Genet 1992; 1:3–6.

13. Lander ES, Schork NJ. Genetic dissection of complex traits. Science 1994; 265:2037–2048.

14. Young RP, Dekker JW, Wordsworth BP, et al. HLA-DR and HLA-DP genotypes and immunoglobulin E responses to common major allergens. Clin Exp Allergy 1994; 24:431–439.

15. Moffatt MF, Hill MR, Cornelis F, et al. Genetic linkage of the TCR-α/δ complex to specific immunoglobulin E responses. Lancet 1994; 343:1597–1600.

16. Cookson WOCM, Sharp PA, Faux JA, Hopkin JM. Linkage between immunoglobulin E responses underlying asthma and rhinitis and chromosome 11q. Lancet 1989; i: 1292–1295.

17. Shirakawa TS, Li A, Dubowitz M, et al. Association between atopy and variants of the β subunit of the high-affinity immunoglobulin E receptor. Nature Genet 1994; 7: 125–129.

18. Marsh DG, Neely JD, Breazeale DR, et al. Linkage analysis of IL-4 and other chromosome 5q31.1 markers and total serum IgE concentrations. Science 1994; 264: 1152–1156.

19. Meyers DA, Postma DS, Panhuysen CIM, et al. Evidence for a locus regulating total serum IgE levels mapping to chromosome 5. Genomics 1994; 23:464–470.

20. Borish L, Mascali JJ, Klinnert M, Leppert M, Rosenwasser LJ. SSC polymorphisms in interleukin genes. Hum Mol Genet 1994; 3:1710.

21. Rosenwasser LJ, Klemm DJ, Dresback JK, et al. Promoter polymorphisms in the chromosome 5 gene cluster in asthma and atopy. Clin Exp Allergy 1995; 25:74.

22. Postma DS, Bleecker ER, Amelung PJ, et al. Genetic susceptibility to asthma-bronchial hyperresponsiveness coinherited with a major gene for atopy. N Engl J Med 1995; 333:894–900.

23. Orit M, Zuzuki Y, Sekiya T, Hayashi K. Rapid and sensitive detection of point mutations and DNA polymorphisms using polymerase chain reaction. Genomics 1989; 5:874–879.

24. Orita M, Iwahana H, Kanazawa H, Hayashi K, Sekiya T. Detection of polymorphisms of human DNA by gel electrophoresis as a single-stranded conformation polymorphism. Proc Natl Acad Sci USA 1989; 86:2766–2770.

25. Rao A. NFATp: a transcription factor required for the coordinate induction of several cytokine genes. Immunol Today 1994; 15:274–281.

8

The Genetics of Mouse Mast Cell Proteases

RICHARD L. STEVENS

Harvard Medical School
Boston, Massachusetts

I. Introduction

The mast cell is a tissue-localized effector cell of the immune response that releases diverse types of cytokines, arachidonic acid metabolites, and preformed mediators when activated. Because most mast cells in the bronchial mucosa of individuals with asthma are either partially or completely degranulated, mast cells have been implicated in this disease. The mast cell can be distinguished from all other immune cells by the number, type, and amount of proteases in its secretory granules. As much as 50% of the total protein of the mast cell consists of granule proteases that are enzymatically active at neutral pH. Thus, mast cells are the major source of neutral protease in the lung. Proteases have been purified from in-vivo- and in-vitro-differentiated mouse, rat, dog, and human mast cells. Based on their N-terminal amino acid sequences, nucleic acid libraries have been screened with relevant synthetic oligonucleotides to obtain cDNAs and genes that encode these proteases. Although mast cell proteases have been implicated in the catabolism of extracellular matrix proteins, membrane proteins, serum proteins, and cytokines, the specific substrates of these proteases remain to be elucidated. Each protease has a novel set of amino acids in its substrate-binding cleft, and thus probably catabolizes a limited number of proteins. X-ray crystallographic studies and three-dimensional protein modeling studies have provided understanding of how mast cell proteases are packaged in the granule; genomic organization studies have yielded knowledge about how their genes probably evolved. The development of gene-specific probes and specific antibodies directed against mast cell proteases have also contributed greatly to our understanding of the factors that regulate the growth, differentiation, and maturation of this important effector cell. In this review, mouse mast cell proteases, their genes, and the cytokines that regulate their expression are discussed.

II. Mouse Mast Cell Proteases

A. Identification, Cloning, and Characterization

Mouse mast cells express varied combinations of seven distinct serine proteases [designated mouse mast cell protease (mMCP) 1 to mMCP-7] and two exopeptidases [designated mouse mast cell carboxypeptidase A (mMC-CPA) and leucine aminopeptidase] [1–15]. The derivation of relatively mature, but transformed, mouse mast cells by co-culturing hematopoietic progenitor cells with fibroblasts producing Kirsten sarcoma virus and the leukemia helper virus 4070 [16] was essential for obtaining the protein sequence data that enabled the cloning of the cDNAs and genes for these proteases. When secretory granule proteins from immortalized mouse mast cells were separated by sodium dodecyl sulfate-polyacrylamide gel electrophoresis (SDS-PAGE), transblotted to polyvinylidene difluoride membranes, and subjected to N-terminal amino acid sequencing, mMC-CPA and four distinct serine proteases were identified [1,5]. None of these proteases possessed the amino terminus of mMCP-1, a 26-kDa serine protease purified by Newlands and co-workers [2,3] from the mast cells that reside in the intestines of *Trichinella spiralis*-infected mice. cDNA libraries were prepared from phenotypically distinct transformed and nontransformed mouse mast cells. When these libraries were screened with redundant oligonucleotides constructed on the basis of the obtained amino acid sequences, cDNAs were isolated that encode all granule proteases so far identified in mouse mast cells except mMCP-3 [5] and leucine aminopeptidase [11]. The gene for mMCP-7 [12] was obtained before its cDNA by screening a mouse genomic library with a mMCP-6 cDNA [9]. Its cDNA was then isolated by probing a cDNA library with a fragment from the isolated mMCP-7 gene. The amino acid sequence of mMCP-1 was first deduced by means of a classical protein sequencing strategy [3] rather than by cDNA and/or genomic cloning. The mMCP-1 gene was obtained by screening a mouse cosmid genomic library with an oligonucleotide that corresponded to the 5′ region of a rat mast cell protease [10]; a mMCP-1 cDNA was isolated by polymerase chain-reaction methodology from interleukin (IL)-10-treated, mouse bone marrow-derived mast cells (mBMMC) [15].

Based on their deduced amino acid sequences, mMCP-1, mMCP-2, mMCP-4, and mMCP-5 are more homologous to pancreatic chymotrypsin than to trypsin. Thus, even though their substrate specificities still have not been deduced, these proteases are often called chymases. All mMCPs are synthesized as zymogens but are stored in the granule in a mature, enzymatically active state. For example, prepro-mMCP-1 possesses an 18-amino acid signal peptide and a Glu-Glu activation peptide [3,10,15]. Presumably, the hydrophobic signal peptide is removed in the endoplasmic reticulum, but the site where the activation peptide is removed is not known. Mature mMCP-1 consists of 206 amino acids and has a net +3 charge at pH 7.0. mMCP-2 is an ~28-kDa serine protease and has a net +7 charge at pH 7.0 [5,6]. Whether or not any of the mast cell chymases are glycoproteins has not been determined, but mMCP-1, mMCP-2, and mMCP-5 all possess at least one Asn-linked glycosylation site. mMCP-4 has a net +15 charge at pH 7.0 and is the only chymase that lacks an Asn-linked glycosylation site [7]. In the course of cloning the mMCP-4 gene, a gene was also isolated that encodes a serine protease (designated mMCP-L) that is ~70% identical to mMCP-4 [7]. mMCP-L has not yet been found in any population of in-vivo-differentiated mast cells, but it may be expressed by an immature Abelson virus-transformed mouse mast cell line [13]. If mMCP-L is expressed in vivo, it would represent the eighth serine protease expressed by nontransformed mouse mast cells. Based on its cDNA and gene [8], prepro-mMCP-5 contains a distinct 19-residue hydrophobic signal peptide and a Gly-Glu activation peptide rather than a Glu-Glu activation peptide as found in mMCP-1, mMCP-2, and mMCP-4. Mature mMCP-5 is ~30 kDa, consists of 226 amino acids, and like mMCP-4 has a high net charge of +12 at pH 7.0. Models of their three-dimensional structures have revealed that mMCP-4 and mMCP-5 have two regions with net charges ranging from +6 to +10 on their surfaces located far from the substrate-binding clefts at diametrically opposite ends of the folded proteases [17]. These positively charged regions are probably heparin-binding sites. The overall amino acid sequence homology of mMCP-5 with mMCP-1, mMCP-2, and mMCP-4 is only 49–59%, but the near identity of their prepro-amino acid sequences suggests that a common proteolytic mechanism activates all of them.

The mouse mast cell chymase family of serine proteases resembles granzymes B, C, E, and F in that they all contain three disulfide bonds rather than four as found in the mast cell tryptases and most other serine proteases. Data obtained from the X-ray crystallographic structures of rat mast cell protease II [18] and bovine chymotrypsin [19] and from the three-dimensional modeling of mMCP-1, mMCP-2, mMCP-4, and mMCP-5 [17] have revealed that the insertion of three additional amino acids near the N terminus and the deletion of seven to eight amino acids in the C terminus resulted in the loss of a disulfide bond and subtle but potentially important changes in the overall tertiary structures of these proteases. Because rat mast cell protease II, mMCP-1, mMCP-2, mMCP-4, and mMCP-5 all possess a loop of amino acids which extends out into their substrate-binding clefts, these seriene protease probably exhibit more limited substrate specificity than pancreatic chymotrypsin. This conclusion suggests that the immune system tightly regulates the activities of its serine proteases.

mMCP-6 [9] and mMCP-7 [12] are more similar to pancreatic trypsin than to chymotrypsin, and thus these two mast cell-derived serine proteases are often called tryptases. mMCP-6 and mMCP-7 are also initially translated as zymogens, but they both contain activation peptides of Ala-Pro-Arg-Pro-Ala-Asn-Gln-Arg-Val-Gly rather than Gly-Glu or Glu-Glu. Since the 10-residue activation peptide is conserved, a proteolytic mechanism distinct from that which activates the chymases must convert both pro-mMCP-6 and pro-mMCP-7 to mature, biologically active enzymes. Mature mMCP-7 is 71–76% homologous with mMCP-6 [9] and with dog [20] and human [21–23] mast cell tryptases. mMCP-7 contains Asn-linked oligosaccharides [24], but the structures of its glycans remain to be deduced. At pH 5.6, the pH of the secretory granule, mMCP-6 and mMCP-7 have net charges of +6 and +4, respectively, and thus are probably ionically bound to serglycin proteoglycans like mMCP-1 to mMCP-5. However, because mMCP-6 and mMCP-7 are histidine-rich proteins, they are acidic at pH 7.0, possessing net charges of −5 and −10. When exocytosed from the mast cell into a more neutral pH environment, mMCP-7 presumably dissociates from its proteoglycan (Ghildyal et al., unpublished observation), as originally reported for human lung tryptases [25–27].

mMC-CPA [4] is also translated as a zymogen but, unlike the mMCPs, its activation peptide consists of 94 amino acids. This pro-peptide is similar in size to that of pancreatic carboxypeptidases [28–30]. In the pancreatic carboxypeptidases, the pro-peptides inhibit enzymatic activities by physically covering the substrate-binding clefts of the exopeptidases [31]. Despite the fact that its pro-peptide is considerably larger than the two-residue pro-peptides of the mouse mast cell chymases, the amino acid sequences that are cleaved to activate mMC-CPA [4], human MC-CPA [32,33], and the chymase mMCPs [3,5–8,10,14] are nearly identical. Thus, the same processing mechanism may be used in the posttranslational modification of these different granule proteases. After the signal and activation peptides are removed, mature mMC-CPA has a molecular weight of 36 kDa. mMC-CPA is an exopeptidase that attacks C-terminal aromatic and aliphatic amino acids [1]. Because mMC-CPA is expressed together with mMCP-5 [4,5,8,15,34–37] and because both are exocytosed from mast cells as a macromolecular complex with heparin proteoglycan [1,5,38], they likely work in concert to catabolize the same proteins.

B. Genomic Organization

Each mast cell-specific protease gene was isolated from a genomic library derived from the BALB/c mouse. Thus, they represent distinct genes rather than allelic variations or alternative spliced forms of a single gene. The size and exon/intron organization of the mmC-CPA gene has not been determined, but the human gene is 32 kb and contains 11 exons [33]. In contrast, all mMCP genes are <4 kb and contain either 5 or 6 exons. The 5′ flanking region of the mMCP-2 gene immediately upstream of its transcription-initiation site exhibits homology to the corresponding 5′ flanking regions of the mMCP-1, mMCP-4, and mMCP-5 genes of 89%, 93%, and 42%, respectively [39]. This finding suggests that common *trans*-acting factors control transcription of many of these chymase genes. Somewhat of a surprise is the relatively high degree of conservation of intron 1. Whereas the overall amino acid sequences of mMCP-1 and mMCP-2 are only 66% identical, 81% of the nucleotides in the first intron of these two genes are the same. The first intron of the mMCP-4 gene also exhibits substantial homology with the corresponding intron in the mMCP-1 and mMCP-2 genes, suggesting that this intron contains *cis*-acting regulatory elements. The mMCP-6 gene contains six exons [9] rather than five as in the mMCP-7 gene [12]. A comparison of the 5′ end of the transcript with the genomic sequence indicated that the region corresponding to the first intron in the mMCP-6 gene is not spliced during transcription of mMCP-7 mRNA because of a point mutation at the intron 1 acceptor splice site. The 5′ untranslated region of mMCP-7 transcript is 195 nucleotides, and therefore is longer than any other mast cell-specific transcript.

Serine protease genes have been found on numerous chromosomes. For example, the genes that encode pancreatic chymotrypsin and pancreatic trypsin reside on chromosomes 8 and 6, respectively [40,41]. The inheritance patterns of restriction-enzyme fragment length polymorphisms of genes in recombinant in-bred mouse strains and interspecific backcrosses were used to determine the chromosomal locations of the mMCP-1, mMCP-2, mMCP-4, mMCP-5, mMCP-6, and mMC-CPA genes [39]. The mMCP-6 and mMC-CPA genes reside on chromosomes 17 and 3, respectively, whereas the four mast cell chymase genes all reside on chromosome 14 linked to a gene complex that encodes neutrophil cathepsin G [42] and four cytotoxic T lymphocyte granzymes [43,44]. As assessed by pulsed field gel electrophoresis of genomic DNA digests, the mMCP-1, mMCP-2, and mMCP-5 genes are within 850 kb of each other [39]. Mapping studies have revealed that an uncharacterized gene and the mMCP-1 gene are only ~7 kb apart and are aligned end to end on chromosome 14. The significance of the clustering of the mMCP-1, mMCP-2, mMCP-4, and mMCP-5 genes on chromosome 14 in the genome of the mouse is unknown. Nevertheless, the observation that at least two of the mMCP genes are extremely close together raises the possibility that a *cis*-acting element can regulate the transcription of two or more mMCPs. As pointed out above, the substrate specificities of the serine proteases encoded by genes at the chromosome 14 complex are predicted to be more restricted than those of pancreatic chymotrypsin and pancreatic trypsin. Thus, a primordial gene that encoded a serine protease with more restricted substrate specificity than chymotrypsin likely underwent extensive duplication and divergence to form a family of genes on chromosome 14 that are preferentially expressed in hematopoietic cells.

C. Cytokine- and Tissue-Regulated Expression

Mouse mast cells are heterogeneous in tissues despite the fact that they all originate from a multipotential hematopoietic stem cell. Unlike most other hematopoietic-derived cells, mast cells do not circulate as mature cells. Thus, the key events in proliferation, differentiation, maturation, and associated functions are tissue-regulated by cell/cell interactions and encounters with soluble local factors. Because cDNAs have been isolated that encode eight mouse mast cell proteases, the steady-state levels of the various protease transcripts can be monitored in different populations of mast cells. The deduction of the amino acid sequences of these proteases has also resulted in the determination of their tertiary structures [17,45] and identification of hypervariable amino acid sequences on the outer surface of the translated proteases that are suitable for obtaining protease-specific antibodies. Affinity-purified rabbit antibodies have been prepared against synthetic peptides that correspond to novel amino acid sequences in mMCP-2 [36], mMCP-5 [46], mMCP-7 [24], and mMC-CPA [47]. These protease-specific antibodies and cDNAs have permitted the identification of new mast cell subclasses in tissues. They also have been invaluable for elucidating the events by which soluble and cell-associated factors regulate the development of mast cell-committed progenitor cells as they migrate from the bone marrow to their final tissue destination for terminal differentiation and maturation.

The safranin$^+$ serosal mast cells of the BALB/c mouse contain high steady-state levels of the transcripts that encode mMCP-4, mMCP-5, and mMCP-6, but not mMCP-1, mMCP-2, or mMCP-7. In contrast, the safranin$^-$ mucosal mast cells that proliferate in the intestines of helminth-infected BALB/c mice contain high steady-state levels of the mMCP-1 and mMCP-2 transcripts, but not the mMCP-4, mMCP-5, mMCP-6, or mMCP-7 transcripts. Mouse bone marrow cells from BALB/c mice cultured in medium containing IL-3 yield mBMMC that contain high steady-state levels of the mMCP-5, mMCP-6, mMCP-7, and mMC-CPA transcripts, but not the mMCP-1, mMCP-2, or mMCP-4 transcripts. Because the mast cell-deficient WBB6F$_1$-*W/W^v* (*W/W^v*) mouse reconstituted with mBMMC from its normal littermate has cells in its stomach muscularis propria that histochemically resemble serosal mast cells and cells in its stomach mucosa that histochemically resemble mucosal mast cells [48], it has been concluded that mBMMC can function in vivo as a precursor for different subclasses of mast cells. That the mMCP-7 transcript is not present in the serosal and mucosal mast cells of the BALB/c mouse but is present in 3-week-old mBMMC from this strain [12] suggested that if mMCP-7 is expressed in vivo it would define an additional mast cell phenotype. Different tissues of the BALB/c mouse were therefore examined for the expression of mMCP-7. Because high steady-state levels of the mMCP-7 transcript and immunoreactive protein were found in the ear and skin [49], it is now clear that not all safranin⁺ mast cells in the BALB/c mouse express the same granule proteases.

Nontransformed, but immature, mBMMC obtained by culturing bone marrow progenitor cells in conditioned medium containing IL-3 [50–53] provided an excellent in-vitro system for the study of cytokine/factor-dependent regulation of gene expression. Although other cytokines regulate the growth, differentiation, and maturation of mBMMC, IL-3, IL-4, IL-9, IL-10, and c-*kit* ligand (KL) are the five mast cell-regulatory cytokines that have been most extensively studied. Unlike IL-3, KL by itself does not promote the preferential differentiation in vitro of bone marrow cells into mast cells [34]. BALB/c mBMMC exposed to KL for 7 to 14 days in the absence of IL-3 express heparin proteoglycan and high levels of the mMCP-4 transcript, but the resulting mast cells are considerably less mature than serosal mast cells in terms of their granule ultrastructure, histamine content, and level of mMC-CPA enzymatic activity [34,54]. IL-9 and IL-10 both regulate the growth of mast cells [55,56] and induce BALB/c mBMMC to express the mucosal mast cell proteases, mMCP-1 and mMCP-2 [15,35–37]. However, unlike the mast cells in the intestines of helminth-infected BALB/c mice, IL-9- and IL-10-treated mBMMC continue to express mMCP-5, mMCP-6, and mMC-CPA. Neither IL-3 nor IL-4 affects the steady-state levels of the mMCP-5, mMCP-6, and mMC-CPA transcripts in BALB/c mBMMC. Nevertheless, both cytokines suppress the IL-10- and IL-9-induced expression of mMCP-1 and mMCP-2 and the KL-induced expression of mMCP-4.

W/W^v mice and WCB6F$_1$-Sl/Sl^d (Sl/Sl^d) mice have almost no skin mast cells [57,58] because they possess defects in their c-*kit* [59] and KL [60,61] genes, respectively. Thus, whether acting directly or indirectly, KL and its receptor are required for the development of skin mast cells in vivo. Although it was originally concluded that Sl/Sl^d and W/W^v mice had decreased numbers of mast cell-committed progenitor cells in their bone marrow, Yung and Moore [62] showed that large numbers of mBMMC can be generated simply by culturing the hematopoietic cells from these mice in IL-3-enriched conditioned medium. Surprisingly, the mBMMC derived from W/W^v and Sl/Sl^d mice differed from BALB/c mBMMC in that they contained high steady-state levels of every granule protease transcript expressed by the mature ear and skin mast cells of their normal +/+ littermates (i.e., mMC-CPA, mMCP-2, mMCP-4, mMCP-5, mMCP-6, and mMCP-7) [63]. Thus, in these mouse strains, c-*kit*-mediated signal transduction is not essential for inducing transcription of those genes that encode the granule proteases of cutaneous mast cells.

Based on in-vitro studies, it has been proposed that KL regulates many steps in the development of mast cells, but its essential function probably is to retain mast cell-committed progenitor cells in tissues. Flanagan and co-workers [60,61] first noted that, unlike other mast cell regulatory cytokines, KL possesses a membrane-spanning domain that causes it to be retained in the plasma membrane of the KL-producing cell. They therefore proposed that KL might function more as an adherence factor than a growth/differentiation/maturation factor. Adachi and co-workers [64] found that the extracellular domain of c-*kit* promotes the attachment of mBMMC to fibroblasts, and Gordon and Galli [65] found that substantial numbers of mast cells can be transiently elicited in the phorbol ester-treated skin of the W/W^v mouse but not the Sl/Sl^d mouse. The observation that normal numbers of safranin$^+$ mast cells appear in the skin of the W/W^v mouse when high concentrations of IL-3 are perfused into the animal [66] and the observation that IL-3 derived mBMMC exhibit the granule protease phenotype [63] of cutaneous mast cells [49] indicate that high levels of IL-3 can compensate for a signal transduction abnormality in c-*kit* to promote the viability and differentiation of progenitor cells into cutaneous mast cells. Because the ligand-binding domain of c-*kit* is still functional in the W/W^v mouse, presumably its mast cell-committed progenitor cells are retained in the skin by binding to KL on the surface of skin fibroblasts and/or keratinocytes. Normally, these progenitor cells cannot differentiate into mast cells because c-*kit* possesses a defect in its signal-transduction domain. However, during an inflammatory reaction in the W/W^v mouse, it is likely that soluble mast cell regulatory cytokines such as IL-3 are generated and released from activated T cells, fibroblasts, and/or keratinocytes. These cytokines can then act through their specific receptors to induce the progenitor cells to differentiate into mast cells. In the Sl/Sl^d mouse, KL is continuously secreted because it lacks a transmembrane domain. Thus, no mast cell-committed progenitor cells can be retained long enough in the tissue for IL-3 to exert its effects during an inflammatory reaction.

D. Strain-Dependent Expression of mMCP-7

In contrast to ear mast cells of the BALB/c mouse and four other strains of mice [49], the ear mast cells of the C57BL/6 mouse do not contain detectable levels of mMCP-7 transcript or protein [24]. Since mMCP-7 mRNA and protein also were not detected in mBMMC from the C57BL/6 mouse, the mMCP-7 gene may be defective in this strain. Alternatively, there may be an abnormality either in the mast cell-committed progenitor cells themselves or in the bone marrow microenvironment that prevents the mast cell-committed progenitor cell from expressing this tryptase. No matter how it occurs, these data indicate that certain mast cell granule proteases can be expressed in mice in a strain-specific manner. It is therefore possible that genetic differences contribute to the determination of which mast cell proteases are expressed in the lungs of normal individuals and those with asthma. The physiologic consequences of the failure of the mast cells of the C57BL/6 mouse to express mMCP-7 remain to be determined. However, the C57BL/6 mouse differs from the BALB/c mouse in its immunologic response to a variety of inflammatory agents. For example, the airway responsiveness of the BALB/c mouse to intravenous infusion of 5-hydroxytryptamine or acetylcholine is greater than that of the C57BL/6 mouse [67]. Because dog mastocytoma tryptase can cleave the bronchodilator, vasoactive intestinal peptide, but not the bronchoconstrictor, substance P [68], mMCP-7 may play a role in bronchial responsiveness.

E. Transcriptional Regulation of the mMC-CPA Gene

Based on studies of in-vitro-derived mast cells, which protease a mast cell expresses is regulated in part at the level of gene transcription. The GATA family of transcription factors has been detected in several mouse and rat mast cell lines that express mMC-CPA [69,70]. However, GATA-1 mRNA was not detected in P815 cells, a mouse mastocytoma-derived cell line [71] that no longer contains electron-dense granules or high levels of preformed mediators. Because the 5′ flanking regions of the mouse and human MC-CPA genes contain a conserved GATA-binding motif 51-base pairs upstream of their translation-initiation sites, the ability of GATA-binding proteins to regulate the promoter activity of the mMC-CPA gene was investigated with a rat mast cell line. The 160 nucleotides immediately upstream of the transcription-initiation site of the mMC-CPA gene exhibited substantial promoter activity in rat basophilic leukemia cells [70]. Site-directed mutagenesis analysis revealed that the conserved GATA motif in the 5′ flanking region of the mMC-CPA gene was essential for its promoter activity. Although many GATA transcription factors have been identified in the mouse, different cell types express varied combinations of these DNA binding proteins. Studies on the platelet factor 4 gene have revealed that the GATA family of DNA-binding proteins can promote transcription in some cells and suppress transcription in others [72]. Because GATA-2 is widely distributed [73], this transcription factor may suppress transcription of the mMC-CPA gene in nonmast cells.

F. Granule Accumulation of Translated Proteases

The granule phenotype of the mast cell is regulated not only at the mRNA level but also at the protein level. mMCP-specific cDNAs and antibodies have been used to monitor the relationship of mRNA to protein levels when bone marrow progenitor cells differentiate into immature mBMMC in response to IL-3 and when mBMMC differentiate further in response to fibroblast co-culture [74] or exposure to other cytokines [15,34–37]. mMCP-5 and mMC-CPA have been detected in serosal mast cells by N-terminal amino acid analysis of SDS-PAGE-resolved cellular proteins [4,5] and by immunohistochemistry [46,47]; yet serosal mast cells have extremely low levels of total RNA [75]. In contrast, the amounts of mMCP-5

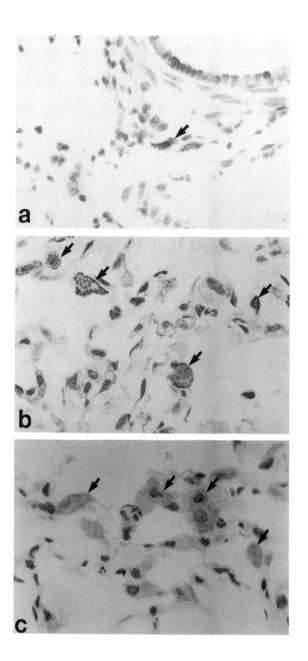

mRNA and mmC-CPA mRNA in mBMMC are substantially greater than those in serosal mast cells, but at no time are the amounts of mMCP-5 or mmC-CPA immunoreactive protein in mBMMC comparable to those in serosal mast cells. Thus, as mBMMC are currently developed in culture, either most of their mMCP-5 and mmC-CPA transcripts are not translated, or if they are translated, the expressed proteases are rapidly degraded or continually exocytosed. The preferential accumulation of proteases in the granule (i.e., granule maturation) during fibroblast coculture [1] might be a consequence of the mesenchymal cell providing a signal or factor that induces mBMMC to form the correct macro-molecular complexes with serglycin proteoglycans in the developing granule or the Golgi, where glycosaminoglycan biosynthesis onto the serglycin peptide core is completed.

Although in-vitro experiments discussed above indicated that BALB/c mBMMC could be induced to express certain granule proteases, it was not clear if a mast cell could reversibly alter its granule phenotype once a particular protein was expressed. The mMCP-2-specific antibody, anti-mMCP-2$_{(56-71)}$ IgG, has been used to study the relationship between mRNA levels and protein accumulation in BALB/c mBMMC stimulated with IL-10 and to study the reversibility of mMCP-2 expression after IL-10 is withdrawn [36]. Time-course analyses revealed that BALB/c mBMMC expressed a high steady-state level of mMCP-2 mRNA 24 h after they are exposed to IL-10. As assessed by SDS-PAGE/immunoblots, a small amount of mMCP-2 protein is present in the cells treated for 24 h, but large amounts of this protease are not obtained until after 7 days of treatment with IL-10. The steady-state level of mMCP-2 mRNA decreases dramatically 24 h after IL-10 is removed, but the level of mMCP-2 protein does not decline measurably until day 5 of culture. The ability to alter reversibly which proteases are expressed by a nontransformed mast cell in vitro now raises the possibility that a mature mast cell residing in a specific tissue can reversibly alter its granule phenotype. These studies indicate the importance of monitoring both protein and mRNA levels before drawing a conclusion about the granule phenotype of a particular mast cell.

Figure 1   Histochemistry and Immunohistochemistry of Mast Cells in the Lungs of a Normal BALB/c Mouse and a V3-Mastocytosis Mouse. Mast cells are rare in the lungs of a normal BALB/c mouse (panel a) but increase in number 2 to 3 weeks after the adoptive transfer of a v-*abl*-immortalized mast cell line (panels b and c). Panels a and b represent tissue sections stained with methylene blue. Panel c depicts a replicate tissue section stained with anti-mMCP-7 Ig. Arrows indicate mast cells. Figure courtesy of Dr. Daniel Friend (Harvard Medical School). (For optimal reproduction, see color plate.)

III. Future Directions

Mast cells are important in pathobiological settings because of their ability to exocytose diverse types of neutral proteases. However, further studies are needed to understand the mechanisms that regulate their expression, to characterize the individual substrate specificities of the proteases, and to relate the protease phenotype of tissue mast cells to their capacity to modulate in-vivo responses. The cloning of the cDNAs and genes that encode eight mouse mast cell proteases now allows the use of different molecular approaches to investigate their biological functions. For example, gene targeting approaches are already underway to ablate specific mast cell protease genes. By disrupting the mast cell protease genes, in-vivo functions related to mast cell distribution and phenotype can be considered and perhaps assessed in transgenic animals that subsequently receive the appropriate pathobiological challenge. Expression studies are also underway to obtain enough of each recombinant protease to elucidate the substrate specificities and metabolism of these proteases. Lastly, because the V3 mastocytosis mouse contains large numbers of mast cells in its lungs 2 weeks after the adoptive transfer of a v-*abl*-immortalized cell line into recipient mice (Fig. 1), it is anticipated that this animal model will be invaluable for investigating the role of specific mast cell mediators in lung function.

References

1. Serafin WE, Dayton ET, Gravallese PM, Austen KF, Stevens RL. Carboxypeptidase A in mouse mast cells: identification, characterization, and use as a differentiation marker. J Immunol 1987; 139:3771–3776.
2. Newlands GFJ, Gibson S, Knox DP, Grencis R, Wakelin D, Miller HRP. Characterization and mast cell origin of a chymotrypsin-like proteinase isolated from intestines of mice infected with *Trichinella spiralis*. Immunology 1987; 62:629–634.
3. Le Trong H, Newlands GFJ, Miller HRP, Charbonneau H, Neurath H, Woodbury RG. Amino acid sequence of a mouse mucosal mast cell protease. Biochemistry 1989; 28: 391–395.
4. Reynolds DS, Stevens RL, Gurley DS, Lane WS, Austen KF, Serafin WE. Isolation and molecular cloning of mast cell carboxypeptidase A: a novel member of the carboxypeptidase gene family. J Biol Chem 1989; 264:20094–20099.
5. Reynolds DS, Stevens RL, Lane WS, Carr MH, Austen KF, Serafin WE. Different mouse mast cell populations express various combinations of at least six distinct mast cell serine proteases. Proc Natl Acad Sci USA 1990; 87:3230–3234.
6. Serafin WE, Reynolds DS, Rogelj S, et al. Identification and molecular cloning of a novel mouse mucosal mast cell serine protease. J Biol Chem 1990; 265:423–429.
7. Serafin WE, Sullivan TP, Conder GA, et al. Cloning of the cDNA and gene for mouse mast cell protease 4. Demonstration of its late transcription in mast cell subclasses and

analysis of its homology to subclass-specific neutral proteases of the mouse and rat. J Biol Chem 1991; 266:1934–1941.

8. McNeil HP, Austen KF, Somerville LL, Gurish MF, Stevens RL. Molecular cloning of the mouse mast cell protease-5 gene. A novel secretory granule protease expressed early in the differentiation of serosal mast cells. J Biol Chem 1991; 266:20316–20322.

9. Reynolds DS, Gurley DS, Austen KF, Serafin WE. Cloning of the cDNA and gene of mouse mast cell protease-6. Transcription by progenitor mast cells and mast cells of the connective tissue subclass. J Biol Chem 1991; 266:3847–3853.

10. Huang R, Blom T, Hellman L. Cloning and structural analysis of mMCP-1, mMCP-4 and mMCP-5, three mouse mast cell-specific serine proteases. Eur J Immunol 1991; 21:1611–1621.

11. Serafin WE, Guidry UA, Dayton ET, Kamada MM, Stevens RL, Austen KF. Identification of aminopeptidase activity in the secretory granules of mouse mast cells. Proc Natl Acad Sci USA 1991; 88:5984–5988.

12. McNeil HP, Reynolds DS, Schiller V, et al. Isolation, characterization, and transcription of the gene encoding mouse mast cell protease 7. Proc Natl Acad Sci USA 1992; 89:11174–11178.

13. Johnson DA, Barton GJ. Mast cell tryptases: examination of unusual characteristics by multiple sequence alignment and molecular modeling. Protein Sci 1992; 1: 370–377.

14. Chu W, Johnson DA, Musich PR. Molecular cloning and characterization of mouse mast cell chymases. Biochim Biophys Acta 1992; 1121:83–87.

15. Ghildyal N, McNeil HP, Stechschulte S, et al. IL-10 induces transcription of the gene for mouse mast cell protease-1, a serine protease preferentially expressed in mucosal mast cells of *Trichinella spiralis*-infected mice. J Immunol 1992; 149:2123–2129.

16. Reynolds DS, Serafin WE, Faller DV, et al. Immortalization of murine connective tissue-type mast cells at multiple stages of their differentiation by coculture of splenocytes with fibroblasts that produce Kirsten sarcoma virus. J Biol Chem 1988; 263:12783–12791.

17. Šali A, Matsumoto R, McNeil HP, Karplus M, Stevens RL. Three-dimensional models of four mouse mast cell chymases. Identification of proteoglycan binding regions and protease-specific antigenic epitopes. J Biol Chem 1993; 268:9023–9034.

18. Remington SJ, Woodbury RG, Reynolds RA, Matthews BW, Neurath H. The structure of rat mast cell protease II at 1.9-Å resolution. Biochemistry 1988; 27:8097–8105.

19. Tsukada H, Blow DM. Structure of α-chymotrypsin refined at 1.68 Å resolution. J Mol Biol 1985; 184:703–711.

20. Vanderslice P, Craik CS, Nadel JA, Caughey GH. Molecular cloning of dog mast cell tryptase and a related protease: structural evidence of a unique mode of serine protease activation. Biochemistry 1989; 28:4148–4155.

21. Miller JS, Westin EH, Schwartz LB. Cloning and characterization of complementary DNA for human tryptase. J Clin Invest 1989; 84:1188–1195.

22. Miller JS, Moxley G, Schwartz LB. Cloning and characterization of a second complementary DNA for human tryptase. J Clin Invest 1990; 86:864–870.

23. Vanderslice P, Ballinger SM, Tam EK, Goldstein SM, Craik CS, Caughey GH. Human mast cell tryptase: multiple cDNAs and genes reveal a multigene serine protease family. Proc Natl Acad Sci USA 1990; 87:3811–3815.

24. Ghildyal N, Friend DS, Freelund R, Austen KF, McNeil HP, Schiller V, Stevens RL. Lack of expression of the tryptase mouse mast cell protease 7 in mast cells of the C57BL/6J mouse. J Immunol 1994; 153:2624–2630.

25. Schwartz LB, Lewis RA, Austen KF. Tryptase from human pulmonary mast cells: purification and characterization. J Biol Chem 1981; 256:11939–11943.

26. Schwartz LB, Bradford TR. Regulation of tryptase from human lung mast cells by heparin. Stabilization of the active tetramer. J Biol Chem 1986; 261:7372–7379.

27. Schechter NM, Eng GY, McCaslin DR. Human skin tryptase: kinetic characterization of its spontaneous inactivation. Biochemistry 1993; 32:2617–2625.

28. Quinto C, Quiroga M, Swain WF, et al. Rat preprocarboxypeptidase A: cDNA sequence and preliminary characterization of the gene. Proc Natl Acad Sci USA 1982; 79:31–35.

29. Gardell SJ, Craik CS, Clauser E, et al. A novel rat carboxypeptidase, CPA2: characterization, molecular cloning, and evolutionary implications on substrate specificity in the carboxypeptidase gene family. J Biol Chem 1988; 33:17828–17836.

30. Clauser E, Gardell SJ, Craik CS, MacDonald RJ, Rutter WJ. Structural characterization of the rat carboxypeptidase A1 and B genes. J Biol Chem 1988; 263:17837–17845.

31. Guasch A, Coll M, Avilés FX, Huber R. Three-dimensional structure of porcine pancreatic procarboxypeptidase A. A comparison of the A and B zymogens and their determinants for inhibition and activation. J Mol Biol 1992; 224:141–157.

32. Reynolds DS, Gurley DS, Stevens RL, Sugarbaker DJ, Austen KF, Serafin WE. 1989. Cloning of cDNAs that encode human mast cell carboxypeptidase A, and comparison of the protein with mouse mast cell carboxypeptidase A and rat pancreatic carboxypeptidases. Proc Natl Acad Sci USA 1989; 86:9480–9484.

33. Reynolds DS, Gurley DS, Austen KF. Cloning and characterization of the novel gene for mast cell carboxypeptidase A. J Clin Invest 1992; 89:273–282.

34. Gurish MF, Ghildyal N, McNeil HP, Austen KF, Gillis S, Stevens RL. Differential expression of secretory granule proteases in mouse mast cells exposed to interleukin 3 and c-*kit* ligand. J Exp Med 1992; 175:1003–1012.

35. Ghildyal N, McNeil HP, Gurish MF, Austen KF, Stevens RL. Transcriptional regulation of the mucosal mast cell-specific protease gene, mMCP-2, by interleukin 10 and interleukin 3. J Biol Chem 1992; 267:8473–8477.

36. Ghildyal N, Friend DS, Nicodemus CF, Austen KF, Stevens RL. Reversible expression of mouse mast cell protease 2 mRNA and protein in cultured mast cells exposed to interleukin 10. J Immunol 1993; 151:3206–3214.

37. Eklund KK, Ghildyal N, Austen KF, Stevens RL. Induction by IL-9 and suppression by IL-3 and IL-4 of the levels of chromosome 14-derived transcripts that encode late-expressed mouse mast cell proteases. J Immunol 1993; 151:4266–4273.

38. Serafin WE, Katz HR, Austen KF, Stevens RL. Complexes of heparin proteoglycans, chondroitin sulfate E proteoglycans, and [^{3}H]diisopropyl fluorophosphate-binding

proteins are exocytosed from activated mouse bone marrow-derived mast cells. J Biol Chem 1986; 261:15017–15021.

39. Gurish MF, Nadeau JH, Johnson KR, et al. A closely linked complex of mouse mast cell-specific chymase genes on chromosome 14. J Biol Chem 1993; 268:11372–11379.

40. Watanabe T, Ogasawara N, Goto H. Genetic study of pancreatic proteinase in mice (*Mus musculus*): linkage of the Prt-2 locus on chromosome 8. Biochem Genet 1976; 14:999–1002.

41. Honey NK, Sakaguchi AY, Lalley PA, et al. Chromosomal assignments of genes for trypsin, chymotrypinogen B, and elastase in mouse. Somat Cell Molec Genet 1984; 10:377–383.

42. Heusel JW, Scarpati EM, Jenkins NA, et al. Molecular cloning, chromosomal location, and tissue-specific expression of the murine cathepsin G gene. Blood 1993; 81: 1614–1623.

43. Brunet JF, Dosseto M, Denizot F, et al. The inducible cytotoxic T-lymphocyte-associated gene transcript CTLA-1 sequence and gene localization to mouse chromosome 14. Nature 1986; 322:268–271.

44. Crosby JL, Bleackley RC, Nadeau JH. A complex of serine protease genes expressed preferentially in cytotoxic T-lymphocytes is closely linked to the T-cell receptor α- and δ-chain genes on mouse chromosome 14. Genomics 1990; 6:252–259.

45. Johnson DA, Barton GJ. Mast cell tryptases: examination of unusual characteristics by multiple sequence alignment and molecular modeling. Protein Sci 1992; 1: 370–377.

46. McNeil HP, Frenkel DP, Austen KF, Friend DS, Stevens RL. Translation and granule localization of mouse mast cell protease-5: Immunodetection with specific antipeptide Ig. J Immunol 1992; 149:2466–2472.

47. Gurish MF, Nicodemus CF, Ghildyal N, Austen KF, Stevens RL. Anti-peptide antibodies against the exopeptidase, mouse mast cell carboxypeptidase A (mMC-CPA). J Allergy Clin Immunol 1993; 89:309 (abstr).

48. Nakano T, Sonoda T, Hayashi C, et al. Fate of bone marrow-derived cultured mast cells after intracutaneous, intraperitoneal, and intravenous transfer into genetically mast cell-deficient *W/W^v* mice. J Exp Med 1985; 162:1025–1043.

49. Stevens RL, Friend DS, McNeil HP, Schiller V, Ghildyal N, Austen KR. Strain-specific and tissue-specific expression of mouse mast cell secretory granule proteases. Proc Natl Acad Sci USA 1994; 91:128–132.

50. Tertian G, Yung Y-P, Guy-Grand D, Moore MAS. Long-term *in vitro* culture of murine mast cells. I. Description of a growth factor-dependent culture technique. J Immunol 1981; 127:788–794.

51. Razin E, Cordon-Cardo C, Good RA. Growth of a pure population of mouse mast cells *in vitro* with conditioned medium derived from concanavalin A-stimulated splenocytes. Proc Natl Acad Sci USA 1981; 78:2559–2561.

52. Schrader JW, Lewis SJ, Clark-Lewis I, Culvenor JG. The persisting (P) cell: histamine content, regulation by a T cell-derived factor, origin from a bone marrow precursor, and relationship to mast cells. Proc Natl Acad Sci USA 1981; 78:323–327.

53. Razin E, Ihle JN, Seldin D, et al. Interleukin 3: a differentiation and growth factor for the mouse mast cell that contains chondroitin sulfate E proteoglycan. J Immunol 1984; 132:1479–1486.

54. Tsai M, Takeishi T, Thompson H, et al. Induction of mast cell proliferation, maturation, and heparin synthesis by the rat c-*kit* ligand, stem cell factor. Proc Natl Acad Sci USA 1991; 88:6382–6386.

55. Thompson-Snipes L, Dhar V, Bond MW, Mosmann TR, Moore KW, Rennick DM. Interleukin-10: a novel stimulatory factor for mast cells and their progenitors. J Exp Med 1991; 173:507–510.

56. Hültner L, Druez C, Moeller J, et al. Mast cell growth-enhancing activity (MEA) is structurally related and functionally identical to the novel mouse T cell growth factor P40/TCGFIII (interleukin 9). Eur J Immunol 1990; 20:1413–1416.

57. Kitamura Y, Go S, Hatanaka K. Decrease of mast cells in *W/W^v* mice and their increase by bone marrow transplantation. Blood 1978; 52:447–452.

58. Kitamura Y, Go S. Decreased production of mast cells in *Sl/Sl^d* anemic mice. Blood 1979; 53:492–497.

59. Geissler EN, Ryan MA, Housman DE. The dominant-white spotting (W) locus of the mouse encodes the c-*kit* proto-oncogene. Cell 1988; 55:185–192.

60. Flanagan JG, Leder P. The *kit* ligand: a cell surface molecule altered in steel mutant fibroblasts. Cell 1990; 63:185–194.

61. Flanagan JG, Chan DC, Leder P. Transmembrane form of the *kit* ligand growth factor is determined by alternative splicing and is missing in the *Sl^d* mutant. Cell 1991; 64: 1025–1035.

62. Yung Y-P, Moore MAS. Long-term *in vitro* culture of murine mast cells. III. Discrimination of mast cell growth factor and granulocyte-CSF. J Immunol 1992; 129:1256–1261.

63. Eklund KK, Ghildyal N, Austen KF, Friend DS, Schiller V, Stevens RL. Mouse bone marrow-derived mast cells (mBMMC) obtained *in vitro* from mice that are mast cell-deficient *in vivo* express the same panel of granule proteases as mBMMC and serosal mast cells from their normal littermates. J Exp Med 1994; 180:67–73.

64. Adachi S, Ebi Y, Nishikawa S, et al. Necessity of extracellular domain of W (c-*kit*) receptors for attachment of murine cultured mast cells to fibroblasts. Blood 1992; 79: 650–656.

65. Gordon JR, Galli SJ. Phorbol 12-myristate 13-acetate-induced development of functionally active mast cells in *W/W^v* but not *Sl/Sl^d* genetically mast cell-deficient mice. Blood 1990; 75:1637–1645.

66. Ody C, Kindler V, Vassalli R. Interleukin 3 perfusion in *W/W^v* mice allows the development of macroscopic hematopoietic spleen colonies and restores cutaneous mast cell number. J Exp Med 1990; 172:403–406.

67. Levitt RC, Mitzner W. Autosomal recessive inheritance of airway hyperreactivity to 5-hydroxytryptamine. J Appl Physiol 1989; 67:1125–1132.

68. Caughey GH, Leidig F, Viro NF, Nadel JA. Substance P and vasoactive intestinal peptide degradation by mast cell tryptase and chymase. J Pharmacol Exp Ther 1988; 244:133–137.

69. Martin DIK, Zon LI, Mutter G, Orkin SH. Expression of an erythroid transcription factor in megakaryocytic and mast cell lineages. Nature 1990; 344:444–437.

70. Zon LI, Gurish MF, Stevens RL, et al. GATA-binding transcription factors in mast cells regulate the promoter of the mast cell carboxypeptidase A gene. J Biol Chem 1991; 266:22948–22953.

71. Dunn TB, Potter M. A transplantable mast-cell neoplasm in the mouse. J Natl Cancer Inst 1957; 18:587–601.

72. Aird WC, Parvin JD, Sharp PA, Rosenberg RD. The interaction of GATA-binding proteins and basal transcription factors with GATA box-containing core promoters. J Biol Chem 1994; 269:883–889.

73. Yamamoto M, Ko LJ, Leonard MW, Beug H, Orkin SH, Engel JD. Activity and tissue specific expression of the transcription factor NF-E1 multigene family. Genes Dev 1990; 4:1650–1662.

74. Levi-Schaffer F, Austen KF, Gravallese PM, Stevens RL. Coculture of interleukin 3-dependent mouse mast cells with fibroblasts results in a phenotypic change of the mast cells. Proc Natl Acad Sci USA 1986; 83:6485–6488.

75. Benfey PN, Yin FH, Leder P. Cloning of the mast cell protease, RMCP II. Evidence for cell-specific expression and a multi-gene family. J Biol Chem 1987; 262:5377–5384.

9

The Regulation of IgE Synthesis

DONATA VERCELLI

San Raffaele Scientific Institute
Milan, Italy

Immunoglobulin (Ig) E plays a key role in the pathogenesis of asthma and allergic disease (reviewed in Refs. 1 and 2). The studies on the cellular basis of IgE regulation have provided important insights into a disease which affects a considerable proportion of the population, worldwide. More recently, the molecular events underlying IgE synthesis have been actively investigated, inasmuch as they represent an ideal model to characterize the signals involved in isotype-specific regulation of Ig synthesis.

In this chapter we discuss the cells, the cytokines, and the molecular mechanisms involved in human IgE synthesis.

I. Induction of IgE Synthesis: The Role of Cells and Cytokines

A. The Two-Signal Model for the Induction of IgE Synthesis

During an immune response, a B lymphocyte can express different immunoglobulin (Ig) heavy-chain isotypes sharing the same VDJ region. This phenomenon (isotype switching) allows a single B-cell clone to produce antibodies with the same fine specificity but different effector functions. In order to switch to a particular isotype, a B cell needs to receive two signals: Signal 1 is cytokine-dependent and results in the activation of transcription at a specific region of the Ig locus, thus determining isotype specificity. Signal 2 activates the recombination machinery, resulting in DNA switch recombination.

The two signals required for switching to IgE are delivered to B cells by T cells through a complex series of interactions. Allergen-specific B cells capture the antigen via their surface Ig molecules, internalize it, and process it into peptides which are then presented on the B-cell surface in association with MHC class II molecules. Recognition of the antigen/MHC class II complex by the T-cell receptor leads to two crucial events: the secretion of lymphokines, in particular IL-4, which provides the first signal for IgE induction, and the expression of CD40 ligand (CD40L). Notably, CD40L is absent on resting T cells, and it is the expression of this molecule following activation that renders T cells fully competent to induce IgE. Engagement of CD40 on B cells by its ligand on T cells delivers the signal that triggers switch recombination to IgE. Amplification circuits involving accessory molecules then lead to high-rate IgE synthesis.

Signal 1: IL-4 and IL-13

The interaction between IL-4 and IL-4 receptors (R) delivers the first signal for switching to IgE (Fig. 1). Evidence from different lines of inquiry consistently shows that IL-4 is essential for IgE production:

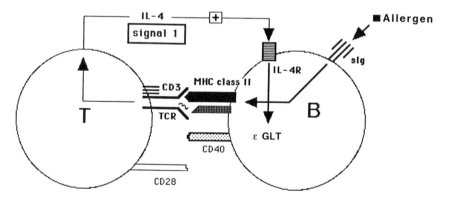

Figure 1 Steps in the induction of IgE synthesis. Engagement of the T-cell receptor/CD3 complex by the allergen presented on B cells triggers an initial wave of IL-4 production. The interaction between IL-4 and IL-4 receptor induces ε germline transcription, and delivers the first signal for switching to IgE.

IL-4 was the only cytokine able to induce IgE synthesis in vitro when added in recombinant form; injection of an anti-IL-4 antibody abolished IgE production in parasite-infected mice [3].

IL-4R exist in vivo not only as cell-bound molecules, but also in a soluble, circulating form. A recombinant extracellular IL-4R domain blocked switching to IgE by blocking IL-4/IL-4R interactions [4].

The same result was obtained using an IL-4 mutant in which a tyrosine at position 124 was replaced by aspartic acid [5]. The mutation preserves the ability to bind IL-4R, but destroys the capacity to transmit a signal upon receptor binding [6]. Both these experiments show that it is sufficient to block the IL-4 signal in order to block isotype switching to IgE, and IgE production.

The most compelling evidence for the central role of IL-4 in IgE induction comes from gene targeting experiments. Mice in which the IL-4 gene had been knocked out by homologous recombination (IL-4 KO mice) were unable to mount an antiparasite IgE response; the IgG1 response was also suppressed, although to a lesser extent, whereas the production of other isotypes was unaffected [7].

Furthermore, as detailed elsewhere in this book, genetic linkage analysis has shown that IL-4, or a nearby gene in the 5q31.1 region (e.g., IL-13, IL-5, IL-9), is responsible for the regulation of overall IgE production [8]. Polymorphism(s) in the regulatory region of these gene(s) may result in a predisposition to secrete abnormally high levels of IgE-inducing cytokines in response to antigen.

More recently, it has become clear that another cytokine, IL-13, shares many of the functional properties of IL-4, including the ability to induce IgE synthesis [9]. Although the sequence homology between IL-13 and IL-4 is only of ~30%, all residues that contribute to the hydrophobic core of IL-4 are conserved or have conservative hydrophobic replacements in IL-13 [6]. Furthermore, receptors for IL-4 and IL-13 share a subunit [6]. Indeed, an IL-4 mutant protein, which binds IL-4R with high affinity, competitively inhibits receptor binding of both IL-4 and IL-13, and blocks induction of IgE synthesis by both cytokines [5]. However, IL-4 and IL-13, as well as their receptors, are by no means identical. IL-13 does not bind to COS-3 cells transfected either with cDNAs for the 130-kDa IL-4R and/or the γ chain [10], and, unlike IL-4, has no effects on human T cells [6]. The elucidation of the respective roles of IL-4 and IL-13 in physiologic conditions will require information about the structure and distribution of IL-13R, as well as a detailed analysis of the mechanisms that control the expression of these cytokines. Preliminary data indicate that the kinetics of IL-4 and IL-13 production following antigen stimulation are quite different (J. de Vries, personal communication). Furthermore, it has recently been shown that naive CD4$^+$CD45R0$^-$ human T cells develop into effector cells that secrete IL-13, IL-5, and interferon (IFN)-γ, but not IL-4 upon T-cell receptor cross linking. These cells are able to efficiently help IgE production [11]. These findings suggest the intriguing possibility that, at least at certain stages of T-helper differentiation, the production of IL-13 and IL-4 may be independently regulated.

Signal 2: CD40/CD40L Interactions

The engagement of CD40 on B cells by CD40L expressed on T cells provides the second signal required for switching to IgE (Fig. 2). CD40L can be replaced in vitro by anti-CD40 monoclonal antibodies (mAbs). Indeed, this was the first experimental system in which the B-cell activating signal for human IgE synthesis was delivered by antibody-induced engagement of a discrete B-cell surface antigen.

CD40 is a 50-kDa surface glycoprotein expressed on human B lymphocytes [12], cytokine-activated monocytes [13], follicular dendritic cells [14], epithelial cells (including thymic epithelium) [15], and by certain carcinomas and melanomas, but not by T cells [16,17]. CD40 plays a key role in the survival, growth, and differentiation of B cells. Signaling through CD40 rescues B cells from apoptosis induced by Fas (CD95) or by cross-linking of the IgM complex [18,19]. Selected anti-CD40 mAbs trigger significant proliferation of highly purified resting B cells, in the absence of other co-stimuli [20].

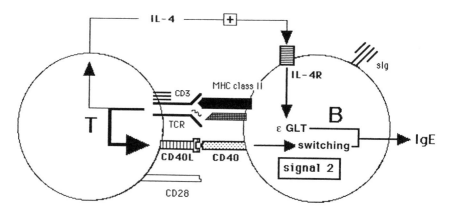

Figure 2 Steps in the induction of IgE synthesis. Engagement of the T-cell receptor/CD3 complex by the allergen presented on B cells results in the rapid expression of CD40 ligand. The engagement of CD40 on B cells by CD40 ligand provides the second signal required for switch recombination to IgE.

CD40 belongs to the TNFR superfamily, that includes TNFRI and TNFRII, NGFR, CD30, CD27, and Fas (CD95) (reviewed in Ref. 21). Members within this family share sequence similarity through their extracellular regions that contain multiple cysteine-rich repeats. The common structural framework of the extracellular domain is reflected by the ability of the TNFR superfamily members to interact with a parallel family of TNF-related molecules, which includes the ligands for CD40, CD27 and CD30, TNF-α, and lymphotoxin. CD40L is a 261-aa type 2 membrane glycoprotein, which is transiently expressed on activated, but not on resting, Th1 and Th2 cells [22]. Cells transfected with CD40L induced IgE synthesis by both murine [22] and human B cells [23], in the presence of IL-4, whereas a soluble CD40-Ig fusion protein inhibited IL-4-dependent IgE synthesis in human PBMC [24]. These results clearly indicated that CD40/CD40L interactions are critical in delivering the second signal required for IgE production. The central role of the CD40/CD40L pathway in IgE synthesis, and more generally, in isotype switching, was confirmed by the finding that defective switching in patients with X-linked hyper-IgM (HIM) syndrome is due to mutations in CD40L, which result in impaired CD40/CD40L interactions [25,26]. Furthermore, no IgG, IgA and IgE response to thymus-dependent antigens was detectable in CD40 [27,28] and CD40L [29] KO mice, and no germinal centers were recognizable in lymphoid organs. In contrast, responses to thymus-independent antigens were preserved. Finally, the inability of human newborn B cells to switch, and the consequent transient immunodeficiency observed in human neonates, has been ascribed to the decrease observed in both CD40L expression [30,31] and responses to CD40 agonists [32]. Thus, data from a number of in-vitro and in-vivo models consistently point to the crucial role of CD40/CD40L interactions in germinal center formation, B-cell activation, isotype switching, and antibody production. The molecular events that lead to isotype switching following CD40 engagement will be discussed below.

The interactions between CD40 and CD40L are tightly regulated. T cells become competent to activate B cells via CD40 only after they express CD40L, and this in turn requires TCR-dependent T-cell activation. The latter process seems to be anatomically constrained, i.e., CD40L is only expressed in secondary lymphoid tissues, at the site of cognate T/B-cell interactions. Interestingly, a subset of CD4$^+$ memory T cells in germinal centers contains preformed CD40L that is rapidly (within minutes), but transiently, expressed on the cell surface after TCR-mediated activation [33]. The speed at which T cells can express CD40L on their surface may be crucial in germinal centers, because centrocytes either leave the light zone within a few hours of activation, or die by apoptosis in situ. On the other hand, the availability of CD40L is drastically limited, because the interaction with CD40 induces rapid endocytosis of surface CD40L [34], and release of soluble CD40 by B cells downregulates CD40L mRNA [35].

CD40L, γ/δ T Cells, and IgE Regulation

CD40L has been shown to be expressed by both α/β and γ/δ activated T cells [36,37]. Because CD40L expression is lower on γ/δ than on α/β T cells, γ/δ T cells are less efficient in inducing IgE synthesis, but they are competent to induce isotype switching to IgE in vitro, in the presence of exogenous IL-4. The recent finding that mice congenitally deficient in α/β T cells produce Ig of all isotypes, with high levels of IgE and IgG1 [38], suggests that γ/δ T cells play a role in directing isotope switching in vivo, as well. The potential role of γ/δ T cells in the induction of IgE responses is further stressed by the recent observation that γ/δ T cells are able to discriminate early in infection between Th1- and Th2-inducing pathogens, and produce cytokines associated with the appropriate pattern of response. Cytokines produced by γ/δ T cells may not only aid in the direct elimination of certain pathogens, but also contribute to the cytokine milieu that influences the differentiation of CD4+ T cells into either Th1 or Th2 [39].

Interestingly, adoptive transfer of small numbers of γ/δ T cells from OVA-tolerant mice selectively suppressed Th2-dependent IgE synthesis, without affecting IgG responses. These γ/δ cells were CD8+, and produced large amounts of IFN-γ. These findings confirm the potential role of γ/δ T cells in the regulation of IgE responses, pointing to potentially different roles in different models.

Accessory Molecules and Amplification Circuits

Several pairs of accessory molecules (CD28/B7, LFA-1/ICAM-1, CD2/CD58) have been shown to participate in T/B-cell interactions conducive to IgE synthesis. Interactions within these ligand/receptor pairs complement and/or upregulate the T-cell-dependent activation of B cells that follows the engagement of CD40 by CD40L (Fig. 3). A major accessory role is likely to be played by the CD28/B7 ligand–receptor pair. CD28 KO mice have reduced basal Ig levels, and decreased class switching after infection with viruses [40]. Both CD28 on T cells and its B-cell counterreceptor, B7, are part of a reciprocal amplification mechanism that amplifies T/B-cell interactions mediated via CD40/CD40L. Engagement of CD40 is known to result in B7 expression on B cells [41]. On the other hand, engagement of CD28 results in increased expression of CD40L on T cells [42], and most importantly, in increased IL-4 secretion [42] and Th2 differentiation [43]. IL-4 in turn upregulates B7 expression [44]. Thus, CD28/B7 interactions may enhance both IL-4 secretion and CD40-mediated B-cell activation, and would ultimately potentiate both signal 1 and signal 2. Consistent with this view, IgE synthesis has recently been shown to be inhibited by anti-CD28 blocking mABs [45].

A marked increase in B7 expression is also induced by cross-linking MHC class II molecules on B cells, particularly when ICAM-1 is engaged simultaneously. Thus, interactions through MHC class II and ICAM-1 complement

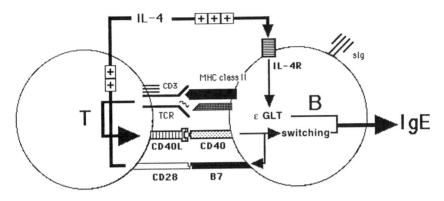

Figure 3   Steps in the induction of IgE synthesis. Engagement of CD40 on B cells results in the upregulation of B7. The interaction of B7 with CD28 on T cells provides the signal required for high-rate IL-4 secretion.

T-cell help provided via CD40/CD40L interactions [46]. In contrast, the weak IgE-inducing signal provided by engagement of CD58 (LFA-3) seems to be independent of the CD40 pathway [47].

Amplification of IgE Synthesis

Human basophils and mast cells have been recently reported to secrete IL-4 [48,49], and to express CD40L [50]. Thus, basophils and mast cells may in principle provide both signal 1 and signal 2 for IgE synthesis. However, these non-T cells conceivably play a role in IgE amplification, rather than in IgE induction. The optimal physiologic stimulus for secretion of IL-4 and IL-13 seems to be allergen-dependent cross-linking of receptor-bound, allergen-specific IgE [48,49]. Thus, cytokine secretion would be predicated on the production of allergen-specific IgE, and this in turn requires the signals and the cells (including allergen-specific T cells) discussed above. Once IgE has been produced, it can recruit basophils and mast cells by binding to their IgE receptors, thus inducing IL-4/IL-13 secretion and CD40L expression. Only at this point may non-T cells trigger an IgE response, which would not necessarily be allergen-specific, but may be polyclonal as well. This scenario is consistent with the observation that a significant proportion of the IgE response in hyper-IgE states is frequently polyclonal, rather than allergen-specific (Fig. 4).

CD40L was recently found to be constitutively expressed on eosinophils from one patient with the hypereosinophilic syndrome. However, these cells were not able to induce IgE synthesis in the presence of exogenous IL-4 [51]. The significance of this isolated observation therefore remains to be understood.

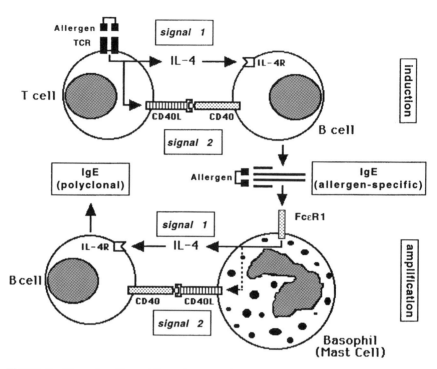

Figure 4   The role of basophils and mast cells in IgE regulation.

Conclusion: From a B Cell's Point of View

The complexity in the interplay among T cells, B cells, and cytokines involved in IgE induction makes it difficult to establish unambiguously a chronology of the events leading to IgE synthesis. On the other hand, the molecular studies discussed below clearly point to a hierarchy in the steps to IgE induction, and in the signals that trigger such steps. The initial event in switching to IgE is the determination of isotype specificity through cytokine (IL-4, IL-13)-dependent induction of ε germ-line transcription, which is followed by CD40-mediated DNA switch recombination. Our terminology of "signal 1" and "signal 2" therefore reflects a B-cell-centered perspective, although high-rate IL-4 secretion (signal 1) and full B-cell activation via CD40/CD40L (signal 2) may well enhance each other, and require CD28/B7 interactions.

B.   The Th1/Th2 Dichotomy and Potential T_H Markers

Studies with T-cell clones obtained from patients with atopic disease and parasitic infections clearly indicate that the lymphokine profile of T-cell clones specific for an antigen is determined both by the nature of the antigen and by the genetic background of the individual (reviewed in Ref. 52). The majority of helper T-cell clones specific for parasitic antigens, isolated from patients with no history of atopic disease, had a Th2 lymphokine profile; i.e., they produced high levels of IL-4, low IL-2 and IFN-γ, and induced vigorous IgE synthesis. On the other hand, allergen-specific CD4$^+$ T-cell clones established from atopic patients had a Th2 lymphokine profile and provided help for IgE synthesis, whereas helper T-cell clones from the same patients, specific for nonallergenic antigens, or CD4$^+$ clones from nonatopic individuals, had a Th1 profile [53–55]. Thus, antigens such as those expressed on parasites seem to be able to evoke a Th2/IgE response regardless of the genetic background. In contrast, the genetic background seems to be critical for the generation of a Th2/IgE response against allergens.

The factors ultimately responsible for skewing the T-helper repertoire toward Th1 or Th2 are discussed elsewhere in this book. Here, it is important to underline the existence of complex cytokine amplification loops, which significantly influence both T-helper differentiation and IgE regulation. Th2-derived IL-4 markedly inhibits IFN-γ production by human T cells [56,57], and furthermore directs the differentiation of precursor T cells into Th2 cells, which will secrete more IL-4 [58,59]. By contrast, IFN-γ promotes the differentiation of CD4$^+$ T cells into Th1 cells [58]. Thus, once an antigen has initially triggered a response—which will be Th1 or Th2 depending on the nature of the antigen and the genetic background of the individual—the antigen-specific T-cell repertoire will be progressively skewed, and more T cells with the same lymphokine profile will be recruited. IL-13, an IgE-inducing Th2 lymphokine, may represent an exception, in that it is not active on T cells [6], and therefore it does not contribute to Th2 skewing. The inability of IL-13 to promote Th2 differentiation may explain why Th2 responses were severely impaired in mice in which the IL-4 gene had been disrupted but the IL-13 gene was intact [7,60].

IL-12 may provide a link between natural and specific immune responses. IL-12 has been shown to skew the profile of the Th response toward Th1 [61]. The effects of IL-12 on Th differentiation seem to be in part direct, and in part mediated by the ability of IL-12 to induce IFN-γ production by both T cells and NK cells [61], because some viruses and intracellular bacteria have the ability to stimulate macrophages to produce IL-12, which in turn induces IFN-γ production by both T cells and NK cells. Thus, Th cells may be simultaneously presented with processed antigen plus cytokines that induce them to differentiate toward a Th1 phenotype [62].

Further understanding of the mechanisms underlying the Th1/Th2 dichotomy may be provided by ongoing studies aimed at identifying potential markers for Th1 and Th2 cells. It has recently been proposed that the ability of Th clones to produce Th-2-type lymphokines may correlate positively or negatively with the expression of two molecules, CD30 and CD27, that belong to the TNFR superfamily. The majority of human Th2 clones stimulated with the relevant allergen express CD30, and concomitantly secrete IL-4 and IL-5 [63], suggesting that CD30 may be associated with the differentiation/activation pathway of human T cells producing Th2-type cytokines. Furthermore, CD30 was expressed on Th2-like T-cell clones isolated from HIV patients with hyper-IgE syndrome [64]. These clones produced IL-4 and provided help for IgE synthesis, in spite of their CD8 phenotype [65,66]. These findings suggest that CD30 may be a marker for CD8$^+$ T cells that have switched to the production of type-2 helper cytokines.

A marker for Th1 cells has not been clearly identified, although this role has been recently proposed for LAG-3, a member of the immunoglobulin gene superfamily (S. Romagnani, personal communication). Because little is known about Th2 physiology, it is not yet clear how the expression of CD30 may result in a Th2 phenotype.

Recent findings have added further complexity to the already difficult issue of T-helper differentiation. A novel receptor involved in T-cell activation, SLAM, has been recently identified on memory human T cells and on a proportion of B cells [67]. Notably, engagement of SLAM resulted in a strong preferential induction of IFN-γ production, even in allergen-specific CD4$^+$ Th2 clones, thereby reversing the phenotype of those cells to a Th0 cytokine production profile. In contrast, the cytokine production pattern of Th1 clones was not altered by stimulation via SLAM [67]. The functional implications of these findings need to be investigated further.

C. T-Cell Independent IgE Induction: The Role of Epstein-Barr Virus (EBV) and Glucocorticoids

It has recently been shown that stimulation with IL-4 and EBV induces T-cell-independent IgE synthesis in human B cells [68,69]. IgE production results from de-novo induction of isotype switching, rather than from expansion of a precommitted sIgE$^+$ B-cell population that has switched to IgE in vivo [69].

The role played by EBV in IgE induction is not entirely clear. However, a clue was recently provided by the characterization of CD40 receptor-associated factor-1 (CRAF-1), a novel component of the CD40 signaling pathway [70,71]. The C terminus of CRAF-1 interacts directly and specifically with the cytoplasmic tail of CD40; overexpression of CRAF-1 interferes with CD40 signaling. Interestingly, the C terminus of CRAF-1 is homologous to the TNF-α receptor-associated factors 1 and 2 (TRAF1 and TRAF2), which can complex with the cytoplasmic tail of the related TNF-α receptor II [72]. The TRAF-C (for COOH-terminal) domain shared by CRAF-1, TRAF1, and TRAF2 is necessary and sufficient for CD40 binding, and for homodimerization. It is likely that other members of the TNFR superfamily use CRAF-related proteins in their signal transduction process. Interestingly, CRAF-1 also interacts with the cytoplasmic domain of EBV latent infection membrane protein 1 (LMP1) [73], an EBV-encoded integral membrane protein that is critical for B-lymphocyte transformation, and, most importantly, is the only EBV gene that has transforming effects in nonlymphoid cells. The IgE-inducing properties of EBV may indeed result from the ability of EBV-encoded protein(s) to activate the CD40 signaling pathway, thus providing B cells with signal 2.

IgE synthesis can be induced in highly purified, sIgE-normal [74] and leukemic [75] B cells by a combination of IL-4 and glucocorticoids (hydrocortisone). The effects of hydrocortisone are specific, inasmuch as steroid sex hormones have no influence on IL-4-dependent IgE synthesis [76]. The mechanisms by which hydrocortisone synergizes with IL-4 in vitro remain unknown. The observation that hormone–receptor interactions can provide a second signal for IgE synthesis warrants further investigation. Paradoxically, in-vivo prolonged topical steroid treatment strongly decreases the number of cells containing IL-4 mRNA in the nasal mucosa of patients with allergen-induced rhinitis [77]. Suppression of IL-4 expression may in the long run contribute critically to the beneficial effects of corticosteroids in the treatment of hyper-IgE states.

II. Molecular Events in the Induction of IgE Synthesis

A. The Role of Germline Transcripts in Isotype Switching

Isotype switching results from a DNA recombination event that juxtaposes different downstream C_H genes to the expressed V(D)J gene. Considerable evidence indicates that isotype switching is not a random event, but is "directed" by cytokines in conjunction with the regulation of B-cell proliferation and differentiation. Molecular analysis has shown that induction of isotype switching to a particular C_H gene almost invariably correlates with the transcriptional activation of the same gene in its germline configuration (reviewed in Refs. 78 and 79) (Fig. 5). The germline transcripts (GLT) that result from this process initiate a few kilobases (kb) upstream of the switch (S) region, and proceed through one or more short exons (I exons) that are spliced to the first exon of the C_H gene. GLT are unable to code for any mature protein of significant length, because the I exon contains multiple stop codons in all three reading frames. Therefore, GLT are also referred to as "sterile" transcripts. Alternatively, GLT are referred to as "truncated" transcripts, because the I exon is usually 200–300 base pairs (bp) shorter than the VDJ exon present in mature transcripts. Although there is no significant conservation of the sequences of GLT of different isotypes, their overall structure is conserved [79].

Expression of GLT is thought to play a key role in modulating the accessibility of a particular S region to a putative common switch recombinase, thus directing switching to the corresponding isotype. The role of GLT in the regulation

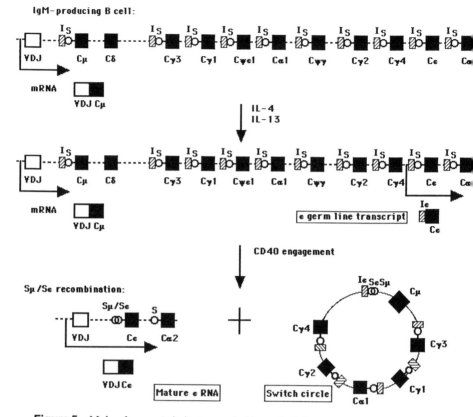

Figure 5 Molecular events in isotype switching to IgE. IL-4 or IL-13 induces ε germline transcription and makes the Sε region accessible for switch recombination. CD40 engagement activates the recombination machinery, and results in Sμ/Sε switch recombination. Intervening sequences are deleted as switch circles.

of isotype switching has recently been tested by gene knock-out experiments. Deletion of the Iγ1 [80] or Iγ2b [81] exons and their promoter resulted in inhibition of class switching to the corresponding genes, indicating that transcription in the S region is necessary to direct switch recombination. However, it is apparently not sufficient: replacement of Iε with a B-cell-specific promoter cassette containing the murine Eμ intronic enhancer and a V_H promoter, without the Iε splice donor site, resulted in only marginal switch recombination to IgE, at about 1% of the frequency induced by IL-4 [82]. In contrast, replacement of all known IL-4-inducible control elements in the Sγ1 region with the heterologous human metallothionein IIA promoter did not impair switch recombination to IgG1, provided that the Iγ1 splice donor site was included in the construct, thus allowing for the induction of artificial, but processed, GLT [83]. These data indicate that (1) artificial induction of structurally conserved, splice GLT can target switch recombination, whereas transcription in the S region as such cannot; (2) spliced switch transcripts (or the process of splicing) have a functional role in switch recombination [83]. The most intriguing speculation is that GLT are part of the switch recombinase, providing the specificity to target distinct S regions.

The 3' enhancer, located several kilobases downstream of the most 3' C_H gene, has been recently identified as a novel regulatory region that controls GLT expression and Ig heavy-chain class switching. 3' Enhancer KO mice showed a global defect in the ability to express GLT and switch to all C_H genes, except γ1 [84]. Notably, the deletion affected germline transcription and class switch recombination of five different C_H genes spread over a 120-kb locus. Based on these data, it has been proposed that sequences within the 3' enhancer deletion may be an essential part of a locus control region that regulates germline transcription and/or the accessibility of downstream C_H genes. Further studies of this region may provide insights into the pathogenesis of human isotype deficiencies.

B. Nuclear Factors Involved in the Regulation of ε Germline Transcription

Nuclear factors bind specifically to relatively short (10–20 bp) DNA sequences, functionally defined as responsive elements (RE). The general paradigm for promoters is that all slots for nuclear transcription factors need to be filled in order for a gene to "fire." This implies a level of tight combinatorial control. Like all weak promoters, the I_H promoters are likely to be limited at multiple steps of the transcription reaction. Thus, the activation function of different transcription factors can operate at different limiting steps in the initiation reaction.

Because transcription through the I_H exon and the S region seems to be required to target the appropriate S region for recombination and switching, the induction of GLT is a key step in determining the isotype specificity of the switching event. Different cytokines specifically induce different nuclear factors that activate transcription at the appropriate GLT promoter. The specificity in the induction of transcription factors is essential for the specificity of cytokine-induced GLT expression and isotype switching.

Expression of ε-GLT is regulated at the transcriptional level by nuclear factors that bind to the Iε promoter and adjacent regions. The requirements for the induction of ε-GLT seem to be somewhat different in mice and humans. Two signals, IL-4 (or IL-13) and LPS, are required for ε-GLT expression in most murine B-cell lines, whereas IL-4 alone is sufficient in humans. A number of transcription factors have been found to bind to ε-GLT promoter (Fig. 6):

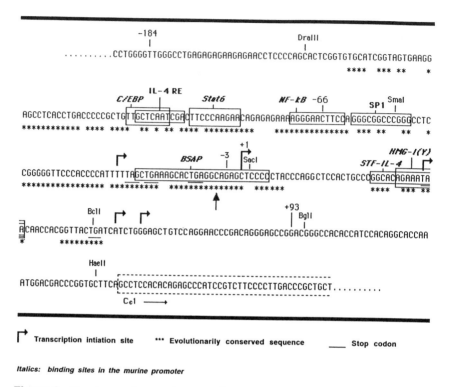

Figure 6   Regulatory elements in ε germline transcript promoter.

The B-cell-specific activator protein (BSAP, Pax-5) is a homeodomain-class transcription factor expressed specifically in the B-cell lineage from the pro-B to the mature B-cell stage. However, BSAP is not found in terminally differentiated plasma cells [85,86]. Binding sites for BSAP have been found in a variety of promoters of B-cell-related genes, including CD19, $V_{preB1,}$ λ5, and the tyrosine kinase blk, and furthermore, in the Ig gene locus (reviewed in Ref 87). Interestingly, although BSAP binding positively regulates transcription from various promoters, binding of BSAP to sites in the Ig 3′ α enhancer has a negative effect [88]. Negative regulation of enhancer activity seems to be due to the ability of BSAP to suppress binding of NF-αP, a protein that positively controls enhancer activity and heavy-chain transcription [89]. BSAP binds to a highly conserved region immediately upstream of the major Iε transcription initiation site in both murine [90] and human (C. Thienes, in preparation) B cells. The role played by BSAP in the regulation of GLT expression remains controversial. Interestingly, murine BSAP has been reported to be upregulated by proliferative stimuli (mitogens, cross-linking of sIgD or CD40) [91], and downregulated by OX40 ligand cross-linking [92]. In contrast, IL-4 has no effect on human BSAP-binding activity (C. Thienes, in preparation).

An IL-4 RE located upstream of the BSAP site has been shown to bind a complex formed by a member of the C/EBP family, NF-κB p50, and the IL-4-inducible factor Stat6 (NF-IL-4, IL-4 NAF: see below) [93]. It has been proposed that these factors may have to interact physically in order to induce ε-GLT expression [93]. The importance of NF-κB for the induction of murine GLT has been recently confirmed by the finding that expression of GLT for several isotypes, including IgE, and switching to the same isotypes, is severely impaired in NF-κB p50 KO mice ([94] and Snapper, personal communication). NF-κB has been found to be essential for human ε-GLT expression, as well (M. Woisetschläger, in preparation).

Stat6 [95,96] belongs to the newly identified family of signal transducers and activators of transcription (Stat) [97,98]. Binding of IL-4 to its receptor leads to activation by tyrosine phosphorylation of two receptor-associated cytoplasmic tyrosine kinases, Janus kinase (JAK)-3 and, to a lesser extent, JAK-1 [99]. These kinases are believed to rapidly (within minutes) induce tyrosine phosphorylation of Stat6, a latent cytoplasmic factor. The phosphorylated Stat6 homodimerizes, translocates to the nucleus, and binds to the promoter of a number of genes, contributing to the activation of transcription [95]. Stat6 preferentially binds dyad symmetric half-sites separated by 4 base pairs (TTCNNNNGAA). DNA binding specificity is localized to a region of 180 amino acids at the N-terminal side of the putative SH3 domain [100]. The discovery of JAKs and Stats has finally provided an explanation for the apparent paradox that the IL-4R, as well as the receptors for a number of other cytokines, lacks kinase domains, and yet couples ligand binding to tyrosine phosphorylation [97]. Stat6 is not B-cell-specific, and is induced by IL-4 in monocytes where it participates in the transcriptional regulation of the IL-4-inducible CD23b promoter, and possibly of the FcγR1 promoter [101]. Stat6-binding sites have been identified in the promoters of a number of other IL-4-responsive genes, such as Cε [93,102–104], Cγ1, FcγR1, MHC class II [101,103]. The presence of homologous RE in the promoter of different genes underlies the concerted regulation of these genes by a single cytokine. Thus, the concerted modulation in the expression of ε-GLT, CD23, and MHC class II in B cells stimulated with IL-4 is mediated by IL-4 RE located in the promoters of these genes.

The minimal set of elements in the human ε-GLT promoter required to confer full IL-4 inducibility to a heterologous promoter has not been determined.

In the mouse, a region containing the binding sites for Stat6 and a C/EBP factor seems to be sufficient to transfer IL-4 inducibility to a minimal c-fos promoter [93]. Interestingly, the Stat6 binding site in the murine and human ε-GLT promoter [102] shares a peculiar functional property with the site that binds the non-histone chromosomal protein HMG-I(Y) [105] in the mouse. Indeed, deletion or mutation of either site results in the loss of IL-4 inducibility, but in a marked increase in basal promoter activity [102,104]. Thus, these elements seem to have a bifunctional activity, i.e., they are required for IL-4-induced promoter activation, but they repress the activity of the promoter in the absence of IL-4. These findings suggest that expression of ε-GLT and IgE in resting B cells is low in part because the GLT promoter is kept in a state of repression that requires depression through specific pathways.

C. DNA Switch Recombination

Although IL-4 (signal 1) is by itself sufficient for the initiation of transcription through the ε locus, switching and expression of mature Cε transcripts (containing VDJ spliced to Cε1–4) require signal 2 (engagement of CD40 by CD40 ligand). The molecular events that follow the delivery of the second signal for switching to IgE have been characterized only recently (Fig. 5). The classical model, according to which switching occurs via loop-out and deletional recombination between highly repetitive S regions (reviewed in Ref. 106), was challenged in the late 1980s, at least for the IgE isotype. Indeed, it was reported that IgE could be produced by B cells in which the immunoglobulin locus was retained in germline configuration [107,108]. Thus, it became important to characterize the molecular mechanisms that underlie the expression of mature VDJ-Cε mRNA in normal human B cells. This issue was investigated using polymerase chain reaction (PCR)-based approaches that allow for amplification, cloning, and sequencing of chimeric Sμ/Sε switch fragments composed of the 5′ Sμ joined to the 3′ portion of the targeted Sε region, or of switch circles, their reciprocal products. DNA sequencing of Sμ/Sε switch fragments amplified from IgE-producing B-cell cultures formally proved that deletional switch recombination had occurred. Most of the switch fragments represented direct joining of Sμ to Sε [109–111] (Fig. 7).

Interestingly, some fragments amplified from B cells stimulated with IL-4 and hydrocortisone contained insertions at the Sμ/Sε junction which were derived from Sγ4 [111]. The presence of an Sγ4-derived insertion suggested that some B cells had undergone sequential isotype switching from IgM to IgG4 to IgE. Indeed, IL-4 has been shown to induce isotype switching to IgG4 [112], as well as to IgE, and single B cells can give rise to clones that secrete IgG4 and IgE [113].

Sequential switching and direct switching coexist. Sequencing of switch circles generated in B cells triggered to switch to IgE by IL-4 and anti-CD40 mAb showed the presence of μ–γ–ε switching, and of sequential events even more

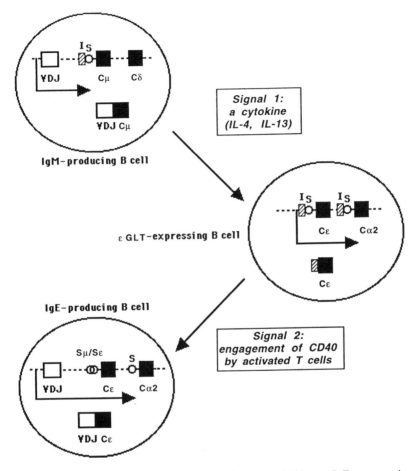

Figure 7 Molecular steps in the induction of isotype switching to IgE: an overview.

complex (μ–α1–γ–ϵ). However, μ–ϵ circles representing direct switching events were also found at high frequency [114]. Likewise, sequence analysis of Sμ/Sϵ switch fragments from patients with atopic dermatitis showed a predominance of direct Sμ/Sϵ joining [115].

More recently, it has been shown that a chimeric Sμ/Sγ1 region resulting from a switching event between μ and γ1 can undergo a secondary recombination between the very 5′ end of Sμ and the very 3′ end of Sγ1. The secondary recombination removes essentially all the tandemly repeated S region sequences from the corresponding chromosome [116]. The mechanisms responsible for secondary recombination events in previously rearranged, chimeric S regions are still unknown. In particular, it is unclear whether secondary recombination requires retargeting of the recombinase. This would be problematic, because of the deletion of the region encompassing the I_H exon and the GLT promoter. Secondary recombination may, however, represent a mechanism to prevent continued switching to downstream isotypes, and ensure isotype stabilization of switched B cells. Upon secondary recombination, in fact, the S sequences retained by the active Ig gene may be insufficient to serve as a substrate for further S/S recombination.

The importance of sequential switching in vivo was investigated by examining switching to IgE in mutant mice which lacked the $S\gamma1$ region [80], and were therefore unable to support sequential switching via IgG1. In these mice, the frequency of switching to IgE was not affected [117]. These results indicated that sequential switching may merely reflect the simultaneous accessibility of two acceptor S regions for switch recombination induced by one cytokine. The apparent dominance of sequential switching observed in the generation of murine IgE-expressing cells following IL-4 stimulation may be due to the parallel activation of $S\gamma1$ and $S\varepsilon$ by IL-4, $S\gamma1$ being intrinsically more accessible to recombination with $S\mu$ [80,117]. Thus, the overall low frequency of IgE switching is an autonomously determined intrinsic feature of $S\varepsilon$ and its control elements. This may explain why, in the presence of saturating concentrations of IL-4 in vitro, the frequency of IgE switching reaches at most 10% of frequency of switching to IgG1, which is also induced by IL-4.

III. Cytokine-Dependent Modulation of IL-4-Induced IgE Synthesis

Cellular studies have shown that, although IL-4 and IL-13 are the only cytokines capable of inducing IgE synthesis, IL-4/IL-13-induced IgE production can be further enhanced, or inhibited, by a number of cytokines (Table 1). However, the mechanisms responsible for the effects of these cytokines, and the event(s) that are targeted, are still mostly unclear.

TNF-α, IL-6, and IL-9 enhance IL-4-dependent IgE synthesis [118–120]. IgE potentiation by TNF-α and IL-6 is detectable in both T-cell-dependent and T-cell-independent systems. The increase in IgE synthesis induced by TNF-α is mediated by enhanced ε-GLT expression, whereas this step is not affected by IL-6 and IL-9 [119]. IL-6 is not isotype-specific [121], and induces IgG secretion by selective accumulation of mRNA for the secreted form of the molecule, and possibly through differential mRNA stabilization [122]. IgE secretion might be amplified by similar mechanisms, but no direct evidence is available. Notably, engagement of CD40 triggers IL-6 and TNF-α secretion by B cells [123] and monocytes [13].

Table 1 Cytokines Modulate Molecular Events in IgE Induction

	T-cell-independent			T-cell-dependent		
	GLT	Mature RNA	IgE	GLT	Mature RNA	IgE
TNF-α	↑	↑	↑	↑	↑	↑
IL-6	↔	↑	↑	↔	↑	↑
IL-9	↔	ND	ND	ND	ND	↑
TGF-β	↓	↓	↓	↓	↓	↓
IFN-γ	↔	↔	↔	↓	↓	↓
IFN-α	↔	↔	↔	↓	↓	↓
IL-8	ND	ND	↓	ND	ND	↓
IL-12	ND	ND	↔	↔	↓	↓
PAF-acether	ND	ND	ND	↓	↓	↓
IL-10[a]	↔	↔	↔	↓	↓	↓

[a]Monocyte-dependent.

All the other cytokines listed in Table 1 inhibit IgE synthesis. Interestingly, only TGF-β has been shown to act on B cells, by targeting ε-GLT expression [119]. IL-8 also inhibits IgE production by purified B cells [124], but the molecular targets remain unknown. The other cytokines are either inactive on germline transcription, or uncharacterized so far. Interestingly, IFN-α, IFN-γ, and IL-12 inhibit IgE secretion only when tested in T-cell-dependent systems [119,125,126], and IL-10 suppresses IgE synthesis only in the presence of monocytes [127]. Thus, none of these cytokines acts directly on B cells.

References

1. Vercelli D, Geha RS. Regulation of IgE synthesis in man. J Clin Immunol 1989; 9: 75–83.
2. Vercelli D, Geha RS. Regulation of IgE synthesis in humans: a tale of two signals. J Allergy Clin Immunol 1991; 88:285–295.
3. Finkelman FD, Katona IM, Urban JF, Snapper CM, Ohara J, Paul WE. Suppression of in vivo polyclonal IgE responses by monoclonal antibody to the lymphokine B-cell stimulatory factor 1. Proc Natl Acad Sci USA 1986; 83:9675–9678.
4. Garrone P, Djossou O, Galizzi J-P, Banchereau J. A recombinant extracellular domain of the human interleukin 4 receptor inhibits the biological effects of interleukin 4 on T and B lymphocytes. Eur J Immunol 1991; 21:1365–1369.
5. Aversa G, Punnonen J, Cocks BG, et al. An IL-4 mutant protein inhibits IL-4 or IL-13 induced human IgG4 and IgE synthesis and B cell proliferation: support for a common component shared by IL-4 and IL-13 receptors. J Exp Med 1993; 178: 2213–2216.

6. Zurawski SM, Vega F, Huyghe B, Zurawski G. Receptors for interleukin-13 and interleukin-4 are complex and share a novel component that functions in signal transduction. EMBO J 1993; 12:2663–2670.

7. Kühn R, Rajewsky KR, Müller W. Generation and analysis of interleukin-4 deficient mice. Science 1991; 254:707–710.

8. Marsh DG, Neely JD, Breazeale DR, et al. Linkage analysis of IL4 and other chromosome 5q31.1 markers and total serum immunoglobulin E concentrations. Science 1994; 264:1152–1156.

9. McKenzie ANJ, Culpepper JA, de Waal Malefyt R, et al. Interleukin 13, a T-cell-derived cytokine that regulates human monocyte and B-cell function. Proc Natl Acad Sci USA 1993; 90:3735–3739.

10. Vita N, Lefort S, Laurent P, Caput D, Ferrara P. Characterization and comparison of the interleukin 13 receptor with the interleukin 4 receptor on several cell types. J Biol Chem 1995; 270:3512–3517.

11. Brinkmann V, Kristofic C. TCR-stimulated naive human CD4+ 45RO− T cells develop into effector cells that secrete IL-13, IL-5, and IFN-γ, but no IL-4, and help efficiently IgE production by B cells. J Immunol 1995; 154:3078–3087.

12. Wang CY, Fu SM, Kunkel HG. Isolation and immunological characterization of a major surface glycoprotein (gp54) preferentially expressed on certain human B cells. J Exp Med 1979; 149:1424–1437.

13. Alderson MR, Armitage RJ, Tough TW, Strockbine L, Fanslow WC, Spriggs MK. CD40 expression by human monocytes: regulation by cytokines and activation of monocytes by the ligand for CD40. J Exp Med 1993; 178:669–674.

14. Caux C, Massacrier C, Vandervliet B, et al. Activation of human dendritic cells through CD40 cross-linking. J Exp Med 1994; 180:1263–1272.

15. Galy AH, Spits H. CD40 is functionally expressed on human thymic cells. J Immunol 1992; 149:775–782.

16. Paulie S, Ehlin-Henriksson B, Mellstedt H, Koho H, Aissa HB, Perlmann P. A p50 surface antigen restricted to human urinary bladder carcinomas and B-lymphocytes. Cancer Immunol Immunother 1985; 20:23–30.

17. Ledbetter JA, Clark EA, Norris NA, Shu G, Hellström I. Expression of a functional B-cell receptor CDw40 (Bp50) on carcinomas. In: McMichael AJ, ed. Leukocyte Typing III. White Cell Differentiation Antigens. Oxford: Oxford University Press, 1987: 432.

18. Liu Y-J, Joshua DE, Williams GT, Smith CA, Gordon J, MacLennan ICM. Mechanism of antigen-driven selection in germinal centres. Nature 1989; 342:929–931.

19. Tsubata T, Wu J, Honjo T. B-cell apoptosis induced by antigen receptor crosslinking is blocked by a T-cell signal through CD40. Nature 1993; 364:645–648.

20. Gruber MF, Bjorndahl JM, Nakamura S, Fu SM. Anti-CD45 inhibition of human B cell proliferation depends on the nature of activation signals and the state of B cell activation. J Immunol 1989; 142:4144–4152.

21. Banchereau J, Bazan F, Blanchard D, et al. The CD40 antigen and its ligand. Annu Rev Immunol 1994; 12:881–922.

22. Armitage RJ, Fanslow WC, Strockbine L, et al. Molecular and biological characterization of a murine ligand for CD40. Nature 1992; 357:80–82.

23. Spriggs MK, Armitage RJ, Strockbine L, et al. Recombinant human CD40 ligand stimulates B cell proliferation and immunoglobulin E secretion. J Exp Med 1992; 176:1543–1550.

24. Fanslow WC, Anderson DM, Grabstein KH, Clark EA, Cosman D, Armitage RJ. Soluble forms of CD40 inhibit biologic responses of human B cells. J Immunol 1992; 149:655–660.

25. Fuleihan R, Ramesh N, Loh R, et al. Defective expression of the CD40 ligand in X-chromosome-linked immunoglobulin deficiency with normal or elevated IgM. Proc Natl Acad Sci USA 1993; 90:2170–2173.

26. Allen RC, Armitage RJ, Conley ME, et al. CD40 ligand gene defects responsible for X-linked hyper-IgM syndrome. Science 1993; 259:990–993.

27. Kawabe T, Naka T, Yoshida K, et al. The immune responses in CD40-deficient mice: impaired immunoglobulin class switching and germinal center formation. Immunity 1994; 1:167–178.

28. Castigli E, Alt FW, Davidson L, et al. CD40 deficient mice generated by RAG-2 deficient blastocyst complementation. Proc Natl Acad Sci USA 1994; 91:12135–12139.

29. Xu J, Foy TM, Laman JD, et al. Mice deficient for the CD40 ligand. Immunity 1994; 1:423–431.

30. Fuleihan R, Ahern D, Geha RS. Decreased expression of the ligand for CD40 in newborn lymphocytes. Eur J Immunol 1994; 24:1925.

31. Nonoyama S, Penix LA, Edwards CP, et al. Diminished expression of CD40 ligand by activated neonatal T cells. J Clin Invest 1995; 95:66–75.

32. Durandy A, de Saint Basile G, Lisowska-Grospierre B, et al. Undetectable CD40 ligand expression on T cells and low B cell responses to CD40 binding agonists in human newborns. J Immunol 1995; 154:1560–1568.

33. Casamayor-Palleja M, Khan M, MacLennan ICM. A subset of CD4+ memory T cells contains preformed CD40 ligand that is rapidly but transiently expressed on their surface after activation through the T cell receptor complex. J Exp Med 1995; 181:1293–1301.

34. Yellin MJ, Sippel K, Inghirami G, et al. CD40 molecules induce down-modulation and endocytosis of T cell surface T cell-B cell activating molecule/CD40 ligand. Potential role in regulating helper effector function. J Immunol 1994; 152:598–608.

35. van Kooten C, Gaillard C, Galizzi J-P, et al. B cells regulate expression of CD40 ligand on activated T cells by lowering the mRNA level and through the release of soluble CD40. Eur J Immunol 1994; 24:787–792.

36. Gascan H, Aversa GC, Gauchat J-F, et al. Membranes of activated CD4+ T cells expressing T cell receptor (TcR) αβ or TcR γδ induce IgE synthesis by human B cells in the presence of interleukin-4. Eur J Immunol 1992; 22:1133–1141.

37. Horner AA, Jabara H, Ramesh N, Geha RS. γ/δ T lymphocytes express CD40 ligand and induce isotype switching in B lymphocytes. J Exp Med 1995; 181:1239–1244.

38. Wen L, Roberts SJ, Viney JL, et al. Immunoglobulin synthesis and generalized autoimmunity in mice congenitally deficient in αβ(+) cells. Nature 1994; 369:654–658.

39. Ferrick DA, Schrenzel MD, Mulvania T, Hsieh B, Ferlin WG, Lepper H. Differential

production of interferon-γ and interleukin-4 in response to Th1- and Th2-stimulating pathogens by γδ T cells in vivo. Nature 1995; 373:255–257.

40. Shahinian A, Pfeffer K, Lee KP, et al. Differential T cell costimulatory requirements in CD28-deficient mice. Science 1993; 261:609–612.

41. Ranheim EA, Kipps TJ. Activated T cells induce expression of B7/BB1 on normal or leukemic B cells through a CD40-dependent signal. J Exp Med 1993; 177:925–935.

42. Klaus SJ, Pinchuk LM, Ochs HD, et al. Costimulation through CD28 enhances T cell-dependent B cell activation via CD40-CD40L interaction. J Immunol 1994; 152:5643–5652.

43. King CL, Stupi RJ, Craighead N, June CH, Thyphronitis G. CD28 activation promotes Th2 subset differentiation by human CD4+ cells. Eur J Immunol 1995; 25: 587–595.

44. Vallé A, Aubry J-P, Durand I, Banchereau J. IL-4 and IL-2 upregulate the expression of antigen B7, the B cell counterstructure to T cell CD28: an amplification mechanism for T-B cell interactions. Int Immunol 1991; 3:229–235.

45. Life P, Aubry J-P, Estoppey S, Schnuriger V, Bonnefoy J-Y. CD28 functions as an adhesion molecule and is involved in the regulation of human IgE synthesis. Eur J Immunol 1995; 25:333–339.

46. Poudrier J, Owens T. CD54/intercellular adhesion molecule 1 and major histocompatibility complex II signaling induces B cells to express interleukin 2 receptors and complements help provided through CD40 ligation. J Exp Med 1994; 179:1417–1427.

47. Diaz-Sanchez D, Chegini S, Zhang K, Saxon A. CD58 (LFA-3) stimulation provides a signal for human isotype switching and IgE production distinct from CD40. J Immunol 1994; 153:10–20.

48. Schroeder JT, MacGlashan DW, Kagey-Sobotka A, White JM, Lichtenstein LM. IgE-dependent IL-4-secretion by human basophils—the relationship between cytokine production and histamine release in mixed leukocyte cultures. J Immunol 1994; 153:1808–1817.

49. Burd PR, Thompson WC, Max EE, Mills FC. Activated mast cells produce interleukin 13. J Exp Med 1995; 1373–1380.

50. Gauchat J-F, Henchoz S, Mazzei G, et al. Induction of human IgE synthesis in B cells by mast cells and basophils. Nature 1993; 365:340–343.

51. Gauchat J-F, Henchoz S, Fattah D, et al. CD40 ligand is functionally expressed on human eosinophils. Eur J Immunol 1995; 25:863–865.

52. Romagnani S. Lymphokine production by human T cells in disease states. Annu Rev Immunol 1994; 12:227–257.

53. Parronchi P, Macchia D, Piccinni M-P, et al. Allergen- and bacterial antigen-specific T-cell clones established from atopic donors show a different profile of cytokine production. Proc Natl Acad Sci USA 1991; 88:4538–4542.

54. Kapsenberg ML, Wierenga EA, Bos JD, Jansen HM. Functional subsets of allergen-reactive human CD4+ T cells. Immunol Today 1991; 12:392–395.

55. Del Prete GF, De Carli M, Mastromauro C, et al. Purified protein derivative of *Mycobacterium tuberculosis* and excretory-secretary antigen(s) of *Toxocara canis*

expand in vitro human T cells with stable and opposite (type 1 T helper or type 2 T helper) profile of cytokine production. J Clin Invest 1991; 88:346–350.

56. Peleman R, Wu J, Fargeas C, Delespesse G. Recombinant interleukin 4 suppresses the production of interferon γ by human mononuclear cells. J Exp Med 1989; 170: 1751–1756.

57. Vercelli D, Jabara HH, Lauener RP, Geha RS. Interleukin-4 inhibits the synthesis of interferon-γ and induces the synthesis of IgE in mixed lymphocyte cultures. J Immunol 1990; 144:570–573.

58. Maggi E, Parronchi P, Manetti R, et al. Reciprocal regulatory effects of IFN-γ and IL-4 on the in vitro development of human Th1 and Th2 clones. J Immunol 1992; 148:2142–2147.

59. Schmitz J, Thiel A, Kühn R, et al. Induction of interleukin-4 (IL-4) expression in T helper (Th) cells is not dependent on IL-4 from non Th-cells. J Exp Med 1994; 179:1349–1353.

60. Kopf M, Le Gros G, Bachmann M, Lamers MC, Bluethmann H, Köhler G. Disruption of the murine IL-4 gene blocks Th2 cytokine responses. Nature 1993; 362:245–248.

61. Manetti R, Parronchi P, Giudizi MG, et al. Natural killer cell stimulatory factor (interleukin 12) induces T helper type 1-specific immune responses and inhibits the development of IL-4-producing Th cells. J Exp Med 1993; 177:1199–1204.

62. Romagnani S. Induction of TH1 and TH2 responses: a key role for the "natural" immune response? Immunol Today 1992; 13:379–381.

63. Del Prete G, De Carli M, Almerigogna F, et al. Preferential expression of CD30 by human CD4+ T cells producing Th2-type cytokines. FASEB J 1995; 9:81–86.

64. Manetti R, Annunziato F, Biagiotti R, et al. CD30 expression by CD8+ T cells producing type 2 helper cytokines. Evidence for large numbers of CD8+CD30+ T cell clones in human immunodeficiency virus infection. J Exp Med 1994; 180:2407–2411.

65. Maggi E, Giudizi MG, Biagiotti R, et al. Th2-like CD8+ T cells showing B cell helper function and reduced cytolytic activity in human immunodeficiency virus type 1 infection. J Exp Med 1994; 180:489–495.

66. Paganelli R, Scala E, Ansotegui IJ, et al. CD8+ T lymphocytes provide helper activity for IgE synthesis in human immunodeficiency virus-infected patients with hyper-IgE. J Exp Med 1995; 181:423–428.

67. Cocks BG, Chang C-CJ, Carballido JM, Yssel H, de Vries JE, Aversa G. A novel receptor involved in T-cell activation, Nature 1995; 376:260–263.

68. Thyphronitis G, Tsokos GC, June CH, Levine AD, Finkelman FD. IgE secretion by Epstein-Barr virus-infected purified human B lymphocytes is stimulated by interleukin 4 and suppressed by interferon-γ. Proc Natl Acad Sci USA 1989; 86:5580–5584.

69. Jabara HH, Schneider LC, Shapira SK, et al. Induction of germ-line and mature Cε transcripts in human B cells stimulated with rIL-4 and EBV. J Immunol 1990; 145: 3468–3473.

70. Hu HM, O'Rourke K, Boguski MS, Dixit VM. A novel RING finger protein interacts with the cytoplasmic domain of CD40. J Biol Chem 1994; 269:30069–30072.

71. Cheng G, Cleary AM, Ye Z-S, Hong DI, Lederman S, Baltimore D. Involvement of CRAF1, a relative of TRAF, in CD40 signaling. Science 1995; 267: 1494–1498.

72. Rothe M, Wong SC, Henzel WJ, Goeddel DV. A novel family of putative signal transducers associated with the cytoplasmic domain of the 75 kDa tumor necrosis factor receptor. Cell 1994; 78:681–692.

73. Mosialos G, Birkenbach M, Yalamanchili R, VanArsdale T, Ware C, Kieff E. The Epstein-Barr virus transforming protein LMP1 engages signaling proteins for the tumor necrosis factor receptor family. Cell 1995; 80:389–399.

74. Jabara HH, Ahern DJ, Vercelli D, Geha RS. Hydrocortisone and IL-4 induce IgE isotype switching in human B cells. J Immunol 1991; 147:1557–1560.

75. Sarfati M, Luo H, Delespesse G. IgE synthesis by chronic lymphocytic leukemia cells. J Exp Med 1989; 170:1775–1780.

76. Wu CY, Sarfati M, Heusser C, et al. Glucocorticoids increase the synthesis of Immunoglobulin E by interleukin-4-stimulated human lymphocytes. J Clin Invest 1991; 87:870–877.

77. Masuyama K, Jacobson MR, Rak S, et al. Typical glucocorticosteroid (fluticasone propionate) inhibits cells expressing cytokine mRNA for interleukin-4 in the nasal mucosa in allergen-induced rhinitis. Immunology 1994; 82:192–199.

78. Vercelli D, Geha RS. Regulation of isotype switching. Curr Opin Immun 1992; 4: 794–797.

79. Coffman RL, Lebman DA, Rothman P. The mechanism and regulation of immuno-globulin isotype switching. Adv Immunol 1993; 54:229–269.

80. Jung S, Rajewsky K, Radbruch A. Shutdown of class switch recombination by deletion of a switch region control element. Science 1993; 259:984–987.

81. Zhang J, Bottaro A, Li S, Stewart V, Alt FW. Targeted mutation in the Ig2b exon results in a selective Iγ2b deficiency in mice. EMBO J 1993; 12:3529–3537.

82. Bottaro A, Lansford R, Xu L, Zhang J, Rothman P, Alt FW. S region transcription *per se* promotes basal IgE class switch recombination but additional factors regulate the efficiency of the process. EMBO J 1994; 13:665–674.

83. Lorenz M, Jung S, Radbruch A. Switch transcripts in immunoglobulin class switch-ing. Science 1995; 267:1825–1828.

84. Cogné M, Lansford R, Bottaro A, et al. A class switch control region at the 3′ end of the immunoglobulin heavy chain locus. Cell 1994; 77:737–747.

85. Adams B, Dörfler P, Aguzzi A, et al. Pax-5 encodes the transcription factor BSAP and is expressed in B lymphocytes, the developing CNS, and adult testis. Genes & Dev 1992; 6:1589–1607.

86. Urbanek P, Wang Z-Q, Fetka I, Wagner EF, Busslinger M. Complete block of early B cell differentiation and altered patterning of the posterior midbrain in mice lacking Pax5/BSAP. Cell 1994; 79:901–912.

87. Hagman J, Grosschedl R. Regulation of gene expression at early stages of B-cell differentiation. Curr Opin Immun 1994; 6:222–230.

88. Nuerath MF, Strober W, Wakatsuki Y. The murine Ig 3′ α enhancer is a target site with repressor function for the B cell lineage-specific transcription factor BSAP (NF-HB, Sα-BP). J Immunol 1994; 153:730–742.

89. Neurath MF, Max EE, Strober W. Pax5 (BSAP) regulates the murine immunoglobu-

lin 3'α enhancer by suppressing binding of NF-αP, a protein that controls heavy chain transcription. Proc Natl Acad Sci USA 1995; 92:5336–5340.

90. Liao F, Birshtein BK, Busslinger M, Rothman P. The transcription factor BSAP (NF-HB) is essential for immunoglobulin germ-line ε transcription. J Immunol 1994; 152:2904–2911.

91. Wakatsuki Y, Neurath MF, Max EE, Strober W. The B cell-specific transcription factor BSAP regulates B cell proliferation. J Exp Med 1994; 179:1099–1108.

92. Stüber E, Neurath M, Calderhead D, Perry Fell H, Strober W. Cross-linking of OX40 ligand, a member of the TNF/NGF cytokine family, induces proliferation and differentiation in murine splenic B cells. Immunity 1995; 2:507–521.

93. Delphin S, Stavnezer J. Characterization of an IL-4 responsive region in the immunoglobulin heavy chain germline ε promoter: regulation by NF-IL-4, a C/EBP family member, and NF-kB/p50. J Exp Med 1995; 181:181–192.

94. Sha WC, Liou H-C., Tuomanen EI, Baltimore D. Targeted disruption of the p50 subunit of NF-κB leads to multifocal defects in immune responses. Cell 1995; 80: 321–330.

95. Hou J, Schindler U, Henzel WJ, Ho TC, Brasseur M, McKnight SL. An interleukin-4-induced transcription factor: IL-4 Stat. Science 1994; 265:1701–1706.

96. Quelle FW, Shimoda K, Thierfelder W, et al. Cloning of murine and human Stat6, Stat proteins that are tyrosine phosphorylated in response to IL-4 and IL-3 but are not required for mitogenesis. Mol Cell Biol 1995; 15:3336–3343.

97. Ihle JN, Kerr IM. Jaks and Stats in signaling by the cytokine receptor superfamily. Trends in Genetics 1995; 11:69–74.

98. Ivashkiv LB. Cytokines and STATs: How can signals achieve specificity? Immunity 1995; 3:1–4.

99. Malabarba MG, Kirken RA, Rui H, et al. Activation of JAK3, but not JAK1, is critical to interleukin-4 stimulated proliferation and requires a membrane proximal region of IL-4 receptor α. J Biol Chem 1995; 270:9630–9637.

100. Schindler U, Wu P, Rothe M, Brasseur M, McKnight SL. Components of a Stat recognition code: evidence for two layers of molecular selectivity. Immunity 1995; 2:689–697.

101. Kotanides H, Reich NC. Requirement of tyrosine phosphorylation for rapid activation of a DNA binding factor by IL-4. Science 1993; 262:1265–1267.

102. Albrecht B, Peiritsch S, Woisetschläger M. A bifunctional control element in the human IgE germline promoter involved in repression and IL-4 activation. Int Immunol 1994; 6:1143–1151.

103. Köhler I, Rieber EP. Allergy-associated Iε and Fcε receptor II (CD23b) genes activated via binding of an interleukin-4-induced transcription factor to a novel responsive element. Eur J Immunol 1993; 23:3066–3071.

104. Wang D-Z, Cherrington A, Famakin-Mosuro B, Boothby M. Independent pathways for de-repression of the mouse immunoglobulin heavy chain germline epsilon promoter: an NF-IL4 site as a context-dependent negative element. Submitted.

105. Kim J, Reeves R, Rothman P, Boothby M. The non-histone chromosomal protein HMG-I(Y) contributes to repression of the immunoglobulin heavy chain germ-line ε RNA promoter. Eur J Immunol 1995; 25:798–807.

106. Max EE. Immunoglobulins: molecular genetics. In: Paul WE, ed. Fundamental Immunology. New York: Raven Press, 1989:235–290.

107. MacKenzie T, Dosch HM. Clonal and molecular characteristics of the human IgE-committed B cell subset. J Exp Med 1989; 169:407–430.

108. Chan MA, Benedict SH, Dosch H-M, Huy MF, Stein LD. Expression of IgE from a nonrearranged ε locus in cloned B-lymphoblastoid cells that also express IgM. J Immunol 1990; 144:3563–3568.

109. Shapira SK, Jabara HH, Thienes CP, et al. Deletional switch recombination occurs in IL-4 induced isotype switching to IgE expression by human B cells. Proc Natl Acad Sci USA 1991; 88:7528–7532.

110. Shapira SK, Vercelli D, Jabara HH, Fu SM, Geha RS. Molecular analysis of the induction of IgE synthesis in human B cells by IL-4 and engagement of CD40 antigen. J Exp Med 1992; 175:289–292.

111. Jabara HH, Loh R, Ramesh N, Vercelli D, Geha RS. Sequential switching from μ to ε via γ4 in human B cells stimulated with IL-4 and hydrocortisone. J Immunol 1993; 151:4528–4533.

112. Lundgren M, Persson U, Larsson P, et al. Interleukin 4 induces synthesis of IgE and IgG4 in human B cells. Eur J Immunol 1989; 19:1311–1315.

113. Gascan H, Gauchat J-F, Aversa G, van Vlasselaer P, de Vries JE. Anti-CD40 monoclonal antibodies or CD4+ T cell clones and IL-4 induce IgG4 and IgE switching in purified human B cells via different signaling pathways. J Immunol 1991; 147:8–13.

114. Zhang K, Mills FC, Saxon A. Switch circles from IL-4-directed ε class switching from human B lymphocytes—evidence for direct, sequential and multiple step sequential switch from μ to ε Ig heavy chain gene. J Immunol 1994; 152:3427–3435.

115. van der Stoep N, Korver W, Logtenberg T. In vivo and in vitro IgE isotype switching in human B lymphocytes: evidence for a predominantly direct IgM to IgE class switch program. Eur J Immunol 1994; 24:1307–1311.

116. Zhang K, Cheah H-K, Saxon A. Secondary deletional recombination of rearranged switch region in Ig isotype-switched B cells. A mechanism for isotype stabilization. J Immunol 1995; 154:2237–2247.

117. Jung S, Siebenkotten G, Radbruch A. Frequency of Immunoglobulin E class switching is autonomously determined and independent of prior switching to other classes. J Exp Med 1994; 179:2023–2026.

118. Vercelli D, Jabara HH, Arai K, Yokota T, Geha RS. Endogenous IL-6 plays an obligatory role in IL-4 induced human IgE synthesis. Eur J Immunol 1989; 19:1419–1424.

119. Gauchat J-F, Aversa G, Gascan H, de Vries JE. Modulation of IL-4 induced germline ε RNA synthesis in human B cells by tumor necrosis factor-α, anti-CD40 monoclonal antibodies or transforming growth factor-β correlates with levels of IgE production. Int Immunol 1992; 4:397–406.

120. Dugas B, Renauld JC, Péne J, et al. Interleukin-9 potentiates the interleukin-4-induced immunoglobulin (IgG, IgM, and IgE) production by normal human B lymphocytes. Eur J Immunol 1993; 1687–1692.

121. Muraguchi A, Hirano T, Tang B, et al. The essential role of B cell stimulatory factor 2 (BSF-2/IL-6) for the terminal differentiation of B cells. J Exp Med 1988; 167: 332–344.

122. Raynal M-C, Liu Z, Hirano T, Mayer L, Kishimoto T, Chen-Kiang S. Interleukin 6 induces secretion of IgG1 by coordinated transcriptional activation and differential mRNA accumulation. Proc Natl Acad Sci USA 1989; 86:8024–8028.

123. Clark EA, Shu G. Association between IL-6 and CD40 signaling. IL-6 induces phosphorylation of CD40 receptors. J Immunol 1990; 145:1400–1406.

124. Kimata H, Yoshida A, Ishioka C, Lindley I, Mikawa H. Interleukin-8 selectively inhibits Immunoglobulin E production induced by IL-4 in human B cells. J Exp Med 1992; 176:1227–1231.

125. Gauchat J-F, Lebman DA, Coffman RL, Gascan H, de Vries JE. Structure and expression of germline ε transcripts in human B cells induced by interleukin 4 to switch to IgE production. J Exp Med 1990; 172:463–473.

126. Kiniwa M, Gately M, Gubler U, Chizzonite R, Fargeas C, Delespesse G. Recombinant interleukin-12 suppresses the synthesis of immunoglobulin E by interleukin-4 stimulated human lymphocytes. J Clin Invest 1992; 90:262–266.

127. Punnonen J, de Waal Malefyt R, van Vlasselaer P, Gauchat J-F, De Vries JE. IL-10 and viral IL-10 prevent IL-4-induced IgE synthesis by inhibiting the accessory cell function of monocytes. J Immunol 1993; 151:1280–1289.

Part Two

ANIMAL MODELS OF ASTHMA, INFLAMMATION, AND BRONCHIAL HYPERREACTIVITY

10

Animal Models of Asthma

PHILIP PADRID

University of Chicago
Chicago, Illinois

Introduction

Bronchial asthma is an inflammatory airway disease which is manifested clinically as episodic cough and wheeze, and is characterized by spontaneous reversible airflow limitation. Recent data regarding the inflammatory component of asthmatic airways have brought us closer toward understanding the pathophysiology of this chronic and sometimes disabling disorder. Nevertheless, the fundamental mechanisms which underlie the development and perturbation of the asthmatic state remain elusive. For many reasons, invasive studies designed to elucidate mechanisms of asthma or test the efficacy of potential therapeutic agents are not possible in asthmatic humans. Because of these limitations, invasive studies of the pathological changes in structure and function in asthmatic airways have focused on experimentally induced bronchoconstriction, airway inflammation, and airway hyperreactivity in animals. There are a number of advantages to this approach. First, the components of an airway inflammatory response (edema, cell infiltration) may be correlated with physiologic events. Second, inflammatory cells, ligands, mediators, etc., may be manipulated in various ways. Additionally, stimulation of isolated cell types and/or tissues can be done in vitro, thus allowing assessment of their respective potential contribution to changes in respiratory function.

It has been the hope that features of human asthma, including abnormal anatomy, physiology, cell biology, molecular genetics, and function, can be mimicked in animal models. Further, it has been assumed that results of such studies can be applied directly to our understanding of asthma in humans. A great deal of information arising from animal studies has been accumulated; these data have profoundly influenced the direction and scope of treatment of humans with asthma. Nevertheless, extrapolation of data from animal studies to the human disease should be pursued with caution, as there are many more species differences than similarities in airway anatomy, cell biology, etc. For example, if mucus hypersecretion is a significant component of the asthmatic airway of humans, we should appreciate that goblet cells comprise 20% of the epithelial cells within trachea of cat, 5% in sheep, 1% in rabbits, and are virtually absent in rats. Similarly, while the airways of humans, sheep, monkeys, dogs, and cats have well-developed submucosal glands, these structures are absent in rats, rabbits, and mice [1].

This chapter presents an overview of various animal models of asthma, with particular emphasis on atopic asthma, the form of human asthma most often mimicked in animal models. Species differences in airway structure and function are highlighted, and speculation focuses on the potential importance of these differences when attempting to apply results of these animal studies to the disease in humans.

II. Naturally Occurring Asthma in Nonhuman Animals

The ideal animal model would experience a human-type airway disease, including cough, wheeze, reversible airflow obstruction manifest by increased lung resistance (R_L) and residual volume which is exacerbated by beta blockade, nonspecific airway hyperreactivity (AHR), a decrease in the mid-expiratory flow rate throughout the vital capacity, and airway inflammation with a late-phase inflammatory response (LAR) to antigen for which eosinophils are prominent infiltrating cells. Only two nonhuman animal species, equine and feline, experience a naturally occurring syndrome of spontaneous bronchoconstriction associated with chronic airway inflammation.

A. Equine Heaves

Heavey horses were described by Aristotle as early as 33 B.C. [2]. More recently, heaves has been characterized as a naturally occurring respiratory disease of equids manifest by episodic airflow obstruction and exercise limitation. Airway hyperreactivity is associated with a neutrophilic and lymphocytic infiltrate in bronchoalveolar lavage (BAL) fluid and is demonstrable only when the animals are exposed to a barn environment; AHR resolves when the animals are put out to pasture. Affected animals are tachypneic, have a reduced tidal volume, and may be hypoxemic. Radiographs demonstrate hyperinflation, and nitrogen washout studies are prolonged, findings consistent with air trapping and diffuse airway obstruction. Administration of propranalol exacerbates the static airflow limitation in heavey horses but not normal horses or heavey horses in remission. Airway hyperreactivity and abnormal BAL cell composition may return to normal within 1 week after the animal is removed from the barn [3].

In many ways the equine syndrome resembles occupational asthma in humans. There are also some important differences. Histologically, while there is mucus hypersecretion and increased airway smooth muscle thickness, heaves is a disease of the bronchioles with a predominantly neutrophilic infiltrate. Lesions within central airways are not usually described [4]. This is in contrast to humans, for whom the larger airways are commonly affected and infiltrated with eosinophils. Additionally, airflow limitation in these horses is reversible with atropine, suggesting a (primarily) reflex vagal mechanism responsible for airway smooth muscle constriction [5]. This also is significantly different than for humans with asthma, for whom anticholinergic therapy is generally ineffective.

B. Feline Asthma

Cats with clinical signs of chronic cough, wheeze, and episodic, acute, life-threatening bronchoconstriction have been recognized in the veterinary literature (feline asthma) for more than 80 years [6]. Bronchoconstriction is usually reversible with beta agonists, and the chronic syndrome is remarkably responsive to corticosteroids. Airway hyperresponsiveness to methacholine is documented in affected cats [7]. Radiographic findings include thickened bronchial walls and pulmonary hyperinflation, the latter presumed to be the result of air trapping. Commonly, the right middle lung lobe is collapsed and atelectatic. Bronchoscopic findings include large amounts of tenacious and thick mucus within airways [8]. Small and large airways of asthmatic cats have been characterized histologically to include epithelial desquamation, goblet cell and submucosal hypertrophy and hyperplasia, and smooth muscle hyperplasia [9] (Fig. 1). Thickened basement membrane, or increased collagen deposition beneath basement membrane, is not a feature of the feline disease. Eosinophils are the predominant inflammatory cell and are found within the submucosa, extending through epithelium to the lumen of the airway. In most respects, then, feline asthma fulfills the criteria for the diagnosis of asthma in humans. It thus appears that cats with asthma would be a scientifically attractive animal model of the human disorder. Interestingly, how-

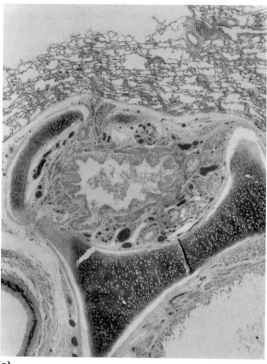

(a)

Figure 1 (a) Medium-sized cartilaginous bronchus from 62-year-old patient with chronic asthma. (Courtesy of Department of Pathology, University of Chicago, Chicago, IL.) (b) Medium-sized cartilagenous bronchus from 11-year-old Siamese cat with chronic asthma. (c) Small bronchiole from horse with "heaves." (Courtesy of Dr. Laurent Viel, Firestone Equine Respiratory Research Laboratory, Ontario Veterinary College, University of Guelph, Guelph, Ontario, Canada.) Note involution of bronchial mucosa, luminal exudate, and smooth muscle thickening and contraction in all three tissues. Additionally, note submucosal gland hyperplasia in cat and human airways.

ever, cats have not been used to study the pathogenesis of asthma in humans, for a number of reasons. First, although the naturally occurring disease is well described in the veterinary literature, it is basically unrecognized in the nonveterinary medical literature. Second, cats resist physical manipulation, and they are relatively difficult to instrument for survival studies. Additionally and critically important is the fact that there are few reagents available with which to study the immunologic aspects of the disease, presumably because there has not yet been a recognized need to develop such reagents.

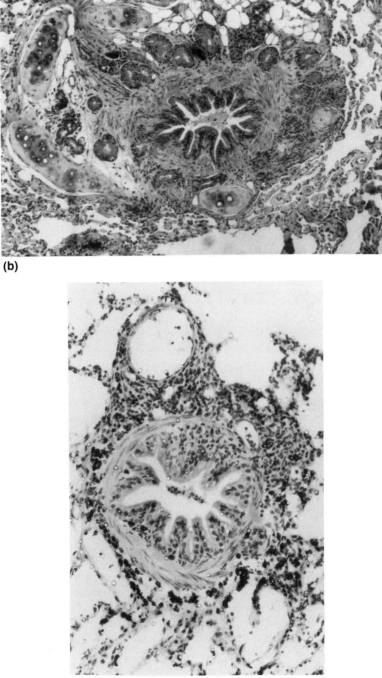

(b)

(c)

III. Experimentally Induced Asthma

Many antigen-sensitized and challenged animal species have been used to model atopic asthma, including rodent (mouse, rat, guinea pig), lagamorph (rabbit), canine, feline, ovine (sheep), and nonhuman primate (cynomolgus, rhesus). As noted by Patterson and Kelly [10] and by others, there are many physiologic limitations inherent in these studies. For example, most methods of determining airflow limitation in humans require active participation of the subject. Animal studies are effort-independent. Therefore, vital capacity, FEV_1, and mid-expiratory flow rates, for example, are not easily determined. Additionally, most animal subjects are anesthetized prior to study (sheep and some guinea pig studies are notable exceptions). Therefore the potential effects of specific anesthetic agents on bronchomotor tone and cellular biology must be appreciated. Consequently, comparisons of study results within and among species must recognize differences in anesthetics used, dosages, routes of administration, duration of effect, etc.

A. Cats

Cats have infrequently been used to study mechanisms of human asthma. Katsumata et al. [11] showed that reactive oxygen species can induce AHR in cats, and suggested that superoxide released from alveolar macrophages may play a role in the development of AHR in human asthmatics. The feline species was also one of the first in which a nonadrenergic, noncholinergic inhibitory nervous control of airway caliber was demonstrated [12]. Our group [13] have recently reported the effects of acute and chronic antigen challenge in sensitized cats. In these animals challenge with *Ascaris suum* results in an immediate increase in R_L and a decrease in dynamic compliance (C_{DYN}), changes which are accompanied by musical wheezes. Bronchoconstriction is completely reversible with terbutaline. Twenty-four hours following antigen challenge, there is a shift to the left in the dose–response curve to acetylcholine (ACh) and an influx of eosinophils into BAL fluid. Significantly, up to 40% of these airway eosinophils are hypodense.

These animals were subsequently exposed to nebulized antigen while awake, for 5 min, 3 times weekly for an additional 6 weeks. Changes in BAL cytology and airway reactivity persisted for at least 72 h following the completion of this 6-week antigen challenge period. Additionally, chronic antigen challenge resulted in a constellation of changes in airway wall structure, including an eosinophil infiltrate within epithelium, occasional foci of ulceration, hypertrophy and hyperplasia of epithelial goblet cells, hyperplasia of submucosal glands, and an increase in airway smooth muscle thickness.

To test the contribution of activated lymphocytes to changes in airway structure and function, an additional series of cats was then treated with high doses of cyclosporine A (CsA) prior to antigen challenge. Cats treated with CsA developed an equivalent early-phase response (EAR) compared to cats not given CsA. However, in CsA-treated cats the development of AHR, BAL eosinophilia, and the structural changes in airway wall that would otherwise occur in antigen-sensitized and challenged cats was abolished or significantly attenuated [14,15]. Thus, immune sensitization and challenge alone resulted in changes in airway wall structure and function which seem dependent upon T-cell activation.

There are unique features of this animal model. First, it is the only species other than human to develop *spontaneous* airflow limitation associated with eosinophilic airway inflammation. Second, the cat is the first reported species besides human in which antigen challenge results in a phenotypic change in the airway eosinophil to a hypodense state. Lastly, and perhaps most important, is the development of pathologic histologic derangements in airway epithelium, the mucus-secreting apparati, and airway smooth muscle which occur following chronic antigen challenge.

B. Dogs

In dogs a defined hypersensitivity disease related to aeroallergens has been recognized in the veterinary medical literature for many years, as noted by Patterson and Kelly [10]. The clinical disease is due to a ragweed pollinosis, although hypersensitivity to grass, house dust, etc., has also been identified. The target organ is the skin, and the disease is manifest primarily as a pruritic allergic dermatitis, while conjunctivitis and rhinitis occur less frequently. A clinical syndrome in pollen-sensitive dogs including cough, dyspnea, and production of thick, ropey mucus was reported by Patterson, but is not recognized in veterinary medicine.

Antigen challenge in sensitized dogs results in increased R_L, decreased C_{DYN}, decreased static compliance, and arterial hypoxemia without a change in functional residual capacity [16]. Additionally, wheezing is never reported. (These latter findings are perhaps not surprising given the degree of collateral circulation and the relatively enormous diameter of the conducting airways in this species [17]. Increased R_L in response to antigen is blocked by pretreatment with atropine, reversed by later administration of atropine, and inhibited by sectioning or cooling the vagus [10,18]. Unilateral antigen challenge of one lung lobe produces constriction in all lobes, which is prevented if the vagus on the side of the exposure is cooled. The generally accepted interpretation is that in the dog, antigen exposure causes changes which are reflex (vagal) in nature, to the level of at least 1 mm in diameter in the airways [16].

Chung et al. [19] showed that mongrel dogs neonatally sensitized with ragweed developed airway hyperreactivity to inhaled ACh. Interestingly, AHR developed in these animals despite the absence of a LAR following antigen challenge [19]. Airway reactivity to ACh in sensitized dogs increased over a 15-month period, while littermate controls had a decreased responsiveness of ACh over the same period of time. Airway hyperreactivity was (transiently) further increased by repeat exposure to antigen [20,21].

Hirshman et al. crossed Basenji and greyhound breeds to produce a barkless animal with great venous architecture and thus an easily instrumented and quiet dog. Routine screening resulted in the finding of AHR in a small number of these dogs. Controlled breeding of the Basenji-greyhound (B-G) cross resulted in a colony of dogs with naturally occurring AHR. Offspring of Basenji-greyhound dogs are also very susceptible to *Ascaris* and have nonspecific AHR to methacholine, citric acid, histamine, and leukotriene D_4. Importantly, AHR in the B-G cross is independent of exposure to antigen [22]. Beta blockers do not increase the nonspecific AHR in sensitized mongrel dogs, but do increase AHR in this strain of dog [23–25]. Airway inflammation is not present in these animals, and no clinical signs related to the laboratory finding of AHR have been reported in this unusual cross. Nevertheless, because AHR in the Basenji-greyhound is an inherited trait, this suggests the existence of a gene locus responsible for conferring AHR. An important implication, obviously, is the possibility of a specific genetic abnormality in humans as well.

In addition to antigen, dogs exposed to viral parasites or ozone also develop AHR in association with neutrophil accumulation within airways [26]. Ozone exposure leads to AHR to ACh within 1 h of exposure and returns to controls levels within about 1 week. Neutrophil depletion by hydroxyurea prevented the development of AHR. Indomethacin inhibited the development of AHR even though the neutrophils were still present [27,28]. These studies suggest an important role for cyclooxygenase products in the development of airway hyperreactivity following ozone exposure in dogs.

Development of the canine model of the EAR to antigen was initially hampered by a syndrome of sudden death in a small but significant number of *Ascaris suum*-sensitized and paralyzed dogs after acute *Ascaris* or ragweed exposure by aerosol [10]. It should be recalled that the target organ during anaphylaxis in dogs is the liver and not the lung. Following system antigen challenge in sensitized individuals, the hepatic vein becomes profoundly constricted, resulting in engorgement of the splanchnic pool and liver and intestinal hemorrhage.

Because (in part) airway responses are variable from one challenge to the next in individual animals as well as between animals, the dog has not been used in recent years to study pharmacological interventions.

C. Guinea Pigs

Guinea pigs are a very frequently used animal model to study the relationship between airway inflammation and airway hyperreactivity. Smith reported in 1904 that actively sensitized guinea pigs develop acute anaphylaxis after systemic reexposure to antigen and succumb soon afterward [29]. Death was secondary to bronchoconstriction and pulmonary vascular congestion. Later studies determined that these terminal responses are the result of the guinea pig's unusual sensitivity to histamine [10]. For this reason, guinea pigs are routinely treated with anti-histamine drugs prior to antigen challenge. The guinea pig has been sensitized and challenged with many antigens, including trimetallic anhydride and toluene diiso-cyanate (TDI) [30], agents associated with the development of occupational asthmatic symptoms in humans. In antigen-sensitized guinea pigs pretreated with antihistamines, antigen challenge results in an increased R_L and a decreased C_{DYN}. Maximal response occurs 2–10 min following exposure, is associated with pul-monary hyperinflation, and resolves within about 30 min [23]. Lung resistance returns to normal but C_{DYN} remains low, suggesting persistent peripheral airway obstruction [16]. Pretreatment with atropine or vagal blockage attenuates the increase in R_L but does not alter the decrease in C_{DYN} [16]. Airway hyperrespon-siveness develops within 24 h and is correlated with an increase in BAL eosino-phils and neutrophils, but not lymphocytes. However, increased numbers of lymphocytes are found in the bronchial mucosa and adventitia 1–2 days following antigen challenge.

Ovalbumin challenge in sensitized awake guinea pigs results in an acute decrease in specific conductance and two separate LARs, at 17 and 72 h post-challenge. Treatment with cromolyn 6 h post-antigen challenge inhibits both LARs. In these studies, the LARs are associated with an early neutrophil infiltrate followed by a progressive increase of eosinophils into airways [31,32].

Nevertheless, the association between airway inflammation (especially air-way neutrophils) and airway hyperreactivity is not so clear in guinea pigs. Sensi-tized guinea pigs exposed to TDI develop AHR to ACh which is associated with an influx of neutrophils into BAL. Hydroxyurea or neutrophil-depleting serum prevents the neutrophil influx without affecting the development of AHR [26,30, 33]. Ozone exposure results in the development of AHR within 2 h following exposure and lasts 3 days. Neutrophilic inflammation occurs *after* the develop-ment of AHR and persists past the time that AHR returns to normal. Neutrophil depletion with cyclophosphamide inhibits the influx of neutrophils but does not inhibit the development of AHR [27]. Taken together, these studies suggest a lack of importance of the neutrophil in the development of AHR in this animal model.

Mauser et al. [34] reported recently the effect of administration of anti-interleukin-5 antibody to sensitized guinea pigs to attenuate the influx of eosino-phils into airways following antigen challenge with ovalbumin. Inhibition of eosinophil influx into airways coincides with inhibition of the development of AHR to substance P only in animals given the highest dose of antibody. Lower doses of antibody ablated the influx of eosinophils but did not prevent the induction of AHR. Again, there may be a dissociation between airway inflammation and airway hyperreactivity in this animal species.

Guinea pigs have also been the primary animal model in which to study the pathogenesis of exercise-induced bronchoconstriction. Anesthetized guinea pigs develop mild increases in airway resistance after, but not during, 10 min of mechanical hyperventilation of room air or after exposure to dry gas hyperpnea. This response occurs in a time course similar to hyperpnea-induced bronchoconstriction in humans. This response is unaffected by drugs which block cholinergic transmission, histamine, serotonin, eicosanoids, or calcium channels, but is attenuated by treatment with salbutamol or aminophylline. Although Garland et al. [35] demonstrated that eicosanoids do play a modulating role in the guinea pig bronchoconstrictor response to dry gas hyperpnea, perhaps the most important mechanisms involve endogenous sensory neuropeptide release. Thus, guinea pigs pretreated with capsaicin to deplete C-fiber neuropeptides do not bronchoconstrict, while animals pretreated with phosphoramidon to inhibit neutral endopeptidase and thus prolong the existence of neuropeptides have a more pathologic bronchoconstriction. Solway et al. [36] reported that both NK1 and NK2 tachykinin receptor antagonist drugs can block this response.

Overall, there are many unique features about the guinea pig used to study mechanisms of bronchoconstriction, airway inflammation, and airway hyperreactivity in humans. They are easy to handle, relatively easy to sensitize, and have a very brisk and predictable response to antigen challenge. Their small size makes pharmacologic studies economically attractive. They have large numbers of goblet cells, and airway smooth muscle extending to the distal bronchi which is more prominent than in any other mammal studied [1,37]. Central airways of the guinea pig are very responsive to manipulation by agonists; they are more sensitive to the bronchoconstrictive actions of ACh than rat, rabbit, cat, dog, monkey, and human [38]. Mikami et al. [39] reported a strain of guinea pigs which is naturally hypersensitive to ACh and has a higher density of muscarinic receptors. There are also some limitations and differences which should be recognized. Although the primary reagenic antibody in humans is IgE, the primary anaphylactic antibody in the guinea pig may be IgG1 [29]. The guinea pig is the only species other than cat to have a large number of eosinophils within airways in health, thus limiting the interpretation of finding eosinophils in BAL after antigen challenge. Additionally, antigen challenge in this species results in a decrease rather than an increase in hypodense eosinophils recovered in BAL fluid [40]. Guinea pigs are also very difficult to intubate and are often exposed to antigen or bronchoconstricting agents while awake and breathing spontaneously. Because they are obligate nose breathers, less than 12% of aerosol is deposited in lungs and > 80% stays in the nose [29]. Interpretation of in-vitro smooth muscle studies of guinea pig distal airways within strips of lung parenchyma may be compromised by the presence of extensive smooth muscle in the pleura compared to other species, including human [41]. Additionally, there are more mast cells in the pleura than in the lung in this species only [42].

D. Nonhuman Primates

The rhesus monkey has been used as a model of human asthma for more than 35 years [43]. Initial studies by Patterson and Kelly [10] focused on the transfer from humans to monkeys of sensitivity to *Ascaris* after exposure to IgE-enriched human serum. In these animals, injection of *Ascaris* led to anaphylaxis; this reaction required repeated IgE exposure prior to each antigen challenge for a respiratory response to be seen. Because of this limitation, monkeys were screened for natural sensitivity to *Ascaris*. In general, some monkeys identified as naturally sensitized to *Ascaris* develop both early and late responses after experimental exposure to *Ascaris* by inhalation. This is usually associated with an increase in BAL eosinophils and nonspecific airways hyperreactivity to agonists including histamine and carbachol. Pretreatment with atropine, or the H_1 antagonist pyrillamine, does not inhibit the early-phase response [23]. In contrast, the 5-lipoxygenase inhibitor L-651,392 inhibited both the early- and late-phase responses to antigen in *Ascaris*-sensitized squirrel monkeys [44]. Although antigen challenge results in mild to moderate hypoxemia, wheezing is rare and pretreatment with beta agonists does not enhance the response to antigen. Additionally, antigen exposure does not cause a reproducible significant change in total lung capacity, functional residual capacity, or residual volume in these animals [16,23].

More recently, Patterson and Harris [45] summarized 20 years of experience with this rhesus model. The observation was made that there was a pronounced variation in the type and magnitude of responses among different animals over time. Thus, three groups of animals with different responses were categorized. Monkeys in group I have consistently positive results to cutaneous antigen testing and bronchoconstrict after each exposure to antigen. These responses have persisted for 5–13 years. Group II animals lost the characteristic of airway hyperreactivity within 1 year after initial exposure to antigen in spite of chronic intermittent exposure. This was associated with a loss of cutaneous reactivity in the majority of animals within 1 year as well. Group III consists of animals that have never responded to antigen. Patterson and Harris also note that animals without natural exposure to antigen which were sensitized in the laboratory setting had positive responses which in general lasted for a much shorter period of time (< 1.0 year) than that in animals with naturally occurring sensitivity to *Ascaris*.

Gundel et al. [46] used a cynomolgus model of *Ascaris*-induced airway hyperreactivity and airway inflammation to test the effect of an adhesion receptor antibody on subsequent inflammatory cell influx into airways, and airway response to cholinergic stimulation. Animals with naturally occurring sensitivity to *Ascaris* were challenged with antigen, and BAL and respiratory resistance was measured 6 h post-challenge. Pretreatment with antibody to ELAM-1 inhibited both the influx of inflammatory cells and the increase in respiratory resistance which occurred in the non-antibody-treated animals. Interestingly, the number of eosinophils *decreased* 6 h after challenge. In contrast, the number of neutrophils recovered in BAL increased > 12-fold in this same time period, and was significantly and positively correlated with the increase in respiratory resistance.

In this and other studies using nonhuman primates (NHP), *baseline* numbers of eosinophils recovered in BAL are often significantly elevated. Although unreported in these studies, lung infestation by the lung mite *Pneumonyssus simicola* is exceedingly common in both rhesus [47] and cynomolgus species. Typical response to the presence of this parasite is a mild to moderate parenchymal eosinophilia in asymptomatic monkeys. The potential effect of this complicating variable on results of antigen challenge studies in nonhuman primates has not been evaluated.

An additional complicating variable is the use of the phencyclidine drug *ketamine*, the most commonly used to induce and maintain anesthesia in the NHP. Ketamine is a potent bronchodilator [48], and it is reasonable to conclude that bronchoconstricter effects reported in these species might have been even more dramatic if a drug without significant effects on bronchomotor tone had been chosen as the anesthetic.

Because of the phylogenetic similarly between NHP and humans, it is tempting to assume that a NHP model would most closely mimic the structural and functional aspects of human airways. However, this assumption is not necessarily warranted. Recall that in this species there is no natural syndrome of asthma. Less than 5% of wild-caught rhesus monkeys are naturally sensitive to *Ascaris* [10], and an even lower percentage of captive-bred animals would be expected to be naturally sensitized. Similarly, nonhuman primates exposed to chronic antigen challenge developed structural changes in airway walls which are mild and limited to eosinophilic infiltration of the superficial airways. Additionally, on a practical level, the NHP are relatively protected species, and cannot be routinely handled without being first anesthetized (except by experienced handlers). On the other hand, to the extent that reagents developed to study immunologic aspects of asthma in humans cross-react with NHP species, these animals may be well suited for study of certain cell and molecular mechanisms involved in the pathogenesis of airway inflammation.

E. Rabbits

The rabbit was the first nonhuman animal species in which a LAR to antigen challenge was reported [49] and it has been used to study the relationship between LAR and the development of antigen-specific IgE. Thus, neonatal rabbits exposed to the mold *Alternaria tenuis* developed both early- and late-phase airway obstruction which was associated with systemic production of IgE. Passive sensitization with sera containing antigen-specific IgE resulted in the development of LAR in a separate series of rabbits. The development of anti-*Alternaria* IgG was associated with a blunting of airway responses, suggesting that antigen-specific IgE is important in the induction of antigen-induced late-phase responses in the rabbit.

Airway hyperreactivity has been induced in adult rabbits by inhalation of antigen, and in juvenile animals immunized from birth. Adult rabbits which are first sensitized and then antigen-challenged develop a modest ($< 50\%$) increase in R_L and a decrease in C_{DYN} which is temporally related to the development of airway wall edema and vessel dilation. Pretreatment with atropine but not adrenergic drugs ablates the increase in R_L but has only a minor effect on the decrease in C_{DYN} [16,49,50]. Cromolyn pretreatment blocks both the early and LAR, while corticosteroids block only the LAR [49,51]. Airway inflammation continues to evolve as late as 3 days following antigen challenge, consists of an early increase in neutrophils and eosinophils followed later by an increase in mononuclear cells in BAL, and is associated with airway hyperreactivity to histamine challenge. Airway hyperreactivity and BAL cell counts return to normal within 1 week of antigen challenge, although there is no direct correlation between the number of cells in BAL and the degree of AHR found in individual animals. Ragweed-sensitized rabbits treated with nitrogen mustard to deplete neutrophils have only an early but not a LAR to antigen challenge. If these same animals are again antigen-challenged after neutrophil repletion by transfusion with neutrophil-rich serum, the LAR occurs in temporal sequence with the development of AHR. Similarly, aerosolization of $C5_a$ produced an influx of neutrophils and the development of AHR in rabbit airways which was ablated by neutrophil depletion [52]. In this animal model, then, the development of the LAR and AHR seems to be dependent on the presence of circulating neutrophils [26]. It should be noted, however, that neutrophil repletion was associated with the development of AHR even though airway inflammation could not be documented.

An unpublished observation by Behrens and Larsen suggested that anesthesia may attenuate the development of the LAR in this model. Thus, rabbits may need to be lightly sedated and spontaneously breathing when lung function is measured [53].

It has been noted that isoproterenol, isoetharane, and epinephrine all fail to reverse airway obstruction associated with the LAR in rabbits [49,50]. The lack of efficacy of adrenergic agents to reverse bronchoconstriction in this species has been interpreted as being consistent with clinical studies of the LAR in humans [50]. Perhaps, too, this is the result of species differences in airway neuroanatomy; neural density is lower in rabbits than other animals examined, there is no adrenergic nerve supply to rabbit bronchial muscle, and rabbit bronchioles are vagotonic compared to humans, dog, cat, sheep, and farm animals in which the bronchioles are sympathotonic [54,55]. An additional important species differ-ence is the presence of atropine esterase in about 60% of rabbits, which efficiently inactivates atropine. Thus, approximately a 10-fold increase in the dose of atro-pine commonly used in other species is required to produce very short-acting vagal blockade. The rabbit lung is also deficient in histamine while having a high serotonin content [56]. However, rabbit pulmonary vessels are exquisitely sensi-tive to histamine; 10 μm will collapse the pulmonary arterial lumen and result in acute right ventricular failure and death [57].

F. Sheep

As noted by Wanner and Abraham [23], most sheep have a natural cutaneous sensitivity to *Ascaris suum* which can be boosted by repeat aerosol antigen challenge. Acute exposure to *Ascaris* results in an increase in lung resistance and respiratory rate, and a decrease in dynamic compliance and tidal volume. These changes are associated with pulmonary hyperinflation, an increase in arterial histamine, and arterial hypoxemia, although hypercarbia is rare. These early responses peak shortly after the termination of the antigen challenge and last 1–3 h. In a subset of these animals (dual responders), a late response occurs generally within 6–8 h of the initial challenge. There is also a decrease in tracheomucocili-ary transport which may last for days. This late response is associated with the development of nonspecific airway hyperreactivity to methacholine, carbachol, and histamine [58,59]. This LAR is also reported to result in an increase in eosinophils recovered in BAL [60], although the finding of 14 eosinophils/1000 BAL cells from late responders versus 4 eosinophils/1000 BAL cells in animals with only an early response should prompt a question as to the biological signifi-cance of this finding. Allergic animals also respond to propranolol with a 150% increase in lung resistance, compared to a 50% increase in lung resistance after propranolol in nonallergic sheep. While there is a great deal of variation in these responses to antigen from animal to animal, within a given animal they are quite consistent.

Sheep have been a frequently used animal model to study pharmacological control of both the early- and the late-phase response to antigen. Thus, it has been demonstrated in sheep that pretreatment with chlorpheneramine blunts 90% of the EAR to antigen, but only partially protects against the LAR in dual responders. Cromolyn or nedocromil sodium pretreatment inhibits both the EAR and the LAR, suggesting a role for products of mast cell activation in generating a LAR. Inter-estingly the 5-lipoxygenase antagonist FPL-55712 blocked only the LAR, sug-gesting a role for products of 5-LO in the LAR but not the EAR. Additional studies with multiple additional antagonists of either 5-LO or specific leukotrienes (LT $C_4, D_4 E_4$) support the hypothesis that leukotrienes mediate the LAR in sheep, and that there may be a differential pattern of leukotriene release during the EAR to explain the phenomenon of both single- and dual-responding sheep [61].

Because sheep have H_2 receptors within airways which modulate bronchodilation, it was proposed that this bronchodilating function is abnormal in allergic sheep, thus accounting for the effects of antihistamine and mast cell-stabilizing drugs to inhibit the EAR. Later studies demonstrated that the development of AHR following the LAR can be inhibited or blocked by drugs which bock cyclooxygenase or 5-lipoxygenase. However, only leukotriene antagonists blocks the LAR to antigen. Thus, in this animal model of atopic asthma, it seems that different eicosanoids may be responsible for the development of the LAR and the development of AHR following antigen challenge [62].

Sheep are one of only a few animals for which the effects of chronic antigen challenge on airway wall structure have been reported. Interestingly, in allergic sheep undergoing 6 weeks of antigen challenge (20 challenges), there was a modest decrease in the number of ciliated cells in the tracheobronchial tree; however, no other significant structural changes similar to human bronchial asthma were found [63].

One unique feature of this model is that airway responses are studied in fully instrumented yet nonanesthetized animals, thus avoiding potentially confounding interactions between anesthetic drugs and cortical transmission of neural reflexes.

G.   Rats/Mice

Mice and rats are frequently used animal models to study physiologic and immunologic phenomena associated with antigen challenge. For example, early- and late-phase responses following antigen challenge commonly develop in inbred brown Norway rats. Fairly unusual to this strain, some of these animals have late but not early responses, suggesting an uncoupling of mechanisms which may be responsible for each of these responses. The LAR subsequent to a single antigen challenge does not lead to AHR, but multiple antigen challenge in the same animal results in the development of AHR to MCh [64]. The development of AHR in this setting is not limited to morphologic changes in airways but is also dependent on changes in lung tissue mechanics [65]. Rats which are first passively sensitized using anti-IgE antibody and subsequently challenged by aerosolization of antigen develop an acute (within 1 h) BAL neutrophilia and a later (2 h) mononuclear cell peribronchiolitis. The EAR does not generally result in a LAR, suggesting that anti-IgE-mediated mast cell degranulation is not sufficient to cause a late response in this strain under these experimental conditions [66,67]. Similarly, sensitized BALB/C mice develop IgE responses but no change in AHR (response of trachealis to electric field stimulation in vitro) unless they are first antigen-challenged by aerosolization into airways [68].

Rats and mice are also frequently used models to study possible genetic loci associated with airway hyperreactivity. Studies using trachealis from one strain of Sprague-Dawley rat which are hyperresponsive to allergen, serotonin, and other bronchospasminogens in vivo failed to demonstrate AHR in vitro. However, lung parenchymal strips were hyperreactive to leukotrienes and mildly hyperreactive to serotonin [24]. Levitt and Mitzner [69,70] produced a strain of inbred mice (AJ) that are specifically hyperresponsive to serotonin and ACh, and strains (C57B/6 and C3H) that are hyporesponsive. The hyperresponsiveness trait is latent in the heterozygous state and consistent with a recessive genotype. These animals, like the Basenji-greyhound cross, suggest the possibility that a specific gene or gene locus may be located which confers AHR to specific stimuli [20]. DBA mice are also hyperresponsive to ACh but not to serotonin, suggesting that the AHR which is inherited is associated with separate gene loci.

Murine asthma models have most recently been used to study the immunologic phenomenon underlying the association between airway inflammation and airway hyperreactivity. This is due in part to an explosion of information detailing the potential role of eosinophils and T cells in the pathogenesis of asthma [71] Mossman et al. were the first to report that at least two different subsets of CD_4 T cells are present in the mouse, distinguished by a differential pattern of cytokine secretion [72]. Thus, after appropriate activation TH_1 cells secrete IL-2 and interferon gamma, while TH_2 clones secrete IL-4,5,6 and IL-10. Both clones secrete IL-3 and GM-CSF. Wierenga et al. [73] have speculated that a similar functional subset of helper T cells occurs in atopic human patients. Because T-cell clones from atopic and asthmatic humans seem to be primarily the TH_2 subset, attention has focused on the role of cytokines released from this population of lymphocytes. Particular emphasis has been placed on IL-4 and IL-5 due to the roles these cytokines play in IgE synthesis, and eosinophilopoiesis, activation, and recruitment. Thus, Gavett et al. [74], employing a mouse (A/J) model of antigen (sheep RBC) sensitization and challenge, depleted the CD_4 T-cell population from one group of animals using anti-CD_4 antibody GK1.5. Animals not given GK1.5 prior to antigen challenge developed airway hyperreactivity, an increase in eosinophils and lymphocytes recovered by BAL, and increased numbers of eosinophils within pulmonary interstitium. Prior treatment with GK1.5 abolished the development of AHR and abolished the cellular infiltrate into BAL and lung parenchyma. Brusselle et al. [75] actively immunized mice with ovalbumin and found a large influx of eosinophils and a lesser increase of lymphocytes into airways following antigen challenge. In these mice this was associated with detectable levels of IgE in serum. Mice of the same strain made deficient in IL-4 ("knockout mice") did not develop a similar degree of airway eosinophilia, and serum IgE was not detectable following antigen challenge. The authors of this study speculated that the induced IL-4 deficiency may have caused a reduction in

TH$_2$ lymphocytes (and their secretion products including IL-5), which depend on IL-4 as a growth factor.

Mice are particularly attractive models for these studies due to their defined genetic background, the wealth of immunologic reagents available which are species-specific, and the rapidly expanding field of transgenics. However, because of their size, individual animals cannot be used for longitudinal or serial studies over time; data from an individual animal must be viewed as a "snapshot" of events. Their size also precludes obtaining large amounts of cells or tissues. It should also be recalled that the structure of murine airways is in some way profoundly different from human airways. For example, it is not clear that mice can generate the tidal volume required to generate a cough. There is no cartilage in the respiratory tree beyond the primary bronchi, which in mice are the only airways as large as 1 mm. The epithelial layer is simple columnar instead of pseudo-stratified. Goblet cells are rare ($<$ 1% of tracheobronchial epithelial cells), and submucosal glands are absent [76]. The primary mediator of the early-phase response to antigen in the mouse and rat is serotonin; mouse (and rat) mast cells have a high serotonin content and are relatively deficient in histamine [77].

Murine models will continue to be used with great frequency to study the cellular and molecular mechanisms involved in airway inflammation. Causal assumptions between these immunologic phenomena and changes in airway function in the mouse will precede and prompt assumptions about similar relationships in human airways. Review of these species differences in airway structure and function may assist in putting these extrapolations in their proper perspective.

IV. Limitations in the Study of Animal Models of Human Asthma

Bronchial asthma in humans is a disease of episodic airflow obstruction which reverses spontaneously or in response to therapy. Some patients may cough as the only clinical sign, and may have an unremarkable physical examination at the time of their clinic appointment. A methacholine challenge study may then be performed in these patients to determine the presence and degree of AHR. Airway hyperreactivity is a defining feature of asthma and helps to explain the phenomenon of spontaneous airflow limitation, wheeze, and cough. Thus, a positive methacholine challenge test in a patient with vague clinical signs helps to confirm the diagnosis of asthma. For the patient with no cough, wheeze, exercise intolerance, or other clinical signs of bronchoconstriction, a positive methacholine challenge test may suggest the *potential to develop* clinical symptoms of asthma. Thus, airway hyperresponsiveness, as determined in the laboratory, is *not* the clinical disease asthma.

Many antigen-sensitized animals bronchoconstrict when exposed (by injection, direct aerosol, or nebulization) to large doses of the sensitizing antigen. A subpopulation of these animals will develop nonspecific AHR within 24 h of antigen challenge. A critical distinction between these animal models and humans with asthma is the finding that no experimentally induced animal model of asthma described to date manifests clinical signs of *spontaneous* bronchoconstriction, such as cough or wheeze. Said in another way, the development of experimentally induced AHR in animals is *not linked* to the phenomenon of spontaneous airflow limitation. If our scientific focus is the pathogenesis of human airway hyperreactivity, we must recognized the uncoupling of AHR and spontaneous bronchoconstriction in these animal models, and thus the uncertainty in extrapolating from these models to the pathogenesis of AHR in human asthma.

A related and perhaps even more telling limitation in the use of animal models of human asthma is the lack of naturally occurring disease in the species chosen for study. As noted by Maurer et al. [63], perhaps we should to be surprised that none of the animal species studied (except cat and NHP?) develops experimentally induced *chronic* airflow limitation and airway inflammation, even after multiple exposure to antigen. With the exception of equine and feline, no other animal nonhuman species develops a naturally occurring chronic airway disorder with any resemblance to asthma. Predictably, then, almost all experiments using animals have been designed to study the *onset* of airways inflammation and hyperreactivity. Critically important to this discussion, patients with asthma have *already established* airway inflammation and hyperreactivity in addition to variable airflow limitation. It is not intuitively obvious that investigating mechanisms involved in the *onset* of a disorder, or treatments designed to inhibit the *onset* of disease, are directly relevant to the study of established and ongoing asthma.

Lastly, because of the limited availability of tissues from asthmatic humans, airway tissues from animal models of asthma have been used to study smooth muscle responses in vitro. However, as pointed out by Macklem [78], it is not at all clear that in-vitro isometric force measurements of airway smooth muscle have any relevance to asthma. Because smooth muscle contraction in vitro is studied in terms of force exerted at a fixed length, it is not analogous to bronchospasm, where smooth muscle exerts force by contracting and changes its length.

V. Conclusions

Pulmonary disorders which result from viral infection, exposure to high doses of ozone, or inhalation of antigen are characterized by airway inflammation and are associated with the development of AHR in persons and animals. Animal studies have clearly shown that AHR can also develop in the absence of an inflammatory cell infiltrate, and that airway inflammation does not necessarily result in AHR. As noted by Larsen [26], the mechanisms resulting in AHR may thus be inflammatory cell-dependent or -independent, as well as both stimulus- and species-specific.

We use animal models to address questions about the pathogenesis of human asthma that cannot be answered directly in humans. Animal models are required for invasive and hazardous studies which test hypotheses related to the immunologic, cellular, molecular, and pharmacologic mechanisms responsible for the development and exacerbation of AHR. However, experimental animal models of asthma do not spontaneously bronchoconstrict and do not (except perhaps the cat), develop a constellation of significant structural abnormalities of epithelium, the mucus-secreting apparatus, and smooth muscle which characterize the airways of human asthmatics. Therefore, the scientist developing an animal model and the clinician attempting to determine the relevance of experiments using animal models should both be aware of the strengths and weaknesses of the models being used. No animal species other than human should be considered a complete model of human asthma. Instead, animal models of asthma are most likely to be of value when they are chosen to test a specific hypothesis concerning the pathogenesis of human asthma. A working knowledge of the biologic profile of each animal model is therefore critical.

Acknowledgments

The author gratefully acknowledges the assistance of Paul Schumacker, Ph.D., for his review of the manuscript, and Ms. Millie Maleckar for typing the manuscript.

References

1. St. George JA, et al. Cell populations and structure-function relationships of cells in the airways. In: Gardner DE, Crapo JD, Massaro J, eds. Toxicology of the Lung. New York: Raven Press, 1988:71–101.
2. McPherson EA, Thomson JR. Chronic obstructive pulmonary disease in the horse. Eq Vet J 1983; 15:203–206.
3. Derksen FJ, et al. Airway reactivity in ponies with recurrent airway obstruction (heaves). J Appl Physiol 1985; 58:598–604.
4. Jubb KV, et al. Pathology of Domestic Animals. Vol. 2. San Diego, CA: Academic Press, 1985.
5. Derksen FJ, et al. Pulmonary function tests in standing ponies: reproducibility and effects of vagal blockade. Am J Vet Res 1982; 43:598–602.
6. Dye, JA. Feline bronchopulmonary disease. Vet Clin N Am 1992; 22:1187–1201.
7. McKiernan BC, Johnson LR. Clinical pulmonary function testing in dogs and cats. Vet Clin N Am 1992; 22:1187–1201.

8. Moise NS, et al. Clinical radiographic and bronchial cytologic features of cats with bronchial disease: 65 cases (1980–1986). J Am Vet Med Assoc 1989; 194:1467–1473.

9. Howard EB, Ryan CP. Chronic obstructive pulmonary disease in the domestic cat. California Vet 1982; 6:7–11.

10. Patterson R, Kelly JF. Animal models of the asthmatic state. Annu Rev Med 1974; 25:53–68.

11. Katsumata U, et al. Oxygen radicals produce airway constriction and hyperresponsiveness in anesthetized cats. Am Rev Respir Dis 1990; 141:1158–1161.

12. Diamond L, O'Donnell M. A nonadrenergic vagal inhibitory pathway to feline airways. Science 1980; 208:185–188.

13. Padrid PA, et al. Persistent airway hyperresponsiveness and histologic alterations after chronic antigen challenge in cats. Am J Respir Crit Care Med 1994; in press.

14. Padrid PA, et al. Cyclosporine treatment in vivo inhibits the development of airway hyperresponsiveness and histologic alterations after chronic antigen challenge in cats. Am Rev Respir Dis 1994; 149:A771.

15. Padrid PA, et al. Cyclosporine treatment in vivo does not attenuate the Schultz-Dale contraction of airway smooth muscle from immune sensitized cats. Am Rev Respir Dis 1994; 149:A771.

16. Drazen JM. Pulmonary physiologic abnormalities in animal models of acute asthma. In: Austen LR, Lichtenstein LM, eds. Asthma: Physiology, Immunology, and Treatment. New York: Academic Press, 1973; 249–264.

17. Robinson NE. Some functional consequences of species differences in lung anatomy. In: Dungworth DL, ed. Advances in Veterinary Science and Comparative Medicine. New York: Academic Press, 1982:2–33.

18. Gold WM, et al. Role of vagus nerves in experimental asthma in allergic dogs. J Appl Physiol 1972; 33:719.

19. Chung KF, et al. Antigen induced airway hyperreactivity and pulmonary inflammation in the allergic dog. J Appl Physiol 1985; 58:1347.

20. Wanner A, et al. Models of airway hyperresponsiveness. Am Rev Respir Dis 1990; 141:253–257.

21. Becker AB, et al. Development of chronic airway hyperresponsiveness in ragweed-sensitized dogs. J Appl Physiol 1989; 66:2691–2697.

22. Hirshman CA. Basenji-greyhound models of asthma. Chest 1985; 87:172s–178s.

23. Wanner A, Abraham WM. Experimental models of asthma. Lung 1982; 160: 231–243.

24. Wanner A. Utility of animal models in the study of human airway disease. Chest 1990; 98:211–217.

25. Hirshman CA. Experimental asthma in animals. In: Weiss EB, Stein M, eds. Bronchial Asthma. Mechanisms and Therapeutics. Boston: Little, Brown, 1993; 382–404.

26. Larsen GL. Experimental models of reversible airway obstruction. In: Crystal RG, West JD, eds. The Lung. New York: Raven Press, 1991; 953–965.

27. Pauwels R. Effect of inflammation in bronchial responsiveness. In: Nadel JA, Pauwels R, Snashall PD, eds. Bronchial Hyperresponsiveness. Oxford: Blackwell 1987; 315–321.

28. O'Byrne PM. Neutrophil depletion inhibits airway hyperreactivity induced by ozone exposure. Am Rev Respir Dis 1984; 130:214.

29. Campos MG, Church MK. How useful are guinea-pig models of asthma? Clin Exp Allergy 1992; 22:665–666.

30. Cibulas, W. Toluene diisocyanate induced airway hyperreactivity in guinea pigs depleted of granulocytes. J Appl Physiol 1988; 64:1773.

31. Hutson PA, et al. Early and late phase bronchoconstriction after allergen challenge of non anesthetized guinea pigs. I. The association of disordered airway physiology to leukocyte infiltration. Am Rev Respir Dis 1988; 137:548–557.

32. Hutson PA, et al. The effect of cromolyn sodium and albuterol on early and late phase bronchoconstriction and airway leukocyte infiltration after allergen challenge of nonanesthetized guinea pigs. Am Rev Respir Dis 1988; 138:1157–1163.

33. Withnall MT, de Brito FB. Asthma as an Inflammatory Disease: are Animal Models Relevant. British Inflammation Research Association, 1990.

34. Mauser PJ, et al. Inhibitory effect of the TRFK-5 anti IL-5 antibody in a guinea pig model of asthma. Am Rev Respir Dis 1993; 148:1623–1627.

35. Garland A, et al. Role of eicosanoids in hyperpnea-induced airway responses in guinea pigs. J Appl Physiol 1993; 75:2797–2804.

36. Solway J, et al. Tachykinin receptor antagonists inhibit hyperpnea-induced broncho-constriction in guinea pigs. J Clin Invest 1993; 92:315–323.

37. Breazile JE, Brown EM. Anatomy. In: Wagner JE, Manning PJ, eds. The Biology of the Guinea Pig. New York: Academic Press, 1976:59–60.

38. Daly IB, Hebb C. Pulmonary and Bronchial Vascular Systems. Baltimore: Williams & Wilkins, 1966.

39. Mikami H, et al. Characteristics of two lines of guinea pigs (BHS and BHR) differing in bronchial sensitivity to acetylcholine and histamine exposure. Exp Anim (Tokyo) 1991; 40:453–460.

40. Rimmer SJ, et al. Density profile of bronchoalveolar lavage eosinophils in the guinea pig model of allergen-induced late phase allergic responses. Am J Respir Cell Mol Biol 1992; 6:340–348.

41. Halonen M, et al. Anatomic basis for species differences in peripheral lung strip contraction to PAF. Am J Physiol Lung Cell Mol Physiol 1990; 3:L81–L86.

42. Brewer NR. The comparative physiology of the guinea pig respiratory system. Chicago: University of Chicago, unpublished.

43. Weiszer I, et al. Ascaris hypersensitivity in the rhesus monkey. I. A model for the study of immediate hypersensitivity in the primate. J Allergy 1968; 41:14–22.

44. McFarlane CS, et al. Effects of a 5-lipoxygenase inhibitor (L651,392) on primary and late responses to Ascaris antigen in the squirrel monkey. Agents Actions 1987; 2: 63–68.

45. Patterson R, Harris KE. IgE-mediated rhesus monkey asthma: natural history and individual animal variation. Int Arch Allergy Immunol 1992; 97:154–159.

46. Gundel RH, et al. Endothelial leukocyte adhesion molecule mediates antigen-induced acute airway inflammation and late-phase airway obstruction in monkeys. J Clin Invest 1991; 88:1407–1411.

47. Georgi JR. Parasitology for Veterinarians. Philadelphia: W. B. Saunders, 1980.

48. Hirshman CA, et al. Ketamine block of bronchospasm in experimental canine asthma. Br J Anaesthesiol 1974; 51:713–717.
49. Shampain MP, et al. An animal model of the late pulmonary responses to *Alternaria* challenge. Am Rev Respir Dis 1982; 126:493–498.
50. Larsen GL. The rabbit model of the late asthmatic response. Chest 1985; 87:184s–188s.
51. Larsen GL, et al. An animal model of the late asthmatic response to antigen challenge. In: Kay AB, Austen KF, Lichtenstein LM, eds. Asthma Physiology, Immunopharmacology and Treatment. London: Academic Press, 1984; 245–262.
52. Irvin CG, et al. Acute effects of airways inflammation on airways function and reactivity. Fed Proc 1982; 41:1358.
53. Larsen GL, et al. Neutrophils and late-phase reaction. In: Kay AB, ed. Allergy and Inflammation. London: Academic Press, 1987:225–244.
54. Hebb C. Motor innervation of pulmonary blood vessels of mammals. In: Fishman AP, Hecht HH, eds. The Pulmonary Circulation and Interstitial Space. Chicago: University of Chicago Press, 1969.
55. Brewer NR. Morphophysiology of the rabbit lung. Proc Inst Med Chgo 1993; 45:7–9.
56. Parrat JR, West GB. 5-Hydroxytryptamine and tissue mast cells. J Physiol 1957; 137:169–192.
57. Gilbert AJ. Microscopic observations of pulmonary artery reactions. J Pharm 1938; 62:228–235.
58. Abraham WM, et al. Characterization of a late phase pulmonary response after antigen challenge in allergic sheep. Am Rev Respir Dis 1983; 128:839–844.
59. Larsen GL, et al. Granulocytes and airway reactivity. Am Rev Respir Dis 1991; 143:S64–S65.
60. Abraham WM, et al. Cellular markers of inflammation in the airways of allergic sheep with and without allergen induced late responses. Am Rev Respir Dis 1988; 138:1565–1571.
61. Abraham WM. Pharmacology of allergen-induced early and late airway responses and antigen-induced airway hyperresponsiveness in allergic sheep. Pulmonary Pharmacol. 1989; 2:33–40.
62. Lanes S, et al. Indomethacin and FPL-57231 inhibit antigen-induced airway hyperresponsiveness in sheep. J Appl Physiol 1986; 61:864–872.
63. Maurer DR, et al. Airway morphology in normal allergic and SO_2 exposed sheep. Physiologist 1981; 24:1105.
64. Bellofiore S, Martin JG. Antigen challenge of sensitized rats increase airway responsiveness to methacholine. J Appl Physiol 1988; 65:1642–1646.
65. Nagase T, et al. Airway and tissue responses to antigen challenge in sensitized brown Norway rats. Am J Respir Crit Care Med 1994; 150:218–226.
66. Blythe S, et al. IgE antibody mediated inflammation of rat lung: histologic and bronchoalveolar lavage assessment. Am Rev Respir Dis 1986; 134:1246–1251.
67. Sorkness R, et al. Pulmonary antigen challenge in rats passively sensitized with a monoclonal IgE antibody induces immediate but not late changes in airway mechanics. Am Rev Respir Dis 1988; 138:1152–1156.

68. Saloga J, et al. Increased airway responsiveness in mice depends on local challenge with antigen. Am J Respir Crit Care Med 1994; 149:65–70.

69. Levitt RC, Mitzner W. Expression of airway hyperreactivity to acetylcholine as a simple autosomal recessive trait in mice. FASEB 1988; 2:2605–2608.

70. Levitt RC, Mitzner W. Autosomal recessived inheritance of airway reactivity to 5-hydroxytryptamine. J Appl Physiol 1989; 67:1125–1132.

71. Berman JS, Weller PF. Airway eosinophils and lymphocytes in asthma. Am Rev Respir Dis 1992; 145:1246–1248.

72. Mossman, et al. Two types of murine helper T cell clone. I. Definition according to profiles of lymphokine activities and secreted proteins. J Immunol 1986; 136:2348–2357.

73. Wierenga EA, et al. Evidence for compartmentalization of functional subsets of CD4 T lymphocytes in atopic patients. J Immunol 1990; 144:4651–4656.

74. Gavett SH, et al. Depletion of murine CD4+ T lymphocytes prevent antigen-induced airway hyperreactivity and pulmonary eosinophilia. Am J Respir Cell Mol Biol 1994; 10:587–593.

75. Brusselle GG, et al. Attenuation of allergic airway inflammation in IL-4 deficient mice. Clin Exp Allergy 1994; 24:73–80.

76. Kaplan HM, et al. Respiratory physiology. In: Foster HL, Small DJ, Fox JG, eds. The Mouse in Biomedical Research. Boston: Academic Press, 1983:252–256.

77. Bivin WS, et al. Respiratory System. In: Baker HJ, Lindsey JR, Weisbroth SH, eds. The Laboratory Rat. New York: Academic Press, 1979:83–86.

78. Macklem PT. Bronchial hyporesponsiveness. Chest 1985; 87:158s–159s.

11

Transgenic Mice for the Study of Lung Disease

**STEPHEN W. GLASSER, THOMAS R. KORFHAGEN,
and JEFFREY A. WHITSETT**

Children's Hospital Medical Center
Cincinnati, Ohio

I. Introduction

Transgenic mice are now used extensively in biomedical research to determine the role of specific genes in normal growth and differentiation and in the pathogenesis of disease. Transgenic animals are produced by the permanent insertion of cloned DNA into the genome of a fertilized egg or early developing embryo. The high efficiency of the embryo transfer and short gestation period facilitates the introduction of genes into the mouse. Transgenic mice are most frequently made by microinjection of a recombinant DNA (transgene) into the male pronucleus of fertilized eggs. The injected DNA randomly and stably integrates into the host chromosome, resulting in a permanent addition of DNA to the mouse genome. Microinjected eggs are returned to a surrogate female mouse and the embryos proceed through development. Transgenic offspring are identified by Southern blot or PCR analysis of DNA extracted from tissue of the transgenic founder animals [1,2]. The transgenic founder animals are bred to establish permanent mouse lines containing the transgene. In mice produced by these manipulations, the integrated transgene has been subjected to the complex regulatory signals present in the cells of the developing mouse. The transgenic offspring are used to determine the consequences of the foreign DNA gene product. Genes may also be

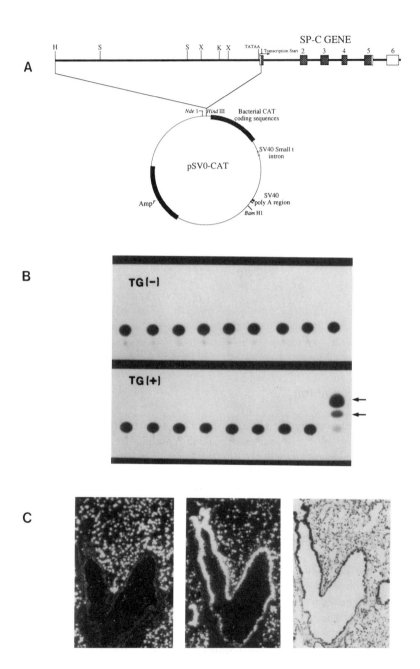

transferred to totipotent embryonic stem cells (ES) using plasmid or viral constructs; the recombinant ES cells are injected into mouse blastocysts from which a chimeric mouse is produced. The latter technique is generally used to produce mutations within the endogenous gene by the process of gene targeting.

A. Generation of Transgenic Mice

The ability of transgenic mice can be placed into the categories of gene addition and gene ablation. Gene addition has been widely used to determine the effect of altered expression of the gene of interest and to identify and map cis-active regions of genes that determine cell-specific expression. Regulatory regions of the transgene are used to control expression of a reporter gene that is monitored by biochemical or immunologic assays. These types of analyses provide insight into the function of cis-active regulatory elements that may determine temporal-spatial expression. The precise pattern of transgene mRNA is readily detected by in situ hybridization or immunochemistry to localize the mRNA or protein produced from the transgene (Fig. 1).

Transgenic mice are used routinely to produce permanent genetic models for study of human disease and development [3,4]. Prior to the emergence of

---

Figure 1 Design and expression of a transgene construct containing the human SP-C promoter region. (A) Illustrates the subcloning of human SP-C genomic DNA extending 5′ of the gene body (top line) into a conventional promoterless reporter plasmid. Features to note are the reporter gene (bacterial chloramphenicol acetyl transferase, CAT) positioned adjacent to the SP-C encoded transcription start site; sequences for correct transgene mRNA processing including the intronic and polyadenylation sequences downstream of the CAT sequences. Unique restriction sites denoted as Nde I and Bam HI are used to release the assembled experimental transgene from the bacterial plasmid vector. Amp^R denotes bacterial ampicillin resistance used in plasmid selection-growth during assembly of the construct. S, X, and K are restriction sites in the SP-C genomic DNA used to orient the promoter sequences. (B) Represents enzyme assays of tissue extracts prepared from transgenic (TG+) and nontransgenic (TG−) SP-C-CAT mice to detect organ specific expression of the CAT reporter. Assays have been normalized to uniform protein from tissue preparations, incubated with acetyl CoA and ^{14}C-chloramphenicol substrate. Reaction products are separated from substrate by thin-layer chromatography and detected by autoradiography (arrows). Tissue extract preparations are (left to right) kidney, liver, spleen, heart, brain, muscle, thymus, trachea, and lung. CAT activity is detected only in lung extract of the TG+ animal. (C) Localization of endogenous SP-C and SP-C-CAT transgene expression by in-situ hybridization. Serial sections of lung probed with antisense riboprobe to SP-C (left), which hybridizes in a pattern consistent with the alveolar distribution of type II cells in the lung. Antisense CAT riboprobe (center) hybridizing along the bronchiolar epithelium and focally throughout the alveolar region. The bright-field photomicrograph (right) depicts lung morphology.

transgenic technology, mice with naturally occurring or induced mutations provided models for study of genetic disease [5]. Transgenic mice now provide the ability to mutate the gene and then assess the role of the gene in vivo. By targeting gene expression with promoters restricted to specific organs and cell types, the role of a gene product in development or disease in specific organs can be assessed.

B.   Gene Deletion-Homologous Recombination

Homologous recombination is now used routinely to inactivate or mutate the endogenous gene. The molecular basis underlying this approach depends on homologous recombination of modified genes with the endogenous gene to create mutations. Recombination vectors are designed to insert a selectable marker (usually resistance to neomycin) to replace endogenous sequences or terminate transcription of the target gene. This rearranged gene is microinjected into pluripotent embryonic stem cells (ES). Homologous recombination between the mutated DNA and identical sequences in the ES cell genome replaces the ES cell gene with the mutated gene. The targeted ES cells are cloned and injected into host embryos wherein ES cells associate with the inner cell mass, resume normal development, and therefore contribute cells to a portion of all developing tissues in the embryo to produce chimeric mice. By using coat color differences between the ES cell strain and the host embryo and Southern blot or PCR analysis of mouse DNA, mice with the inserted gene can be identified. When bred to homozygosity, the targeted mice display the phenotype conferred by the mutation [6,7].

The recent cloning of genes that are selectively expressed in lung cells has provided reagents useful in directing gene expression to specific pulmonary cells. The present chapter reviews experiments generating transgenic models for study of pulmonary disease and development. The reader is referred to current reviews of lung-specific gene expression [8,9], and the use of transgenic mice [10,11].

II.   Genes Expressed Selectively in the Pulmonary Epithelium

Several genes are expressed in a highly selective manner in respiratory epithelial cells. These genes include pulmonary surfactant protein SP-A, B, and C and the Clara cell secretory protein CCSP (also termed CC10 or uteroglobin) genes.

Pulmonary surfactant proteins contribute to both the surface tension-reducing properties of surfactant and to the regulation of surfactant phospholipid metabolism [12–14]. The surfactant protein genes are transcribed in distinct but overlapping subsets of respiratory epithelial cells including alveolar type II, bronchial, bronchiolar cells and in epithelial cells of the tracheal-bronchial glands. Surfactant protein gene expression is influenced by distinct humoral, temporal, and spatial signals. Developmental studies indicate that SP-C is expressed early in embryonic lung development [15–18]. SP-A and SP-B expression begins slightly later, in association with the appearance of cuboidal respiratory epithelial cells [17,19,20]. With advancing gestation, the abundance of SP-A, B, and C mRNAs and proteins increases in association with increased numbers of epithelial cells. In adult lungs of both humans and rodents, SP-C mRNA is detected only in type II cells [21,22]. In contrast, SP-A and SP-B mRNA are detected in both type II and bronchiolar epithelial cells.

Originally identified as a Clara cell marker, the CCSP gene encodes a homodimeric protein that binds hydrophobic xenobiotic molecules. CCSP inhibits phospholipase A_2 activity, which may in turn regulate antiinflammatory responses of the conducting airways [23]. The pattern of CCSP expression differs from the expression of surfactant protein genes. CCSP is expressed primarily at high levels in airway epithelial cells and also at low but detectable levels in the uterus of progesterone-treated rats [24–26]. CCSP and CCSP mRNA are detected within subsets of nonciliated epithelial cells of the conducting airways from the trachea extending to the respiratory bronchioles. In the mouse, CCSP mRNA and protein are not expressed in the alveolus. CCSP expression is detected late in rodent lung development (p.c. day 15–16), in a pattern distinct from surfactant proteins. The promoters from these genes can therefore be used to express genes in distinct populations of cells and at distinct developmental stages in transgenic mice.

III. In-Vivo Mapping of cis-Active DNA Elements That Control Lung-Specific Transcription

A. CCSP Promoter Function

DNA from the CCSP and SP-C gene loci that include candidate regulatory regions have been tested in transgenic mice to identify DNA sequences that direct gene transcription in the pulmonary epithelium. From sequence analysis of these two genes, regions of highly conserved DNA sequence between rodent and human genes were identified. Transgenic mice were generated with 2.3 kb of genomic DNA 5′ to the transcriptional start site of rat CCSP gene controlling chloramphenicol acetyl transferase (CAT) expression. High levels of CAT activity were detected in tissue extracts of trachea and lung but not in extracts from other organs from the transgenic mice. In-situ hybridization analysis demonstrated co-localization of endogenous murine CCSP mRNA and the CAT mRNA produced by 2.3 CCSP-CAT transgene expression [24]. Endogenous CCSP mRNA and CCSP-CAT transgene mRNA were detected along the tracheal, bronchial, and bronchiolar epithelium. Both the CAT and CCSP mRNA diminished abruptly at the alveolar ducts, consistent with the distribution of Clara cells in the mouse. In a separate analysis, the 2.3-kb rat CCSP DNA was used to drive expression of human growth hormone (hGH) in transgenic mice [27,28]. Expression of the hGH reporter was identified using immunocytochemistry with antibodies directed to hGH demonstrating hGH immunostaining similar to that of the endogenous CCSP. Thus the 2.3 kb of CCSP DNA contains cis-active regulatory elements that respond to lung-specific and perhaps cell-specific transcription factors in the lung. The location of CCSP transcriptional control elements were mapped by deletion mutagenesis of the 2.3 kb of 5'-flanking CCSP gene sequence. Selective CAT expression was seen in H441 cells, a Clara cell-like pulmonary adenocarcinoma cell line. Cell-selective CAT expression was maintained in H441 cells with CCSP-CAT constructs retaining only 175 bp from the original 2.3 kb tested [24].

B. SP-C Promoter Function

A similar experimental design has been used to analyze the regulation of SP-C gene transcription in vivo. Approximately 3.7 kb of the 5' region of the human SP-C DNA was used to drive CAT expression in transgenic mice. High levels of CAT activity were detected in lung but not other tissues (Fig. 1B). Lung-specific CAT activity was detected in multiple independent 3.7 SP-C-CAT founder lines, indicating that cis-active regulatory elements within the 3.7-kb fragment direct lung-specific transcription [29]. Localization of CAT mRNA was not identical to that of the endogenous SP-C mRNA in the transgenic mice. Messenger RNA derived from the human SP-C-CAT transgene was present at high levels in bronchiolar and alveolar epithelial cells, while endogenous murine SP-C was detected only in alveolar type II cells [30]. The discordance between the human SP-C-CAT transgene and the murine SP-C gene expression may reflect subtle species differences between human and mouse cis-active elements or transcription factors (Fig. 1C).

IV. Developmental Expression of the SP-C-CAT Transgene

The ontogeny of SP-C and CAT mRNA was determined in the fetal lung of SP-C-CAT transgenic mice. SP-C-CAT expression was detected early in embryogenesis and increased with advancing gestation [30]. The pattern of CAT mRNA closely paralleled that of the endogenous mouse SP-C gene. Expression of the transgene was detected in the earliest epithelial buds of the lung primordium on day 10 of gestation. Endogenous SP-C and the SP-C-CAT mRNA were located in the distal tips of the developing lung buds. As lung development progressed, CAT and SP-C mRNAs were extinguished in the developing lobar and segmental bronchi and were progressively restricted to the distal edge of the respiratory epithelium [31]. These experiments demonstrated that the 5' region of the human SP-C DNA contains cis-active nucleotide sequences that determine developmental and pulmonary type II cell-specific gene expression. Biochemical analysis of the regions of genomic DNA that have been functionally defined are in progress to discern the nuclear transcription factors that initiate and regulate cell-specific expression of SP-C.

V. Identification of Transcription Factors That Activate Lung-Specific Gene Transcription

The promoter regions of SP-A, B, C, and CCSP genes have been analyzed in vitro to identify specific transcription factors that bind their target DNA recognition site to stimulate transcription in pulmonary epithelial cells. Several identified transcription factors are expressed in a spatially restricted organ pattern that include the lung. Members of the hepatocyte nuclear factor (HNF) family are expressed in a variety of tissues including the lung [32]. The thyroid transcription factor (TTF-1) is expressed primarily in thyroid and lung. TTF-1 is expressed from the onset of lung development in the distal growing epithelium of the lung buds [33]. Co-transfection assays of cells in culture with TTF-1 expression plasmids and 5' flanking sequences from lung-specific genes demonstrate that TTF-1 activates expression of the lung gene sequences. SP-A, B, C, or CCSP flanking sequences were transactivated with TTF-1. Electrophoretic mobility shift assays and DNAase 1 footprint analyses demonstrate the specific target binding sites for TTF-1 and HNF-3 on the SP-B promoter [34]. Mutation of these binding sites dissociated TTF-1 or HNF-3 binding to the SP-B promoter. The transactivation experiments and binding studies indicate that the precise cell-selective expression of these genes is the result of combinatorial interactions of transcription factors at multiple DNA binding sites in the 5' flanking sequences of the SP-B gene. Recent studies support the importance of HNF-3α in bronchiolar and HFH-8 in alveolar selective gene expression [35].

VI. Transgenic Models of Lung Development and Disease

The lung-specific promoter elements have been incorporated into a series of transgenes to express biologically active molecules in the lung. The ectopic production of bioactive molecules is intended to disturb the balance of regulatory factors that guide normal lung development and function (Table 1).

A. Cell Ablation in the Study of Pulmonary Development

The expression of a toxic reporter gene under the direction of precise transcriptional control elements has been used to ablate subsets of cells in developing organ

Table 1 Applications of in-Vivo Transgenic Technology

Experimental	Outcome
I. Dominant transgenes—phenotype detectable in heterozygotes	
Cell-specific expression of toxigene	Eliminates cells; useful for cell lineage studies of cell to cell interactions [40]
Cell-specific expression of reporter genes	Identifies cellular sites of gene expression; useful for identifying cell-specific promoter/enhancer elements [24,27,29–31]
Cell-specific expression of bioactive genes	Identifies function of overexpressed growth factors, enzymes, cytokines, or oncogenes [44,47,55,59]
II. Recessive transgenes—phenotype detectable in homozygotes	
Gene ablation	Locus-specific mutation leads to a deficiency or absence of gene product, useful for identifying role of gene product in the developing or adult lung [61–66,68,69]
III. Bitransgenic	
Insert dominant transgene in gene-ablated mice	Compensate for deleterious tissue-specific effects of null mutation [67]
	Role of cell-specific gene expression in null background
Cross-breed transgenic lines	Regulated or conditional transgene expression [73–77]

systems. The diphtheria toxin A (DT-A) and ricin genes have been used successfully in toxigene constructs in transgenic mice. The temporal and spatial expression of the transgene results in expression of DT or ricin that leads to cell death. The promoters of several tissue-specific genes have been utilized to ablate specific cells in the developing eye [36], pancreas [37], and brown fat [38]. These in-vivo cell ablation models have been used to demonstrate the presence of tissue-specific transcriptional control elements and to map cell lineage relationships during development. Cell lineage analysis by genetic cell ablation has been assessed using regulatory regions of genes expressed in subsets of pancreatic islet cells to direct DT-A expression. The promoters from the pancreatic polypeptide, insulin, and glucagon genes were used to analyze developmental fates of cells with a common origin. The analysis of altered pancreatic development from the three DT-A constructs demonstrated that insulin- and glucagon-producing cells are not required for differentiation of islets of Langerhans, while ablation with the pancreatic polypeptide DT-A vector eliminated the mature insulin- and somatostatin-producing cells [39]. Insulin and glucagon DT-A expression ablated only the targeted cell type. These studies demonstrate the utility of the approach to discern progenitor cell relationships.

Korfhagen et al. [40] produced transgenic mice in which the DT-A gene was driven by the 3.7 SP-C promoter region. Transgenic pups bearing the 3.7 SP-C-DT-A transgene died from respiratory failure within 20 min of birth. In nine independent transgene pups, developmental abnormalities were confined to the lung, while the lung development in nontransgenic littermates appeared normal. Lung pathology varied from atelectasis and epithelial cell death to more severely impaired organ development characterized by loss of all organized lung parenchyma. The proximal tracheal-bronchial tree was unaffected by the transgene. These findings and the developmental pattern of SP-C-CAT expression in distal epithelial lung buds support the concept that at least two distinct epithelial cell lineages are determined early in lung development. One set of progenitor cells, expressing SP-C early in fetal development, represent the precursor cells of the distal epithelium that ultimately produce the distal bronchioles and alveoli. Progenitor cells of the tracheal and lobar bronchi are not influenced by the SP-C-DTA transgene and likely represent a subset of proximal respiratory epithelial cells that are distinguished early in lung morphogenesis.

B. Expression of TGF-α During Pulmonary Growth and Remodeling

A complex interplay of growth and differentiation signals must occur in order to sustain the process of normal lung development. The lung-specific promoter elements have been used to alter growth factor-dependent processes. Several reports indicate that the epidermal growth factor (EGF), transforming growth factor-α (TGF-α) family have a role in lung development and in recovery from pulmonary injury. EGF accelerates lung maturation and stimulates surfactant synthesis in primates [41]. Both EGF and TGF-α initiate signal transduction by binding to the EGF receptor. The importance of EGF/TGF-α in lung disease is supported by reports of both TGF-α and EGF receptor expression increasing in epithelial cells after bleomycin treatment [42] and increased EGF in the bronchiolar epithelium of infants with bronchopulmonary dysplasia [43]. Pulmonary fibrosis is a frequent outcome associated with recovery from bleomycin injury and BPD.

Transgenic mice were generated with the human 3.7 SP-C promoter directing human TGF-α expression in order to define the role of TGF-α expression by selectively increasing TGF-α levels in pulmonary epithelial cells and then assessing altered lung morphogenesis. Analysis of founder 3.7 SP-C-TGF-α mice by Northern blot hybridization demonstrated that human TGF-α was expressed only in the lung. The 3.7 SP-C-TGF-α mice developed progressive pulmonary fibrosis (Fig. 2) [44]. Histological findings included a thickened pleural surface and extensive interstitial fibrotic lesions associated with marked collagen deposition. In-situ hybridization identified TGF-α mRNA in the lung parenchyma and

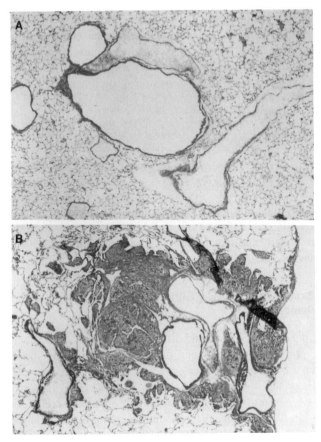

Figure 2 Overexpression of TGF-α in SP-C-TGF-α transgenic mice induces pulmonary fibrosis. (A) Bright-field photomicrograph of a lung section from a nontransgenic mouse showing normal architecture of the bronchiolar, vascular, and alveolar structures. (B) Photomicrograph of a trichrome stain of lung tissue from an SP-C-TGF-α transgenic mouse, illustrating the extensive central and peripheral fibrotic lesions which stain positive for collagen. Also visible is a thickened pleural surface. TGF-α was detected by in-situ hybridization in lung parenchyma adjacent to the fibrotic lesions. Fibrotic lesions were confined to the lung. Reproduced by permission of the authors.

pockets of clustered epithelial cells within the fibrotic lesions. Increased EGF receptors and increased cdk-1 synthesis in the interstitium were consistent with the hypothesis that TGF-α produced by the epithelial cells stimulated proliferation of adjacent interstitial cells [45]. The 3.7 SP-C-TGF-α transgenic lines varied in the severity of phenotype, the severity correlating with the level of hTGF-α mRNA. Analysis of the pulmonary fibrosis among these distinct 3.7 SP-C-TGF-α lines may provide a useful model to assess therapeutic modalities for pulmonary fibrosis.

C. Alteration of Lung Development by a Dominant Negative Transgene

The role of the fibroblast growth factor (FGF) family in lung development was assessed by expressing a SP-C-dominant negative FGF receptor transgene construct. FGF family members are expressed in a variety of embryonic tissues with FGF receptor expression in fetal epithelia. One of the FGF receptor genes FGF^{R2}, is expressed in the epithelium of the developing lung. Furthermore, KGF (keratinocyte growth factor) which is a member of the FGF growth factor family, stimulates DNA synthesis in cultured type II cells in vitro [46]. The human 3.7 SP-C promoter was used to express a deletion mutant of the FGF^{R2} in the developing lung. Dimerization of the truncated mutant FGF^{R2} with endogenous wild-type FGF^R produced a nonfunctional hybrid receptor rendering the pulmonary epithelial cells unresponsive to FGF stimulation [47].

The 3.7 SP-C-FGF^R transgenic founder mice died of respiratory failure at birth. Examination of the animals identified developmental abnormalities in the lung without gross morphologic alterations of other organs. As with the 3.7 SP-C-DT-A mice, lung growth was reduced. Histological analysis demonstrated that within the lungs there was a complete absence of bronchiolar branching and alveolarization. Airway development was restricted to tubule outgrowth from the tracheal bifurcation that extended as two simple bronchi. The bronchi were lined by epithelial cells that expressed the Clara cell marker CCSP, but lacked endogenous SP-C mRNA. These data support the conclusion that the kinase-deficient FGF^R dimers inhibited the effects of FGF stimulation that normally modulates epithelial cell proliferation and branching morphogenesis. The finding that the tracheo-bronchial tree was intact provide further support for the concept that distinct subsets of airway progenitor epithelial cells form the proximal and distal respiratory tract.

D. Identification of New Lung-Specific Genes by Insertional Mutagenesis

The production of transgenic mice offers an alternative to the otherwise lengthy process of identifying/isolating new lung-specific genes by what has been termed "enhancer traps" or "promoter traps." This approach exploits the fact that permanent integration of the microinjected transgene DNA is an uncontrolled event. In a small percentage of transgenic mice, the integrated transgene disrupts a functioning structural or regulatory gene. The result is a transgenic mouse with an altered phenotype based on the insertional mutagenesis of an essential gene [48]. In order to selectively identify such integrations, transgenic mice are made with a promoterless bacterial β-galactosidase (β-gal) transgene as the transcriptionally inactive trap. Production of β-gal in tissue sections of transgenic animals identifies the fortuitous integration of the β-gal gene adjacent to a functional promoter. The tissue distribution of β-gal staining reveals the specificity of the "trapped" promoter detected by expression of β-gal [49]. Allen and co-workers demonstrated various different organ-specific patterns of β-gal transgene activation in 11 β-gal positive out of 52 founder transgenic pups. One of the 11 founder animals expressed β-gal in a fetal lung restricted pattern [50]. In a separate study, Hansborough et al. reported a detailed characterization of a transgenic mouse line with lung-specific β-gal expression resulting from the site of insertion. Expression of the β-gal transgene was initiated early in fetal lung growth (fetal day 11), with a pattern of expression that followed the proximal to distal growth into the most peripheral airways. In adult mice, expression of the β-gal transgene was restricted to alveolar type II cells, producing an overall pattern of expression similar to that of the SP-C promoter [51]. In this specific example, the transgene integrated adjacent to dominant, cis-active genomic DNA that determined lung specificity. Identification of the regulatory element now requires molecular "backtracking." The β-gal DNA can be used to clone the genomic insertion site of the transgene, which can be used ultimately to clone the intact wild-type gene that originally directed β-gal expression in the lung.

E. Pulmonary Adenocarcinoma

Transgenic models of cancer have been developed using tissue-specific promoters to express oncogenic proteins. Transgenic mice generated with an oncogene construct develop tumors in target organ(s), identifying the pattern of organ-specific gene transcription. Tumors from the transgenic mice can be utilized to define the role of specific oncogenes, develop models of carcinogenesis, and generate immortalized cell lines from specific tissues [52].

Organ-specific and nonspecific promoters have been used to produce models of pulmonary carcinogenesis. Adenocarcinomas were detected in the lung and other organs of transgenic mice wherein portions of the albumin gene were used to direct expression of the H-ras oncogene [53]. Expression of the SV40 large TAg produced lung tumors from transgenes using the rabbit uteroglobin (homolog of CCSP) and human SP-C promoter. Lung and urogenital tumors were produced from the uteroglobin-TAg construct, consistent with the tissue specificity of the rabbit uteroglobin promoter. Morphology of these lung tumors was consistent with the characteristics of pulmonary adenocarcinoma [54]. In the 3.7 SP-C-TAg mice, tumors were confined to the lungs, leading to death by 4–6 months of age. Solid, papillary, and lepidic patterns of tumor growth were observed in histological sections of lungs from the 3.7 SP-C-TAg mice, with the solid tumors morphologically indistinguishable from human pulmonary adenocarcinomas. In-situ hybridization analysis with TAg probe precisely overlaps the pattern of tumor formation seen in the 3.7 SP-C-TAg lungs. In-situ hybridization using probes for markers of differentiated respiratory epithelial cells detected heterologous patterns of SP-A, B, C, and CCSP expression in the tumors from the 3.7 SP-C-TAg mice [55]. This finding of heterogeneity in markers expressed among the tumors is consistent with the origin of the tumors from distinct cell types along the airway epithelium or reflect differentiation of a common progenitor cell.

F. Immortalization of Mouse Lung Epithelial Cell Lines (MLE Cells)

Explants from lung tumors of 3.7 SP-C-TAg mice were used to establish immortalized epithelial cell lines. The epithelial cell lines were screened by Northern blot analysis to identify specific cell lines that sustained expression of a marker or differentially expressed markers for pulmonary epithelial cells. MLE cell lines were identified that expressed different combinations of the surfactant protein A, B, and C mRNA. While CCSP expression was specifically detected in the 3.7 SP-C-TAg lung tumors, no cell lines were identified that sustained CCSP expression [56]. All cell lines sustained expression of the ApoJ (murine clusterin) gene. Apo J is consistently expressed at high levels in early murine fetal lung development and is completely extinguished in the murine lung by fd 18.5 of development, thus serving as a marker of cells immortalized at early stages of differentiation [57]. At the ultrastructural level, MLE cells displayed microvilli, multivesicular bodies, with multilamellar bodies present in some MLE cell lines [56]. Cell lines produced by transformation with lung-specific promoters may provide useful in-vitro models for distinct lung cell types.

G. Transgenic Models of Pulmonary Oxygen Injury

Oxygen supplementation is used therapeutically to treat a variety of acute pulmonary disorders. However, the elevated oxygen levels can cause lung injury mediated by reactive oxygen intermediates. A number of proteins, including superoxide dismutases, catalase, glutathione peroxidase, and others, protect against oxidant injury. Enhanced survival in oxygen was noted in mice that express the human copper/zinc superoxide dismutase (Cu/Zn-SOD) cDNA [58]. Expression of human Mn-SOD mRNA and protein was demonstrated in mice bearing the human 3.7 SP-C Mn-SOD gene construct. Human Mn-SOD mRNA was confined to the lungs, and immunogold electron microscopy demonstrated correct subcellular localization of huMn-SOD protein in the mitochondria of type II cells. SP-C-Mn-SOD transgenic mice survived 95% oxygen exposure longer than the non-transgenic mice. Histological assessment of the lungs from nontransgenic litter-mates demonstrated pulmonary edema, atelectasis, a disorganized pattern of alveolar septae formation, and the presence of thickened hyaline membrane-like structures. This severe acute lung pathology was absent in the lungs of the 3.7 SP-C-Mn-SOD mice exposed to oxygen [59]. These experiments indicated that increased mitochondrial Mn-SOD was protective against oxygen injury and demonstrated the importance of distal respiratory epithelial cells in oxygen injury to the lung.

VII. Gene Targeting and Pulmonary Development

Recent advances in molecular embryology make feasible the experimental inactivation or mutation of a specific endogenous gene by homologous recombination. Selective markers can be included in DNA used to alter a gene in pluripotent stem cells for in-vitro manipulation. Modified ES cells are implanted into developing blastocysts and the blastocysts transferred to surrogate mothers. The intrauterine growth and development of the embryo from the altered embryonic stem cells must then proceed in the absence of the targeted gene product.

Several genes that have been selectively inactivated by homologous recombination produce alterations in organogenesis including the lung. Targeted disruption of the homeodomain gene, GSH-4, produced mice that died of respiratory failure within 30 min of birth [60]. Histological examination of the GSH-4 pups revealed no anatomical abnormalities. The only discernible phenotype was that of delayed type II cell maturation but no overall alteration of lung growth. The spatial restrictions of GSH-4 in utero in the developing hindbrain and spinal cord supports the concept that GSH-4 contributes to essential steps in formation of respiratory center and its associated signal pathways.

Targeted disruption of the n-myc oncogene produced a more profound alteration of lung development [61–63]. The myc family of protooncogenes have structural motifs in common with helix-loop-helix transcription factors and regulate growth and differentiation. In the analysis of lung growth and development, in-situ studies localizing the transcripts of c-myc and n-myc to distinct compartments of epithelialized organs. C-myc transcripts localized over pulmonary mesenchyme, while N-myc mRNA was detected over airway epithelium. Investigators from three independent laboratories have disrupted the n-myc gene by homologous recombination. Pups homozygous for the inactivated n-myc gene died of respiratory failure at birth. The major organ pathology was the reduction of fetal lung growth. The lungs were hypoplastic, with severely reduced branching of the conducting airways and poor alveolar septation.

VIII. Gene Targeting and Models of Pulmonary Disease

Homologous recombination has been used to produce animal models of cystic fibrosis and alveolar proteinosis by disruption of the cystic fibrosis transmembrane regulator (CFTR) and of granulocyte-macrophage colony-stimulating factor (GM-CSF), respectively.

A. Cystic Fibrosis Knockout Mice

Cystic fibrosis (CF) is a common recessive genetic disease seen primarily in the Caucasian population and is due to a single gene defect. Cystic fibrosis is caused by mutations in the membrane protein CFTR causing defective cAMP-dependent Cl^- secretory activity in epithelial cells. Morbidity and mortality in CF is caused by the mucus accumulation and recurrent infections in the lung. The murine CFTR gene has been mutated in ES cells to produce CFTR-deficient animals [64–66]. CFTR-deficient animals do not have prominent pulmonary disease or pancreatic insufficiency as seen in humans, but die in the weaning period from intestinal atrophy and obstruction. Physiological studies of the CFTR mice demonstrate the loss of cAMP-dependent chloride secretion in the intestinal epithelia. The CFTR knockout mice may be useful for modeling the multiorgan involvement in CF but also point out the limitations that may be encountered in attempting to model the molecular basis of a human disease in mice.

B. Animal Model of Alveolar Proteinosis

Inactivation of the granulocyte-macrophage colony-stimulating factor (GM-CSF) gene defined the unexpected role of this molecule in pulmonary surfactant homeostasis. The GM-CSF molecule stimulates proliferation and activation of hematopoietic cells. Analysis of GM-CSF knockout mice demonstrated normal hematopoietic development and immune function. Mice homozygous for the GM-CSF mutation appeared healthy, but developed a progressive accumulation of pulmonary surfactant lipid and proteins similar to that seen in human alveolar proteinosis [68,69]. Analysis of bronchoalveolar lavage from the GM-CSF mice identified increased surfactant proteins A, B, and C and surfactant phospholipids. The abundance of surfactant protein mRNA was indistinguishable from mRNA levels in the lungs of control mice, suggesting that the transcriptional control of surfactant components is appropriately maintained in the GM-CSF mice but that the clearance of pulmonary surfactant is disrupted.

A second example of altered pulmonary surfactant homeostasis resulting from a specific mutation has been identified in human infants. Nogee et al. have reported a hereditary neonatal alveolar proteinosis in full-term infants that manifest respiratory distress syndrome [70]. Lavage from affected infants have both an altered surfactant phospholipid profile and an absence of SP-B. Sequence analysis of the SP-B gene from these infants identified a frame-shift mutation that results in a translation stop, terminating the synthesis of the SP-B protein [71]. Vorbroker et al. extended these studies to demonstrate an aberrant processing of the proSP-C protein in lungs of affected individuals [72]. Bronchoalveolar lavage of SP-B-deficient patients was analyzed by Western blot analysis with antibodies raised to the amino terminus of proSP-C. A unique 12-kDa form of SP-C containing amino-terminus and active peptide regions was identified only in the lavage from SP-B-deficient infants [77].

These data indicate that gene knockout experiments, eliminating genes expressed in pulmonary epithelial cells, will define the role that a specific protein product contributes to lung function but may also reveal unknown roles that the target gene fulfills in lung homeostasis and how the lung compensates for altered levels of the targeted gene product.

IX. Temporal and Spatial Control of Transgenes in Bitransgenic Mice

Gene ablation may cause fetal or neonatal lethality that obviates the study of gene function late in development. For example, lethal intestinal obstruction is caused by gene targeting of the CFTR in transgenic mice. Strategies to conditionally express potential lethal transgenes have therefore been developed, wherein the onset of transgene expression can be manipulated by the investigator. The two successful approaches use the cre-lox and tet-operon systems. The conditional expression with cre/lox is based on controlled DNA recombination. The bacterial recombinase enzyme, cre, has the capacity to remove DNA sequences that are flanked by 34 bp cre binding sites, the lox element. The cre and lox transgenes are established as independent lines, with condition expression achieved only when both transgenes are present. In one transgenic mouse the DNA construct flanks the bioactive reporter molecule (a growth factor or transcription factor) with lox elements. In a second, separate transgenic line cre recombinase expression is driven by a tissue/cell-specific promoter. Breeding of the two mice produces a hybrid bitransgenic mouse in which cell-specific cre production excises the target transgene DNA bounded by lox sites, resulting in the desired activation or inactivation of the bioactive molecule [73,74]. A similar use of a binary system to regulate transgene expression in vivo has been achieved with tetracycline responsive transgenes, based on tetracycline-sensitive tet transactivator to tet operator site binding. The tet transactivator-operator binding in the bitransgenic mice results in transgenic expression. Injection of tetracycline dissociates the tet transactivator-operator complex, extinguishing the expression of the tet operator transgene. Tetracycline-dependent regulation of transgene expression has been recently achieved with tissue-specific promoters [75,76].

An example of innovative cancer therapy was achieved from breeding of two liver-specific transgenic lines. An albumin promoter-driven SV40 TAg reporter (Al-TAg) produced a transgenic model of hepatocarcinoma. A second transgenic line in which the alpha-fetoprotein promoter expressed the Herpes thymidine kinase gene (Afp-TK) was bred to the hepatocarcinoma line. The treatment of AFP-TK/Al-TAg bitransgenic mice with the Herpes-specific antiviral drug, gancyclovir, has shown gancyclovir-dependent suppression of tumor formation [77]. Such examples of precise cell-specific activation or inactivation support the use of this approach with the described lung-specific promoters.

Bitransgenic mice have been generated in an effort to exploit more fully the CFTR null mice to model cystic fibrosis. Transgenic mice have been established with the promoter of the intestinal fatty acid-binding protein (FABP) expressing the CFTR cDNA as reporter. Breeding the FABP-CFTR line to the CFTR null-mutation mouse restores appropriate cAMP-dependent chloride channel expression in cells of the intestinal epithelium, correcting the lethal intestinal obstruction in the original CFTR null mouse [67]. The bitransgenic animals represent a surviving, long-lived model that retains the CFTR null mutation and allows both extended investigation of cellular and transport defects and development of the CFTR null mouse for further study of pulmonary infection and inflammation associated with cystic fibrosis. In designing future models of lung disease, this bitransgenic approach may be useful to correct lethal or undesired outcomes of a gene knockout model.

X. Expression of Inflammatory Cytokines in the Respiratory Epithelium of Transgenic Mice

Transgenic mice have been used to express specific proinflammatory molecules that are components of the complex web of cellular and biochemical signals resulting in airway inflammation. Some of the proinflammatory mediators that may contribute to inflammation associated with the asthmatic responses include tumor necrosis factor alpha (TNF-α), interleukin 1β (IL-1β), and interleukin 6 (IL-6). These cytokines have been shown to be released by macrophages and from the bronchiolar epithelial cells of asthmatic patients [78–81]. These same cytokines stimulate synthesis of intercellular adhesion molecules, and at least one (TNF-α) downregulates expression of the surfactant proteins SP-A, B, and C contributing to surfactant dysfunction [82].

To define the role of specific cytokines in the pathogenesis of airway inflammation, transgenic mice were generated in which expression of TNF-α and IL-6 was directed to airway epithelial cells. The human SP-C promoter was used to express TNF-α in transgenic mice, producing severe pathology confined to the lung. The severity of lung disease was correlated directly with TNF mRNA levels.

The lungs of several transgenic pups dying at birth were hypoplastic. Lungs from surviving transgenic lines bearing the SP-C-TNF transgene developed lymphocytic infiltrates, alterations in alveolar septation, and progressive alveolar fibrosis [83], which were distinct from the fibrotic lesions found in SP-C-TGF-α transgenic mice [44]. The extent of lymphocyte accumulation and fibrosis was correlated with levels of TNF produced in the lungs. In a separate study, the CCSP promoter was used to express IL-6 in the bronchial and bronchiolar epithelium. Lungs from CCSP-IL-6 mice contained lymphocytic infiltrates but lacked pulmonary fibrosis [84]. Challenge with methacholine demonstrated that the CCSP-IL-6 mice were less responsive to induced bronchoconstriction than control mice. These findings suggest that mediators which affect inflammation may not directly account for airway hyperresponsiveness in asthma.

XI. Conclusions

The models described in this chapter illustrate the utility of transgenic mice to determine the role of specific genes in lung development and disease. At present these experiments are limited to a small number of epithelial-specific elements to direct gene expression in a precise, lung-specific manner. More precise models may be generated by identifying elements that target expression in other subsets of the 40 distinct respiratory cells. Promoters specific for other pulmonary cells, including pulmonary vascular cells, endothelium, fibroblasts, etc., will be useful in defining the role of nonepithelial cells in lung growth, development, and disease.

The use of gene ablation and addition in transgenic mice may provide insight into the pathogenesis of complex lung disorders such as asthma, pulmonary idiopathic fibrosis, cystic fibrosis, bronchopulmonary dysplasia, and others, providing animal models that will be useful in developing new therapies for acute and chronic lung diseases.

Acknowledgments

This work was supported by Program of Excellence HL41496 and Center for Gene Therapy for Cystic Fibrosis and Other Lung Diseases HL51832.

References

1. Hogan B, Constantini F, Lacy E. Manipulating the Mouse Embryo. Cold Spring Harbor, NY: Cold Spring Harbor Lab, 1986.

2. Gordon JW, Ruddle FH. Gene transfer into mouse embryos: production of transgenic mice by pronuclear injection. Meth Enzymol 1983; 101:411–433.

3. Lathe R, Mullins JJ. Transgenic animals as models for human disease—report of an EC study group. Trans Res 1993; 2:286–299.

4. Hanahan D. Transgenic mice as probes into complex systems. Science 1989; 246: 1265–1275.

5. Reith AD, Bernstein A. Molecular basis of mouse developmental mutants. Gene Develop 1991; 5:1115–1123.

6. Koller BH, Smithes O. Altering genes in animals by gene targeting. Annu Rev Immunol 1992; 10:705–730.

7. Bronson SK, Smithies D. Altering mice by homologous recombination using embryonic stem cells. J Biol Chem 1994; 269:27155–27158.

8. Stripp BR, Whitsett JA, Lattier DL. Strategies for analysis of gene expression: pulmonary surfactant proteins. Am J Physiol (Lung Cell Mol Physiol) 1990; 259: L185–L197.

9. Korfhagen TR, Glasser SW, Stripp BR. Regulation of gene expression in the lung. Curr Opin Pediatr 1994; 6:255–261.

10. Ho YS. Transgenic models for the study of lung biology and disease. Am J Physiol (Lung Cell Mol Physiol) 1994; 266:L319–L353.

11. Glasser SW, Korfhagen TR, Wert SE, Whitsett JA. Transgenic models for study of pulmonary development and disease. Am J Physiol (Lung Cell Mol Physiol 11) 1994; 267:L489–L497.

12. Kuroki Y, Voelker DR. Pulmonary surfactant proteins. J Biol Chem 1994; 42:25943–25946.

13. Weaver TE, Whitsett JA. Function and regulation of expression of pulmonary surfactant-associated proteins. Biochem J 1991; 273:249–264.

14. Johansson J, Curstedt T, Robertson B. The proteins of the surfactant system. Eur Respir J 1994; 7:372–391.

15. Whitsett JA, Weaver TE, Clark JC, et al. Glucocorticoid enhances surfactant proteolipid Phe and pVal synthesis and RNA in fetal lung. J Biol Chem 1987; 262:15618–15623.

16. Khoor A, Stahlman MT, Gray ME, Whitsett JA. Temporal-spatial distribution of SP-B and SP-C proteins and mRNAs in the developing respiratory epithelium of the human lung. J Histochem Cytochem 1994; 42:1187–1199.

17. Schellhase DE, Emrie PA, Fisher JH, Shannon JM. Ontogeny of surfactant proteins in the rat. Pediatr Res 1989; 26:167–174.

18. Wohlford-Lenane CL, Durham PL, Snyder JM. Localization of surfactant-associated protein C (SP-C) mRNA in fetal rabbit lung tissue by *in situ* hybridization. Am J Respir Cell Mol Biol 1992; 6:225–234.

19. Wohlford-Lenane CL, Snyder JM. Localization of surfactant-associated proteins SP-A and SP-B mRNA in rabbit fetal lung tissue by *in situ* hybridization. Am J Respir Cell Mol Biol 1992; 7:335–343.

20. D'Amore-Bruno MA, Wikenheiser KA, Carter JE, Clark JC, Whitsett JA. Sequence, ontogeny and cellular localization of murine surfactant protein SP-B mRNA. Am J Physiol (Lung Cell Mol Physiol) 1992; 262:L40–L47.

51. Hansbrough JR, Fine SM, Gordon JI. A transgenic mouse model for studying the lineage relationships and differentiation program of type-II pneumocytes at various stages of lung development. J Biol Chem 1993; 268(13):9762–9770.

52. Compere SJ, Baldacci P, Jaenisch R. Oncogenes in transgenic mice. Biochim Biophys Acta 1988; 948:129–149.

53. Maronpot RR, Palmiter RD, Brinster RL, Sandgren EP. Pulmonary carcinogenesis in transgenic mice. Exp Lung Res 1991; 17:305–320.

54. Demayo FJ, Finegold MJ, Hansen TN, Stanley LA, Smith B, Bullock DW. Expression of SV40 T-antigen under control of rabbit uteroglobin promoter in transgenic mice. Am J Physiol 1991; 261(2):L70–L76.

55. Wikenheiser KA, Clark JC, Linnoila RI, Stahlman MT, Whitsett JA. Simian virus-40 large T-antigen directed by transcriptional elements of the human surfactant protein-C gene produces pulmonary adenocarcinomas in transgenic mice. Cancer Res 1992; 52 (19):5342–5352.

56. Wikenheiser KA, Vorbroker DK, Rice WR, et al. Production of immortalized distal respiratory epithelial cell lines from surfactant protein C/simian virus 40 large T antigen transgenic mice. Proc Natl Acad Sci USA 1993; 90:11029–11033.

57. Ikeda K, Clark JC, Bachurski CJ, et al. Immortalization of subpopulations of respiratory epithelial cells from transgenic mice bearing SV 40 large T antigen. Am J Physiol (Lung Cell Mol Physiol) 1994; 267:L309–L317.

58. White CW, Avraham KB, Shanley PF, Groner Y. Transgenic mice with expression of elevated levels of copper-zinc superoxide dismutase in the lung are resistant to pulmonary oxygen toxicity. J Clin Invest 1991; 87:2162–2168.

59. Wispe JR, Warner BB, Clark JC, et al. Human Mn-superoxide dismutase in pulmonary epithelial cells of transgenic mice confers protection from oxygen injury. J Biol Chem 1992; 267(33):23937–23941.

60. Li H, Witte DP, Branford WW, et al. Gsh-4 encodes a LIM-type homeodomain, is expressed in the developing central nervous system, and is required for early postnatal survival. EMBO J 1994; 13:2876–2885.

61. Moens CB, Auerbach AB, Conlon RA, Joyner AL. Rossant J. A targeted mutation reveals a role for N-myc in branching morphogenesis in the embryonic mouse lung. Gene Dev 1992; 6:691–704.

62. Sawai S, Shimono A, Wakamatsu Y, Palmes C, Hanaoka K, Kondoh H. Defects of embryonic organogenesis resulting from targeted disruption of the N-myc gene in the mouse. Development 1993; 117:1445–1455.

63. Stanton BR, Perkins AS, Tessarollo L, Sassoon DA, Parada LF. Loss of N-myc function results in embryonic lethality and failure of the epithelial component of the embryo to develop. Gene Dev 1992; 6:2235–2247.

64. Clarke LL, Grubb BR, Gabriel SE, Smithies O, Koller BH, Boucher RC. Defective epithelial chloride transport in a gene-targeted mouse model of cystic fibrosis. Science 1992; 257:1125–1128.

65. Dorin JR, Dickinson P, Alton EWF, et al. Cystic fibrosis in the mouse by targeted insertional mutagenesis. Nature 1992; 359:211–215.

66. Snouwaert JN, Brigman KK, Latour AM, et al. An animal model for cystic fibrosis made by gene targeting. Science 1992; 257:1083–1088.

67. Zhou L, Dey CR, Wert SE, DuVall MD, Frizzell RA, Whitsett JA. Correction of lethal intestinal defect in a mouse model of cystic fibrosis by human *CFTR*. Science 1994; 266:1705–1708.

68. Dranoff G, Crawford AD, Sadelain M, et al. Involvement of granulocyte-macrophage colony-stimulating factor in pulmonary homeostasis. Science 1994; 264:713–716.

69. Stanley E, Lieshka GJ, Grail D, et al. Granulocyte/macrophage colony stimulating factor-deficient mice show no major perturbation of hematopoiesis but develop a characteristic pulmonary pathology. Proc Natl Acad Sci USA 1994; 91:5592–5594.

70. Nogee LM, deMello DE, Dehner LP, Colten HR. Brief report: deficiency of pulmonary surfactant protein B in congenital alveolar proteinosis. N Engl J Med 1993; 328: 406–410.

71. Nogee LM, Garnier G, Dietz HC, et al. A mutation in the surfactant protein B gene responsible for fatal neonatal respiratory disease in multiple kindreds. J Clin Invest 1994; 93:1860–1863.

72. Vorbroker DK, Profitt SA, Nogee LM, Whitsett JA. Aberrant processing of surfactant protein C (SP-C) in hereditary SP-B deficiency. Am J Physiol 1995; 268:L647–L656.

73. Furth PA, St. Onge L, Böger H, et al. Temporal control of gene expression in transgenic mice by a tetracycline-responsive promoter. Proc Natl Acad Sci USA 1994; 91:9302–9306.

74. Passman RS, Fishman GI. Regulated expression of foreign genes in vivo after germline transfer. J Clin Invest 1994; 94:2421–2425.

75. Lakso M, Sauer B, Mosinger B, et al. Targeted oncogene activation by site-specific recombination in transgenic mice. Proc Natl Acad Sci USA 1992; 89:6232–6236.

76. Orban PC, Chui D, Marth JD. Tissue- and site-specific DNA recombination in transgenic mice. Proc Natl Acad Sci USA 1992; 89:6861–6865.

77. Macri P, Gordon JW. Delayed morbidity and mortality of albumin/SV40 T-antigen transgenic mice after insertion of an a-fetoprotein/herpes virus thymidine kinase transgene and treatment with ganciclovir. Human Gene Ther 1994; 5:175–182.

78. Lassalle P, Gosset P, Delneste Y, et al. Modulation of adhesion molecule expression on endothelial cells during the late asthmatic reaction: role of macrophage-derived tumour necrosis factor-alpha. Clin Exp Immunol 1993; 94:105–110.

79. Marini M, Vittori E, Hollembourg J, Mattoli S. Expression of the potent inflammatory cytokines, granulocyte-macrophage-colony-stimulating factor and interleukin-6 and interleukin-8, in bronchial epithelial cells of patients with asthma. J Allergy Clin Immunol 1992; 89:1001–1009.

80. Gosset P, Tsicopoulos A, Wallaert B, Joseph M, Capron A, Tonnel A-B. Tumor necrosis factor alpha and interleukin-6 production by human mononuclear phagocytes from allergic asthmatics after IgE-dependent stimulation. Am Rev Respir Dis 1992; 146:768–774.

81. Gosset P, Tsicopoulos A, Wallaert B, et al. Increased secretion of tumor necrosis factor α and interleukin-6 by alveolar macrophages consecutive to the development of the late asthmatic reaction. J Allergy Clin Immunol 1991; 88:561–571.

82. Bachurski CJ, Pryhuber GS, Glasser SW, Kelly SE, Whitsett JA. Tumor necrosis factor-α inhibits surfactant protein C gene transcription. J Biol Chem 1995; 270: 19402–19407.

83. Miyazaki Y, Araki K, Vesin C, et al. Expression of a tumor necrosis factor-α transgene in murine lung causes lymphocytic and fibrosing alveolitis. J Clin Invest 1995; 96: 250–259.

84. DiCosmo BF, Geba GP, Picarella D, et al. Airway epithelial cell expression of interleukin-6 in transgenic mice: uncoupling of airway inflammation and bronchial hyperreactivity. J Clin Invest 1994; 94:2028–2035.

12

Inbred Animal Models of Genetic Susceptibility to Bronchial Hyperresponsiveness

SUSAN L. EWART

Michigan State University
East Lansing, Michigan

ROY CLIFFORD LEVITT

Magaining Institute of Molecular Medicine
Plymouth Meeting, Pennsylvania

I. Introduction

Asthma is an inflammatory disorder of the airways characterized by intermittent airway obstruction. Although asthma can be difficult to characterize, several features closely associated with this disorder are easily measured and objectively defined. Recently, the basis for genetic susceptibility to bronchial hyperresponsiveness, which is a heightened response to bronchoconstrictors, has been the focus of intensive study because it is considered important in the pathogenesis of asthma. Evidence suggests that there is a strong heritable predisposition to bronchial hyperresponsiveness [1–6]. Longitudinal studies in children show that bronchial hyperresponsiveness precedes asthma and constitutes a risk factor for the development of this disorder [3,4]. Analysis of the inheritance of bronchial hyperresponsiveness is complicated by the tremendous genetic diversity that characterizes outbred human populations. In addition, variation in exposure to environmental factors that influence the expression of asthma, such as air quality, allergens, diet, toxins, and pharmaceuticals, further confounds the analysis. For these reasons animal models have been developed to facilitate the study of asthma.

II. Asthma and Bronchial Hyperresponsiveness in Animals

Many animal systems may be uniquely relevant to the study of asthma; however, no animal species mimics precisely the clinical and pathological features of this disease. Only the cat and the horse have naturally occurring recurrent airway obstruction. Cats affected with feline asthma have attacks of dyspnea, wheezing, and cyanosis which are associated with peripheral and bronchoalveolar lavage eosinophilia [7,8]. While an allergic component to feline asthma has been suggested, the pathophysiology of naturally occurring feline asthma has not been extensively explored. In horses or ponies with heaves, bronchial hyperresponsiveness develops after exposure to environmental allergens, such as *Micropolyspora faeni*, that are present in hay. When affected horses are removed from the inciting environment, the level of bronchial responsiveness returns to normal [9,10]. A neutrophilic airway inflammation is present in horses with heaves [11], in contrast to the primarily eosinophilic inflammation found in human asthmatics.

While asthma per se is not widely recognized in animals, there are many animal models of bronchial hyperresponsiveness, a prevailing feature of asthma. In select strains of mice [12–17], rats [18–20], and breeds of dogs [21], bronchial hyperresponsiveness does not occur spontaneously but rather can be elicited by intravenous or inhaled challenge with mediators such as acetylcholine (ACh), methacholine (MCh), 5-hydroxytryptamine (5HT), substance P analogs (subP), histamine, adenosine, or neuromuscular blockers. Additionally, bronchoconstriction can be elicited in many of these models by antigen sensitization and subsequent challenge [21–26]. Thus, while several animal models have phenotypic characteristics which are similar to those of asthma, no animal model mimics precisely the spontaneous recurrent airway obstruction with underlying chronic airway inflammation, eosinophilic infiltration, and epithelial damage which describes asthma in humans [27–29].

A unifying characteristic of the above-mentioned animal models is that they each demonstrate some degree of genetic predisposition to bronchial hyperresponsiveness. As in asthma, genetic makeup appears to be critical to the bronchial responsiveness phenotype. As we gain appreciation for the genetic contribution to bronchial hyperresponsiveness, it becomes apparent that in order to understand fully the pathogenesis of this risk factor for asthma, we must search for the underlying mechanisms which provide genetic susceptibility to this trait.

III. Inbred Laboratory Animals

A. Characteristics and Advantages over Outbred Species

Inbred strains of laboratory animals have tremendously facilitated all fields of biomedical research and are used extensively in genetic, immunologic, physiologic, and cancer research. There are numerous advantages to studying inbred laboratory animals as compared to outbred animal populations [30] or humans. This discussion will be limited to inbred mice (*Mus musculus*) and rats (*Rattus norvegicus*), as extensive genetic databases are available for these species, making them excellent biologic resources. The mouse is the most commonly used species for genetic studies because a large number of highly standardized inbred mouse strains are readily available. Over 200 inbred strains and substrains of mice exist [31,32], and the genetic map of the mouse is highly detailed, with over 6000 loci mapped [33–35]. The mouse genome database is expanding rapidly and closely parallels that for humans. While fewer inbred rat strains have been developed as compared to the mouse, the physiological database for the rat is especially well characterized. The rat has often been preferred over the mouse in physiologic studies because its 10-fold larger size allows for greater ease of in-vivo manipulations. The usefulness of the rat in physiologic studies has stimulated interest in the genetic aspects of inbred rat strains and has helped to expedite the development of the rat genome database [36,37]. Similarly, with the elaborate characterization of the mouse genome, many physiologic measurements have been adapted for the mouse [38].

Animal models are particularly useful when invasive techniques are required that cannot be performed in humans. In addition, a wide variety of biological reagents and assays have been described for mice and rats, and many are commercially available. Rodents have short gestation periods and large litter sizes, making genetic manipulations and breeding experiments rapid and economical. Environmental conditions, which are critical to control in genetic studies, can readily be made uniform in rodent populations. Sterilized cage environments, microisolator or laminar-flow hood housing systems, and automated control of ambient temperature and dark:light periods makes strict control of macroenvironmental conditions readily achievable for large groups of laboratory animals.

B. Genetic Characteristics of Inbred Strains

The objective of inbreeding is to reduce genetic variability within strains to near zero. This is accomplished by full-sibling matings which over time effectively eliminates heterozygosity at every locus. Two or more forms of a gene (polymorphism) are designated alleles. The probability that two alleles at any locus are identical by descent, that is, derived from a common ancestor, is termed the coefficient of inbreeding (F). Although the coefficient of inbreeding never reaches 100%, after 20 generations of full-sibling matings, F should be 98.6% [39]. It is at this point that a strain is designated as inbred [40]. Inbred strains are characterized by two important and distinct features: isogenicity and homozygosity. Isogenicity implies that all individuals within an inbred strain are genetically identical, while homozygosity is the state of carrying identical alleles at all loci. The distinctness of these characteristics is illustrated in the first filial (F1) generation produced by

crossing two inbred strains. The F1 progeny are isogeneic, but they are heterozygous at all loci which differ in the parental strains. Absolute isogenicity and
homozygosity are never realistically achieved as a result of random mutations and
residual segregation due to incomplete inbreeding. The result of isogenicity and
homozygosity is that all animals within an inbred strain will be phenotypically
identical in traits that are not under environmental influence.

C. Recombinant Inbred and Congenic Strains

The development of recombinant inbred and congenic strains through the selective crossing of established inbred progenitor strains has facilitated advances in
the field of mammalian genetics. Recombinant inbred strains are sets of inbred
strains derived from the cross of two unique inbred strains and are maintained by
full-sibling mating for at least 20 generations (until homozygosity and isogenicity
are achieved) after the second filial (F2) generation [41,42]. Because inbreeding is
maintained independently within each recombinant inbred line from the first
segregating generation, F2, the result is a number of recombinant inbred lines,
each with a unique genotype derived from the progenitor strains. All the recombinant inbred strains that are derived from one pair of progenitor strains are used as a
set. The pattern of characteristics displayed in a set of recombinant inbred strains,
the strain distribution pattern, is determined by the genotype and the number of
genes which determine the trait.

Congenic strains are used to study the effect of genetic background on the
expression of a locus. A congenic strain differs genetically from its background
strain at only one locus and a surrounding segment of chromosome. Congenic
strains can be developed by back-crossing mice which carry a "unique" gene of
interest (donor strain) into an inbred strain of the desired genetic background
(background strain or inbred partner) [43,44]. Offspring carrying the gene of
interest in each successive generation are selected to be back-crossed to the
background strain. After a number of generations of mating to the background
strain, the new congenic strain and the background strain are likely to differ only
at the selected locus and a linked segment of chromosome. At this point the
congenic strain can be maintained by full-sibling mating. Congenic strains can be
especially useful in dissecting the genetic contribution made by specific genes to
complex phenotypes.

IV. Nongenetic Factors Influencing Bronchial
Hyperresponsiveness

The phenotype characterizes the observable properties of an organism that result
from the interaction between the environment and the genotype. Thus, phenotypic
expression of most traits is under both genetic and environmental influence.

Because inbred strains are isogeneic, variation within inbred strains is due to nongenetic factors such as environmental and methodological factors. Therefore, when environmental conditions are uniform and methodology is strictly controlled, phenotypic variation between inbred strains is considered to be genetic in origin. The proportion of the total variation that is accounted for by genetic differences between strains can be determined when nongenetic variation is minimized. In the case of bronchial hyperresponsiveness, it is essential to control exposure to allergens, toxins [45], and certain drugs [46] which may influence the expression of the phenotype. Additionally, variation in ambient air quality and diet may further confound the analysis.

V. Human–Animal Genetic Homologies

Genetic loci, the chromosomal location of genes, are arranged in a linear fashion along the chromosomes. Many chromosomal segments have been evolutionarily conserved between species. These conserved chromosomal regions are identical in their genetic content, thus they encode the same proteins in different species, and are termed homologous. The genetic homologies between humans and mice have been extensively characterized such that most portions of the mouse genome can now be assigned a human homolog [47]. In addition, over 1300 specific loci with mouse–human homologies have been reported [48]. Rat–human and rat–mouse homologies are being established as well. Yamada and colleagues [37] described rat linkage maps with 218 human genes and over 150 mouse genes homologous to the rat. Homologous map information can be used to predict the chromosomal location of genes that are mapped in one species but are unmapped in another species for which chromosomal homology information is available. Animal models of human diseases can be identified based on known chromosomal homologies between species. In addition, mapping information can be conferred from chromosomal areas that are well described to those less well characterized. While biologic variability may be explained by the same gene in two species, different genes in the same pathway may also produce a similar phenotype. In either case, insight may be gained by studying an animal model of human pathophysiology. Thus, mouse–human or rat–human homologies may be able to identify not only animal models of human disease, but we may find that the same genetic mechanism explains a similar phenotype in both species.

VI. Genetic Linkage Methods for Inbred Strains

An association between a phenotype under genetic control in the whole animal and a putative cellular mechanism in vitro can be established using co-segregation (linkage) analysis. Linkage analysis is an approach used to discover genes that produce significant biologic variability when the gene identity is unknown [49]. Coinheritance of a phenotype with a DNA sequence of known chromosomal location implies co-localization of these loci. Conversely, when the phenotype does not co-segregate with markers at a particular locus, that site can be ruled out from containing the genes which determine the phenotype. In this manner, linkage analysis can be used to identify the primary molecular defects responsible for bronchial hyperresponsiveness, as well as to exclude possible candidate genes and their role in pathophysiologic mechanisms. The availability of large numbers of isogeneic animals and the ease with which crosses can be produced, make inbred mice (or rats) an ideal system in which to conduct linkage studies. The phenotype of interest must first be established in a large population of segregating offspring (F2 or backcross) which derive from progenitors known to differ in the trait under study. DNA markers of known chromosomal location which differ in the parental strains, referred to as informative, are then identified. The genotypes at these informative markers are established in the phenotyped segregating offspring. Comparisons are then made to identify if the phenotype and genotype for each DNA marker are coinherited. When a marker allele is consistently inherited with a phenotype, the marker and the gene which controls the phenotype should co-localize to the same chromosomal region. In this event the marker and the gene of interest are genetically linked. If alleles at a marker do not segregate with the bronchial hyperresponsiveness phenotype, the marker is referred to as unlinked because it arises from a chromosomal location that assorts independently from bronchial hyperresponsiveness at meiosis. Any genes that map in close association with an unlinked marker can be excluded as primary candidates for controlling the phenotype under study in the whole animal. Each unlinked locus evaluated ultimately contributes to the exclusion map and narrows the possibilities for the chromosomal location of the loci controlling bronchial hyperresponsiveness. A great advantage to this approach is that genes hypothesized to produce this phenotype which do not map in close proximity to the bronchial hyperresponsiveness loci can be eliminated as potentially important in the etiology.

VII. Mediator-Induced Bronchial Hyperresponsiveness in Mice

To ascertain the importance of genetic makeup in the determination of a physiologic trait, significant phenotypic variability between strains and minimal intrastrain variability must be demonstrated for the trait of interest (Fig. 1). This has been accomplished for bronchial responsiveness by evaluating differences between and within inbred strains for the magnitude of response to bronchoprovocation. Studies of this nature have demonstrated a significant difference in bronchial responsiveness between multiple inbred strains of mice to various mediators

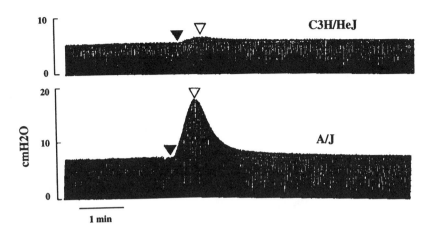

Figure 1 Pressure tracing after acetylcholine administration of 50 μg/kg i.v. (filled arrows) in C3H/HeJ (top) and A/J mice (bottom). Bronchial responsiveness was measured during end-inflation occlusion performed at baseline and at peak of response (open arrows) after challenge. (From Ewart et al., 1995b.)

including ACh, MCh, 5HT, subP, and the neuromuscular blocker atracurium (Fig. 2). The A/J strain was among the most responsive to ACh [12,38,50], MCh [17,51], 5HT [13], and atracurium [16]. The DBA/2 strain was the most responsive to subP [14], 5HT [13], and atracurium [16]. The C57BL/6 [17,51], SJL, and C3H/HeJ strains were consistently the least responsive to any agent [12–14,16]. Minimal within-strain biologic variability in the response to bronchoconstrictors suggested that the differential responsiveness of these strains was due to variation in genetic makeup. In addition, significant differences were noted between the strain distribution patterns for the majority of the agents tested, which supported the hypothesis that the responses to individual mediators are determined by unique gene(s). The ACh-induced bronchial responses measured in a population of 23 outbred mice were all phenotypically hyporesponsive (R.C. Levitt, unpublished observations). This suggests that the magnitude of the average response to ACh in an outbred population may be similar to that of the least responsive inbred strains.

The significant variability in bronchial responsiveness demonstrated between inbred strains of mice can be attributed to differences in genetic makeup when all other variables are controlled. A difference in any measured variable between inbred strains may be due to a single gene (Mendelian inheritance) or any number of genes working in combination. Non-Mendelian traits may be inherited in a relatively simple manner if only two or three major loci interact to determine the phenotype. However, when a large number of genes control the expression

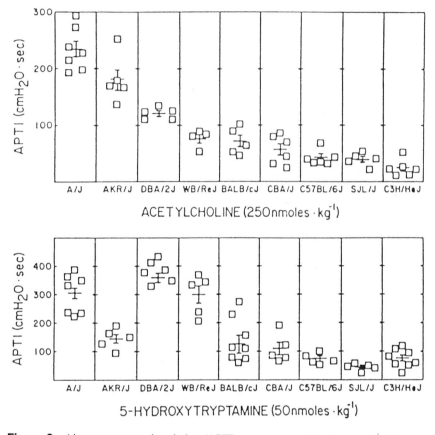

Figure 2 Airway pressure time index (APTI) response to either i.v. acetylcholine or 5-hydroxytryptamine in different strains of inbred mice. APTI refers to integrated change in peak airway pressure over time. Symbols represent the APTI response for an individual mouse. Cross-hatches indicate the means ± SE. (From Levitt and Mitzner, 1989.)

of a trait, the genetic interactions may be very complex (polygenic inheritance). Preliminary information concerning the mode of inheritance of a trait can be inferred from the strain distribution pattern, which is determined by evaluating the trait in a number of different inbred strains. The presence of a major locus is suggested by a bimodal distribution in the strain distribution pattern. Similarly, when a number of recombinant inbred strains are typed, bimodality indicates a major locus [41]. Significant variation in a trait between inbred strains cannot be used alone to characterize a genetic relationship fully. Ideally, classical crosses derived from two inbred strains which differ significantly for the trait of interest are used to ascertain the trait's mode of inheritance. The two parental strains (P1 and P2) and the F1 generation, derived from crossing the parental strains, are uniform in their genetic makeup and are thus referred to as nonsegregating. The three segregating groups are the F2 intercross, produced by crossing F1 × F1, and the two back-crosses obtained by crossing F1 × P1, and F1 × P2. The F2 and back-cross progeny are referred to as segregating because they differ at numerous loci along each chromosome, which assort independently at meiosis. The division of genetic material and independent assortment of chromosomes in the gametes allows for a limited number of combinations of genotypes in the offspring of these crosses. The frequency with which animals in the segregating generations resemble either progenitor strain or an intermediate response is genetically determined. From this information, conclusions can be drawn regarding the genetic basis for the difference in bronchial responsiveness (Fig. 3).

Multiple investigators have found that A/J mice represent the high extreme of the phenotypic range for bronchial responsiveness to cholinergic agonists, while C3H/HeJ and C57BL/6J mice are typically among the least responsive strains (Fig. 4) [12,17,38,50,51]. However, different modes of inheritance for bronchial hyperresponsiveness have been suggested in these strains. In the ACh-induced model originally described by Levitt and Mitzner [12], an autosomal recessive mode of inheritance was suggested for the hyperresponsive phenotype based on the segregation of this trait in (C3H/HeJ × A/J)F1, F2, and back-cross generations. Subsequent studies by investigators in the same laboratory determined that the segregation data obtained from these crosses were best described by a two locus model [15]. These investigators concluded that the use of new genetic modeling techniques which permitted critical comparisons of multiple segregation models resulted in refinement of the original segregation analysis, and that while the inheritance of cholinergic-induced bronchial responsiveness was relatively simply (two genes), it was not likely to be strictly Mendelian. De Sanctis and colleagues [17] found a similar differential responsiveness between the high-responding A/J and low-responding C57BL/6J strains; however, the (C57BL/6J × A/J)F2 animals resembled the A/J parent, suggesting a dominant mode of inheritance for the hyperresponsive phenotype. This is in contrast to the studies by Levitt and Mitzner [12] in which the hyperresponsive phenotype appeared to be recessive. De Sanctis et al. [17] also reported a wide dispersion of phenotypes in 14 AXB recombinant inbred strains (derived from A/J and C57BL/6J progenitor strains), suggesting a non-Mendelian mode of inheritance.

Several factors are likely to contribute to the differential results of genetic analysis in these studies. Levitt and co-workers studied crosses derived from the A/J × C3H/HeJ strains because these two strains were phenotypically the highest (A/J) and lowest (C3H/HeJ) of all strains tested. De Sanctis and colleagues took advantage of the available AXB recombinant inbred strains by studying the A/J C57BL/6J crosses. Identical crosses were not studied by these two groups, thus

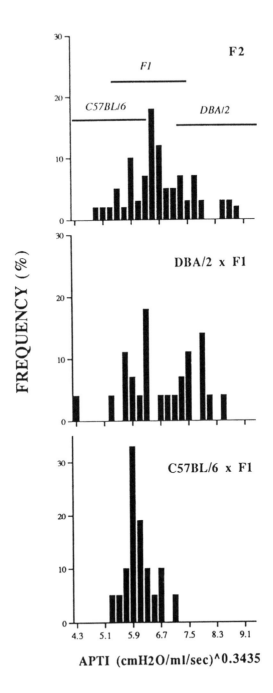

APTI (cmH2O/ml/sec)^0.3435

direct comparisons of these results must be made cautiously. In addition, different techniques for measuring parameters of bronchial hyperresponsiveness were employed. Levitt and Mitzner [12] developed a low-dead-space ventilatory system in which they measured the time-integrated change in peak inflation pressure following intravenous agonist challenge. Ewart and colleagues [38] used the end-inflation occlusion technique in the same ventilatory system to measure respiratory resistance and elastance at baseline and following intravenous single-dose challenge. In this system, serial ACh challenges resulted in progressive augmentation of mediator-induced bronchial hyperresponsiveness which was most marked in hyperresponsive strains (Fig. 5) [38]. De Sanctis and colleagues [17] used plethysmography to measure airway resistance and dynamic compliance following repeated intravenous MCh challenges. These methodologic differences, particularly single-dose versus multiple-dose challenges, may have contributed to the differential results of the above-described studies. Additionally, the bronchial hyperresponsiveness phenotype may be uniquely derived in individual inbred strains, precluding direct comparisons of crosses between different strains of mice.

Linkage analyses for bronchial hyperresponsiveness have been reported in inbred strains of mice. Using quantitative trait locus (QTL) analysis, De Sanctis and colleagues [51] demonstrated two regions which co-segregated with bronchial hyperresponsiveness (LOD > 3.0) in crosses derived from the A/J and C57BL/6J strains. Ewart and co-workers [50] studied markers on mouse chromosome 11 which surrounded the genes encoding IL-3, IL-4, IL-5, and GM-CSF and excluded the region near this cytokine gene cluster from containing ACh-induced bronchial hyperresponsiveness loci in A/J × C3H/HeJ crosses. It is anticipated that continued linkage studies will ultimately identify specific loci which determine cholinergic-induced bronchoconstriction.

Linkage studies have also been performed in an atracurium-induced model of bronchial hyperresponsiveness [52]. Using a candidate gene approach, QTL analysis was performed in 24 BXD recombinant inbred strains which derive from strains hyperresponsive (DBA/2J) and hyporesponsive (C57BL/6J) to intravenous atracurium challenge. Based on evidence that bronchial hyperresponsiveness and

---

Figure 3 Frequency distribution of bronchial responsiveness to atracurium (10 mg/kg, i.v.) in DBA/2 ($n = 10$) and C57BL/6 ($n = 15$) mice and progeny of crosses between them. The dispersion of progenitor and progeny responses suggests that this trait is genetically determined in a relatively simple (two-gene) manner. F1 ($n = 17$) are the offspring of crosses between female C57BL/6 and male DBA/2 mice. F2 ($n = 60$) are the offspring of the intercross between F1 mice. DBA/2 × F1 ($n = 28$) and C57BL/6 × F1 ($n = 21$) are the backcross generations. Data are presented as the airway pressure time index (APTI) following power transformation ($x = y^p$, $P = 0.3435$).

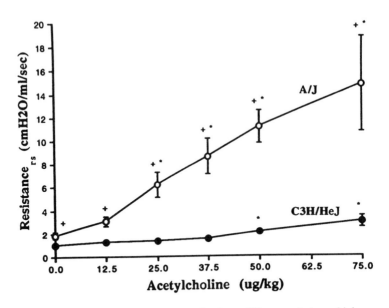

Figure 4   Dose–response curve demonstrating large differences in bronchial responsiveness between hyperresponsive (A/J) and hyporesponsive (C3H/HeJ) inbred mouse strains. Respiratory system resistance was measured in mice after challenge with 12.5 to 75 µg/kg i.v. acetylcholine; $n = 3$–6 mice per strain per dose. + difference between strains; * difference between doses at $P < 0.05$. (From Ewart et al., 1995.)

serum total IgE, as indices of allergic asthma, map to human chromosome 5q31-q33 [5,6,53], the mouse homologs of human chromosome 5q31-q33 were evaluated for linkage; four regions of mouse chromosomes 11, 13, and 18 are homologous with human chromosome 5q31-q33 [48,54]. Atracurium-induced bronchoconstriction mapped to mouse chromosome 13 near the *Il9* locus [52], thus demonstrating a conserved linkage between bronchial hyperresponsiveness in humans on chromosome 5q31-q33 and the mouse on chromosome 13. The gene encoding IL-9 is a candidate gene for this trait because, as a T-cell growth factor, it relates logically to the hypothesis of inflammation-associated bronchial hyperresponsiveness, and it maps to the chromosomal regions linked to this phenotype in both humans (chromosome 5q31-q33) and mice (chromosome 13).

The refined localization and ultimate identification of loci which contribute to inherited bronchial hyperresponsiveness in mice will enhance tremendously our knowledge of the pathophysiology of this phenotype. Information gained regarding bronchial hyperresponsiveness loci in mice may be used to direct homologous mapping studies of the genetics of asthma. Dissection of the molecular mechanisms which determine bronchial hyperresponsiveness is paramount to under-

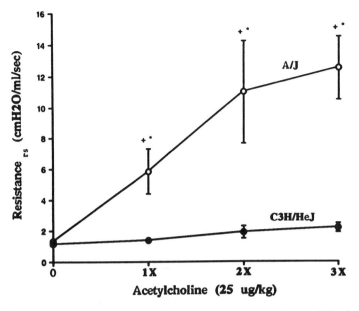

Figure 5 Progressive augmentation of bronchial responsiveness is seen following serial cholinergic challenges. Respiratory system resistance was measured after 1, 2, and 3 serial challenges of 25 μg/kg i.v. acetylcholine. Challenges were administered at 5-min intervals; $n = 3–6$ mice per strain per dose. + difference between strains; * difference between doses at $P < 0.5$. (From Ewart et al., 1995.)

standing fully how genetic predisposition and environmental factors interact to produce asthma.

VIII. Mediator-Induced Bronchial Hyperresponsiveness in Rats

Martin and colleagues [19] tested the hypothesis that bronchial responsiveness in the rat is a strain-related characteristic by determining dose–response curves to inhaled aerosols of MCh in the following highly inbred rat strains; Lewis, ACI, BN, WF, BUF, WKY, and three batches of F344. Aerosols of saline or progressively doubling concentrations of MCh were delivered to anesthetized mice and measurements of total pulmonary resistance were made by plethysmography. Strain-related differences in bronchial responsiveness were detected, and the variability between strains was significantly greater than that within strains (Table 1) ($P < 0.001$). The Lewis rat was most resistant to the bronchial effects of MCh; the mean concentration required to produce a twofold increase in pulmonary

Table 1 Strain Distribution Pattern for MCh-Induced Airway
Responsiveness in Inbred Rat Strains

Strain	Lewis	ACI	BN	WF	BUF	WKY	F344
$ED_{200}R_L{}^a$ (mg/mL)							
Mean	6.92	6.61	4.68	3.55	2.45	1.35	0.35
Range min	3.25	2.00	3.25	1.15	0.81	0.52	0.07
Range max	19.7	12.13	6.96	18.38	13.00	2.16	1.06

[a]Airway responsiveness is expressed as the concentration of MCh required to produce a
twofold increase in lung resistance; $ED_{200}R_L$. (From Ref. 19.)

resistance ($EC_{200}R_L$) was 6.92 mg/mL. In contrast, the F344 strain demonstrated
the greatest bronchial responsiveness, with a mean $EC_{200}R_L$ of 0.35 mg/mL. The
response of the three groups of F344 rats did not differ significantly from each
other. These authors concluded that bronchial responsiveness to MCh in inbred
rats is strain-related, suggesting that genetic factors are important determinants of
this trait. Pauwels and colleagues [18] characterized the bronchial reactivity of
the Lewis rat and five additional strains to single intravenous challenge with 5HT
or carbachol. In contrast to what would be predicted from the findings of Martin,
Lewis rats were poor responders to carbachol and 5HT. BN rats did not respond to
either agent, and DA rats were poor responders to 5HT. RA rats were intermediate
responders to both agents. OM/N rats were strong reactors to 5HT but not to
carbachol, and IC rats were good responders to both agents. The discrepancy in
responsiveness of the Lewis strains to two cholinergic agonists may be related to
genetic variation in the two Lewis populations, which were presumably obtained
from different sources. However, methodological differences, including intravenous versus aerosol and single versus multiple progressive challenges, were
factors which could significantly affect these results. Nevertheless, significant
genetic variation was observed in the response to bronchoconstrictors among
inbred strains of rats.

The strain-related airway differences in the strains identified by Martin to
have the greatest (F344) and least (Lewis) sensitivity to MCh challenge were
further characterized by quantitating the airway smooth muscle as a fraction of
total lung tissue [20]. The higher-responding F344 strain had significantly more
airway smooth muscle than did Lewis rats (3.22 ± 0.176 versus $2.48 \pm 0.185\%$,
mean $\pm$ SE, $P < 0.001$) suggesting that the quantity of airway smooth muscle may
contribute to interstrain variability in bronchial responsiveness. In a separate study
[55], interleukin-2 (IL-2) administered intravenously to Lewis and F344 rat strains
produced greater increase in MCh-induced bronchial responsiveness in Lewis rats
as compared to controls ($EC_{200}R_L = 0.6 \pm 0.2$ and 4.3 ± 1.4 for Lewis rats
receiving IL-2 and vehicle, respectively; $P = 0.003$) than in the F344 strain

(EC$_{200}$R$_L$ = 0.13 ± 0.03 and 0.35 ± 0.25 for F344 rats receiving IL-2 and vehicle, respectively; P = 0.09). IL-2 caused similar pathologic changes in the lungs of both strains characterized by significant bronchial epithelial detachment and peribronchial and perivascular edema. It is interesting to note that there was little, if any, cellular infiltration. In this study, increased bronchial responsiveness prior to treatment with IL-2 did not predispose to the induction of further bronchial responsiveness. The proportionally smaller change in the F344 animals may have reflected a relative plateau in bronchial responsiveness of this strain, making further augmentation of the phenotype difficult to measure.

The results of studies on inherent, or baseline, bronchial responsiveness in the rat are similar to those found in inbred mice strains and suggest that comparable mechanisms may determine baseline bronchial hyperresponsiveness in both inbred rats and mice. Additional studies to confirm the inheritance of this trait in the rat and further define its genetic complexity would be valuable for the purposes of both comparative physiology and genetics. Gene mapping studies underway in the mouse, and homology mapping information, may be useful to identify chromosomal regions and specific loci that determine bronchial responsiveness in the rat.

IX. Antigen-Induced Bronchial Hyperresponsiveness in Mice and Rats

Bronchial hyperresponsiveness has long been known to be a factor in asthma; however, it has only recently become clear that asthma is a chronic inflammatory disease involving interactions among multiple cell types. Airway infiltration with eosinophils and lymphocytes, and epithelial cell sloughing, is characteristic of asthma, regardless of whether asthma is allergic or apparently nonallergic in origin. Airway inflammation and bronchial hyperresponsiveness have been induced in many animal models by antigen sensitization with subsequent antigen challenge. Gavett and Wills-Karp [25] demonstrated in an antigen-sensitized inbred mouse model that compromise in lung function concurrent with airway inflammation was dependent on preexisting bronchial hyperresponsiveness. Pulmonary inflammation was induced by intraperitoneal immunization and intratracheal challenge with sheep red blood cells (SRBC) in inbred strains of mice which were inherently hyperresponsive (A/J) or hyporesponsive (C3H/HeJ) to ACh challenge. Both strains responded to SRBC challenge with a vigorous lung inflammatory response characterized by increased numbers of lavaged alveolar macrophages, neutrophils, lymphocytes, and eosinophils compared to controls. The total number of alveolar macrophages and neutrophils were significantly greater in SRBC-challenged C3H/HeJ mice as compared to SRBC-challenged A/J mice. While airway inflammation was somewhat greater in the C3H/HeJ than the

A/J strain, ACh-induced bronchial responsiveness was unchanged in SRBC-challenged C3H/HeJ mice but was significantly augmented in SRBC-challenged A/J mice as compared to controls. Postinflammatory bronchial responsiveness may depend on a genetic predisposition that may result in differences in the response of lung tissue to mediators of inflammation or differences in the type of inflammatory mediator elaborated.

Early studies of the respiratory response of the rat to aerosolized antigen challenge were reported by Holme, Piechuta, and colleagues [56,57]. In their original work they characterized the respiratory pattern induced by aerosol challenge with ovalbumin 14 to 18 days following sensitization in conscious Sprague-Dawley, Long-Evans, Wistar, and Fisher 344 rats [56]. Respiratory pattern changes were categorized as mild, moderate, or severe based on the extent and duration of apnea, increased airflow, dyspnea, and pronounced movement of thoracic and abdominal muscles. Rats experiencing a severe response had continuous dyspnea and evidence of distress. Fisher 344 rats had only mild responses to antigen challenge without evidence of dyspnea, despite their ability to make IgE antibodies to the ovalbumin. The remaining three strains exhibited large variation in their phenotypic response to antigen challenge in that only a portion of the rats in each strain had a severe response (20–70%). The magnitude of response was not correlated with serum IgE levels in any strain.

These investigators recognized the value of having a homogeneous population in which animals of a like genetic makeup demonstrate uniform responses to antigen challenge. In a subsequent study, Holme and Piechuta [57] selectively crossed only Sprague-Dawley rats which developed severe respiratory impairment after sensitization and aerosolized antigen challenge. The initial incidence of dyspnea noted in Sprague-Dawley rats was 44%. In the "F1" generation, produced by crossing severe-responding progenitor rats, the incidence of a severe response increased to 55%, and was greater than 90% in the "F2" and "F3" generations. Thus, selective breeding resulted in a significant increase in the incidence of antigen-induced dyspnea and yielded an "inbred" population that was homogeneous for that trait. The results of these studies highlight the degree of genetic impurity which characterized some inbred rat strains at the time of this work [58–60]. Because genetic contamination, residual heterozygosity, and the occurrence of new mutations with subline divergence can contribute to genetic, and thus phenotypic, variability within strains, strict genetic monitoring must be maintained in all inbred species to ensure the authentication of genetically defined animals. Recent efforts to expand the rat genome database, along with our increased knowledge of genetic monitoring, have greatly enhanced the genetic stringency of many commercially available inbred rat strains.

Because an inflammatory component underlies the development of asthma, it is important to investigate animal models in which bronchial hyperresponsiveness is accompanied by airway inflammation. The studies described here suggest a heritable component to antigen-induced bronchial hyperresponsiveness. Additional studies are currently underway to characterize further the inheritance of inflammatory-mediated bronchial hyperresponsiveness and pursue identification of specific loci which contribute to this trait. It will be interesting to see whether the antigen-induced bronchial hyperresponsiveness is inherited independently of baseline bronchial hyperresponsiveness or whether overlapping genes contribute to both inflammatory and noninflammatory bronchoconstrictor phenotypes.

X. Future Directions

While the genetic analysis of complex diseases is a relatively new field, much progress has already been made toward describing the inheritance of asthma-related phenotypes in several animal models. The results of bronchial hyperresponsiveness linkage analyses have suggested candidate regions for further study, and have also been used to exclude chromosomal regions from containing bronchial hyperresponsiveness loci. Continued work should aim to refine the genetic map position and ultimately identify loci that determine the hyperresponsive phenotype. This information will aid in deciphering the molecular mechanisms predisposing to bronchial hyperresponsiveness and should lead to more rational and less palliative therapies.

References

1. Konig P, Godfrey S. Exercise induced bronchial lability in monozygotic (identical) and dizygotic (non-identical) twins. J Allergy Clin Immunol 1974; 54:280–287.
2. Townley RG, Guirgis H, Bewtra A, Watt G, Burke K, Carney K. IgE levels and methacholine inhalation responses in monozygous and dizygous twins. J Allergy Clin Immunol 1976; 57:227.
3. Hopp RJ, Bewtra AK, Biven R, Nair NM, Townley RG. Bronchial reactivity pattern in nonasthmatic parents of asthmatics. Ann Allergy 1988; 61:184–186.
4. Hopp RJ, Townley RG, Biven RE, Bewtra AK, Nair NM. The presence of airway reactivity before the development of asthma. Am Rev Respir Dis 1990; 141:2–8.
5. Meyers DA, Postma DS, Panhuysen CIM, et al. Evidence for a locus regulating total serum IgE levels mapping to chromosome 5. Genomics 1994; 23:464–470.
6. Postma DS, Bleecker ER, Amelung PJ, et al. Linkage analyses of bronchial hyperresponsiveness with markers on human chromosome 5q31-q33. N Engl J Med 1995; 333:894–900.
7. Moses BL, Spaulding GL. Chronic bronchial disease of the cat. Vet Clin North Am [Small Anim Prac] 1985; 15:929–948.
8. Moise NS, Wiedenkeller D, Yeager AE, Blue JT, Scarlett J. Clinical, radiographic, and bronchial cytologic features of cats with bronchial disease: 65 cases (1980–1986). J Am Vet Med Assoc 1989; 194:1467–1473.

9. Derksen FJ, Robinson NE, Armstrong PJ, Stick JA, Slocombe RF. Airway reactivity in ponies with recurrent airway obstruction (heaves). J Appl Physiol 1985; 58: 598–604.

10. Armstrong PJ, Derksen FJ, Slocombe RF, Robinson NE. Airway responses to aerosolized methacholine and citric acid in ponies with recurrent airway obstruction (heaves). Am Rev Respir Dis 1986; 133:357–361.

11. Derksen FJ, Scott JS, Miller DS, Slocombe RF, Robinson NE. Bronchoalveolar lavage in ponies with recurrent airway obstruction (heaves). Am Rev Respir Dis 1985; 132:1066–1070.

12. Levitt RC, Mitzner W. Expression of airway hyperreactivity to acetylcholine as a simple autosomal recessive trait in mice. FASEB J 1988; 2:2605–2608.

13. Levitt RC, Mitzner W. Autosomal recessive inheritance of airway hyperreactivity to 5-hydroxytryptamine. J Appl Physiol 1989; 67(3):1125–1132.

14. Levitt RC. Understanding biologic variability in susceptibility to respiratory disease. Pharmacogenetics 1991; 1:94–97.

15. Ewart SL, Meyers DA, Mitzner W, Levitt RC. Two loci genetic regulation of airway resistance in a mouse model of airway hyperresponsiveness. Am J Human Genetics 1994; 55(3):A184.

16. Levitt RC, Ewart SL. Genetic susceptibility to atracurium-induced bronchoconstriction. Am J Respir Crit Care Med 1995; 151:1537–1542.

17. De Sanctis GT, Martin TR, Beier DR, Drazen JM. Airway responsiveness in C57BL/6J, A/J and AXB/BXA recombinant inbred mice: evidence for genetic control of airway responsiveness. Am J Respir Crit Care Med 1994; 149(4):A755.

18. Pauwels R, Van Der Straeten M, Weyne J, Bazin H. Genetic factors in non-specific bronchial reactivity in rats. Eur J Respir Dis 1985; 66(2):98–104.

19. Martin JG, Bellofiore S, Guttman RD. Strain-related differences in airway reactivity amongst highly inbred rats. Am Rev Respir Dis 1987; 135:A473.

20. Eidelman DH, DiMaria GU, Bellofiore S, Wang NS, Guttman RD, Martin JG. Strain-related differences in airway smooth muscle and airway responsiveness in the rat. Am Rev Respir Dis 1991; 144:792–796.

21. Hirshman CA, Malley A, Downes H. Basenji-greyhound dog model of asthma: reactivity to Ascaris suum, citric acid, and methacholine. J Appl Physiol 1980; 49(6): 953–957.

22. Peters JE, Hirshman CA, Malley A. The Basenji-greyhound dog model of asthma: leukocyte histamine release, serum IgE, and airway response to inhaled antigen. J Immunol 1982; 129(3):1245–1249.

23. Bellofiore S, Martin JG. Antigen challenge of sensitized rats increases airway responsiveness to methacholine. J Appl Physiol 1988; 65(4):1642–1646.

24. Kips JC, Cuvelier CA, Pauwels RA. Effect of acute and chronic antigen inhalation on airway morphology and responsiveness in actively sensitized rats. Am Rev Respir Dis 1992; 145:1306–1310.

25. Gavett SH, Wills-Karp M. Pulmonary inflammation increases airway reactivity to acetylcholine challenge in genetically hyperresponsive, but not hyporesponsive mice. Am Rev Respir Dis 1993; 147(4):A572.

26. Gavett SH, Chen X, Finkelman F, Wills-Karp M. Depletion of murine CD4+ T

lymphocytes prevents antigen-induced airway hyperreactivity and pulmonary eosino-philia. Am J Respir Cell Mol Biol 1994; 10:587–593.

27. Bousquet J, Chanez P, Lacoste JY, et al. Eosinophilic inflammation in asthma. N Engl J Med 1990; 323:1033–1039.

28. Hogg JC, James AL, Pare PD. Evidence for inflammation in asthma. Am Rev Respir Dis 1991; 143:S39–S42.

29. Lacoste J-Y, Bousquet J, Chanez P, et al. Eosinophilic and neutrophilic inflammation in asthma, chronic bronchitis, and chronic obstructive pulmonary disease. J Allergy Clin Immunol 1993; 92:537–548.

30. Bonhomme F, Guénet J-L. The wild house mouse and its relatives. In: Lyon MF, Searle AG, eds. Genetic Variants and Strains of the Laboratory Mouse. 2d ed. New York: Oxford University Press, 1989:649–662.

31. Festing MW. Inbred strains of mice. In: Lyon MF, Searle AG, eds. Genetic Variants and Strains of the Laboratory Mouse. 2d ed. New York: Oxford University Press, 1989:636–648.

32. Green MC, Witham BA. Inbred strains and F1 hybrids. In: Handbook on Genetically Standardized JAX mice. 4 ed. Bar Harbor, ME: The Jackson Laboratory, 1991:3–40.

33. Elliott RW. DNA polymorphisms. In: Lyon MF, Searle AG, eds. Genetic Variants and Strains of the Laboratory Mouse. 2d ed. New York: Oxford University Press, 1989: 537–558.

34. Silver LM. Master locus list. Mamm Genome 1993; 4:S2–S9.

35. Dietrich WF, Miller JC, Steen RG, et al. A genetic map of the mouse with 4,006 simple sequence length polymorphisms. Nat Genetics 1994; 7(2):220–245.

36. Kunieda T, Kobayashi E, Tachibana M, Ikadai H, Imamichi T. Polymorphic micro-satellite loci of the rat (*Rattus norvegicus*). Mamm Genome 1992; 3:564–567.

37. Yamada J, Kuramoto T, Serikawa T. A rat genetic linkage map and comparative maps for mouse or human homologous rat genes. Mamm Genome 1994; 5:63–83.

38. Ewart S, Levitt R, Mitzner W. Respiratory system mechanics in mice measured by end-inflation occlusion. J Appl Physiol 1995; 79(2):560–566.

39. Festing MFW. Characteristics common to all inbred strains. In: Inbred Strains in Biomedical Research. New York: Oxford University Press, 1979:54–62.

40. Committee on Standardized Nomenclature for Inbred Strains of Mice. Standardized nomenclature for inbred strains of mice. Cancer Res 1952; 12:602.

41. Festing MFW. Recombinant inbred strains. In: Inbred Strains in Biomedical Re-search. New York: Oxford University Press, 1979:115–121.

42. Taylor BA. Recombinant inbred strains. In: Lyon MF, Searle AG, eds. Genetic Variants and Strains of the Laboratory Mouse. 2d ed. New York: Oxford University Press, 1989:773–798.

43. Festing MFW. Congenic, coisogenic and segregating inbred strains. In: Inbred Strains in Biomedical Research. New York: Oxford University Press, 1979:104–114.

44. Lane PW, Lyon MF. Congenic and segregating inbred strains: mutant genes and biochemical loci. In: Lyon MF, Searle AG, eds. Genetic Variants and Strains of the Laboratory Mouse. 2d ed. New York: Oxford University Press, 1989:825–842.

45. Kleeberger SR, Levitt RC. Animal models for studies on genetic predisposition to adverse effects of chemical exposure. In: Ecogenetics: Predisposition to the Toxic

Effects of Chemicals. World Health Organization Consultation. London: Chapman & Hall, 1991:91–110.

46. McDonald JR, Mathison DA, Stevenson DD. Aspirin intolerance in asthma: detection by oral challenge. J Allergy Clin Immunol 1972; 50:198–207.

47. Nadeau JH, Davisson MT, Doolittle DP, et al. Comparative map for mice and humans. Mamm Genome 1992; 3:480–536.

48. Mammalian Comparative Mapping Data. Mouse Genome Database. Mouse Genome Informatics Project. Bar Harbor, ME: The Jackson Laboratories, 1995; World Wide Web (URL:http://www.informatics.jax.org).

49. Ott J. Methods of linkage analysis. In: Analysis of Human Genetic Linkage. Baltimore: Johns Hopkins University Press, 1991:54–81.

50. Ewart SL, Levitt RC, Wills-Karp M, Mitzner W. Genetic regulation of airway hyperresponsiveness: the role of IL-4 and IL-5 determined by linkage analysis. Am J Respir Crit Care Med 1994; 149(4):A755.

51. De Sanctis GT, Merchant M, Lander ES, Beier DR, Drazen JM. Genetics of airway responsiveness in C57BL/6 and A/J mice: a segregation and quantitative trait locus analysis. Am J Respir Crit Care Med 1995; 151(4):A341.

52. Ewart SL, Zhang L-Y, Kleeberger SR, Levitt RC. Atracurium-induced bronchial hyperresponsiveness in mice maps to chromosome 13 homologous to a region important in asthma. Am J Respir Crit Care Med 1995; 151(4):A341.

53. Marsh DG, Neely JD, Breazeale DR, et al. Linkage analysis of IL4 and other chromosome 5q31.1 markers and total serum immunoglobulin E concentrations. Science 1994; 264:1152–1156.

54. Nadeau JH, Reiner AH. Linkage and synteny homologies in mouse and man. In: Lyon MF, Searle AG, eds. Genetic Variants and Strains of the Laboratory Mouse. 2d ed. New York: Oxford University Press, 1989:506–536.

55. Renzi PM, Du T, Sapienza S, Wang NS, Martin JG. Acute effects of interleukin-2 on lung mechanics and airway responsiveness in rats. Am Rev Respir Dis 1991; 143: 380–385.

56. Piechuta H, Smith ME, Share NN, Holme G. The respiratory response of sensitized rats to challenge with antigen aerosols. Immunology 1979; 38:385–392.

57. Holme G, Piechuta H. The derivation of an inbred line of rats which develop asthma-like symptoms following challenge with aerosolized antigen. Immunology 1981; 42: 19–24.

58. Sharp DW. Rejection of islet <isografts> in a strain of Lewis rats. Transplantation 1981; 31:229–230.

59. Pennline KJ, Smith JP, Bitter-Suermann H. My kingdom for an inbred rat. Transplantation 1982; 34:70.

60. Festing MFW. Genetic contamination of laboratory animal colonies: an increasingly serious problem. ILAR News 1982; 25(4):6–10.

Part Three

GENETIC APPROACHES: FAMILY STUDIES, MOLECULAR TECHNIQUES, AND ANALYSIS

13

Molecular Approaches to the Identification of Disease Genes

JOANNA GRODEN

University of Cincinnati College of Medicine
Cincinnati, Ohio

HANS ALBERTSEN

Huntsman Cancer Institute
Eccles Institute of Human Genetics
University of Utah
Salt Lake City, Utah

I. Introduction

The identification of "disease" genes—genes whose aberrant alleles are responsible for defined clinical syndromes—has been a major focus of human genetics over the past 10 years as a natural consequence of significant improvements in DNA technology and genetic resources. In particular, these improvements have derived from the development of better genetic marker systems for linkage analysis, the construction of large-insert libraries of genomic clones, and the genetic mapping and characterization of an ever-growing number of human genes. To identify genes involved in inherited disease or predispositions, two general strategies are being applied that take advantage of these resources: One is known as positional cloning and the other as a candidate-gene approach. Both strategies are based on knowledge of the approximate genomic location of the disease allele. It follows that the more narrowly the chromosomal region is defined, the simpler will be the task of identifying the gene.

In the case of positional cloning, a physical map of the region must be developed. Overlapping genomic clones covering an entire region are isolated and ordered linearly, expressed sequences (i.e., fragments of genes) from the region are identified by means of the genomic clones from the physical map, and expressed sequences are assembled into full-length genes. All genes located within the mapped region are considered as candidates for the disease gene and are subject to screening for mutations in constitutional DNA from patients. In the candidate-gene approach, prior knowledge of genes located in the target region is exploited by analyzing these genes for mutations, the order of priority being based on their biological function rather than the status of the physical map of the region. Obviously, these two strategies are not mutually exclusive; in fact, both approaches are applied in the hunt for a disease gene whenever possible. Table 1 is a partial list of many of the disease genes recently cloned by either of these approaches [1].

Methods of screening for aberrant genes also have improved dramatically in recent years. Certainly, as technologies for direct sequencing for DNA and for analysis and storage of these sequences are improved, it is inevitable that these techniques will become the most rapid, cost-effective, and reliable choice for the detection of DNA alterations that disrupt genes in consequential ways. In the meantime, however, numerous methods are available for identifying DNA sequence alterations. These techniques range from long-range restriction mapping by pulsed-field gel electrophoresis (PFGE), which can identify gross alterations in the structure or length of large regions of a chromosome, to techniques that detect single base-pair alterations in coding or noncoding regions of a gene, such as single-strand conformation polymorphism (SSCP) or RNase-protection analyses. Each of these techniques has features that are suited to particular projects and to the inheritance pattern (dominant or recessive) of the disease of interest. Generally, a combination of approaches to the evaluation of a chromosomal region or a candidate gene in affected individuals is the most logical choice for ultimately pinpointing a disease gene.

The identification of disease genes has been greatly accelerated by the Human Genome Project. One of the immediate goals of the Genome Project is to produce descriptive maps of each human chromosome at increasingly finer resolution. A map is the linear order of elements in the genome; the elements may be genes, polymorphic markers, DNA fragments, or any other distinguishable feature on a chromosome. Several different technologies exist by which maps can be developed. The earliest maps of the human genome were genetic linkage maps based on the phenomenon of meiotic recombination between chromosomal homologs and the detection of the resulting segregation patterns of genetic markers in large families. The measurable feature of genetic linkage maps is the frequency of meiotic recombination between genetic markers, the number of recombinational events determining genetic distance. These genetic distances are measured in centimorgans (cM). Each cM represents an observed recombination frequency of 1%; that is, a single meiotic recombination event observed between a pair of markers in a set of 100 chromosomes. In genetic maps, the linear order of three or more markers is based on a statistically determined likelihood for a specific order

Table 1 Selected Disease Genes Cloned by Positional Cloning, Functional Complementation, and Candidate-Gene Approaches [1]

A. Positional cloning approach
   Aarskog-Scott syndrome
   Acondroplasia
   Adenomatous polyposis coli
   Adrenoleukodystrophy
   Agammaglobulinaemia, X-linked
   Aniridia
   Ataxia telangiectasia
   Becker muscular dystrophy
   Bloom's syndrome
   Breast/ovarian cancer predisposition
   Chondrodysplasia punctata
   Choroideraemia
   Chronic granulomatous disease
   Congenital adrenal hypoplasia
   Cystic fibrosis
   Dentatorubral pallidoluysian atrophy
   Diastophic dysplasia
   Duchenne muscular dystrophy
   Emory-Dreifuss muscular dystrophy
   Fragile X syndrome
   Glycerol kinase deficiency
   Huntington disease
   Kallmann syndrome
   Limb-Girdle muscular dystrophy
   Lissencephaly
   Lowe syndrome
   Machado-Joseph disease
   McLeod syndrome
   Menkes disease
   Myotonic dystrophy
   Neurofibromatosis type I
   Neurofibromatosis type II
   Norrie syndrome
   Ocular albinism
   Polycystic kidney disease

   Spinal muscular dystrophy
   Spinocerebellar ataxia I
   Retinoblastoma
   Tuberous sclerosis
   von Hippel-Lindau disease
   Werner's syndrome
   Wilms tumor
   Wilson disease
   Wiskott Aldrich syndrome
   Xeroderma pigmentosum,
      complementation group B
B. Functional complementation approach
   Cockaynes syndrome A
   Fanconi anemia
C. Candidate gene approach
   Alzheimer's disease
   Amyotrophic lateral sclerosis
   Charcot-Marie Tooth disease type 1A
   Charcot-Marie Tooth disease type 1B
   Crouzon syndrome
   Familial hypertrophic cardiomyopathy
   Familial melanoma
   Hereditary hemorrhagic telegiectasia
      type I
   Hereditary nonpolyposis colon cancer
      or Lynch syndrome
   Hyperekplexia
   Jackson-Weiss syndrome
   Long QT syndrome
   Malignant hypothermia
   Marfan syndrome
   Multiple endocrine neoplasia type 2A
   Pfeiffer syndrome
   Supravalvular aortic stenosis
   Retinitis pigmentosa
   Waardenburg syndrome

compared to another order. Sometimes, when very closely linked markers are involved, the correct linear order cannot be determined by linkage analysis with an acceptable or significant likelihood.

Very different from genetic linkage mapping, which reflects or infers distances on a chromosome as the frequency of meiotic recombination between particular DNA characteristics or markers, physical mapping techniques attempt to determine the exact linear order of markers and to measure chromosomal distance exactly in DNA base pairs. Physical mapping techniques vary with respect to their fields of vision and their degrees of resolution. The most global view of the genome is obtained by means of microscopic analysis of metaphase chromosomes. This kind of analysis, also known as cytogenetic analysis, reveals the entire nuclear genome in a single view and allows the assessment of individual chromosomes based on distinctive banding patterns. Using fluorescent in-situ hybridization, or FISH, one can visualize DNA markers as discrete fluorescent signals emanating from a small region of a banded chromosome; this technique indicates directly the genomic location of the marker.

Particular DNA markers or sequences can be mapped with finer resolution using panels of somatic-cell hybrids or rodent cells that contain small fragments of the human chromosome in question. Often the chromosomal fragments have a known origin, being derived from translocation chromosomes; at other times they are randomly generated before incorporation into host cells, using γ-irradiation to break a chromosome along its length. Panels composed of numerous individual hybrid cells (each containing different human chromosomal fragments) are analyzed with appropriate primers for the polymerase chain reaction (PCR) to identify which members are positive for particular PCR products and which are not. In this way, the somatic-cell hybrid panel provides information that associates the presence of a particular PCR marker with the presence of other PCR markers, as well as with a narrow chromosomal location. The level of resolution obtained by means of cytogenetics or cell-hybrid studies range from entire chromosomes down to large chromosomal fragments—in other words, from hundreds of millions of base pairs down to only a few million.

The next level of resolution for mapping is defined by gel electrophoresis of DNA fragments generated from restriction enzyme-digested genomic DNA or maintained as cloned DNA segments in particular vectors. Different applications of the gel electrophoresis technique permit visualization of DNA fragments ranging from the million-base-pair level down to single nucleotides. A restriction map describes the order and physical distance between very short, defined DNA sequences (4–8 base pairs) that are sensitive to cleavage by restriction enzymes. Human DNA fragments can be cloned and propagated in living hosts such as yeast or bacteria. Depending on the vector and the host, such fragments may range in size from a few nucleotides to several million.

Physical maps of chromosomal regions are developed using one or more of the techniques described above. They are often composed of numerous, ordered, partially overlapping DNA fragments on which genetic and physical landmarks have been located. Most biologists consider physical maps a tool rather than a goal, for the simple reason that the truly interesting features of biology lie in the genes themselves. Physical maps are useful in that they extend help for the identification and characterization of genes. The expression maps that in turn are generated from physical maps show the locations of expressed DNA segments, i.e., exons, relative to known physical or genetic landmarks. The highest level of resolution of the physical map—and the ultimate goal of the Human Genome Project—is the complete DNA base-pair sequence of all chromosomes in the human genome and the identification of all the genes within that sequence. Its purpose is to permit development of diagnostic and therapeutic tools for the study of human biology and disease. An overview of the process of physical mapping and disease-gene identification is shown in Fig. 1 and described in the figure legend.

II. Genomes, Genes, and Base Pairs

The haploid human genome is estimated to be slightly more than 3 billion base pairs in total length [2,3]. From experience, we know that the average gene contains 2000 base pairs of coding sequence and that the average distance between genes is 40,000 base pairs. In general, genes do not exist as single continuous stretches of coding DNA, but rather as several small, sequentially arranged, but discontinuous sections known as exons, which are interrupted by noncoding sequence known as introns. Only after transcription of a gene will its introns be excised and the exons spliced together into a single, continuous coding sequence. The sizes of exons can vary greatly. Some are as small as 15 base pairs and others continue for several thousand base pairs. On average, exons are about 130 base pairs long; introns vary even more widely in length.

Although recombination events are more common in some regions of the genome than in others, a general relationship does exist between genetic and physical distance. Therefore, a simple calculation can estimate the amplitude of a positional cloning project, given a genetic distance, by calculating expected numbers of genes within a region based on average gene sizes and average gene densities. Thus, in the case of gene X, mapped with 95% likelihood to a 4.2-cM region, we would expect the physical extent of the region to be in the neighborhood of 4,200,000 base pairs. Given this estimated physical size of the region, we would expect to find 105 different genes distributed in more than 1600 exons. It should be clear that the establishment of a complete expression map of this magnitude is a costly and labor-intensive undertaking.

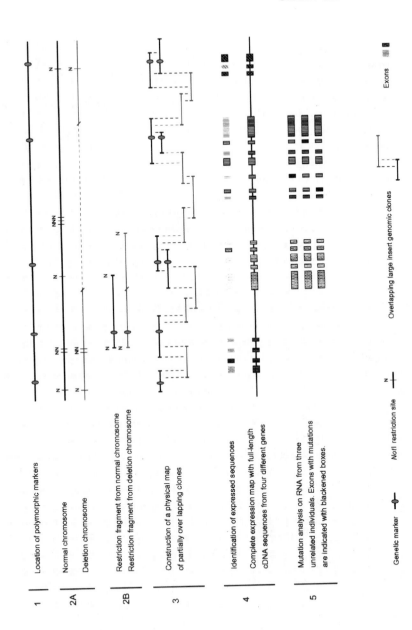

1   Location of polymorphic markers

2A   Normal chromosome
     Deletion chromosome

2B   Restriction fragment from normal chromosome
     Restriction fragment from deletion chromosome

3   Construction of a physical map
     of partially over lapping clones

4   Identification of expressed sequences
     Complete expression map with full-length
     cDNA sequences from four different genes

5   Mutation analysis on RNA from three
     unrelated individuals. Exons with mutations
     are indicated with blackened boxes.

Genetic marker ⬥   NotI restriction site ⊢   Overlapping large insert genomic clones   Exons

Figure 1 Techniques in physical mapping. The physical mapping of a genomic region is a cumulative process which combines mapping results from different techniques into a single map. This generalized example of the physical mapping process demonstrates the stepwise refinement of the map from the initial location of DNA markers to the identification of a complete expression map and detection of mutations in a candidate gene. The initial genomic localization of a disease gene is usually obtained by genetic linkage analysis. In the top of the schematic (1), the relative locations of five genetic markers are indicated by grayed ovals on a chromosomal DNA segment. In the following section (2A), two lines show chromosomal DNA segments with several *Not*I restriction sites indicated with the letter N. The top line represents a normal chromosome, while the bottom line represents a chromosome with a deletion (indicated with a stippled line). Comparison of restriction-digested DNAs from the normal and the deleted chromosomes (2B) reveals two differently sized restriction fragments suggestive of a chromosomal rearrangement of the abnormal chromosome. The assembly of a "contig" of partially overlapping genomic clones (3) is a very important step in the isolation of genes by physical mapping, since the genomic clones provide the resources for isolating expressed sequences by any of several different strategies. In (4) the individual exons identified are completed into full-length consensus cDNA sequences. Individual exons are coded here in patterns indicating to which of the four genes each belongs. On the basis of their locations with respect to the genetic markers in (1) (and on meiotic breakpoints derived from pedigrees where the disease segregates), and considering information from other deletion chromosomes, we can classify the two central genes of this series as candidate genes. Mutational analysis of the two candidate genes (5) reveals no mutations in the first candidate, while the second gene shows mutations (blackened boxes) in different exons among three unrelated patients. This result confirms the second candidate as the disease gene.

A. Refinement of Genomic Location

The success of finding a disease gene depends critically on several factors. First, how well defined are the phenotype and genetic pattern of the disease? Is the disease homogenic or heterogenic, and is it a mono- or multifactorial disease? Is the appropriate genetic material available for detection of mutations in patients? How precisely has the disease locus been mapped in the genome? How extensive are the genetic and genomic resources available for this region? What is the current status of the chromosomal map for this region? Lastly, can critical observations be verified in biological test systems?

As described in other chapters of this book, statistical methods exist by which simple and multifactorial genetic traits in families can be mapped. After DNA samples are collected from appropriately characterized affected individuals and their families, the key resources for these types of analyses are genetic markers that detect polymorphic loci in the human genome. Several types of genetic markers have been developed since 1980, when it was first proposed that a genetic map of DNA markers for the human genome be developed. The seminal paper by Botstein et al. (1980) suggested that 300 polymorphic markers spaced 10cM apart would be sufficient to map most hereditary traits by linkage analysis [4].

The first type of marker proposed for mapping in humans was the restriction-fragment length polymorphism, or RFLP [4]. Variation that alters the nucleotide sequence recognized by a restriction enzyme results in the failure of cleavage at that site, which is seen as a change in the length of the particular DNA fragment being analyzed. These length variations are detected by Southern blotting and hybridization of genomic DNA to a radioactively labeled DNA probe for that particular DNA fragment. Although useful in practice, polymorphisms of this kind were not always present or "informative" in particular individuals; nor were they easy to find in great numbers throughout the genome. Variable number of tandem repeat (VNTR) loci were the next major improvement in the development of DNA markers [5]. Those loci, which contained repeated blocks of sequence, showed tremendously more variation (i.e., in the number of repeated sequence blocks) among individuals than simple RFLPs; most VNTR markers could even distinguish between the maternal and paternal chromosomes in any one individual, allowing better resolution of recombination events. Like RFLPs, VNTR loci were evaluated by Southern blotting and hybridization to radioactively labeled probes. Finally, the introduction of the polymerase chain reaction (PCR) allowed the detection of polymorphisms involving very small repetitive blocks in the genome, when the unique sequences flanking such loci were used as primers. These repetitive blocks, of two to four nucleotides, have revolutionized our ability to map the genome, because the numbers of repeats at these so-called micro-satellite loci vary considerably within the population. These PCR-based, simple tandem-repeat, polymorphic markers are known as STRPs [6]. In addition to their high degree of polymorphism, also known as a PIC value, STRP loci have the advantage of being detectable by polyacrylamide gel electrophoresis. Genotyping requires only minute amounts of DNA from the individual being studied. Currently, about 10,000 genetic markers are available for mapping, the majority of which are STRPs. As the number of markers has increased, genetic maps of ever higher resolution have been developed; the average genetic distance between markers on chromosomal maps is now less than 1 cM. This 1-cM genetic distance represents approximately 1 million base pairs.

Fluorescent in-situ hybridization (FISH) complements genetic mapping as a method to determine genomic locations and the linear order of genomic landmarks. Because FISH relies on hybridization of fluorescently labeled DNA fragments to metaphase or interphase chromosomes, it does not require that the locus be polymorphic. The probes best suited for FISH are large genomic DNA fragments 10–100 kilobase pairs (kb) long. Representative images of FISH are shown in Fig. 2.

For the success of a positional-cloning strategy, the chromosomal region harboring the gene must be localized with a high degree of likelihood between two landmarks. (Usually such a landmark would be a genetic marker, but a translocation junction or the boundaries of a small deletion can be just as useful.) The goal of physical mapping is to identify overlapping genomic clones that bridge the genomic segment between two genetic markers. Therefore the closer the two genetic markers are to one another, the shorter is the physical distance; consequently, the task of identifying a complete set of overlapping clones becomes simpler. The upper limit for the physical distance between landmarks should not exceed 4–5 million base pairs.

B. Chromosomal Anomalies: An Alternative Way to Determine the Location of Disease Genes

Chromosomal anomalies present in germline DNA, such as translocations, duplications, expansions, and deletions, are found either as de-novo mutations or are transmitted in ova or sperm from parents to their offspring. In either case the chromosomal abnormality can be associated with a genetic disease; its presence implies a direct correlation between the location of the chromosome change and the location of the disease gene. Some examples of diseases mapped on the basis of these types of anomalies include neurofibromatosis type 1, fragile-X syndrome, and Duchenne muscular dystrophy [7–9]. In each of these diseases, a chromosomal rearrangement detected by microscopic observation provided a clue to the location of the disease gene. Chromosomal rearrangements may permit localizing specific genes within approximately 2 million base pairs, a limit corresponding to the resolution obtainable by cytogenetic analysis of metaphase chromosomes.

Not all chromosome anomalies are carried in the germline, however. Those

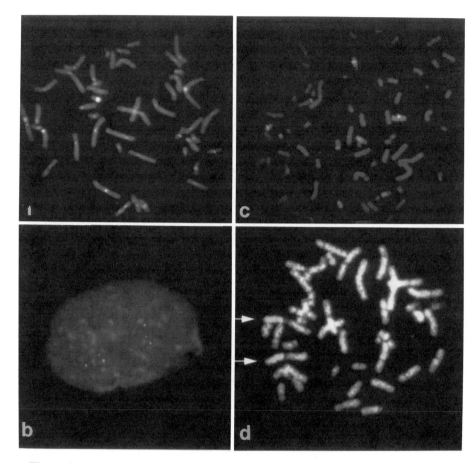

Figure 2   Fluorescent in situ hybridization and comparative genome hybridization. These pseudo-colored images illustrate mapping techniques using dual-color fluorescence in situ hybridization (FISH) and comparative genomic hybridization (CGH). (a) Normal male metaphase chromosomes hybridized with a digoxigenin-labeled α-satellite probe (green) specific for the pericentromeric region of chromosome 17 (Oncor, Inc.; detected using an anti-digoxigenin FITC-conjugated antibody) and with the biotinylated P1 phage probe, 108B11 (red),which is visualized in the 17q12-21 chromosomal region after treatment with streptavidin-Cy3. (b) Interphase nucleus hybridized with three different P1 clones; two were biotin-labeled probes chosen for their known physical locations and were detected with streptavidin-Cy3 (red). The other P1 clone here is mapped relative to the two of known location, labeled with digoxigenin and detected with an anti-digoxigenin FITC-conjugated antibody (green). (c) Partial metaphase from a prostate tumor cell line, PC-3, hybridized with Spectrum Green-labeled chromosome 5 paint (Vysis, Inc.) and a P1 probe which localizes to the 5q23 chromosomal region. A single apparently normal chromosome 5 is present in the metaphase, along with three other copies of the P1-specific sequence and

that occur somatically can often be associated with particular tumor types; a frequent type of rearrangement found in tumors involves deletion of large chromosomal segments or the loss of genetic complexity. Such chromosomal losses, detected when testing tumor DNA with polymorphic markers, indicate a "loss of heterozygosity" (LOH). Generally it is believed that tumors acquire a growth advantage by losing particular chromosomal regions, based on the assumption that the lost regions harbor genes that normally restrain cellular growth. In other words, regions that show LOH provide clues to the location of tumor-suppressor genes. LOH, and the other techniques described in detail below, can be applied equally to searches for aberrant genes, whether in tumor DNA or in constitutional DNA from patients with inherited clinical syndromes.

C. Chromosomal Anomalies: Pulsed-Field Gel Electrophoresis to Detect Breakpoints, and Marker Development Using Microdissection of Chromosomes

The resolution of metaphase chromosome structure by cytological analysis ranges from a whole chromosome to the order of several megabases. Therefore, by itself, cytological analysis of an aberrant chromosome is unable to determine precisely

---

several derivative translocated fragments of chromosome 5. (d) Partial metaphase illustrating CGH, using a Spectrum Red-labeled (Vysis, Inc.) DNA from a breast cancer cell line (MPE-600) and Spectrum Green-labeled (Vysis, Inc.) normal female DNA, both hybridized to a normal male metaphase. Increased red signal intensity is seen on both copies of chromosome 1p (arrows). The entire p arms (nearest the arrows) appear to be amplified. A small region of increased green signal at the distal end of each copy of chromosome 1q suggests a small chromosomal deletion at this locus in the tumor DNA. (For optimal reproduction, see color plate.)

the location of a disease gene. Several supporting techniques, such as pulsed-field gel electrophoresis (PFGE) and chromosome microdissection, can help in determining more exactly the region containing a significant anomaly.

Pulsed-field gel electrophoresis (PFGE) was developed in the mid-1980s [10,11] to overcome the limited resolution of large DNA fragments in standard gel electrophoresis. In standard gel electrophoresis, smaller DNA fragments are separated as a function of their size in a constant and unidirectional electric field, while larger DNA fragments (>30 kb) are caught in the gel matrices. Exposing the DNA fragments to an alternating electrical field allows large fragments to "get unstuck" and to continue their migration through the gel. The introduction of PFGE yielded a dramatic increase in the range of DNA fragments separable, from some 30 kb up to several million base pairs. Conveniently, a collection of rare-cutting restriction enzymes were discovered during the same period in which PFGE was under development, and they provided the necessary enzymatic tools to generate DNA fragments in the 100-kb to 1000-kb range. PFGE can be used to develop long-range restriction maps; as a result, it enables one to detect restriction-fragment anomalies, such as inversions, deletions, and insertions, that accompany chromosome changes. Once a restriction-fragment alteration is discovered, the location of this alteration can be analyzed more closely. Figure 3 illustrates some of the main electrode arrangements of electrophoresis chambers.

Microdissection techniques allow the investigator to obtain and develop a panel of genomic probes as well as polymorphic markers from a specific chromosomal region. Microdissection involves selectively recovering fragments of DNA from a specific chromosomal region from metaphase spreads, and cloning them into appropriate vectors. Because the probes and markers isolated by microdissection are distributed over a fairly large region (2 to 20 Mb), it is necessary to verify the location of each of them. One way of doing this is to develop a sequence tagged site, or STS, from the probe or marker and to verify the location of the STS on a panel of radiation-hybrid cell lines (discussed in Section II.E). Radiation-hybrid panels are particularly useful for this purpose, as they do not rely on polymorphisms for mapping but only on the presence or absence of a hybridizing band or PCR product. In this way, a large number of probes and markers can be generated for refining the genetic localization of a gene or for expanding the physical map of the region surrounding a gene.

D. Loss of Heterozygosity and Comparative Genome Hybridization as a Means to Define the Genomic Location of a Gene in Tumors

Tumor cells accumulate somatic mutations as the tumor evolves. These changes can often be visualized cytogenetically as tumor karyotypes may include gross chromosomal rearrangements such as duplications and deletions. In addition to

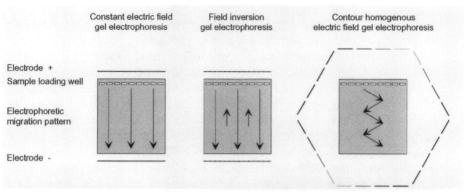

Figure 3 Standard gel electrophoresis, FIGE, and CHEF. Gel electrophoresis is the most commonly used method of separating DNA fragments by size. Traditional gel electrophoresis will only permit separation of DNA fragments within a certain size range, which is determined by the pore size of the gel matrix; very small fragments will not encounter significant resistance from the gel and migrate almost freely in the electric field, whereas very large fragments will be caught and immobilized in the gel matrix. Between these extremes, DNA fragments will migrate in the gel at speeds that vary as a function of their sizes. The leftmost of the three diagrams represents an electrophoresis chamber with a single, constant electric field. This type of electrophoresis chamber is generally used to separate DNA fragments ranging in size from 50 base pairs to 25,000 base pairs. The diagram in the center represents field-inversion gel electrophoresis, or FIGE, and varies form the previous type only by its alternating electric field. In this case the predominant electric field is inverted for brief periods of time (usually at a 3:1 ratio). As a result of this periodic change in the electric field, the large DNA fragments which have been caught in the gel matrix are freed to migrate farther in the gel. Field-inversion gel electrophoresis can be used efficiently to separate DNA fragments 1000 base pairs long up to 700,000 base pairs. The most efficient and versatile electrophoretic system for separating very large DNA fragments is contour-clamped homogeneous electric-field gel electrophoresis, or CHEF, illustrated in the right diagram. In this design, as the gel is surrounded by 24 individually controlled electrodes, the operator can apply alternating electric fields at any angle. The CHEF design has successfully separated the three chromosomes from *Schizosaccharomyces pombe* (a yeast species), the smallest of which is 3 million base pairs and the largest of which is 9 million base pairs.

chromosome microdissection and PFGE, two other major techniques can detect genetic changes in tumors. The first is LOH analysis and the second is comparative genome hybridization (CGH).

LOH is evaluated by comparing the allelic patterns of polymorphic genetic markers in DNA samples extracted from normal and tumor tissues from a given individual. As in genetic linkage studies, polymorphic marker systems can distinguish between the two chromosomal homologs within a cell, but only if the locus is heterozygous in the normal tissue. If a given pair of normal and tumor-tissue samples reveals heterozygosity at the locus in normal tissue, but only one of the two alleles can be detected in tumor tissue, one concludes that the other allele known to harbor the second polymorphic allele has been lost sometime during tumorigenesis. Several large-scale studies have applied LOH analysis to discover which chromosomal arms are deleted most often in different cancers. In breast cancers, for example, not all chromosomal regions are deleted at the same frequency; moreover, the chromosomal regions preferentially lost vary among different kinds of breast cancers. Table 2 indicates the LOH patterns observed in a larger collection of breast tumors. Defining the boundaries of the region(s) on the chromosome that lose heterozygosity can lead to the pinpointing of the position of damaged genes involved in tumor formation. The paradigm for this type of study is that completed by Cavenee et al. in 1983 for the retinoblastoma gene [12].

Genes critical for normal cell control (i.e. negative growth regulators) are likely to be those missing from a cancer cell, because such loss confers a growth advantage to the cell. Conversely, amplification of specific regions that contain positive growth-regulating genes can occur. An elegant technique for detecting chromosomal deletions or amplifications is known as comparative genome hybridization (CGH). In this technique, DNA from a normal cell is "painted" in a specific color with a fluorescent dye (green), while DNA extracted from a tumor is, in a separate experiment, "painted" with another fluorescent dye (red). By simultaneously hybridizing the "painted" DNAs from the normal and the tumor cells to a normal metaphase spread, a uniform mixture of the two colors is expected in regions that show no difference between the two hybridization reagents. However, in deleted regions of the tumor, less or no probe DNA is available to compete with DNA from the normal cell; only green signal from the normal DNA is observed there. On the other hand, if certain regions have been amplified in the tumor, these regions will appear more strongly pigmented red (Fig. 2). CGH can therefore help to pinpoint the positions of genes involved in tumor formation.

E. Somatic-Cell Hybrid Mapping Panels

Culture techniques exist by which single cells from different organisms may be fused. Cells resulting from this type of experiment are called somatic-cell hybrids. When human cells are fused to a rodent cells, most human chromosomes are lost, although one or more may be retained under selective conditions. Cytogenetic analysis of hybrid cells can determine which human chromosomes remain in the hybrid. It also is possible to determine if a hybrid cell line carries a specific piece of human DNA by testing for the presence of an STS by PCR. Using a panel of hybrid cell lines, where each cell line carries a different human chromosome, one can determine which human chromosome carries the STS. Regional localization

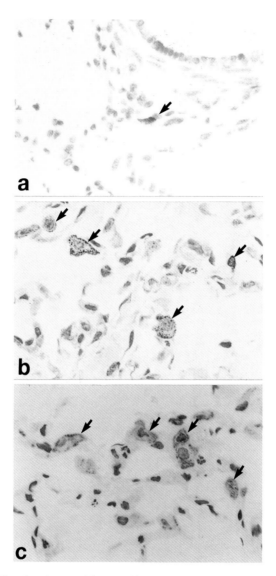

Figure 8.1 Histochemistry and immunohistochemistry of mast cells in the lungs of a normal BALB/c mouse and a V3-mastocytosis mouse. Mast cells are rare in the lungs of a normal BALB/c mouse (panel a) but increase in number 2 to 3 weeks after the adoptive transfer of a v-*abl*-immortalized mast cell line (panels b and c). Panels a and b represent tissue sections stained with methylene blue. Panel c depicts a replicate tissue section stained with anti-mMCP-7 Ig. Arrows indicate mast cells. Figure courtesy of Dr. Daniel Friend (Harvard Medical School).

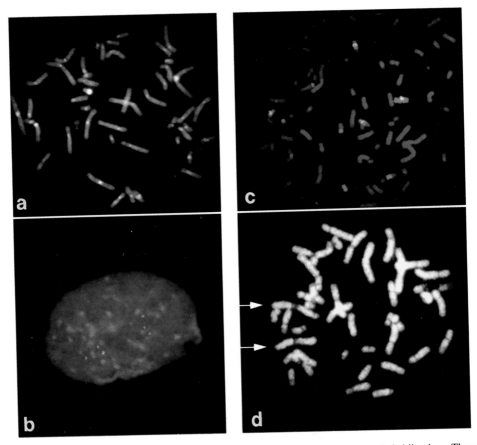

Figure 13.2 Fluorescent in situ hybridization and comparative genome hybridization. These pseudo-colored images illustrate mapping techniques using dual-color fluorescence in situ hybridization (FISH) and comparative genomic hybridization (CGH). (a) Normal male metaphase chromosomes hybridized with a digoxigenin-labeled α-satellite probe (green) specific for the pericentromeric region of chromosome 17 (Oncor, Inc.; detected using an anti-digoxigenin FITC-conjugated antibody) and with the biotinylated P1 phage probe, 108B11 (red), which is visualized in the 17q12-21 chromosomal region after treatment with streptavidin-Cy3. (b) Interphase nucleus hybridized with three different P1 clones; two were biotin-labeled probes chosen for their known physical locations and were detected with streptavidin-Cy3 (red). The other P1 clone here is mapped relative to the two of known location, labeled with digoxigenin and detected with an anti-digoxigenin FITC-conjugated antibody (green). (c) Partial metaphase from a prostate tumor cell line, PC-3, hybridized with Spectrum Green-labeled chromosome 5 paint (Vysis, Inc.) and a P1 probe which localizes to the 5q23 chromosomal region. A single apparently normal chromosome 5 is present in the metaphase, along with three other copies of the P1-specific sequence and several derivative translocated fragments of chromosome 5. (d) Partial metaphase illustrating CGH, using a Spectrum Red-labeled (Vysis, Inc.) DNA from a breast cancer cell line (MPE-600) and Spectrum Green-labeled (Vysis, Inc.) normal female DNA, both hybridized to a normal male metaphase. Increased red signal intensity is seen on both copies of chromosome 1p (arrows). The entire p arms (nearest the arrows) appear to be amplified. A small region of increased green signal at the distal end of each copy of chromosome 1q suggests a small chromosomal deletion at this locus in the tumor DNA.

Table 2 Summary of Observed LOH in Breast Cancers, from the Literature (references below)

Chromosomal arm	Informative tumors	Allelic losses (%)	Chromosomal arm	Informative tumors	Allelic losses (%)
1p	102	10 (10)	11q	37	3 (8)
1q	87	17 (20)	12p	26	2 (7)
2p	60	10 (18)	12q	39	1 (3)
2q	66	9 (14)	13q	101	26 (26)
3p	56	17 (30)	14q	107	21 (20)
3q	53	4 (8)	15q	42	11 (26)
4p	48	1 (2)	16p	79	3 (4)
4q	88	9 (10)	16q	87	36 (41)
5p	11	1 (9)	17p	131	74 (56)
5q	47	5 (11)	17q	86	16 (19)
6p	39	5 (13)	18p	29	6 (21)
6q	65	22 (34)	18q	55	11 (20)
7p	22	1 (5)	19p	51	8 (16)
7q[a]	52	3 (6)	19q	41	5 (12)
8p	22	6 (27)	20p	49	2 (4)
8q	29	7 (24)	20q	57	1 (2)
9p	31	3 (10)	21q	57	9 (16)
9q	79	21 (27)	22p	9	1 (11)
10p	52	6 (12)	22q	33	9 (27)
10q	57	9 (16)	Xp	44	7 (16)
11p	95	16 (17)	Xq	44	4 (9)

[a]The observations made here for chromosome 7q are in striking disagreement with results published by Bieche et al. (1992), where LOH frequency of 40% was observed for the marker p*met*H.

Sato T, Tanigami A, Yamakawa K, et al. Allelotype of breast cancer: cumulative allele losses promote tumor progression in primary breast cancer. Cancer Res 1990; 50:7184–7189.

Devilee P, van Vliet M, van Sloun P, et al. and Cornelisse CJ (1991). Allelotype of human breast carcinoma: a second major site for loss of heterozygosity is on chromosome 6q. Oncogene 1991; 6:1705–1711.

Bieche I, Champame MH, Matifas F, Hacane K, Callahan R, Lidereau R. Loss of heterozygosity on chromosome 7q and aggressive primary breast cancer. Lancet 1992; 339:139–143.

within a specific chromosome also is possible. In that case, the DNA in a rodent cell line carrying a single human chromosome is fragmented by γ-irradiation. The irradiated cell is then fused to a second rodent cell line, effectively mixing the DNA fragments from the irradiated cell with intact rodent chromosomes. Some fragments from the human chromosome will be integrated into the rodent host genome, although most are lost. As a result, a few fragments of the original human chromosome are retained in the new hybrid cell line. Given a panel of these hybrid cell lines, each of which carries a different human DNA fragment(s), it is possible to determine the order of DNA markers on the original intact human chromosome by testing which markers coexist in any given cell line. The closer two markers are to one another, the more frequently will they be found in the same cell lines. This technique allows for the physical co-localization of markers, and provides the potential for isolating closely linked DNA markers through subcloning and identification of human sequences by means of hybridization to human repetitive DNA.

F. Genomic Insert Libraries: YACs, P1s, PACs, BACs, and Jumping and Linking Libraries

The establishment of physical maps is an essential prerequisite for gene isolation by positional cloning. As already mentioned, a physical map is a complete set of partially overlapping genomic fragments. Usually these fragments are carried in a vector that allows the fragment to be stably maintained and propagated. As physical mapping projects often span large genomic segments and sometimes involve more than 100 genomic clones [13], it should be clear that the larger the genomic insert, the fewer clones are necessary to span the region of interest. In the mid-1980s, the largest clonable fragments could not exceed 40 kb in length, since they were propagated in *Escherichia coli* in modified λ-phage vectors known as cosmids. However, in 1987 a new vector system was described by which genomic DNA fragments of up to 1000 kb could be maintained in *Saccharomyces cerevisiae* as yeast artificial chromosomes, or YACs [14]. The introduction of large YAC libraries was a tremendous improvement, as the identification of many disease genes could not have been accomplished rapidly without the use of such large-insert clones [15–18]. However, because a significant portion of YACs are unstable or chimeric, additional vector systems have since been developed to provide alternative large-insert resources for physical mapping. Three systems in particular deserve mentioning: P1 phage clones that will accommodate up to 85 kb inserts [19–22], P1 artificial chromosomes (PAC) that will accommodate inserts of 100 to 300 kb [23], and bacterial artificial chromosomes (BAC) that also can accommodate inserts of 100 to 300 kb [24]. Many of these libraries are available from commercial sources or from laboratories supported by the Human Genome Project.

Several methods have been developed for screening large-insert libraries, but the one most frequently used is PCR screening of arrayed libraries [25]. The term "arrayed libraries" reflects the fact that clones from these libraries are maintained individually, usually in wells of a microtiter plate. Because the library is arrayed, screening results can be recorded and compared to subsequent screenings. This recorded information becomes very valuable for the linear ordering of genomic clones: As more and more clones in the arrayed libraries are identified, the more likely it becomes that important information from previous screenings

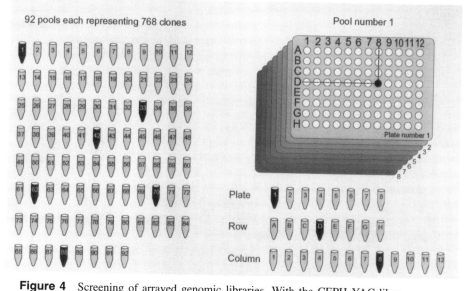

92 pools each representing 768 clones

Pool number 1

Plate

Row

Column

Figure 4 Screening of arrayed genomic libraries. With the CEPH YAC library as an example, a PCR-based procedure for screening of arrayed libraries is illustrated. Because the procedure is performed using PCR, it is fast and consumes only modest amounts of library reagents. The advantage of screening an arrayed library is that positive clones can be rapidly, efficiently, and exhaustively identified. The essential feature of the procedure is the organization of the clones in a three-dimensional array, where each individual clone can be identified by its x, y, and z coordinates. In this scheme all 70,000+ members of the CEPH YAC library are stored in a set of 96-well microtiter plates; the 736-plate library is divided into 92 pools of 8 plates each, with each pool containing 768 YAC clones. As illustrated at left, each of the 92 pools is initially screened by PCR to identify whether it contains a clone positive for a particular PCR marker. In the example, pools numbered 1, 33, 42, 62, 70, and 88 were positive (blackened tubes). For each pool identified as positive, the exact "address" of the positive clone must now be ascertained by a secondary PCR screening. The secondary screening of pool number 1 is illustrated in the right half of the figure. The DNA template for the secondary screening is organized as a three-dimensional array representing the positive pool. The array consists of a total of 28 samples, composed of 8 rows [A ... H], 12 columns [1 ... 12], and 8 plates [1 ... 8]. By testing the 28 samples, one identifies a single address by its plate number, column, and row. In the example the positive clone was first identified in pool number 1; its exact location is on plate number 1 at the coordinates D,8.

already exists for newly identified clones [26–29]. Screening of an arrayed library is outlined in Fig. 4.

An important step in extending and bridging physical islands is the ability to isolate the extremities of a genomic clone and to use those ends to identify overlapping neighbors by rescreening large-insert libraries. Three different PCR-

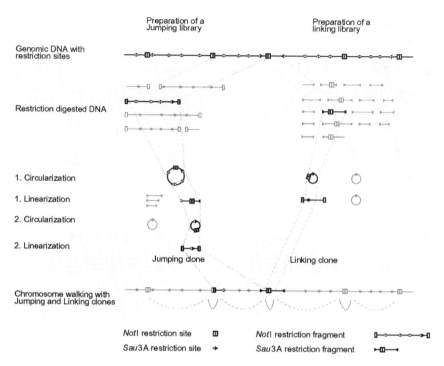

Figure 5 Preparation of jumping and linking libraries. The specialized cloning techniques illustrated in this figure describe the construction of jumping clones and linking clones. The top line represents a segment of genomic DNA with *Not*I and *Sau*3A restriction sites indicated by boxes and diamonds respectively. *Not*I restriction sites are rare in the genome and generate restriction fragments an average of 1 million base pairs long. *Sau*3A restriction sites, however, are frequent and generate restriction fragments averaging 250 base pairs in length. (The figure is not drawn to scale.) To prepare jumping clones, the genomic DNA is digested with *Not*I and circularized by ligating the restriction fragments under very dilute conditions. This brings the two extremities of each restriction fragment together. In the next step the circularized DNA is digested with *Sau*3A to generate a large population of small restriction fragments, of which only a few will contain a *Not*I site. The small restriction fragments are again circularized by ligating the fragments under very dilute conditions and then are cut with *Not*I. At this point only the few circles containing a *Not*I site will be linearized and available for further subcloning and propagation as jumping clones; most circles remain intact, and because they are unclonable they will not be present in the jumping library. Construction of linking clones is illustrated in the right half of the figure. Following digestion of the genomic DNA with *Sau*3A, the restriction fragments are circularized under dilute conditions and digested with *Not*I. Again, the vast majority of DNA circles will not be affected by the treatment with *Not*I, while the circles that did contain the restriction site will have been linearized. The linearized fragments represent linking clones and can be propagated in libraries after subcloning.

based techniques have been described in the literature; each has been applied in our laboratories to generate DNA templates specific to the ends of YAC inserts. These techniques are inverse PCR, originally described by Ochman et al. (1988) and later modified by us [30,31]; Alu-vector PCR [32,33]; and vectorette, or "bubble," PCR [34].

The construction of "jumping" and "linking libraries" complements traditional genomic walking from one genomic clone to another, partially overlapping, genomic clone. This occurs when one jumps from one end of a large restriction fragment to the next using jumping clones and then links one end of the restriction fragment to the end of the neighboring restriction fragment using linking clones [35]. When jumping and linking libraries are screened sequentially, genomic representations of neighboring restriction sites will follow each other like pearls on a string, while the intervening fragments between the extremities are eliminated. Preparation of these libraries is depicted in Fig. 5.

III. Identification of Expressed Sequences

Once a genetic and physical map is established for a region in which a disease gene is known to reside, the next step in identification of the gene of interest is the establishment of an expressed-sequence map. This can be accomplished in a number of ways: by plating and screening expressed sequence libraries with reagents from the physical map, by exon trapping, or by direct sequencing. Another and increasingly more important source for expressed sequences is the collection of publicly accessible sequence databases. The technical challenge in identifying a specific expressed sequence (i.e., gene) in a library of expressed sequences is fully understood when seen in light of the complexity of the aggregate of mRNAs present in the average mammalian cell. It is estimated that approximately 500,000 mRNA molecules are present in the cell at any given time, representing the transcripts from some 30,000 different genes [2,3]. The abundance of message from a specific gene depends on the cell type and may range from just a few copies to hundreds or even thousands of copies.

A. Identifying Expressed Sequences with Expressed-Insert Libraries: cDNA Libraries, Exon Trapping, and Direct Selection

For positional cloning, the primary reagents used to identify expressed sequences are the genomic clones that cover the region determined to contain the disease gene. These genomic clones can be used in different ways, but the most common method for isolating expressed sequences is hybridization-based screening of cDNA libraries. A cDNA library is constructed from mRNA (or total RNA) isolated from a selected tissue. The mRNA is converted into first-strand cDNA using reverse transcriptase, and subsequently converted into double-stranded DNA using a DNA polymerase. Following cloning of the double-stranded DNA in an appropriate cloning vector, the library is ready to be plated and screened. An alternative method to isolate expressed sequences from a cDNA library is known as "direct selection," which involves a combination of DNA hybridization and a PCR technique [36,37]. In this case the cDNA library is specifically prepared with PCR primer sequences attached to the ends of the double-stranded cDNA fragments. As before, a genomic DNA clone is used in the hybridization step, but in this case the clone has been conjugated with magnetic beads. Following hybridization, the heteroduplexes of genomic DNA and cDNA are precipitated with a magnet, while nonspecific cDNA can be washed away. In the process, the cDNA fragments complementary to parts of the genomic DNA ar enriched, and because these cDNA fragments can be amplified by PCR, the cDNA fragments can be further enriched and exposed to additional rounds of purification. After several rounds of enrichment, individual cDNA fragments can be isolated and analyzed.

A disadvantage of both of the hybridization-based methods, however, is their absolute dependency on the target gene being present (expressed) in the cDNA library. The method known as exon trapping does not carry this require-ment, but instead relies on the biological fact that most mammalian genes are spliced following transcription [38,39]. Briefly described, a specially designed cloning vector serves as a recipient for small DNA fragments from the larger genomic clones. The vector is constructed with an RNA transcription initiation site (R_{ini}) followed by two exons (E_1 and E_2) separated by an intron (I_1), in the order R_{ini}-E_1-I_1-E_2. RNA transcribed from this vector can, under special circum-stances, be spliced; excision of the intron gives the order R_{ini}-E_1-E_2. This RNA splicing process is functional even after insertion of a random genomic DNA fragment into a cloning site located in the intron. However, if the genomic DNA fragment contains an exon (E_3) in the proper orientation, the RNA splicing mechanism will recognize the exon and splice the RNA to give the order R_{ini}-E_1-E_3-E_2. Different RNA splice forms with or without novel exons can be detected by variations in length using a combination of reverse transcriptase and PCR.

B. DNA Sequence Maps—Expressed Sequence Tags (ESTs), Sequence Databases, and the Information Highway

Expressed sequences identified by one of the methods described above only rarely result in the ascertainment of a full-length cDNA. It is therefore almost always necessary to go through a repetitive and tedious process of further cDNA isola-tion, DNA sequencing, and sequence comparisons to generate complete transcrip-

Table 3 Medicine- and Biology-Oriented World Wide Web Servers on the Internet

http://www.kumc.edu/instruction/medicine/genetics/prof/geneprof.html
   This home page contains information relevant to clinical and genetic professionals.
http://gdbwww.gdb.org/
   Human Genome Data Base home page includes an on-line version of Victor McKusick's "Mendelian Inheritance in Man," genetic maps of the human genome, and ideograms of the human chromosomes.
http://www.ornl.gov/TechResources/Human_Genome/genetics.html
http://golgi.harvard.edu/biopages/all.html
   These two home pages provide access to a large collection of biosciences-oriented servers.
http://www-mcb.ucdavis.edu/info/bio.html
   This home page provides access to companies that offer biology-related products. It also provides general information and access to biological databases.

tion maps across a genomic region. However, two important resources have significantly reduced this previously time-consuming work. One is the introduction over the past 10 years of specialized tools which facilitate DNA sequencing, sequence comparison and alignment, and protein translation. The other is the result of massive efforts to identify expressed-sequence tags (ESTs) representing partial genes or exons. These sequencing efforts account for the majority of sequences accessible from public databases (also described in another chapter of this book). With the help of this archived information, genetic and physical maps as well as expressed-sequence maps are being developed in laboratories around the world; moreover, to give scientists access to the most recent maps, many are accessible via the Internet. The list in Table 3 shows a few of the Internet starting points which can be visited using browsers on the World Wide Web such as Netscape or Mosaic.

IV. Alternative Techniques for Identifying Disease Genes When the Target Region Is Poorly Characterized

As described above, strategies exist by which a single gene may be identified from a defined chromosomal region. However, it is not always possible to place the target gene(s) in a nicely defined physical region. In such a case the presence of a well-defined cellular phenotype associated with the disease, such as sensitivity to DNA damage, and its correction in affected cells, can be more efficient than positional cloning in the isolation of candidate genes. Finally, the expression of genes in the affected tissue itself may provide the best clue for the identification of a disease gene. For example, there are significant differences in the expression patterns of genes between cells in the basal sheet as opposed to the luminal cells of mammary-duct epithelium, and between cells isolated from tumors as opposed to cells in surrounding normal tissue. To identify effectively which genes display different expression patterns in different tissues, alternate cloning strategies must be applied. At least two techniques can identify critical differences between tissues: The first is a functional test of living tissue; the second allows a comparison of gene expression on the basis of mRNA isolated from different cells.

A. Differential Display and Subtraction Libraries

Changes in the genetic expression patterns of specific genes are the origin of cellular differentiation; such changes are reflected in living systems as differences in the levels of transcription of relevant messenger RNAs. Therefore, although for the majority of genes transcription levels are unaffected by cellular differentiation, expression of a few genes will change significantly following differentiation. Differential display is a technique that detects and reflects expression patterns of mRNA and enables one to compare expression patterns from different tissues. An autoradiogram of a differential display experiment is shown in Fig. 6; its purpose is to obtain the DNA sequences of gene segments that are differentially expressed. Once differentially displayed DNA sequences have been identified, they become subject to completion of the cDNA sequence, database comparisons, and functional studies.

An alternative method for obtaining differentially expressed sequences, known as a subtraction library, is based on competitive hybridization between cDNA from two different tissues, where one is known as the target and the other is known as the driver. The goal of this technique is to deplete the pool of cDNA from the target tissue for all sequences it has in common with the driver, leaving only cDNA species unique to the target tissue available for cloning. To achieve this result, intermediary cDNA libraries are made from each tissue, but only the extremities of the DNA fragments of the target tissue are prepared for further subcloning. DNA samples from the two tissues are mixed and denatured, with the "driver" DNA in large molar excess. Following hybridization, most of the DNA from the target will have hybridized with the DNA from the driver to form unclonable heteroduplexes. Only if a given cDNA is unique to the target will clonable homoduplexes from the target be formed. These homoduplexes, which represent sequences uniquely expressed in the target tissue, provided the DNA for

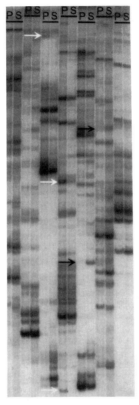

Figure 6 Differential display. There are four major steps in the differential display technique. First, total RNA is isolated from the relevant tissue and reverse-transcribed into cDNA using a poly(T) primer, which specifically allows the reverse transcription of messenger RNA. In the second step an arbitrarily selected pair of oligonucleotide primers is used for PCR with the cDNA as a template. Because the stringency of the PCR conditions are relaxed, a large number of products are generated in such an experiment; and because this step is performed with a collection of 20 different primer pairs in parallel experiments, one obtains an almost complete reflection of the transcriptional activity of the cell. In the third step the PCR products from the two cell types are size-separated on an acrylamide gel to facilitate comparisons and uncover differences in expression. As the last step in the procedure, the differentially displayed PCR products are recovered from the gel, cloned, and sequenced. The cell line used in the experiment pictured is a prostate cancer line, PPC 1 (P in the figure), and its derivative, SF15-2 (S in the figure). SF15-2 was developed by introducing a normal chromosome 17q into PPC1 cells; this resulted in more moderate growth characteristics. The general expression pattern (banding pattern) is very similar between the two cell lines for each pair of oligonucleotide primers tested; in a few places, however, clear evidence of differences in transcription are observed (indicated by arrows).

preparation of the subtraction library. To obtain expressed sequences unique to the driver, a new subtraction library must be prepared, using the tissues in the opposite roles.

B. Functional Complementation Experiments

The basis for functional complementation is the presumption that phenotypic changes that have occurred in a cell as result of a recessively mutant allele can be corrected by the reintroduction of the normal gene or the missing gene product by transfer of a whole or partial normal chromosome or gene into the cells. Successful complementation, as shown by the loss of the disease phenotype in the transfected cells, can lead to determination of the gene responsible through identification of the newly introduced, or wild-type gene. Functional complementation has resulted in the identification of a gene for Fanconi's anemia and the gene for Cockayne's syndrome group [40,41]. This type of gene cloning requires an expression vector that functions efficiently in mammalian cells, and a cDNA library with a large average insert size.

C. Brute-Force Sequencing of Genomic DNA

DNA sequencing, which is becoming more and more economical and efficient, has already proved its value in the sequencing of random cDNA clones and genomic clones. The most highly publicized high-throughput sequencing facility is a not-for-profit organization, the Institute for Genome Research (TIGR), which has submitted more than 55,000 unique expressed-sequence tags (ESTs) to public databases. TIGR also has published the entire DNA sequence of *Haemophilus influenzae*, the first genome of a free-living organism to be sequenced completely [42]. In a similar effort, Merck, Inc., has also begun sequencing random cDNA clones and its researchers are currently submitting more than 5000 ESTs to the public databases on a weekly basis. (A more detailed presentation of this subject can be found elsewhere in this book.) While only a few devoted, high-throughput sequencing facilities can produce DNA sequence on this scale, a growing number of "ordinary" institutions possess sequencing instruments that individually have the potential to produce more than 25,000 bases of DNA sequence per day. Even for a positional cloning project focusing on a region of 1 million base pairs in length, direct sequencing becomes quite appealing. Given that only 5% of the human genome consists of coding sequence, and under the assumption that any segment would only be sequenced once, a throughput of 25,000 base pairs would result in 1250 base pairs of coding DNA per day. With today's computer tools, this raw sequence can be analyzed readily for the presence of exons that potentially are portions of candidate disease genes, and the exonic sequences can be stored in databases for future comparisons.

V. Evaluation of Expressed Sequences for Mutation; Techniques Used to Identify Sequence Alterations in Candidate Genes

Once expressed sequences are identified within the confines of a physical map, they can be evaluated for the presence of alterations that are associated with the disease phenotype. Once again, this is a critical time, as initially in the determination of linkage, for the precise definition of the disease phenotype. The clinical evaluation of patients determined to have a particular disorder is of great importance: If the phenotype is not strictly defined, the genotypic information is also irrelevant or too loosely associated with a disease. Therefore, the astute clinician, following a precise set of parameters to define the disease in affected individuals, is invaluable. The difficulty of sifting through large numbers of genes is obvious; the difficulty encountered in evaluating ambiguous results of sequence analysis when patients exhibit varying disease phenotypes should also be clear.

A variety of techniques are available to assess the sequences or structures of genes that are candidates for involvement in an inherited disease. Most of these techniques will uncover numerous sequence variations that may or may not be related to a particular disease. Generally, DNA polymorphisms are sequence variations that do not contribute to the disease; they must be identified and properly defined as such, in order to separate those variations that are related directly to the disease from those that are not deleterious. Therefore, DNA samples from an adequate number of normal "control" individuals must always be studied in addition to samples from the set of affected individuals. In turn, the identification of novel polymorphisms within the sequence of a candidate gene can provide strategically placed markers for further delimiting the genomic position of the disease gene.

Techniques for detection of mutations in candidate genes must be rapid and reliable. The choice of a particular technique will depend on the resources of a laboratory, the bias of the investigator, and, most importantly, the genetics of the disorder. A disease that is a recessive trait implies a loss of function of a gene; therefore, one would predict that sequence alterations would be those that disrupt or eliminate the function of a gene and its gene product. A disease that is a dominant trait, with the exception of cancer-predisposing diseases which are recessive at the cellular level but dominant at the pedigree level, would imply a gain of function in the candidate gene and therefore suggest a more subtle alteration in its sequence, such as a missense alteration. Obviously, these predictions should not be rigidly adhered to, but they can guide the choice of what resources to study, on what techniques to focus, and how long to pursue a given gene. For example, an investigator may not want to evaluate changes in the long-range restriction map in patients with a dominant disease; but if the disease appears to be a loss-of-function disorder, the restriction map becomes very important because changes in the map in one or many individuals may point directly to a more precise position of the disease gene.

Lastly, inheritance patterns of disease-causing alleles in families and in ethnic groups are important to consider when determining a strategy for mutation screening. Are mutations expected to be identical in a large number of patients? Is there consanguinity in any of the families? Is there evidence from linkage disequilibrium for a founder effect? The epidemiology of the disease is a determining factor in choosing the correct size of the sample set to be evaluated. In general, the greater the number of unrelated individuals included in a mutation study, the better is the chance of rapidly finding sequence alterations in any candidate gene. Once mutations are identified in a certain gene among a small number of affected individuals, a more focused approach can be designed to identify mutations in that gene in all the affected individuals. Family members can also be evaluated for the appropriate inheritance patterns: Obligate heterozygotes should be heterozygous for alterations identified in affected offspring; affected siblings should have identical sequence alterations. When an affected individual has no family history of the disease, the mutation found in that patient's constitutional DNA is probably a novel mutation that one should not expect to find in either parent or in other relatives, although it may have been transmitted to his or her offspring.

A. Techniques That Scan Genes for Structural Alterations: Pulsed-Field Gel Electrophoresis, Southern and Northern Analyses

As described previously, the generation of long-range restriction maps by PFGE when one is establishing the physical map of a region is an important step in the proper ordering of DNA markers and in the mapping of expressed sequences from a particular region of DNA. PFGE also is important in determining the location of any chromosomal breakpoints present in a patient's karyotype that may directly disrupt the gene of interest. PFGE analysis of all patient DNAs, whether a cytogenetic abnormality is present or not, can provide important clues to the exact position of the disease gene by uncovering deletions or insertions. One example of the success of this approach can be found in the positional cloning of the adenomatous polyposis coli gene (*APC*), where the identification of overlapping deletions in DNA from each of two patients among a set of 60 persons with adenomatous polyposis coli was instrumental in identifying the disease gene. One patient carried a 250-kb genomic deletion; the other patient's 100-kb deletion fell wholly within the 250-kb region deleted in the first patient [31,43].

Southern analysis of DNA, using restriction enzymes with four- and six-base-pair recognition sites, is useful for closely scrutinizing small segments of DNA. Likewise, Northern analysis of RNA from patients (if the correct tissue is available for study) probed with isolated expressed sequences can reveal anomalies within genes.

B. Techniques That Scan Genes for Sequence Alterations: RNase Protection, SSCP, DGGE, TGGE, Heteroduplex Analysis, and Chemical Cleavage

RNase protection analysis involves the hybridization of PCR products from affected individuals to sense and anti-sense RNA transcripts corresponding to the normal or expected gene sequence. Segments of the gene to be scanned must therefore be cloned into a vector that allows for transcription of the inserted sequence. The RNA-DNA hybrids then are digested with RNase A, which cleaves at mismatches between the hybrids [44]. This technique is a good choice for the detection of small insertions or deletions, as hybrids with those anomalies will be relatively more sensitive to RNase digestion than those bearing point mutations [45].

Single-strand conformation polymorphism (SSCP) analysis can detect single-base substitutions in DNA as well as short insertions and deletions of DNA. It is based on the observation that denatured single strands of DNA will assume a particular conformation when electrophoresed in nondenaturing gel conditions; this conformation reflects the nucleotide sequence of the single strand of DNA [46,47]. During electrophoresis, homologous single-stranded products will therefore have slightly different mobilities from one another, allowing the variants or "conformers" to be separated and identified. SSCP is easy to execute and is reliable for mutational screening when the DNA sequence being screened is less than 200 base pairs long. DNA samples (genomic or cDNA) can be amplified by PCR, using primers designed from intronic sequences flanking exons or from exons themselves. Radiolabeled PCR products are diluted in a formamide buffer containing dye, and heat-denatured before being loaded on a 5% nondenaturing polyacrylamide gel. Two gel-running conditions are generally used: 10% glycerol at room temperature and no glycerol at 4°C. (Many laboratories currently are using commercially available matrices that replace these two conditions with a single 5% polyacrylamide gel.) Bands then are visualized by autoradiography; if novel conformers are detected, they are isolated directly from the gel and sequenced. Figure 7 shows examples of SSCP analysis and its use in detecting sequence variants. SSCP analysis can also detect the formation of heteroduplexes between mutant and normal alleles, if the double-stranded product that re-forms, or remains after denaturation, can be visualized at the bottom of the nondenaturing gel.

Recently, Liu and Sommer (1995) have modified SSCP analysis to scan segments of genes that are up to 1 kb in length [48]. This technique is called restriction endonuclease fingerprinting (REF) and employs PCR amplification of

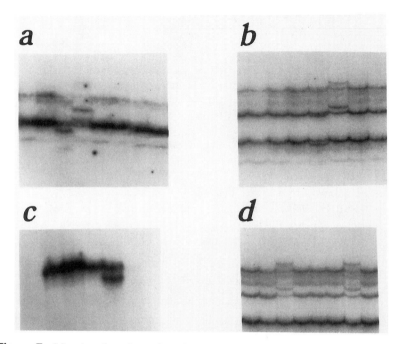

Figure 7 Mutation detection using single-strand conformation polymorphism (SSCP) analysis. SSCP is designed to detect any sequence variation, nonsense or missense, in a denatured (and therefore single-stranded) segment of DNA by nondenaturing gel electrophoresis. Each strand of DNA takes on a characteristic structure, using a particular set of gel conditions, that reflects its sequence. Alterations in sequence are detected by variations in the mobility of the DNA bands. These four panels show SSCP analysis of the *APC* gene in a number of patients with the autosomal-dominant disease adenomatous polyposis coli (APC). Sequence alterations are detected as novel conformers in each panel. Panels A and B show the same set of samples analyzed using two different gel electrophoresis conditions. In panel A, lanes 3 and 4 contain novel DNA conformers that are unique to each of the two unrelated individuals with APC. Each of the novel conformers is different from the others and represent a different sequence alteration. Lane 3 contains a DNA segment that carries a four-base-pair deletion which is associated with the disease. Lane 4 contains a DNA segment that carries a single nucleotide alteration which results in an amino acid change; whether this is a polymorphism or a missense mutation is unknown. Panel C contains DNA from four members of one family: lane 1 contains DNA from a normal male; lane 2 contains DNA from his normal father; lane 3 contains DNA from his normal mother; and lane 4 contains DNA from his brother, affected with APC. The novel conformer represents a new mutation in the *APC* gene (a five-base-pair deletion) that is associated with the sporadic onset of the disease in this individual. Panel D contains eight lanes of DNA from unrelated APC patients. Novel conformers are observed in lanes 3 and 7. These conformers have the identical pattern and were subsequently shown to derive from the same sequence alteration, a five-base-pair deletion, in each of these two individuals with APC.

cDNA, followed by DNA digestion with each of five groups of restriction endo-nucleases. The enzymes in each group are chosen to generate average fragment sizes of about 150 base pairs. Digested DNAs are radioactively labeled by a kinase reaction, denatured and electrophoresed under nondenaturing conditions. On average, a 1-kb DNA segment prepared in this manner will yield 68 segments per lane for analysis by alterations in electrophoretic mobilities [48]. This technique was used to identify the gene for ataxia telangiectasia [49].

Denaturing gradient gel electrophoresis (DGGE) and temperature-gradient gel electrophoresis (TGGE) are techniques that, like SSCP, enable the resolution of DNA fragments that differ by as little as a single nucleotide [50,51]. Both methods utilize a gradient of denaturant (one a chemical gradient, the other a temperature gradient) to vary the electrophoretic mobility of double-stranded DNA. As the strands move through an increasing linear gradient of the denaturing agent, the strands fall apart or "melt" in a manner that reflects the sequence of the DNA duplex. This melting occurs according to the behavior of sequence blocks called melting domains, which vary in length from 25 to several hundred base pairs; these domains generally have different melting temperatures. The melting temperature of a particular domain is the temperature at which the two DNA strands begin to denature, an event that in turn retards the electrophoretic mobility of the DNA duplex. For DGGE, this occurs at the point where the concentration of the denaturant (generally a combination of formamide and urea) is such that the DNA strands in a part of the double-stranded molecule begin to disassociate. The denaturing temperature is determined by the sequence of the DNA fragment. If a nucleotide substitution has occurred in the DNA fragment, the melting temperature of that region changes, altering the motility of the fragment compared to that of a normal DNA fragment. This difference will allow one to discriminate between the mutant sequence and the normal sequence.

One limitation of DGGE and TGGE techniques is that they will detect sequence changes only in the lowest-melting domain of the DNA duplex. Therefore a GC-rich region, or GC clamp, is attached to the PCR fragments when they are generated for screening [52,53]. This procedure allows an increase in the proportion of a fragment that can be screened by DGGE or TGGE. The DNA fragments that can be examined are in the range of 25–500 nucleotides [54].

Two other modifications of DGGE and TGGE have been described; these include the formation of heteroduplexes between mutant and wild-type fragments [55], and enzymatic digestion of the DNA fragment [56]. Since the DNA fragments to be screened are usually generated by PCR, heteroduplexes tend to form during the cycles of denaturation and reannealing. These heteroduplexes are less stable than either of the two homoduplexes that can form; therefore those molecules will generally melt before the homoduplexes. Restriction digestion of the DNA can remove the lowest-melting domain and allow the higher-melting domains to be scanned.

For DNA sequence alterations to be identified, the denaturing or temperature conditions that will enable optimal detection of sequence differences must first be determined. This can be accomplished in either of two ways: by empirically predicting the fragment behavior and varying gradient conditions and run times accordingly; or by invoking a computational mathematical model of the DGGE or TGGE system. For the DGGE system, such models have been worked out by Lerman and Silverstein (1987), who have described three series of computer algorithms that predict the behavior of a DNA fragment under DGGE conditions based on its nucleotide sequence [57]. These programs (MELT 87, MUTRAV, and/or SQHTX) allow one to predict "melt maps" of mutant and normal DNA domains, to select appropriate ranges of denaturant concentration, to set the electrophoresis time for the run, to estimate the number and size of the various melting domains, and to predict whether a particular sequence alteration will be visible under the conditions chosen. Otherwise, DGGE is used to determine the melting behavior of a fragment by using a gradient of denaturants perpendicular to the direction of electrophoresis; in this way one can predict the denaturant concentration at which a shift in electrophoretic mobility will occur. Then, a gel is run for varying lengths of time to establish the time required to electrophorese the fragment into the correct denaturant concentration. A parallel gel contains the appropriate small range of denaturant.

A review of the use of DGGE published by Fodde and Losekoot (1994) includes a list of 26 genes in which DGGE has been used successfully to identify mutations [58]. The advantages of DGGE (and most likely TGGE, although this technique is used less often than DGGE) are (1) sequence alterations are detected frequently, especially if the analysis is optimized by computer simulation; (2) no reagents are radioactive; and (3) the differently migrating band is easily excised from the gel. Obviously, its disadvantages are the need for a detailed computer simulation or for multiple gel runs to determine conditions, the limitation on the size of the fragment that can be analyzed, and the cost of the GC clamp that must be attached to one member of each PCR primer pair to generate DNA fragments for study.

Chemical cleavage and heteroduplex analysis can also detect mutations in potential disease genes. However, each of these techniques is laborious and not extremely sensitive.

C. The Protein Truncation Test

Many disease genes have been shown to be inactivated by chain-terminating mutations almost exclusively. If this is the case, one can use what is known as the protein truncation test or PTT to screen additional patients. When the majority of mutations (or even a significant number) in a gene lead to truncated protein in vivo, an in vitro synthesized-protein assay can detect the production of truncated proteins from RNA isolated from patients. If the gene contains an exon of sufficient size, genomic DNA can also be used. Generally, however, this assay requires RNA isolation, reverse transcription-PCR of that RNA to make cDNA, and a coupled in vitro transcription and translation step followed by gel electrophoresis and autoradiography to identify aberrant proteins and hence mutant alleles of a gene. This relatively simple technique carries a high degree of success in mutation detection, and it allows one to screen larger segments of a gene (2 kb) than any of the other methods described. In a recent study of mutations in the *APC* gene, a human tumor suppressor in which germline mutations lead to an inherited colon cancer syndrome, the PTT detected 82% of the mutations present among 51 unrelated patients [59]. This technique has also played an important role in the detection of mutations in other very large disease genes such as *NF1*, whose mutant alleles cause neurofibromatosis type 1. Both *APC* and *NF1* have open reading frames of more than 8500 base pairs, and known mutations are scattered throughout each of these genes. Therefore, the ability to scan a large gene in five overlapping segments permits investigators to search rapidly for the mutation in any single individual.

D. Direct Sequencing of Candidate Genes in Affected Individuals

As mentioned earlier, direct sequencing of the clones that contribute to the physical map of a genomic region can identify exons of candidate genes. Direct sequencing can then be invaluable in assessing the sequences of these candidate genes in affected individuals. Rather than relying on scanning techniques that may fail to detect all sequence alterations in affected individuals, the investigator can choose manual or automated sequencing of the entire open reading frame of a gene in each affected individual. This option is guaranteed to detect any and all sequence variations, whether polymorphisms or mutations. Once sequence alterations are detected, it becomes much easier to develop rapid screening protocols to identify those particular sequence changes with simple PCR-based assays. The sensitivity of direct sequencing also is an important consideration in the provision of clinical or diagnostic testing services, as well as for the timely identification of human disease genes.

Automated sequencers can reliably read sequence from an average of 400 base pairs to more than 900 base pairs per reaction, depending on the enzymology of the reaction, the electrophoresis run time, and the software of the machine that collects the data. For an Applied Biosystems Inc. sequencer, 36 lanes of sequence can be electrophoresed twice a day; at an average of 400 base pairs of sequence per lane, the number of base pairs that can be evaluated per day is, optimistically, 25,000 base pairs per machine. Sequence can then be rapidly evaluated with software that compares the sequences obtained from unaffected and affected individuals.

Both automated and manual sequencing technologies have the ability to detect heterozygosity at any position in the sequence studied. For the automated facility, computer analysis with specially designed software packages is required to call the heterozygous base pair. These packages also can display the sequences of each allele independently. With the improvements in automated sequencing technology that will undoubtably come from the Genome Project, this approach to evaluation of candidate genes is expected to replace all others mentioned above.

E. Newer Strategies to Detect Mutation

All conventional methods of mutation screening, such as SSCP, DGGE, TGGE, or RNase protection assays, are labor-intensive, gel-based assays that normally are reliable for DNA segments no longer than about 400 nucleotides. The PTT, which allows screening of at least 2 kb at one time, involves the use of radioisotopes and gel electrophoresis. Direct sequencing may not be an option for many smaller laboratories. Methods that are not gel-based, such as allele-specific PCR and the oligo-ligation assay, are directed toward the diagnosis of carriers of known mutations and are not applicable when the specific mutation is unknown.

A functional screen for nonsense and frame-shift mutations has been devised that allows genes to be scanned in large segments [60]. This assay is based on the cloning of these segments in-frame with a colorimetric marker gene (*lacZ*) followed by screening for the level of functional activity from the marker polypeptide (beta-galactosidase). In this way candidate genes can be screened quickly for chain-terminating mutations introduced by stops and frameshifts.

This "blue/white" assay is composed of four steps: (1) PCR amplification of a sequence from genomic DNA or cDNA; (2) cloning of PCR products into a plasmid, upstream, and in-frame, with a beta-galactosidase coding sequence; (3) transformation of bacteria; and (4) plating onto X-gal (5-bromo-4-chloro-3-indolyl β-D-galactopyranoside) medium and differential counting of blue, light blue, and white colonies to indicate the presence or absence of a chain-terminating mutation in the insert. An intense blue colony is produced from in-frame cloning and maintenance of the reading frame in DNA containing a normal sequence; the color results from the production of high levels of functional beta-galactosidase fusion protein. White colonies are produced when plasmids do not carry a cloned DNA insert, and almost no beta-galactosidase is produced. In-frame cloning of an insert that contains a frame shift or a premature stop codon, however, produces a colony of intermediate blue color whose intensity varies with the specific mutation. This result may be due to reinitiation at downstream, in-frame ATGs in the cloned segment or to read-through of the particular stop codon present, and/or may be related to factors specific to the plasmid and bacterial strains used in the assay [60].

Another recently published technique for mutation detection uses the segregation of a disease allele-carrying chromosome from the normal chromosome by the generation of somatic-cell hybrids. Monoallelic mutation analysis (MAMA) allows the unmasking of the disease allele by removing the background of the normal allele [61]. Although this technique requires a significant time period in which to generate the hybrids, separation of the mutant allele can facilitate its identification by either DNA-based techniques or by western blotting.

A review of a recent meeting in Gotland, Sweden (May 18–21, 1995), also describes many of the newer modifications and technologies that can be applied to mutation detection [62].

VI. Summary

The process of identifying disease genes is heavily reliant on constantly evolving technologies of molecular biology and computer science. The impact of the Human Genome Project and separate genome projects for less complex genomes, of research by biotechnology companies, and of the vast power of the Internet or "information superhighway" cannot be underestimated in its importance to the molecular geneticist who is interested in identifying and characterizing disease genes. The techniques in use today will soon be replaced by faster, cheaper, and more reliable techniques. With improvements in the content of databases and their availability to all members of the scientific community, finding genes that cause disease may someday become a trivial exercise. In the meantime, using any and all technology available, we hope to find genes and proteins that contribute to numerous disease processes and to study them further, in the interest of improving medical options for presymptomatic genetic testing, disease diagnostics, and treatment.

Acknowledgments

We greatly appreciate Dr. Briana Williams' contribution of the figure showing fluorescent in-situ hybridization. We are also indebted to Ruth Foltz for editing the manuscript.

References

1. Collins FS. Positional cloning moves from perditional to traditional. Nat Genet 1995; 9:347–350.
2. Morton, NE. Parameters of the human genome. Proc Natl Acad Sci USA 1991; 88: 7474–7476.
3. Liang P, Pardee AB. Parameters of the human genome. Science 1992; 257:967–971.
4. Botstein D, White RL, Skolnick M, Davis RW. Construction of a genetic linkage map

in man using restriction fragment length polymorphisms. Am J Hum Genet 1980; 32: 314–331.

5. Nakamura Y, Leppert M, O'Connell P, et al. Variable number of tandem repeat (VNTR) markers for human gene mapping. Science 1987; 235:1616–1622.

6. Weber JL, May PE. Abundant class of human DNA polymorphins which can be typed using the polymerase chain reaction. Am J Hum Genet 1989; 44:388–396.

7. Viskochil D, Buchberg AM, Xu G, et al. Deletions and a translocation interrupt a cloned gene at the neurofibromatosis type 1 locus. Cell 1990; 62:187–192.

8. Verkerk AJMH, Pieretti M, Sutcliffe JS, et al. Identification of a gene (FMR-1) containing a CGG repeat coincident with a breakpoint cluster region exhibiting length variation in fragile X syndrome. Cell 1995; 65:905–914.

9. Kunkel LM. Analysis of deletions in DNA from patients with Becker and Duchenne muscular dystrophy. Nature 1986; 322:73–77.

10. Schwartz DC, Cantor CR. Separation of yeast chromosome-sized DNAs by pulsed field gradient gel electrophoresis. Cell 1984; 37:67–75.

11. Carle GF, Frank M, Olson MV. Electrophoretic separations of large DNA molecules by periodic inversion of the electric field. Science 1986; 232:65–68.

12. Cavenee WK, Dryja TP, Phillips RA, et al. Expression of recessive alleles by chromosomal mechanisms in retinoblastoma. Nature 1983; 305:779–784.

13. Albertsen HM, Smith SA, Mazoyer S, et al. A physical map and candidate genes in the BRCA1 region on chromosome 17q12-21. Nat Genet 1994; 7:472–479.

14. Burke DT, Carle GF, Olson MV. Cloning of large segments of exogenous DNA into yeast by means of artificial chromosome vectors. Science 1987; 236:806–812.

15. Albertson HM, Abderrahim H, Cann HM, Dausset J, le Paslier D, Cohen D. Construction and characterization of a yeast artificial chromosome library containing seven haploid human genome equivalents. Proc Natl Acad Sci USA 1990; 87:4256–4260.

16. Anand R, Riley JH, Smith JC, Markham, AF. A 3.5 genome equivalent multi access YAC library: construction, characterisation, screening and storage. Nucleic Acids Res 1990; 18:1951–1955.

17. Brownstein BH, Silverman GA, Little RD, et al. Isolation of single-copy human genes from a library of yeast artificial chromosome clones. Science 1989; 244:1348–1351.

18. Garza D, Ajioka JW, Burke DT, Hartl DL. Mapping the *Drosophila* genome with yeast artificial chromosomes. Science 1989; 246:641–646.

19. Pierce JC, Sauer B, Sternberg N. A positive selection vector for cloning high molecular weight DNA by the bacteriophage P1 system: improved cloning efficacy. Proc Natl Acad Sci USA 1992; 89:2056–2060.

20. Pierce JC, Sternberg NL. Using bacteriophage P1 system to clone high molecular weight genomic DNA. Meth Enzymol 1992; 216:549–574.

21. Sternberg N. The P1 cloning system: past and future. Mamm Genome 1994; 5: 397–404.

22. Sternberg N, Smoller D, Braden T. Three new developments in P1 cloning. Increased cloning efficiency, improved clone recovery, and a new P1 mouse library. Genet Anal Tech Appl 1994; 11:171–180.

23. Ioannou PA, Amemiya CT, Garnes J, et al. A new bacteriophage P1-derived vector for the propagation of large human DNA fragments. Nat Genet 1994; 6:84–89.

24. Shizuya H, Birren B, Kim U-J, et al. Cloning and stable maintenance of 300-kilobase-pair fragments of human DNA in *Escherichia coli* using an F-factor-based vector. Proc Natl Acad Sci USA 1992; 89:8794–8797.

25. Green ED, Olson MV. Systemic screening of yeast artificial-chromosome libraries by use of the polymerase chain reaction. Proc Natl Acad Sci USA 1990; 87:1213–1217.

26. Arratia R, Lander ES, Tavare S, Waterman MS. Genomic mapping by anchoring random clones: a mathematical analysis. Genomics 1991; 11:806–827.

27. Barillot E, Lacroix B, Cohen D. Theoretical analysis of library screening using a N-dimensional pooling strategy. Nucleic Acids Res 1991; 19:6241–6247.

28. Ewens WJ, Bell CJ, Donnelly PJ, Dunn P, Matallana E, Ecker JR. Genome mapping with anchored clones: theoretical aspects. Genomics 1991; 11:799–805.

29. Palazzolo MJ, Sawyer SA, Maartin CH, Smoller DA, Hartl DL. Optimized strategies for sequence-tagged-site selection in genome mapping. Proc Natl Acad Sci USA 1991; 88:8034–8038.

30. Ochman H, Gerler AS, Hartl DL. Genetic applications of an inverse polymerase chain reaction. Genetics 1988; 120:621–623.

31. Groden J, Thliveris A, Samowitz W, et al. Identification and characterization of the familial adenomatous polyposis coli gene. Cell 1991; 66:589–600.

32. Nelson DL, Ledbetter SA, Corbo L, et al. Alu polymerase chain reaction: a method for rapid isolation of human-specific sequences from complex DNA sources. Proc Natl Acad Sci USA 1989; 86:6686–6690.

33. Breukel C, Wijnen J, Tops C, Klift H v/d., Dauwerse H, Meera Khan P. Vector-Alu PCR: a rapid step in mapping cosmids and YACs. Nucleic Acids Res 1990; 18:3097.

34. Riley J, Butler R, Ogilvie G, et al. Isolation of cDNA clones using yeast artificial chromosome probes. Nucleic Acids Res 1990; 18:2887–2890.

35. Coulson A, Waterson R, Kiff J, Sulston J, Kohara Y. Genome linking with yeast artificial chromosomes. Nature 1988; 335:184–186.

36. Parimoo S, Patanjali SR, Shukla H, Chaplin DD, Weissman SM. cDNA selection: efficient PCR approach for the selection of cDNAs encoded in large chromosomal DNA fragments. Proc Natl Acad Sci USA 1991; 88:9623–9627.

37. Lovett M, Kere J, Hinton LM. Direct selection: a method for the isolation of cDNAs encoded by large genomic regions. Proc Natl Acad Sci USA 1991; 88:9628–9632.

38. Buckler AJ, Chang DD, Graw SL, et al. Exon amplification: a strategy to isolate mammalian genes based on RNA splicing. Proc Natl Acad Sci USA 1991; 88:4005–4009.

39. Church DM, Stotler CJ, Rutter JL, Murrell JR, Trofatter JA, Buckler AJ. Isolation of genes from complex sources of mammalian genomic DNA using exon amplification. Nat Genet 1994; 6:98–105.

40. Strathdee CA, Gavish H, Shannon WR, Buchwald M. Cloning of cDNAs for Fanconi's anemia by functional complementation. Nature 1992; 356:763–767.

41. Henning KA, Li L, Iyer N, et al. The Cockayne syndrome group A gene encodes a WD repeat protein that interacts with CSB protein and a subunit of RNA polymerase II TFIIH. Cell 1995; 82:555–564.

42. Smith HO, Tomb JF, Dougherty BA, Fleishmann RD, Venter JC. Frequency and distribution of DNA uptake signal sequences in the *Haemophilus influenzae* Rd genome. Science 1995; 269:496–512.

43. Joslyn G, Carlson M, Thliveris A, et al. Identification of deletion mutations and three new genes at the familial polyposis locus.Cell 1991; 66:601–613.

44. Winter E, Yamamoto F, Almoguera C, Perucho M. A method to detect and characterize point mutations in transcribed genes: amplification and overexpression of the mutant c-Ki-ras allele in human tumor cells. Proc Natl Acad Sci USA 1985; 82:7575–7579.

45. Miyoshi Y, Ando H, Nagase H, et al. Germ-line mutations of the APC gene in 53 familial adenomatous polyposis patients. Proc Natl Acad Sci USA 1992; 89:4452–4456.

46. Orita M, Suzuki Y, Sekiya T, Hayashi K. Rapid and sensitive detection of point mutations and DNA polymorphisms using the polymerase chain reaction. Genomics 1989; 5:874–879.

47. Orita M, Iwahana H, Kanazawa H, Hayashi K, Sekiya T. Detection of polymorphisms of human DNA by gel electrophoresis as single-strand conformation polymorphisms. Proc Natl Acad Sci USA 1989; 86:2766–2770.

48. Liu Q, Sommer SS. Restriction endonuclease fingerprinting (REF): a sensitive method for screening mutations in long, contiguous segments of DNA. Biotechniques 1995; 18:470–477.

49. Savitsky K, Bar-Shira A, Gilad S, et al. A single ataxia telangiectasia gene with a product similar to PI-3 kinase. Science 1995; 268:1749–1753.

50. Fisher SG, Lerman LS. Separation of random fragments of DNA according to properties of their sequences. Proc Natl Acad Sci USA 1980; 77:4420–4424.

51. Fischer SG, Lerman LS. DNA fragments differing by single base-pair substitutions are separated in denaturing gradient gels: correspondence with melting theory. Proc Natl Acad Sci USA 1983; 80:1579–1583.

52. Myers RM, Fischer SG, Lerman LS, Maniatis T. Nearly all single base substitutions in DNA fragments joined to a GC-clamp can be detected by denaturing gradient gel electrophoresis. Nucleic Acids Res 1985; 13:3131–3145.

53. Sheffield VC, Cox DR, Lerman LS, Myers RM. Attachment of a 40-base-pair G + C-rich sequence (GC-clamp) to genomic DNA fragments by the polymerase chain reaction results in improved detection of single-base change. Proc Natl Acad Sci USA 1989; 86:232–236.

54. Myers RM, Fischer SG, Maniatis T, Lerman LS. Modification of the melting properties of duplex DNA by attachment of a GC-rich DNA sequence as determined by denaturing gradient gel electrophoresis. Nucleic Acids Res 1985; 13:3111–3129.

55. Myers RM, Lumelsky N, Lerman LS, Maniatis T. Detection of single base substitutions in total genomic DNA. Nature 1985; 313:495–498.

56. Gray MR. Detection of DNA sequence polymorphisms in human genomic DNA by using denaturing gradient gel blots. Am J Hum Genet 1992; 50:331–346.

57. Lerman LS, Silverstein K. Computational simulation of DNA melting and its application to denaturing gradient gel electrophoresis. Meth Enzymol 1987; 155:482–501.

58. Fodde R, Losekoot M. Mutation detection by denaturing gradient gel electrophoresis (DGGE). Hum Mutat 1994; 3:83–94.

59. Powell SM, Petersen GM, Krush AJ, et al. Molecular diagnosis of familial adenomatous polyposis [see comments]. N Engl J Med 1993; 329:1982–1987.

60. Varesco L, Groden J, Spirio L, et al. A rapid screening method to detect nonsense and frameshift mutations: identification of disease-causing APC mutations. Cancer Res 1993; 53:5581–5584.

61. Papadopoulos N, Leach FS, Kinzler KW, Vogelstein B. Monoalleleic mutation analysis (MAMA) for identifying germline mutations. Nature Genet 1995; 11:99–102.

62. Forest S, Cotton R, Landegren U, Southern E. How to find all those mutations. Nat Genet 1995; 10:375–376.

14

Large-Scale Expressed DNA Sequencing for Elucidation of New Drug Targets and Mutations in Disease

CLAIRE M. FRASER

Institute for Genomic Research
Gaithersburg, Maryland

Work in our laboratory during the past two years has been focused on human gene discovery and understanding human gene diversity and expression. To this end, we have sequenced over 200,000 templates from more than 250 new cDNA libraries representing all major organs and tissues [1]. Single-pass, partial sequencing of randomly selected cDNA clones to generate expressed sequence tags (ESTs) has been demonstrated to be a rapid method for gene discovery [2], which has been widely applied in humans [2–11] and other species [12–15]. The EST strategy was developed to permit rapid identification of expressed genes by sequence analysis. The combination of data on gene expression and putative gene functions inferred from sequence similarity provides a powerful means of assessing the transcriptional activity of the genome in the cells and tissues of an organism. The EST approach has revealed that a significant number of transcripts in a cell or tissue are of unknown function [1–15], and thus represent potential new cellular markers and therapeutic targets. Prior to 1991 and the development of the EST method, fewer than 3000 human genes had been characterized by DNA sequence analysis (GenBank release 68, June 1991). The number of ESTs in the public EST database, dbEST [16], has recently exceeded 50,000; 45% of these are from human cDNA libraries and represent approximately 10,000 human genes [16].

A recent search of dbEST with 32 known human disease genes that had been cloned by either positional cloning or positional candidate methods revealed that 38% of these human disease gene sequences had exact matches in dbEST, and another 47% were represented by homologs in other organisms [16]. This finding underscores the utility of EST analysis in human gene discovery and suggests that the EST database is already likely to contain sequences for many other human disease genes. As an example, EST analysis has recently been used as a method for discovering thee new genes implicated in familial colon cancer [17,18] and one gene implicated in familial breast cancer [19], demonstrating the utility of this approach in disease gene identification.

As an extension of the EST method as originally described, comparative EST analysis has recently proven to be a means of surveying global changes in gene expression patterns in response to various biological signals [20]. Application of the comparative EST approach holds tremendous promise for elucidating the qualitative and quantitative alterations in gene expression that are responsible for and associated with physiological and pathological processes such as differentiation, development, homeostasis, cell cycle regulation, apoptosis, cancer progression, and drug treatment. With regard to asthma, the EST strategy is likely to be important in uncovering potential new therapeutic targets, understanding the pathophysiology of the disease, and comparing changes in gene expression in asthma of distinct etiologies.

I. Large-Scale cDNA Sequencing

A. cDNA Library Construction

For an EST project, a cDNA library should be: (1) representative, containing all sequences present in the initial polyA$^+$ RNA population in the same relative frequencies; (2) unidirectionally cloned so that the orientation of each cDNA is known, facilitating subsequent sequence analysis; (3) composed of a high proportion of long or full-length inserts; (4) uncontaminated with genomic, mitochondrial, or rRNA inserts; and (5) composed of a large proportion of inserts with short poly A tails (see Ref. 21 for a review of methodology).

Sequencing of a small number (100–200) of clones has proven to be an excellent way of assessing library quality in terms of gene content and determining problems that may have arisen during library construction. Libraries that are well suited for large-scale EST analysis based on quality control analysis typically exhibit less than 50% exact matches to known human genes, a broad diversity of transcripts (no single gene or genes dominating the distribution), a low percentage of clones with no inserts, mitochondrial transcripts and/or ribosomal RNA species, and no evidence of contamination with another organism. In the case of cDNA libraries with one or more highly abundant transcripts, individual abundant cDNAs can be radiolabeled and used as probes to screen gridded array of clones for the library and nonhybridizing clones selected for sequencing.

The 5' end of each cDNA clone is more likely to contain protein coding sequence than the 3' end, which increases the likelihood that database searches will result in the assignment of putative identification. To further increase the chance that a database match will be significant, it is of benefit if the read length of each DNA template is as long as possible. However, sequence accuracy should not be compromised in order to obtain a longer read length, because accuracy is of paramount importance in evaluating the results from database searching. For example, a database match of 90% identity at the DNA level may represent a new member of a gene family and may be given such putative identification with confidence if EST sequence accuracy is high ($\geq$97%). In contrast, if sequence accuracy is low (<95%), it may be difficult, if not impossible, to distinguish an exact match to a sequence in a public database from a novel sequence.

B. Data Analysis

EST sequences are searched against all nucleotide sequences in GenBank using software for sequence similarity searching such as **graze**, a modification of the Smith-Waterman algorithm [22], which produces an optimal gapped alignment between two similar sequences. Peptide searches are performed with all six possible translations of ESTs against sequences from GenPept, PIR, and Swiss-Prot. Based on our experience, database matches that represent new members of gene families may be significant only at the peptide level and not at the nucleotide level.

Because mRNA species are present at different concentrations in cells and these differences are reflected in the composition of cDNA libraries, random sampling of cDNA libraries results in abundant mRNAs being represented by many ESTs. This redundancy can be used to build longer, contiguous blocks of sequence by assembly of overlapping ESTs. Assembly of ESTs into consensus sequences aids in the assignment of putative gene identifications because the consensus sequences are generally longer than any single ESTs, and facilitate the identification of distinct transcripts that differ only in splicing patterns.

Analysis of more than 250 cDNA libraries, sampled at levels ranging from 100 to several thousand cDNA clones per library, has allowed us to assess the ability of the EST method to identify abundant (several thousand copies per cell), moderately abundant (several hundred copies per cell), and rare (5–25 copies per cell) mRNA species [1]. In the case of cDNA libraries that do not contain one or a few highly abundant transcripts (i.e., the pituitary gland, which expresses growth hormone and prolactin at levels equivalent to a few percent of the total mRNA), DNA sequence analysis of 200–500 randomly selected cDNA clones usually uncovers most abundant mRNA species and a significant number of moderately abundant mRNAs. Additional sequencing to a total of 500–2000 cDNA clones identifies a much larger number of moderately abundant cDNA clones and a sampling of rare mRNA species. In order to identify a large number of rare mRNA species, it is necessary to increase the sampling size from a cDNA library to several thousand clones or to sample from a normalized cDNA library. While the failure to observe a transcript by cDNA sequencing does not prove a lack of gene expression in a particular tissue, the observation that it is expressed in many tissues or in a single tissue at a high level is informative.

Depending on the source of tissue from which a cDNA library was derived, between 40 and 50% of ESTs can be assigned a putative identification based on hits to either human or nonhuman sequences contained in public databases [1–15]. A similar number of ESTs have no clear database matches and thus are classified as unknowns [1–15]. Of particular interest within this category are abundant unknown genes, which may be broadly or narrowly expressed. With each cDNA library, between 5 and 20% of total ESTs analyzed represent mitochondrial or ribosomal sequences or known human repetitive elements. The number of EST sequences deposited in databases has increased exponentially during the past four years. As this dataset expands, our understanding of human gene expression will continue to increase.

II. Analysis of Gene Expression in Human Lung

Because asthma is primarily a disease of the airways, an understanding of the genes expressed in normal lung is an important starting point in elucidating changes in gene expression that may be associated with the pathophysiology of the disease. More than 11,000 ESTs from lung cDNA libraries were analyzed as part of our large-scale human cDNA sequencing effort [1]. Approximately 50% of the ESTs were assigned putative identifications based on matches to human and nonhuman sequences in public databases. The data presented in Table 1 represent a compilation of the putative identifications assigned to ESTs selected from several different human lung cDNA libraries. There is a wide range in the redundancy of gene expression in human lung, indicating that this strategy has identified a variety of abundant, moderately abundant, and rare mRNA species.

The most highly expressed genes in human lung represent "housekeeping" genes, such as ribosomal proteins, elongation factor-1, and Wilm's tumor-related protein, and tissue-specific genes such as pulmonary surfactant-associated proteins (lung) and globin (red blood cells) (Fig. 1). The finding that globins represent 2.6% of lung ESTs reflects the extensive blood supply to the lung, which is critical for facilitating gas exchange. The extracellular matrix is an important structural component of lung, reflected by the abundance of collagens (2.3%) and chondroitin sulfates (0.3%) and other proteoglycans. The abundance of tubulins (1.3%) likely derives from the fact that epithelial cells which lines the human respiratory tract are covered with cilia. The guanine nucleotide-binding protein subunit, $G_{s\alpha}$ (designated as guanine nucleotide-binding protein, G_s, alpha subunit, or adenylate cyclase stimulatory element, alpha), is also one of the more abundant proteins in human lung, representing 1.3% of all identified ESTs. It is far more abundant than any other G-protein alpha subunit; its abundance is not matched in a stoichiometric fashion by either the β or γ subunits of the G proteins. The functional significance of the high abundance of the $G_{s\alpha}$ subunit in lung is not known. Among the ESTs which matched nonhuman sequences are several receptors and GTP-binding proteins, indicating that these genes have not previously been characterized in humans (Table 1).

III. Comparative EST Sequencing as a Method for Evaluating Asthma-Related Changes in Gene Expression

Current methods of comparing gene expression profiles in different cell types, such as two-dimensional gel electrophoresis of cellular proteins [23] and differential screening of cDNA libraries [24–26], are limited in the amount of information they can provide. In contrast, comparative EST analysis allows for assessment of changes in the expression of hundreds of genes and thus serves an efficient means of obtaining steady-state mRNA profiles and identifying differentially regulated mRNAs in a variety of experimental systems [20].

The utility of comparative EST analysis is well illustrated by a recent study from Lee et al. [20] in which more than 600 differentially expressed mRNAs were identified in control and nerve growth factor (NGF)-treated PC12 cells. The line of rat adrenal chromaffin-like PC12 cells differentiates into sympathetic-like neurons in response to NGF. Cellular differentiation to a neuronal phenotype involves mitotic arrest and the appearance of electrical excitability, and has been shown to involve alterations in gene expression [27,28]. Two sets of EST data were generated that contained approximately 3700 ESTs each from control or NGF-treated cells. Many of the mRNAs were found equally in both libraries and represented "housekeeping" genes such as elongation factor 1-alpha, glyceraldehyde-3-phosphate dehydrogenase, and cyclophilin. Other mRNAs associated with cells of neuroendocrine origin were also found equally in both libraries, including the secretory proteins, secretogranin I and II, and the catecholamine synthesizing enzyme, tyrosine hydroxylase.

Of more interest were the more than 600 distinct mRNAs that appeared more than once in a cDNA library and were not equally distributed between the two matched cDNA libraries. Many differentially expressed mRNAs identified

Table 1 Continued

Identification from an exact match to a human DNA sequence	No. total matches	Identification from an exact match to a human DNA sequence	No. total matches
GTP-binding protein, Gs alpha subunit	1	*H. sapiens* hypothetical protein (GB:D21065)	1
GTP-binding protein, alpha subunit	1	*H. sapiens* hypothetical protein (GB:D21261)	3
GTP-binding protein, beta subunit	5	*H. sapiens* hypothetical protein (GB:D21262)	1
GTP-binding protein, ras-related	1	*H. sapiens* hypothetical protein (GB:D21853)	1
GTPase activating protein	3	*H. sapiens* hypothetical protein (GB:D25539)	2
GTPase-activating protein rap1	3		
Gamma-interferon-inducible protein, IP-30	3	*H. sapiens* hypothetical protein (GB:D26068)	2
Globin, beta	1	*H. sapiens* hypothetical protein A9A2BRB5 (GB:U009	2
Glutamine synthase	2		
Glutaminyl-tRNA synthetase	1		
Glutathione S-transferase (GST-Pi)	1	*H. sapiens* hypothetical protein CTG-B33 (GB:L10376	1
Glutathione S-transferase (mu-GST)	1		
Glutathione peroxidase	4	*H. sapiens* hypothetical protein, 49kDa (GP:L22009)	2
Glyceraldehyde 3-phosphate dehydrogenase	7		
Guanine nucleotide-binding protein G(S), alpha sub	7	*H. sapiens* hypothetical protein, liver (GB:L13799)	5
		H19	6
Guanine nucleotide-binding protein, beta subunit	2	HAP1 endonuclease	1
		HLA class I antigen	1
H. sapiens hypothetical protein (GB:D13630)	1	HLA class II histocompatibility antigen, gamma chain	2
H. sapiens hypothetical protein (GB:D13641)	1		
H. sapiens hypothetical protein (GB:D14665)	1	HLA-E heavy chain	1
H. sapiens hypothetical protein (GB:D14696	2	HS1 protein	1
		Heat shock cognate protein 70	1
H. sapiens hypothetical protein (GB:D14811)	1	Heat shock protein 90	2
H. sapiens hypothetical protein (GB:D17793)	1	Heparan sulfate proteaglycan	2
		Heparin cofactor II	1
H. sapiens hypothetical protein (GB:D21063)	1	Heparin-binding EGF-like growth factor	1
		High-mobility group 1 protein	1

Table 1 Continued

Identification from an exact match to a human DNA sequence	No. total matches	Identification from an exact match to a human DNA sequence	No. total matches
High-mobility group box (SSRP1)	2	M4 protein	1
		M6 antigen	3
Hox 1.3	1	MARCKS (myristoylated alanine-rich protein kinase	1
IEF 7442 (GB:X72841)	1		
IEF SSP 9306	2	MGC-24	2
IEF SSP 9306 (GB:X71810)	2	MHC class I	1
Ig heavy-chain V region	1	MHC class I HLA-B	1
Ig kappa chain	1	MHC complex enhancer-binding protein MAD-3	1
IgM heavy chain	1		
Inosine-5′-monophosphate dehydrogenase	2	Mannose 6-phosphate receptor	1
		Mannose receptor	1
Insulinlike growth factor binding protein 5	3	Metalloproteinase inhibitor (TIMP)	1
Intercellular adhesion molecule-2	1	Mitochondrial ADP/ATP translocator	1
Interferon alpha induced transcriptional activator	1	Mitochondrial phosphate carrier protein	1
Interferon-gamma	3	Moesin	1
Interferon-gamma receptor segment	1	Monocyte chemoattractant protein-1	1
Interferon-induced protein 1-8D	1	Myosin heavy chain, alpha	2
Interferon-induced protein 1-8U	3	Myosin heavy chain, smooth muscle	2
Interferon-inducible protein 9-27	1	Myosin light chain isoform MLC2a	3
Interleukin-2 receptor alpha chain kappa B-binding	1	Myosin light chain, alkali	2
		Myosin light chain, smooth muscle	1
KDEL receptor	1	Myotonic dystrophy kinase DMR19-N9	2
LLRep3	2		
Lamin A	1	N-ras (GB:X02751)	1
Laminin B1 chain	1	NK4 protein	2
Laminin B3 chain	1	Na$^+$/K$^+$-ATPase, alpha subunit	1
Laminin receptor	3		
Laminin receptor homolog	1	Nonerythroid band 3-like protein	1
Large fibroblast proteoglycan, versican	3	Nuclear factor IV	1
		Nucleolar phosphoprotein B23	7
Lon proteaselike protein	2	ORF	1
Lysyl hydroxylase	2		

(continued)

Table 1 Continued

Identification from an exact match to a human DNA sequence	No. total matches	Identification from an exact match to a human DNA sequence	No. total matches
Ornithine decarboxylase	1	Pulmonary surfactant-associated protein SP-C	1
Osteonectin/SPARC	2		
PCTAIRE-1 serine/threonine protein kinase	2	Pyruvate dehydrogenase beta subunit	1
Peptidylglycine alpha-amidating monooxygenase	1	Pyruvate kinase isozyme M2	1
		RAB protein, member RAS oncogene family	1
Peripheral myelin protein 22	3		
Phosphatase 2A	1	RING10	1
Phosphatidylserine synthase	1	RNA helicase	3
Phosphoglycerate kinase	2	RNA helicase p68	3
Phospholipase A2	1	RNA-binding protein AUF1	1
Phospholipase C-alpha	1	RSU-1/RSP-1	1
Plasma protease C1 inhibitor	1	Rab5	1
Platelet-derived growth factor (PDGF) receptor	1	Ras inhibitor	1
		Retinoic acid-binding protein II	1
Poly(ADP-ribose) polymerase	1		
Pr22 protein	2	Ribonucleoprotein A1	1
Proalpha 1 (I) procollagen chain	1	Ribosomal phosphoprotein P0	12
Profilin	1	Ribosomal phosphoprotein P1	2
Proliferation-associated gene	2		
Promotor-binding protein	1	Ribosomal phosphoprotein P2	1
Proteasome component C13	1		
Protein phosphatase 2A alpha subunit	1	Ribosomal protein L10e	1
		Ribosomal protein L12	1
Protein-serine kinase PSK-J3	1	Ribosomal protein L17	2
Proteolipid protein	1	Ribosomal protein L18a	11
Prothymosin alpha	1	Ribosomal protein L23	2
Protocadherin 43	1	Ribosomal protein L27	1
Pulmonary surfactant apoprotein (PSAP)	4	Ribosomal protein L3	8
		Ribosomal protein L32	1
Pulmonary surfactant proteolipid (SPL(pVal))	1	Ribosomal protein L37	1
		Ribosomal protein L6	2
Pulmonary surfactant-associated protein B	8	Ribosomal protein L7	5
		Ribosomal protein L7a	7
Pulmonary surfactant-associated protein C	13	Ribosomal protein RPS4Y	1
		Ribosomal protein S17	1
Pulmonary surfactant-associated protein SP-A (SFTP)	1	Ribosomal protein S18	8
		Ribosomal protein S19	2
		Ribosomal protein S26	3

Table 1 Continued

Identification from an exact match to a human DNA sequence	No. total matches	Identification from an exact match to a human DNA sequence	No. total matches
Ribosomal protein S28	1	Tax-responsive enhancer element-binding protein	2
Ribosomal protein S3	4	Tetracycline transporter-like protein	1
Ribosomal protein S4	1		
Ribosomal protein S4, X isoform	3	Tetranectin	1
Ribosomal protein S6	5	Thioredoxin	1
Ribosomal protein S8	1	Thromboxane synthase	1
Ribosomal protein s3	3	Thy-1 glycoprotein	1
S-100 protein, alpha chain	2	Thymosin beta-10	1
S-adenosylmethionine decarboxylase	1	Tissue specific protein GB:X67698	1
S-adenosylmethionine decarboxylase 2	3	Transcription factor BTF3	2
		Transcription factor GATA-3	1
S-laminin	1	Transglutaminase	2
SM22	1	Translationally controlled tumor protein	1
Selenoprotein P	2		
Signal-recognition particle 19-kDa subunit	1	Transplantation antigen P198	2
		Tristetraproline	1
Signal-recognition particle subunit 14	1	Tropomyosin TM1, muscle	1
		Tryptophanyl-tRNA synthetase	2
Signal-transducing protein, beta-subunit	1		
		Tubulin, alpha	3
Sphingolipid activator protein 1	2	Tumor protein, TCTP	1
		Tumor-associated antigen L6	1
Splicing factor, SF2p32	1	Tyrosine phosphatase, alpha	1
Squalene synthetase	2	U1 small nuclear ribonucleoprotein A	3
Stathmin (p18)	2		
Stromyelsin-3	1	U1 small nuclear ribonucleoprotein C	1
Subtilisin-like protein, PACE4	4		
		U1 snRNP A protein	1
Succinate-ubiquinone oxidoreductase iron sulfur	1	U1 snRNP C protein	1
		UNR-gene, upstream of ras	1
Superoxide dismutase (Mn)	2	Ubiquitin	2
T-Plastin	2	Ubiquitin carboxyl-terminal extension protein	1
T-cell surface glycoprotein E2	1		
		Ubiquitin-52 amino acid fusion protein	1
TAPA-1, 26-kDa cell surface protein	4		
		Urokinase plasminogen activator surface receptor	1
TEGT	4		

(continued)

Table 1 Continued

Identification from an exact match to a human DNA sequence	No. total matches	Identification from an exact match to a human DNA sequence	No. total matches
Vacuolar H$^+$ ATPase subunit E	1	Adenylyl cyclase inhibiting GTP-binding protein	1
Villin 2	1	Adenylyl cyclase stimulatory element, alpha S1	34
Vimentin	1		
Voltage-dependent anion channel isoform 2 (VDAC)	1	Alcohol dehydrogenase 2, class I, beta polypeptide	3
Wilm's tumor-related protein	38	Alcohol dehydrogenase 3, class I, gamma polypeptide	1
X (inactive)-specific transcript c	2		
X (inactive)-specific transcript d	2	Aldolase A	3
		Alpha-1-antitrypsin	2
XE169	2	Alpha-1-antitrypsin protease inhibitor 1	2
XE7	1		
XE7, pseudo-autosomal gene	2	Alpha-1-antitrypsin, 5′ end	1
XIST, X chromosome inactive segment a	4	Alpha-2-macroglobulin	6
		Alpha-2-macroglobulin	7
Acid phosphatase 2A, lysosomal	1	Alpha-L-fucosidase	2
		Alpha-N-acetylgalactosamindase	1
Actin, alpha 1, skeletal muscle	2		
		Amyloid A4 (GB:X06989)	2
Actin, alpha, cardiac	2	Amyloid beta (A4) precursor protein	8
Actin, alpha, skeletal muscle	2		
Actin, beta	25	Amyloid protein homolog	2
Actin, beta, cytoskeletal	19	Anion exchanger 2	1
Actin, gamma 1	14	Annexin II	4
Actin, gamma, cytoskeletal	1	Annexin XI, 56 kDa	1
Actin, gamma, smooth muscle, aorta	1	Antiproliferative protein BTG1	2
Adaptin, beta	2	Antigen MIC2	1
Adducin, alpha subunit	2	Apolipoprotein E	1
Adenine nucleotide translocator 1	1	Apurinic/apyrimidinic endonuclease	14
Adenosine receptor A2a	1	Arachidonate 5-lipoxygenase	1
Adenylate cyclase stimulatory element, alpha S1	11	Arginine-rich nuclear protein, 54 kDa	2
		Asialoglycoprotein receptor 2	1
Adenylate cyclase stimulatory element, alpha S2	12	Aspartate aminotransferase, cytosolic	1
		Aspartylglucosaminidase	4

Table 1 Continued

Identification from an exact match to a human DNA sequence	No. total matches	Identification from an exact match to a human DNA sequence	No. total matches
Autoimmune antigen Ku, p70/p80 subunit	1	Chondroitin sulfate proteoglycan core protein	8
Benzodiazepine receptor	2	Chondroitin/dermatan sulfate proteoglycan (PG40) c	8
Beta-galactoside-binding lectin	3	Clathrin, light polypeptide	2
Biglycan	9	Clathrin, light polypeptide a	1
Bone morphogenetic protein 2 (GB:M22490)	1	Clathrin, light polypeptide b	3
Breast basic conserved protein	2	Cofilin	2
		Collagen VII alpha-1	1
Breast basic conserved protein 1	3	Collagen, type 1, alpha 1	45
		Collagen, type I, alpha 2	10
c-syn Protooncogene	1	Collagen, type III, alpha 1	13
cAMP-dependent protein kinase alpha subunit type 1	1	Collagen, type IV, alpha 1	5
		Collagen, type IV, alpha 2	4
Calcium-activated neutral protease, small subunit	2	Collagen, type IV, alpha 2 (GB:X05610)	2
Calgranulin A	1	Collagen, type IV, alpha 5 (GB:M31115)	1
Calmodulin type III	1		
Calreticulin	2	Collagen, type IV, alpha 5 (GB:M58526)	1
Caltractin	1	Collagen, type VI, alpha 2	1
Carboxyl methyltransferase, isozyme II	2	Collagen, type VI, alpha 2 (GB:M34570)	1
Carboxypeptidase E	2	Collagen, type VI, alpha 2, C-terminal globular do	2
Cardiodilatin-atrial natriuretic factor	11	Collagen, type VI, alpha 3	19
Cardiodilatin-atrial natriuretic factor (CDD-ANF)	7	Collagen, type VII, alpha 1 (GB:S62616)	1
		Collagen, type XI, alpha 1	2
Catenin, alpha	1	Collagen, type XVI, alpha 1	1
Catenin, alpha 2(E)	4	Collagenase, type IVA	1
Cathepsin A	3	Colligin	2
Cathepsin B	3	Complement component 1, r subcomponent	1
Cathepsin S	4		
Caveolin, 22kDa	1	Cyclophilin	8
Cell cycle gene RCC1	1	Cyclophilin A	10
Cell surface antigen Thy-1	1	Cyclophilin-related processed pseudogene	2
Cell surface protein TAPA-1, 26 kDa	4		
		Cystatin C	1

(continued)

Table 1 Continued

Identification from an exact match to a human DNA sequence	No. total matches	Identification from an exact match to a human DNA sequence	No. total matches
Cytochrome b-245, beta polypeptide	1	Fibulin D	4
Cytochrome b-5	1	Flightless-I homolog	1
Cytochrome b5	1	Fructose-1,6-bisphosphatase	1
Cytochrome bc-1 complex core protein II	2	Gap junction protein connexin 40	1
Cytochrome-c oxidase, VIIc subunit	2	Globin, alpha	33
Decorin	20	Globin, alpha 1	22
Elastin	6	Globin, alpha 2	20
Elongation factor 1 alpha	6	Globin, beta	1
Endoglin	1	Globin, gamma	24
Endothelin receptor, type A	1	Globin, gamma A	23
Enolase, beta, muscle-specific	2	Globin, gamma G	1
Enoyl-coenzyme A hydratase, short chain, mitochond	1	Glucocerebrosidase	2
		Glutamate ammonia ligase	2
		Glutaminyl-tRNA synthetase	2
		Glutathione S-transferase pi	1
Epican	5	Glutathione S-transferase, mu class, brain and tes	1
Epoxide hydroxylase, microsomal	2	Glutathione peroxidase	1
Epoxide hydroxylase, microsomal (xenobiotic)	1	Gluthatione peroxidase (GB:D00632)	1
Erythrocyte membrane protein 7.2	4	Glutathione peroxidase (GB:M83094)	2
Farnesyl diphosphate synthase	1	Glutathione peroxidase GPx-3	4
Farnesyl pyrophosphate synthetase	1	Glutathione peroxidase, extracellular	7
Ferritin, heavy polypeptide	3	Glyceraldehyde 3-phosphate dehydrogenase	7
Ferritin, light chain	15	gro (growth regulated)	1
Ferritin, light polypeptide	15	Guanine nucleotide-binding protein G(S), alpha sub	12
Fibrillin	1	hAES-1 (GB:X73358)	1
Fibroblast growth factor receptor 3	1	Heat shock protein, 27/28 kDa	1
Fibroblast growth factor receptor 4	2	Heat shock protein, 70 kDa (GB:Y00371)	2
Fibromodulin	1	Heat shock protein, 90 dDa (GB:M16660)	1
Fibronectin 1	16	Heat shock protein, 90 kDa (GB:X15183)	1
Fibronectin, cellular	26		

Table 1 Continued

Identification from an exact match to a human DNA sequence	No. total matches	Identification from an exact match to a human DNA sequence	No. total matches
Heat shock transcription factor 1	1	histone H3.3	3
		hnRNP C protein	1
Heparan sulfate proteoglycan 1, cell surface-asoc	2	hnRNP C-like protein	2
		hnRNP C2 protein	1
Heparan sulfate proteoglycan 3	2	hnRNP L	1
		hnRNP core protein A1	2
Heparin cofactor II	1	hnRNP-E1	2
Heparin-binding EGF-like growth factor	1	Homeobox 1.3	1
		Hyaluronate receptor CD44, epithelial	4
Heterogenous nuclear protein M4	1	Immunoglobin kappa chain, V region	1
Heterogeneous nuclear ribonucleoprotein C-like protein	3	Immunoglobulin C(mu) and C(delta) heavy chain,	1
Heterogeneous nuclear ribonucleoprotein E1	2	Immunoglobulin heavy-chain gene, VDJC regions (GB	1
Heterogeneous nuclear ribonucleoprotein E2	1	Immunoglobulin kappa chain	1
Heterogeneous nuclear ribonucleoprotein G	2	Immunoglobulin kappa chain constant region	1
Heterogeneous nuclear ribonucleoprotein L	1	Immunoglobulin kappa chain, V region	1
Heterogeneous nuclear ribonucleoprotein U21.1	2	Immunoglobulin kappa light chain	2
Heterogeneous nuclear ribonucleoprotein core protein	3	Immunoglobulin kappa light chain, V region (GB:X067)	1
High-density lipoprotein binding protein	2	Immunoglobulin kappa light chain, C region	1
High-mobility group box protein	2	Immunoglobulin kappa light chain, V region	1
High-mobility group protein I, placenta	1	Immunoglobulin mu (GB:X17115)	1
Highly basic protein, 23 kDa	13	Immunoglobulin mu heavy chain (GB:X17115)	2
Histone H3, family 2	2	Immunoglobulin mu heavy chain V,D,J,C regions (GB:	1
Histone H3, family 2 (GB:M11353)	1	
Histone H3, family 2 (GB:M11354)	1	Immunoglobulin mu heavy chain, variable region	1

(continued)

Table 1   Continued

Identification from an exact match to a human DNA sequence	No. total matches	Identification from an exact match to a human DNA sequence	No. total matches
Inosine-5′-monophosphate dehydrogenase	2	Loricrin	1
Insulinlike growth factor 2	3	Lymphocyte-activation gene 2	2
Insulinlike growth factor II-associated protein	1	Lymphocyte-specific protein 1	2
Insulinlike growth factor binding protein 5	3	Lysyl hydroxylase	5
Integrin, beta 1	2	Major histocompatibility complex (class II)-encode	1
Intercellular adhesion molecule 2	1	Major histocompatibility complex enhancer-binding	1
Interferon gamma-induced protein IEF SSP 5111	3	Major histocompatiblity complex, B homolog	8
Interferon, gamma receptor (GB:A09781)	2	Major histocompatibility complex, Bw62.3	1
Interferon, gamma transducer 1	3	Major histocompatibility complex, E	1
Interferon-induced protein 1-8D	2	Major histocompatibility complex, class I antigen	1
Interferon-induced protein 1-8U	4	Major histocompatibility complex, class I, A (GB:M	14
Interferon-inducible protein 9-27	1	Major histocompatibility complex, class I, A (GB:M	2
Interleukin-2 receptor alpha chain kappa B-binding	1	Major histocopmatibility complex, class I, A (GB:M	1
Interleukin-2 receptor, alpha chain, kappa B bindi	2	Major histocompatiblity complex, class I, A (GB:M	1
Lamin A/C	2	Major histocompatibility complex, class I, B (GB:M	8
Lamin A/C (GB:L12399)	1		
Lamin B receptor	1	Major histocompatiblity complex, class I, B35	1
Laminin receptor 1	8		
Laminin, B1	1	Major histocompatibility complex, class I, C (GB:M	1
Laminin, B2 chain	1		
Laminin, B2 polypeptide	1		
Laminin, S polypeptide	2		
Laminin-binding protein	1		
Large fibroblast proteoglycan	3		
Large ribosomal subunit L7a	7		
Lectin, 14 kDa	3	Major histocompatibility complex, class I, C (GB:M	1
Leukocyte antigen-related protein	2		

Table 1 Continued

Identification from an exact match to a human DNA sequence	No. total matches	Identification from an exact match to a human DNA sequence	No. total matches
Major histocompatibility complex, class I, E (GB:M	2	Myosin, light polypeptide, alkali	2
Major histocompatibility complex, class II, DR, in	26	Myosin, light polypeptide, alkali, non-muscle	1
Major histocompatibility complex, class I, HLA-B27	1	Myosin, smooth muscle	4
Man9-mannosidase	2	Natural killer cell protein, transcript 4	2
Mannose 6-phosphate receptor	1	Nonhistone chromosomal protein HMG-17	4
Mannose receptor	3	Nucleolar phosphoprotein B23	11
Mannose-6-phosphate receptor, cation dependent	6	Nucleophosmin-anaplastic lymphoma kinase fusion protein	5
Mannosidase Man9	2		
Melanoma growth stimulatory activity protein	1	Ornithine decarboxylase 1	1
		Osteoinductive factor	1
Metallopanstimulin 1	3	Osteonectin/SPARC	5
Metalloproteinase stromelysin 3	2	Oxoglutarate dehydrogenase	2
		p53 Cellular tumor antigen	1
Moesin	1	Paired basic amino acid cleaving enzyme	1
Myelin proteolipid protein	3		
Myosin light chain 2	4	Parathyroid hormone receptor	1
Myosin regulatory light chain	1		
		Peptidylglycine alpha-amidating monooxygenase	1
Myosin, heavy polypeptide 6, cardiac muscle, alpha	1	Periodic tryptophan protein isolog, 56 kDa	1
Myosin, heavy polypeptide 9, nonmuscle	2	Peripheral myelin protein 22	3
Myosin, heavy polypeptide, nonmuscle, alpha	1	Phosphate carrier protein, mitochondrial	1
Myosin, light chain 2, 20 kDa	4	Phosphatidylserine synthase	1
		Phosphoglycerate kinase	4
Myosin, light polypeptide 1, slow	1	Phosphoglycerate kinase 1	2
Myosin, light polypeptide 2, regulatory	1	Phospholipase A2 (GB:M86400)	1
		Phospholipase C, alpha	1
Myosin, light polypeptide 2, regulatory, atrial	3	Platelet-derived growth factor receptor, beta poly	2
Myosin, light polypeptide 3, alkali; ventricular,	1	Poly(ADP-ribose) synthetase	1
		Polyadenylate-binding protein	2

(continued)

Table 1 Continued

Identification from an exact match to a human DNA sequence	No. total matches	Identification from an exact match to a human DNA sequence	No. total matches
Polyadenylate-binding protein (GB:Y00345)	2	Proto-oncogene src-like kinase	2
Polymeric immunoglobulin receptor	2	Proto-oncogene trk	1
Porin	1	Protocadherin 43	2
Pre-mRNA splicing factor SF2p32	1	Pseudo-autosomal gene XE7	1
pre-mRNA splicing factor SRp20	4	Pulmonary surfactant apoprotein (GB:M30838)	10
Profilin 1	1	Pulmonary surfactant-associated protein B	39
Proliferation-associated gene	2	Pulmonary surfactant-associated protein C	15
Proline-rich protein	1	Pulmonary surfactant-associated protein SP-A	14
Prosaposin	2		
Protease inhibitor C1	1	Pulmonary surfactant-associated protein SP-B	12
Proteasome LMP7	1		
Proteasome, C13 component	4	Putative cytokine HC21	2
Protective protein	3	Pyruvate dehydrogenase, E1 beta polypeptide	1
Protein 59	2		
Protein kinase C inhibitor	1	Pyruvate kinase, M1 type and M2 type	1
Protein kinase C substrate, heavy chain	2		
Protein kinase, cAMP-dependent, regulatory, type I	1	raf Oncogene	4
		Rapamycin-binding protein FKBP25	1
Protein kinase, calcium/calmodulin-dependent	1	ras Inhibitor INX	1
		ras-like Protein TC4	1
Protein phosphatase 2A, alpha catalytic subunit	2	ras-Related G protein Rab1A	1
		Replication protein P1-Cdc46	3
Protein phsophatase 2A, alpha, 55 kDa	1	ret Transforming gene	3
		Retinoblastoma susceptibility protein	2
Proteoglycan 1, secretory granule	1		
		Retinol-binding protein 2, cellular	1
Prothymosin, alpha	9		
Proto-oncogene aml-1	1	rfp Transforming protein	2
Proto-oncogene c-syn	1	rfp Transforming protein (ret finger protein)	2
Proto-oncogene pim-1	2		
Proto-oncogene raf	4	rho C	1
Proto-oncogene rhoA, multidrug resistance protein	4	rhoh12	1
		Ribonuclease A, pancreatic	5
		Ribonuclease, pancreatic	4

Table 1 Continued

Identification from an exact match to a human DNA sequence	No. total matches	Identification from an exact match to a human DNA sequence	No. total matches
Ribosomal S30/ubiquitinlike fusion protein	7	Ribosomal protein L6	5
		Ribosomal protein L7	33
Ribosomal phosphoprotein P0, acidic	15	Ribosomal protein L8	2
		Ribosomal protein S10	2
Ribosomal phosphoprotein P1	2	Ribosomal protein S11	6
		Ribosomal protein S12	2
Ribosomal phosphoprotein P2	1	Ribosomal protein S13	9
		Ribosomal protein S14	12
Ribosomal protein	1	Ribosomal protein S16	4
Ribosomal protein L1 homolog	6	Ribosomal protein S17	1
		Ribosomal protein S18	22
Ribosomal protein L11	4	Ribosomal protein S19	2
Ribosomal protein L11 homolog	2	Ribosomal protein S2	2
		Ribosomal protein S20	6
Ribosomal protein L12	1	Ribosomal proein S21	7
Ribosomal protein L17	2	Ribosomal protein S24	7
Ribosomal protein L18	2	Ribosomal protein S24 homolog	2
Ribosomal protein L18a	11		
Ribosomal protein L19	8	Ribosomal protein S26	3
Ribosomal protein L23	2	Ribosomal protein S3	7
Ribosomal protein L27	3	Ribosomal protein S3a	1
Ribosomal protein L28	2	Ribosomal protein S4, X-linked	3
Ribosomal protein L28 homolog	4		
Ribosomal protein L3	8	Ribosomal protein S4, Y-linked	2
Ribosomal protein L3, isoform 1	3	Ribosomal protein S6	7
		Ribosomal protein S7	6
Ribosomal protein L3, isoform 2	14	Ribosomal protein S8	1
		Ribosomal protein YL41	10
Ribosomal protein L30	9	Secreted protein, acidic, cysteine-rich	7
Ribosomal protein L30 homolog	8		
		Selenoprotein P	4
Ribosomal protein L32	3	Serglycin	1
Ribosomal protein L35a	2	Serine kinase PSK-J3	1
Ribosomal protein L37	3	Serine/threonine kinase ERK1	1
Ribosomal protein L37a	2	Serine/threonine kinase PCTAIRE-1	2
Ribosomal protein L38	4		
Ribosomal protein L4	5	Signal-recognition particle receptor	2
Ribosomal protein L41	3		

(continued)

Table 1   Continued

Identification from an exact match to a human DNA sequence	No. total matches	Identification from an exact match to a human DNA sequence	No. total matches
Signal-recognition particle, 19 kDa	1	Tissue inhibitor of metalloproteinase 1	1
Signal-recognition particle, subunit 14	1	Tissue-specific protein	1
Signal transducing protein, beta subunit	1	Transaldolase	1
		Transcription activator SNFL2	1
Small inducible cytokine A2	6	Transcription factor BTF3b	2
Small nuclear ribonucleoprotein, polypeptide B	1	Transcription factor IIB	1
		Transcription factor ISFG-3, interferon alpha-indu	1
Small nuclear ribonucleoprotein, polypeptide C	2	Transcription factor hGATA3, trans-acting T-cell-	2
Smooth muscle protein SM22	1	Transcription-associated factor II70	2
snRNP protein B	1	Transcriptional activator. ISGF-3, 113 kDa, interfe	2
Splicing factor (GB:L10910)	2	Transcriptional regulator	1
Splicing factor CC1.3	1	Transformation-associated protein p53	1
Splicing factor CC1.3/CC1.4	1		
Squalene synthetase, hepatic	5	Transforming growth factor beta-induced gene BIGH3	1
Subtilisinlike protein PACE4	4		
Succinate-ubiquinone oxidoreductase, iron sulfur s	1	Transforming growth factor beta-induced protein	1
Superoxide dismutase 1, cytosolic	8	Transglutaminase 1	3
		Transketolase	2
Superoxide dismutase 2, mitochondrial	5	Translation elongation factor 1, alpha	54
Tetracycline transporterlike protein	1	Translation elongation factor 1, beta	4
Tetranectin	1	Translation elongation factor 1, delta	1
Thioredoxin	3		
Thrombospondin	1	Translation elongation factor 1, gamma	14
Thrombospondin 1	1		
Thromboxane A synthase	1	Translation elongation factor 2	2
Thromboxane synthase	1		
Thymosin beta-10	1	Translation initiation factor 4A	9
Thymosin beta-10 (GB:S54005)	2		
		Translation initiation factor 4AI	8
Thyroid autoantigen	4		

Table 1 Continued

Identification from an exact match to a human DNA sequence	No. total matches	Identification from an exact match to a human DNA sequence	No. total matches
Translation initiation factor 4B	3	Ubiquinol cytochrome-c	1
Translation initiation factor sui1iso1	1	reductase core I protein, m	
		Ubiquitin	8
Translationally controlled tumor protein	2	Ubiquitin (GB:M17597)	5
		Ubiquitin (GB:M26880)	12
Translocon-associated protein, beta subunit	6	Ubiquitin (GB:X04803)	4
		Ubiquitin carboxyl-terminal	1
Transmembrane 4 protein SAS	1	extension protein	
		Ubiquitin, B subfamily	2
Transmembrane 4 superfamily protein SAS	1	(GB:X04803)	
		Ubiquitin-52 amino acid	1
Triosephosphate isomerase	7	fusion protein	
Triosephosphate isomerase 1	8	Urokinase plasminogen	4
trk Oncogene	1	activator surface receptor	
Tropomyosin TM1, muscle	2	v-fos Transformation effector	1
Tropomyosin TM30, cytoskeletal	1	protein (Fte-1)	
		Villin 2	1
Tropomyosin, beta, skeletal muscle	1	Vimentin	1
		von Willebrand factor	12
Troponin T, cardiac	1		
Troponin T, heart	1	Putative identification from a	No.
Tryptophanyl-tRNA synthetase (GB:X59892)	2	match to a nonexact human or nonhuman DNA sequence	total matches
Tubulin, alpha	17	3-Hydroxyacyl-Coenzyme A	1
Tubulin, b-alpha 1	22	dehydrogenase	
Tubulin, beta	2	3-Methyl-2-oxobutanoate	1
Tubulin, d-beta 1	5	dehydrogenase (lipoamide)	
Tubulin, k-alpha 1	21	ABC1 protein	1
Tumor necrosis factor alpha-inducible primary resp	1	ADP,ATP carrier protein	1
		ADP/ATP carrier protein	1
Tumor-associated antigen L6	1	AHNAK novel protein	1
Tyrosinase-related protein 1	1	ATP synthase epsilon subunit, mitochrondrial	3
Tyrosine phosphatase	1		
Tyrosine phosphatase MEG2	1	ATP synthase, epsilon subunit, mitochondrial	1
Tyrosine phosphatase PAC-1	1		
Tyrosine phosphatase, alpha	1	ATP synthase, gamma chain, mitochondrial	2
Tyrosine phosphatase, receptor-type, c polypeptide	1	ATPase	1

(continued)

Table 1 Continued

Putative identification from a match to a nonexact human or nonhuman DNA sequence	No. total matches	Putative identification from a match to a nonexact human or nonhuman DNA sequence	No. total matches
ATPase, Ca2+ transporting, RT15-1	1	Fibroblast growth factor receptor	1
Acetyl-CoA acetyltransferase	1	G protein	1
Acetylcholine receptor gamma subunit	1	GOS2 gene	2
Acyl-CoA oxidase	1	GTP-binding protein ERA	1
Adenylylsulfate kinase	1	GTP-binding protein GTR1	1
Agrin	1	GTP-binding protein HFLX	1
Annexin XI	1	GTP-bidning protein MMR	1
B-box protein IAI3B	1	GTP-binding protein SPOOB	1
Bet2	1	GTP-binding protein rab18a	1
C. elegans hypothetical protein, cosmid F09G8_3	1	GTP-binding protein rab5c	1
C. elegans hypothetical protein, cosmid ZK688_4	1	GTP-binding protein rab7	2
C. elegans cosmid ZK370 phosphoprotein	1	GTP-binding protein, beta subunit	1
C. elegans cosmid ZK688	1	GTP-binding protein, rab-related	1
C. elegans hypothetical protein 10, cosmid C50C3_10	1	Gelsolin	1
		Glycerate dehydrogenase	1
Cadherin-associated protein, CAP102	1	Glycogenin	1
Calgizzerin	1	Guanine nucleotide dissociation stimulator	1
Caltractin	1	Guanylate kinase family	1
Cathepsin C	1	High-mobility-like group 1 protein NHP2	1
Cell division control protein 46	3	Hypothetical protein	1
Clathrin-associated protein AP19	1	Int-1-related protein	1
Collagen X alpha-1	1	Integrin alpha 1 subunit	1
Collagen family	1	Isocitrate dehydrogenase, NADP-specific, mitochond	1
Connexin 40	1	Kinaselike protein, KLG gene	1
Cytochrome b, mitochondrial	1	LL5 protein	2
DEAD box protein	1	Line-1 reverse transcriptase homolog	1
DNA polymerase alpha (P1)	1	Lon protease	1
Diff6 protein homolog	2	*M. musculus* hypothetical protein (GB:L07063)	1
EGF-inducible gene cMG1	1	M4 protein	1
Erythrocyte membrane protein	1	MER5 protein	1
		Minichromosome maintenance protein	1

Table 1 Continued

Putative identification from a match to a nonexact human or nonhuman DNA sequence	No. total matches	Putative identification from a match to a nonexact human or nonhuman DNA sequence	No. total matches
Myosin light chain kinase	2	Ribosomal protein S29	2
Myosin light chain, smooth muscle	1	Ribosomal protein S5	1
		Ribosomal protein S9	1
N-acetyl-galactosaminyltransferase	1	Ribosomal protein YL10 homologue	2
NADH dehydrogenase	1	*S. cerevisiae* ORF YKL153 from S30133	1
NADH dehydrogenase (ubiquinone) B15 subunit	1	*S. cerevisiae* hypothetical protein 20	1
NADH dehydrogenase (ubiquinone) MLRQ chain	1	*S. cerevisiae* hypothetical protein 29	1
NADH-ubiquinone oxidoreductase, B14.5a subunit	1	*S. cerevisiae* hypothetical protein YKL165	1
NEDD-6	1	SM22	1
P311	1	Seryl-tRNA synthetase	1
Parathyroid hormone receptor	1	Signal-recognition particle SRP72	1
Phospholipase C-alpha	1	Signal sequence receptor beta subunit	5
Procollagen alpha 1 type 3	1	Smooth muscle protein (SM22)	4
RNA helicase	1		
RNA polymerase II, 5.4 kDa subunit	1	Superoxide dismutase	1
RNA-binding protein Raly	1	Superoxide dismutase (Cu-Zn)	1
RNA/DNA-binding protein	1		
RSP-1 for p33 protein	1	T-complex protein 1	2
Retinoid X receptor gamma	1	TC1 mRNA	1
Ribonuclease, pancreatic	1	Transaldolase B	1
Ribosomal protein L1a	1	Transplantation antigen P198	1
Ribosomal protein L21	1	Troponin T, cardiac	1
Ribosomal protein L23a	6	Ubiquinol-cytochrome-c reductase core protein 1	1
Ribosomal protein L28	3		
Ribosomal protein L30	1	Ubiquitin-conjugating enzyme	1
Ribosomal protein L38	1	Vacuolar ATP synthase subunit E	1
Ribosomal protein L5	4		
Ribosomal protein L8	1	Vegetative cell protein X	1
Ribosomal protein S10	1	Zinc finger protein	1
Ribosomal protein S21	8	Zinc finger protein family	1
Ribosomal protein S27	2	Acetylcholine receptor, gamma subunit	5
Ribosomal protein S28	1		

(continued)

Table 1 Continued

Putative identification from a match to a nonexact human or nonhuman DNA sequence	No. total matches	Putative identification from a match to a nonexact human or nonhuman DNA sequence	No. total matches
Aconitase precursor	2	Dishevelled	1
Actin-capping protein, beta chain	1	dsRNA-binding protein 4F.1	1
Actinin, alpha	1	Ecdysone receptor	1
Acyl-coenzymeA dehydrogenase	1	Endopeptidase	1
		Enoyl-coenzyme A hydratase	1
Adducin	2	Estrogen receptor	1
Ankyrin repeat	2	Exoribonuclease	1
cAMP-dependent protein kinase, type II-associated	2	Fibrinogen, alpha chain	1
		Fowlpox virus FP4	1
Calcium/calmodulin-dependent protein kinase, type	1	Glucose-repressible alcohol dehydrogenase transcri	1
		Glutaminyl-tRNA synthetase	2
Calcyphosin	1	Goliath protein	1
Calgranulin B	1	Growth arrest specific protein gas2	1
Carboxypeptidase M, precursor	1	Growth factor-like protein Cyrol	1
Cathepsin D	1	Guanine nucleotide-binding protein	1
Cell division control protein 39	1	Helix-loop-helix phosphoprotein	1
Cell division protein FTSH	1	Histamine N-methyltransferase	1
Chaperonin	1		
Chloride channel protein	2	Histidyl-tRNA synthetase	1
Choline acetyltransferase	1	Histone H2A1	1
Clathrin coat assembly protein AP50	1	hnRNP complex K	1
		Hypoxanthine phosphoribosyl transferase	2
Clathrin-associated protein AP17	1	Immunoglobulin heavy chain, V region	1
Coat protein, beta	1	Immunoglobulin lambda chain	1
Coatomer, zeta-COP subunit	3		
Cofilin	2	Immunoglobulin, kappa chain	1
Collagen, type V, alpha 2	1		
Collagen, type X, alpha 1	1	Interferon-alpha-inducible gene p27	1
Corpuscles of stannius protein	2		
Cysteine-rich fibroblast growth factor receptor	1	Kallikrein family	1
Cytochrome b, mitochondrial	1	Lumican	1
Cytokine	1	Macrophage inflammatory protein	1
Cytosol aminopeptidase	1		
Dihydrodiol dehydrogenase	1		

Table 1 Continued

Putative identification from a match to a nonexact human or nonhuman DNA sequence	No. total matches	Putative identification from a match to a nonexact human or nonhuman DNA sequence	No. total matches
Macrophage inflammatory protein (GOS19-1)	1	Proto-oncogene pim-1	1
Malate dehydrogenase, mitochondrial	1	Pulmonary surfactant-associated protein SP-A	1
Mannosidase, alpha	1	Pumilio	1
Microfibril-associated glycoprotein	1	Putative transmembrane protein	1
Mitotic control protein dis3+	1	ras-Related protein	1
Myosin light chain 1	1	ras-Related protein p23	1
Myosin, light chain kinase	1	Reticulocalbin	1
Nerve terminal protein SNAP 25B	1	Retinal pigment	1
Olfactory receptor	1	Retinoblastoma-binding protein 2	1
Olfactory receptor-like protein DTMT	1	Retinoid X receptor, beta	1
Oligosaccharyltransferase, 48 kDa subunit	2	Retinoid X receptor, gamma	1
Osteopontin	1	Rhombotin family 1	1
p53-Associated protein	1	Ribosomal protein L23a	5
Phospholipase C	2	Ribosomal protein L27a	2
Plasma-cell membrane protein PC-1	1	Ribosomal protein L36	3
Postsynaptic density protein 95	1	Ribosomal protein L44 (L36A)	1
Pre-mRNA splicing factor PRP6	1	Ribosomal protein L8	1
Primary response geneTIS11	1	Ribosomal protein L9	1
Procollagen, alpha 1	1	Ribosomal protein P23	1
Prohibitin	1	Ribosomal protein S10	2
Proline-rich protein Bat2	2	Ribosomal protein S17	1
Proteasome, PUP1 component	1	Ribosomal protein S27	2
Protein disulfide isomerase P5	1	Ribosomal protein S5	4
Protein kinase	1	Ribosomal protein S9	2
Protein transport protein SEC61, gamma subunit	1	Ribosomal protein YL10 homolog	3
Proteosome, PUP1 component	1	Ribosomal protein YL41	2
		Secretory protein translocation SSS1 protein	3
		Selenium-binding protein, liver	1
		Serum-inducible kinase	2
		Seryl-tRNA synthetase	1
		Sex lethal protein, female-specific	1

(continued)

Table 1 Continued

Putative identification from a match to a nonexact human or nonhuman DNA sequence	No. total matches	Putative identification from a match to a nonexact human or nonhuman DNA sequence	No. total matches
Signal-recognition particle, 9-kDa subunit	1	Translation initiation factor SUI1	1
Small nuclear ribonucleoprotein-associated protein	1	Tubulin, alpha	2
		Tubulin, beta	2
		Tyrosine kinase elk/erk/cek	1
Spermidine synthase	1	Ubiquitin-conjugating enzyme	1
Thyroid hormone receptor	1		
Thyroid peroxidase	2	Ubiquitin-conjugating enzyme E2	1
Transcription factor NFATp	1		
Transcription initiation factor TFIID, 42-kDa subu	1	unc-18	1
		von Willebrand factor	1
Transcriptional regulator TSC-22	1	Zinc finger protein	3
		Zinc finger protein 5	1
Transforming growth factor beta-1-binding protein	1	Zinc finger protein ZNF2	1
		Zinc finger protein family	3
Translation initiation factor 4AI	1	Zytin	2
		Zyxin	2
Translation initiation factor 4AII	1		

with EST sequencing have previously been reported to be regulated by NGF, such as neurofilament-L and neurofilament-M (Fig. 2, Table 2). Many of the mRNAs in NGF-treated PC12 cells were not previously identified as differentially regulated (Fig. 2, Table 2). The magnitude of changes in mRNA levels as measured by Northern blot analysis supported results from EST analysis.

The regulated mRNAs represented a broad spectrum of proteins from ribosomal proteins, G-protein-coupled receptors, cell-trafficking proteins kinesin light-chain C and beta-COP, synaptic vesicle proteins, enzymes involved in oxidative stress such as superoxide dismutase, and a large number of novel transcripts without database matches. It is not known whether the regulated mRNAs are directly responsible for cellular differentiation or secondary to it. However, the comparative EST information provides multiple starting points to investigate these questions.

The application of the comparative EST approach can be readily extended to other cellular processes or disease states. Thus, it should be possible to study changes in gene expression in the airways of normal and asthmatic patients, in

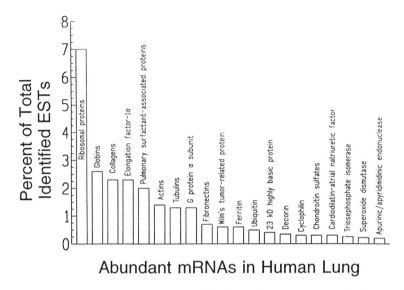

Figure 1 Abundant mRNA species found in human lung. From a total of more than 11,000 ESTs sequenced from libraries derived from human adult and fetal lung, mRNAs representing the most abundant transcripts were identified. The percent abundance was calculated by dividing the number of times a known transcript was hit by the total number of ESTs with putative identifications.

asthma of varying severity or triggered by different external factors, and in response to various therapeutic regimens.

IV. Large-Scale DNA Sequencing in Mutation Screening

The availability of rapid, high-throughput automated DNA sequencing technology has obvious applications in clinical research, including the detection of mutations responsible for various diseases [29,30]. This advance, combined with the exponential increase since the late 1960s on the chromosomal localization of genes, has had an enormous impact on the pace at which associations between genes and genetic diseases have been made.

It has long been postulated that asthma may, in part, be due to an imbalance in the autonomic control of airway diameter due to a decrease in β-adrenergic sensitivity in bronchial smooth muscle, mucus glands, and mucosal blood vessels [31]. The notion that dysfunctional β-adrenergic receptors are responsible for asthma has been supported by findings of reduced β-adrenergic receptor levels and/or responses in patients and animal models of asthma [32–35]; however,

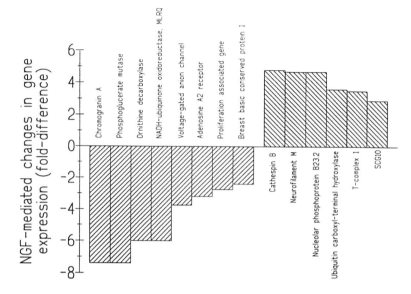

Figure 2   Changes in gene expression in NGF-treated PC12 cells. The fold differences in mRNA levels in control and NGF-treated PC12 cells were calculated by dividing the number of times a known transcript was identified in the untreated control library by the number of times it was identified in the NGF-treated library or vice versa to obtain a number greater than 1. Values with a negative value were expressed as greater abundance in the control cells (i.e., NGF caused a decrease in transcript level), whereas values with a positive value were expressed as greater abundance in NGF-treated cells (i.e., NGF caused an increase in transcript level).

Table 2   Differential Regulation of Distinct mRNAs by NGF in PC12 Cells

Downregulated mRNAs	Upregulated mRNAs
SC2 synaptic glycoprotein	Superoxide dismutase Cu-Zn
Transketolase	Clusterin
Glutaminyl-tRNA synthetase	Macrophage migration inhibitory factor
Cell surface glycoprotein OX47	Kinesin light chain C
MEK kinase	Myelin basic protein-related
TAXREB107	Synapsin 2
MAP kinase kinse	Calcineurin A-beta
Beta-COP	Neurofilament L
ADP-ribosylation factor 5	Developmentally regulated protein TPO

Genes listed in the left column are those that appeared only in the cDNA library constructed from mRNA isolated from untreated PC12 cells. Genes listed in the right column are those that appeared only in the cDNA library constructed from mRNA isolated from NGF-treated PC12 cells.

some instances of reduced responsiveness are thought to be a result of chronic therapy with β-adrenergic agonists [36,37]. Relevant to this question is the recent finding by Reishaus et al. [38] of six different forms of the human β_2-adrenergic receptor. Mutation of Thr[164] to Ile in the fourth transmembrane domain results in a receptor with markedly altered ligand-binding properties and abnormal receptor–G-protein coupling [39]. Two other amino-terminal polymorphisms are associated with altered agonist-mediated receptor regulation have no effect on ligand binding or functional activation, but alter the extent of agonist-promoted downregulation [40]. While the frequency and distribution of β_2-adrenergic receptor polymorphisms are no greater in asthmatics than in the population as a whole, the mutations which confer different functional properties on the receptor may play an accessory role in the pathogenesis of the disease or may affect patient response to therapeutic regimens with β_2-agonists [36–40]. Recently, a coding block polymorphism in the beta chain of the high-affinity receptor for IgE has also been identified [41], which may be associated with atopy [41,42].

Our understanding of the molecular mechanisms involved in asthma has expanded to encompass nonadrenergic, noncholinergic receptors and inflammatory cells and mediators. This raises the possibility that mutations in genes involved in these other signaling pathways may exist and may, in part, be responsible for the manifestations of asthma. The widespread availability of automated DNA sequencing combined with PCR for rapid gene amplification makes it now feasible to consider large-scale DNA screening as a means of identifying gene mutations associated with disease [29,30]. Based on preliminary data obtained from human EST analysis, it appears that the frequency of polymorphisms within the coding regions of genes may be higher than previously assumed [1]. If this is indeed the case, then it may be that such naturally occurring polymorphisms may be responsible for known variations in the human population to therapeutic intervention in various diseases.

V. Summary and Conclusions

The development of the EST method, together with advances in PCR and automated DNA sequence analysis, will likely have a major impact on all fields of research in the coming years. As summarized in this review, it is now feasible to think about biological questions on a global scale and to examine changes in the expression of hundreds or thousands of genes associated with various experimental paradigms. This fundamental change has several implications relevant not only to the understanding of asthma but also to many other diseases and physiological processes.

The EST approach has provided sequence tags for hundreds of novel genes whose function can be inferred by sequence similarity to known genes from humans and other species, and thousands of novel genes and gene families whose biological functions are currently unknown. The large number of new genes discovered to date with the EST approach demonstrates how incomplete our understanding of cellular biology is at this point in time. Furthermore, these novel sequences potentially represent new targets in the therapy of a large number of diseases. In addition to using the EST approach to provide a static picture of cellular physiology, comparative EST studies can reveal temporal changes in gene expression in response to various external signals and/or physiological or pathological processes. Chromosomal mapping of all of the novel genes identified both physically and genetically will be of enormous value, not only to medical genetics but also to the basic understanding of genome structure and function.

References

1. Adams MD, Kerlavage AR, Fleischmann RD, et al. Initial assessment of human gene diversity and expression patterns based upon 52 million basepaires of cDNA sequence. Nature 1995; 377:3–174.
2. Adams MD, Kelley JM, Gocayne JD, et al. Complementary DNA sequencing: Expressed sequence tags and the human genome project. Science 1991; 252:1651–1656.
3. Adams MD, Dubnick M, Kerlavage AR, et al. Sequence identification of 2375 human brain genes. Nature 1992; 355:632–634.
4. Adams MD, Kerlavage AR, Fields C, et al. 3400 new expressed sequence tags identify diversity of transcripts in human brain. Nature Genet 1993; 4:256–267.
5. Adams MD, Soares MB, Kerlavage AR, et al. Rapid cDNA sequencing (expressed sequence tags) from a directionally cloned human infant brain cDNA library. Nature Genet 1993; 4:373–380.
6. Affara N, Bentley E, Davey P, et al. The identification of novel gene sequences from the human adult testis. Genomics 1994; 22:205–210.
7. Geiser L, Swaroop A. ESTs and chromosomal localization of cDNA clones from a subtracted retinal pigment epithelium library. Genomics 1992; 13:873–876.
8. Liew C. A human heart cDNA library—the development of an efficient and simple method for automated DNA sequencing. J Mol Cell Cardiol 1993; 25:891–894.
9. Khan AS, Wilcox AS, Polymeropoulos MH, et al. Single pass sequencing and physical and genetic mapping of human brain cDNAs. Nature Genet 1992; 2:180–185.
10. Okubo K, Hori N, Matoba R, et al. Large-scale cDNA sequencing for analysis of quantitative and qualitative aspects of gene-expression. Nature Genet 1992; 2:173–179.
11. Takeda J, Yano H, Eng S, et al. A molecular inventory of human pancreatic islets: sequence analysis of 1000 cDNA clones. Human Mol Genet 1993; 2:1793–1798.
12. McCombie WR, Adams MD, Kelley JM, et al. *Caenorhabditis elegans* expressed sequence tags identify gene families and potential disease gene homologues. Nature Genet 1992; 1:124–131.
13. Waterson R, Martin C, Craxton M, et al. A survey of expressed genes in *Caenorhabditis elegans*. Nature Genet 1992; 1:114–123.

14. Uchimiya H, Kidou S, Shimazaki T, et al. Random sequencing of cDNA libraries reveals a variety of expressed genes in cultured cell of rice. Plant J 1992; 2:1005–1009.
15. Keith CS, Hoang DO, Barrett BM, et al. Partial sequence analysis of 130 randomly selected maize cDNA clones. Plant Physiol 1993; 101:329–332.
16. Boguski M, Tolstoshev CM, Bassett DE Jr. Gene discovery in dbEST. Science 1994; 265:1993.
17. Papadopoulos N, Nicolaides NC, Wei Y-F, et al. Mutation of a mutL homolog in hereditary colon cancer. Science 1994; 263:1625–1629.
18. Nicolaides NC, Papadopoulos N, Liu B, et al. Mutations of two PMS homologs in hereditary nonpolyposis colon cancer. Nature 1994; 371:75–80.
19. Miki Y, Swensen J, Shattuck-Eidens D, et al. Isolation of BRCA1, the 17q-linked breast and ovarian cancer susceptibility gene. Science 1994; in press.
20. Lee NH, Weinstock KG, Kirkness EF, et al. Comparative EST analysis of differential gene expression profiles in PC12 cells before and after nerve growth factor treatment. Proc Natl Acad Sci USA 1995; 92:8303–8307.
21. Moreno-Palanques RF, Fuldner RA. Construction of cDNA libraries. In: Adams MD, Fields C, Venter JC, eds. Automated DNA Sequencing and Analysis. New York: Academic Press, 1994:102–109.
22. Smith T, Waterman M. Identification of common molecular subsequences. J Mol Biol 1981; 147:195–197.
23. McGuire JC, Greene LA, Furano AV. NGF stimulates incorporation of fucose or glucosamine into an extracellular glycoprotein in cultured rat PC12 pheochromocytoma cells. Cell 1978; 15:357–365.
24. Levi A, Eldridge JD, Paterson BM. Molecular cloning of a gene sequence regulated by nerve growth factor. Science 1985; 229:393–395.
25. Anderson DJ, Axel R. Molecular probes for the development and plasticity of neural crest derivatives. Cell 1985; 42:649–662.
26. Leonard DGB, Ziff EB, Greene LA. Identification and characterization of mRNAs regulated by nerve growth factor in PC12 cells. Mol Cell Biol 1987; 7:3156–3167.
27. McGuire JC, Greene LA. Stimulation by nerve growth factor of specific protein synthesis in rat PC12 pheochromocytoma cells. Neuroscience 1980; 5:179–189.
28. Halegoua S, Armstrong RC, Kremer NE. Dissecting the mode of action of a neuronal growth factor. Curr Top Microbiol Immunol 1991; 165:119–170.
29. Larder BA, Kohli A, Kellam P, et al. Quantitative detection of HIV1 drug resistance mutations by automated DNA sequencing. Nature 1993; 365:671–673.
30. Adams MD, Fields C, Venter JC. Automated DNA Sequencing and Analysis. New York: Academic Press, 1994.
31. Szentivanyi A. The beta-adrenergic theory of atopic abnormality in bronchial asthma. J Allergy 1968; 42:203.
32. Barnes PJ, Dollery CT, MacDermott J. Increased pulmonary α-adrenergic and reduced β-adrenergic receptors in experimental asthma. Nature 1980; 285:569–571.
33. Gatto C, Green TP, Johnson MG, et al. Localization of quantitative changes in pulmonary beta-receptors in ovalbumin-sensitized guinea pigs. Am Rev Respir Dis 1987; 136:150–154.
34. Parker CW, Smith JW. Alterations in cAMP metabolism in bronchial asthma. J Clin Invest 1973; 52:48–59.

35. Sano Y, Watt G, Townley RG. Decreased mononuclear cell beta-adrenergic receptors in bronchial asthma: parallel studies of lymphocyte and granulocyte desensitization. J Allergy Clin Immunol 1983; 72:495–503.

36. Galant SP, Durisetti L, Underwood S, et al. Beta-adrenergic receptors of polymorphonuclear particulates in bronchial asthma. J Clin Invest 1980; 65:577–585.

37. Conolly ME, Greenacre JK. The lymphocyte β-adrenoceptor in normal subjects and patients with bronchial asthma. J Clin Invest 1976; 58:1307–1316.

38. Reishaus E, Innis M, MacIntyre N, et al. Mutations in the gene encoding for the β_2-adrenergic receptor in normal and asthmatic subjects. Am J Respir Cell Mol Biol 1993; 8:334–339.

39. Green SA, Cole G, Jacinto M, et al. A polymorphism of the human β_2-adrenergic receptor within the fourth transmembrane domain alters ligand binding and functional properties of the receptor. J Biol Chem 1991; 268:23117–23121.

40. Green S, Turki J, Innis M, et al. Amino-terminal polymorphisms of the human β_2-adrenergic receptor impart distinct agonist-promoted regulatory properties. Biochemistry 1994; 33:9414–9419.

41. Shirakawa TS, Li A, Dubowitz M, et al. Association between atopy and variants of the β subunit of the high affinity immunoglobulin E receptor. Nature Genet 1994; 7: 125–129.

42. Hill MR, Daniels SE, James AL, et al. A coding polymorphism for FcϵRIβ in a random population sample: associations with atopy. Genet Epidemiol 1994; 11:297.

15

Linkage Analysis in Complex Disorders

JIANFENG XU

Johns Hopkins University School of Medicine
Baltimore, Maryland

DEBORAH A. MEYERS

Johns Hopkins University School
of Medicine
Baltimore, Maryland

I. Introduction

A. Definition

A complex genetic disorder is any disorder that has known evidence of genetic components in its etiology, but does not exhibit a classic Mendelian dominant or recessive inheritance attributable to a single gene locus. Asthma and allergy, some psychiatric disorders such as mood disorders and schizophrenia, and Alzheimer's disease are examples. In general, the complexities arise when the simple correspondence between genotype and phenotype breaks down, due to possible misclassification of phenotype, incomplete and age-dependent penetrance, phenocopies, genetic heterogeneity, and/or oligogenic inheritance. Incomplete and age-dependent penetrance refers to the phenomenon that an individual who inherits a predisposing disease allele may not manifest the disease at all, or the chance of manifesting the disease may depend on his or her age. Phenocopy, on the other hand, is a phenomenon that an individual who does not inherit a predisposing disease allele may show the disease, probably caused by environmental factors. Genetic heterogeneity is a situation where mutations in any one of several genes may result in identical phenotype. Oligogenic inheritance requires the simultaneous presence of mutations in multiple genes.

B. Types of Approaches

The lack of a clear one-to-one relationship between genotype and phenotype makes genetic studies difficult; however, several genetic epidemiology approaches are helpful in searching for a genetic component in complex disorders. These approaches are used to determine whether a disorder is caused by environmental factors, polygenes (several genes affect the disorder, each by a small amount), Mendelian major genes (one or several major genes involved), or mixed polygenic and Mendelian major genes (besides Mendelian genes, there is still a residual polygenic effect).

Familial Aggregation (Relative Risk)

Although familial aggregation of a disorder could be caused by either common environmental factors within a family or genetic components, it is usually the first clue that a disorder may be genetic. In the presence of familial aggregation, the recurrent risk for relatives of an affected person is higher than that of general population. Often, accurate estimates of the recurrent risks in relatives an population are difficult to obtain. Well-designed large-scale epidemiological studies and even longitudinal studies are needed. For example, in a Dutch asthma family study, 92 probands were selected from 1284 patients with obstructive airway disease evaluated in a regional asthma and airway disease referral center hospital near Groningen between 1962 and 1970 by the following criteria: symptomatic asthma at the time of study, < 45 years of age, and bronchial hyperresponsive to histamine [1]. Their offspring were investigated 25 years later for asthma. There are 49 asthmatic offspring out of 265 (incidence rate = 18.5%). This number can be compared to that of control group (the offsprings of nonasthmatic probands) or general population (incidence rate = 4.1%) [2]. Thus a familial aggregation is clearly seen in this study population.

Recently, much attention has been paid to the parameter of relative risk, λ_R, defined as the incidence rate for a relative of an affected person divided by that of the general population. The subscript R denotes the type of relative; for example λ_O and λ_S are the risk to offspring and siblings, respectively. This ratio is related to the ease or difficulty of genetic mapping [3]. Genetic mapping is much easier for traits with high λ (for example, $\lambda_S > 10$) than for those with low (for example $\lambda_S < 2$). Again, it may be difficult to obtain accurate estimates of these risks.

Twin Studies

Twins constitute a unique sample design provided by nature, and are an excellent way to match for age and many environmental factors. The goal of twin studies is to compare similarities (correlation coefficients for quantitative traits and concordance rates for qualitative traits) in monozygotic twins (MZ) and dizygotic twins

(DZ). Since (1) MZ twins are completely identical for all genetic factors and DZ twins, on average, share half their genes, and (2) the environmental components of variance of both types of twins are similar (both types of twin pairs are assumed to have the same environmental variation—for example, they grow up in the same families), the difference of the similarities between MZ and DZ twins suggests genetic components. For example, MZ asthma concordance rate of 19.0%, compared to DZ asthma concordance rate of 4.8% in 7000 same-sex twin pairs [4], suggests a genetic etiology of asthma. Twin studies are very helpful in differential genetic and environmental factors of family aggregations, but they have limited usage in inferring the mode of inheritance of a disorder.

Complex Segregation Analysis

Complex segregation analysis is a useful tool to identify the mode of inheritance of a disorder and to estimate some important parameters. In complex segregation analysis, the fitting of various specified models to the observed inheritance pattern in the pedigrees is compared, that is, how likely it is that we observed the inheritance pattern in the available pedigrees if the inheritance pattern is environmental, polygenic, Mendelian, or mixed. The best-fitting and most parsimonious model (the model with higher likelihood and fewer parameters) suggests that the specified model is the most likely mode of inheritance.

Segregation analysis can be performed on both quantitative and qualitative traits using several computer programs, such as PAP (Pedigree Analysis Package [5] and S.A.G.E.[6]. In PAP, different inheritance patterns (one locus) of a quantitative trait can be modeled by the following parameters. (1) The unobserved genotypes, or more generally, "ousiotype," are the products of one factor with two alternatives, "A" and "a" (in the genetic cases, they are two different alleles). "A" is the factor associated with lower levels of a trait, while "a" is associated with higher levels. If Hardy-Weinberg equilibrium is assumed, the proportions of each possible genotype (*AA*, *Aa*, and *aa*) can be determined by the frequencies of "A" (q_A, $q_a = 1 - q_A$). (2) The transmission probability for each genotype (τ_{AA}, τ_{Aa}, τ_{aa}) is defined as the probability that any individual of a given genotype (ousiotype) transmits a factor "A" to an offspring. The Mendelian models are specified if we set τ to Mendelian expectations, i.e., 1, 1/2, and 0 for genotypes *AA*, *Aa*, and *aa*, respectively. The environment model is specified if we set τ to be the same for all three ousiotypes, since an environmental factor cannot be transmitted. (3) The means for each genotype (μ_{AA}, μ_{Aa}, and μ_{aa}) can also be used. Thus, "A" dominant to "a" can be modeled by forcing $\mu_{AA} = \mu_{Aa}$, which is lower than μ_{aa}. Similarly, we can model "A" recessive and co-dominant. (4) Residual variations within each genotype (σ) can be further partitioned into a polygenic component (h^2) and individual-specific environmental factors.

The parametrization for a qualitative trait is similar to that for a quantitative trait. Instead of estimating means for each genotype, affection probabilities (penetrances) for each genotype (f_{AA}, f_{Aa}, f_{aa}) are used.

As shown above, Mendelian inheritance models, environmental models, polygenic models, and mixed polygenic and Mendelian models can be specified by fixing some of the parameters: τ, μ, and h^2. These models can be compared to a general model where all the parameters are free to be estimated, which by definition should have the highest likelihood. Two criteria can be used to compare these different models. For comparing each submodel to a general model (hierarchical models), twice the difference in log likelihoods ($-2 \ln L$) between a submodel and a general model follows a χ^2 distribution, with the number of degree of freedoms equal to the difference in the number of parameters under the two models. The best-fitting model is the one requiring the fewest estimated parameters and exhibiting a likelihood not significantly smaller than that of the general model. For comparing nonhierarchical models (not nested models), the Akaike's Information Criterion (AIC) can be used, $AIC = 2 \ln L + 2k$, where k is the number of parameters estimated in the model. The most parsimonious model is the one with the minimum AIC.

For example, a complex segregation analysis of adjusted log IgE levels (adjusted for age) in the Dutch asthma family study population [7] was performed to investigate its mode of inheritance, using PAP. The likelihoods of observing the inheritance pattern in these 92 families under several models (hypotheses) were calculated (Table 1). A mixed environmental model, a mixed Mendelian dominant model, and a polygenic model fitted the data significantly worse than the general model ($p < 0.05$), and could be rejected. Both a mixed Mendelian co-dominant model and a mixed Mendelian recessive model fitted the data well, compared to the general model. However, the mixed Mendelian recessive model had fewer parameters, which gave evidence for a major recessive gene with a residual polygenic effect controlling IgE levels. The frequency of an allele (q_a) associated with high IgE level is estimated to be 0.59. Mean log IgE levels for individuals with genotypes AA and Aa were estimated to be 1.36 (23 IU), and for individuals with genotype aa, 2.38 (240 IU). The residual heritability (h^2) was estimated to be 0.49.

Segregation analyses are not limited to one-locus models; two-locus models are also possible. In the two-locus models, unobserved genotypes, or more generally "ousiotypes," are the products of two factors, each with two alternatives (A, a and B, b). Thus there are nine possible different genotypes, $AABB$, $AABb$, $AAbb$, $AaBB$, $AaBb$, $Aabb$, $aaBB$, $aaBb$, and $aabb$. Gene frequencies of factors "a" (q_a) and "b" (q_b), the recombination fraction between the two loci (θ), the transmission probabilities for each genotype, τ (the probability of passing "A" and "B" to offspring for each genotype), the nine means (for a quantitative trait) or affection probabilities (for a qualitative trait), and the residual heritability (h^2) are parametrized. The likelihoods of different models, for example, an environmental model

Table 1 Segregaton Analysis of log(IgE) Levels in 92 Dutch Asthma Families

Model	q_A	τ_{AA}	τ_{Aa}	τ_{aa}	μ_{AA}	μ_{Aa}	μ_{aa}	σ	h^2	$-2\ln(L)$	χ^2	df	p	AIC
General model	0.41	1.00	0.48	0.00	1.46	1.33	2.37	0.51	0.53	1045.62				1059.62
Mixed environmental	0.95	$= q_A$	$= q_A$	$= q_A$	1.72	1.72	3.91	0.70	0.60	1064.35	18.73	1	<0.001	1076.35
Mixed Mendelian codominant	0.40	[1.0]	[0.5]	[0]	1.46	1.33	2.37	0.51	0.53	1045.63	0.01	1	>0.05	1057.63
Mixed Mendelian "a" recessive	0.41	[1.0]	[0.5]	[0]	1.36	$= AA$	2.38	0.51	0.49	1046.22	0.60	2	>0.05	1056.22
Mixed Mendelian "a" dominant	0.81	[1.0]	[0.5]	[0]	1.41	2.32	$= Aa$	0.56	0.42	1063.12	17.50	2	<0.001	1073.12
Polygene	[1]	[1.0]	[0.5]	[0]	1.72	$= AA$	$= AA$	0.70	0.60	1067.61	21.99	4	<0.001	1073.61

(fixing the transmission probabilities for each genotype to be the same), Mendelian two-locus models (the transmission probabilities are fixed to follow the Mendelian expectation), and the Mendelian one-locus model (set factor "A" to be the same as factor "B," which is a special case of two-locus), can be compared using AIC and χ^2. An example is our two-locus segregation analysis of total IgE levels in the Dutch families, which gives evidence for two Mendelian loci involving in the regulation of IgE levels [8]. The segregation analysis modeling for more than two loci is practically very difficult, due to the large number of parameters that would have to be estimated.

Unfortunately, segregation analysis can be extremely sensitive to biases in the ascertainment of families. The common ascertainment scheme for linkage analyses, where usually only pedigrees with multiple affected members are selected from a population, may lead to a false evidence of Mendelian inheritance and also overestimate gene frequency and penetrance. However, if families are selected through a single proband such as in the Dutch families, segregation analysis with adjustment for ascertainment method is possible. Segregation analysis may have little ability to distinguish among many possible modes of inheritance for a complex trait. Moreover, it can be especially difficult to estimate the number of distinct genes influencing a trait [9].

II. Parametric Linkage Analysis

A. Definition

Genetic linkage is a powerful methodology to help elucidate the underlying genetic mechanisms for inherited disorders (traits) and to find chromosomal locations for susceptibility disease genes. The demonstration of a linkage is the highest level of statistical "proof" that a disease is due to a genetic mechanism [10]. At present, there are two major categories of genetic linkage analysis, parametric linkage analysis using family pedigree method and allele-sharing analysis using relative pairs (especially sib pairs).

Genetic linkage is defined as the violation of Mendel's law of independent assortment. The law states that the alleles at two chromosome locations (loci) will assort independently and transmit to offspring in random combinations. Noninde-pendent assortment occurs when genetic loci are positioned near each other on the same chromosome. For example, if parent 1 has the haplotype A_1B_1 and A_2B_2 and parent 2 has the haplotype A_3B_3 and A_4B_4, we would expect the children's haplotypes to be the same as their parents if the loci are tightly linked (that is, no crossover between the two loci). As the distance between two loci increases, crossovers (recombination fraction) between the two loci increase, producing new haplotypes of A_1B_2, B_1A_2, A_3B_4, and A_4B_3.

Parametric linkage analysis involves the comparison of likelihoods of observing the segregation pattern of two loci within the pedigree for several specific hypotheses. First, the likelihood of observing the segregation pattern of two loci assuming the null hypothesis of no genetic linkage to be true is calculated, that is, independent assortment between the two loci. Next, the likelihoods for each of several alternative hypotheses, that is, different extents of crossing over (recombination fraction), are calculated and compared with the likelihood of the null hypothesis by means of an "odds ratio." The odds ratio consists of the likelihood of an alternative hypothesis divided by the likelihood of the null hypothesis. An odds ratio of greater than 1000 to 1 is taken as evidence for linkage. For ease of comparison, the base-10 logarithm of the odds ratio is reported (lod score) at different hypothesis (recombination fractions). The traditional lod score threshold has been 3.0 for Mendelian disorders [11].

If the two loci being studied are both genetic markers, the parametric linkage analysis is straightforward because we know the mode of inheritance of a genetic marker (co-dominant) and there is a 1-to-1 relationship between genotype and phenotype (one band on a gel represents a unique allele). The situation is similar to a simple Mendelian disease locus because, by definition, the disorder is controlled by a major locus with a known mode of inheritance, and it is safe to infer the genotype by the phenotype (no misdiagnosis, no phenocopy). Linkage analysis has been applied successfully to many simple Mendelian traits. The simplest situation is when unequivocal linkage can be demonstrated in a single large pedigree with lod score ≥ 3, even though other families may show no linkage (genetic heterogeneity). This has been done for such diseases as adult polycystic kidney disease and early-onset Alzheimer's disease [12]. If linkage cannot be established on the basis of any single pedigree or is seen in the total sample of families, one can ask whether a subset of pedigrees collectively shows evidence of linkage. Of course, one cannot simply choose those families with positive lod scores, as such an ex-post selection criterion will always produce a positive lod score. However, families can be selected on the basis of a-priori considerations (for example, different clinical presentations).

B. Problems in Complex Disorders

Parametric linkage analysis is difficult for a complex disorder, mainly because of the breakdown of the simple relationship between phenotype and genotype, caused by the following reasons. First is misdiagnosis. The misdiagnosed affected family members are not susceptibility gene carriers, while the misdiagnosed "unaffecteds" actually carry the susceptibility gene. Second is incomplete penetrance. Due to the reduced penetrance, a certain percent of the unaffected family members are susceptibility gene carriers. Third is phenocopy. Individuals with the disorder are affected by some other, nongenetic risk factors and do not have the susceptibility gene under study (although possibly a different gene). Misdiagnosis is one form of phenocopy. Fourth is heterogeneity. Some affected family members have a genetic defect in another locus and thus do not have the susceptibility gene under study. Last is oligogenic inheritance. A disease phenotype is the result of several defect genes, either additive or interactive. Thus the phenotype "affected" may or may not be due to the specific gene under study. Inferring an individual's genotype for the susceptibility gene from his or her phenotype is necessary for linkage studies, and the breakdown in the relationship between phenotype and genotype dramatically decreases the power of finding linkage using parametric linkage analysis.

These factors affect all methods of linkage analysis of complex disorders, including allele-sharing methods, because they create uncertainty. However, they have more impact on parametric linkage analysis [9]. This is because, unlike allele-sharing methods, where no model is assumed, parametric linkage analysis is a model-based method; thus the results are the outcome of two components, the correct specified model and real linkage. As can be seen, the correct specified model is difficult to establish for complex disorders.

C.   Strategies Used in the Analysis of Complex Disorders

Parametric linkage analysis for complex disorders, however, is by no means useless. Understanding of the difficulties may help researchers to overcome these problems, and there are several successful examples, such as early-onset breast cancer [13]. Several strategies can be considered in the parametric linkage analysis of complex disorders.

In the case of an obscure phenotype where there is a relatively high rate of misdiagnosis, various alternative diagnostic schemes can be applied. However, it is then necessary to adjust for the number of disease models used when determining significance. Another approach is first to study a related phenotype for which information on a genetic model may be available. An example of this is total serum IgE level, which is correlated with the presence of asthma [14]. After obtaining evidence for a major locus for IgE regulation mapping to 5q, linkage analysis with the asthma phenotype was performed assuming a dominant model. Evidence for linkage for a susceptibility locus for asthma was obtained [15].

Overestimating the degree of penetrance can lead to spurious evidence against linkage (caused by individuals who inherit a trait-causing allele but are unaffected). "Affected only" parametric linkage analysis is a common practice used to deal with the problem of incomplete and age-dependent penetrance [9]. This kind of analysis might decrease the effective number of meioses, but it also decreases the possible impact of false recombinants from unaffected family members who are gene carriers. The decision should be made based on the knowledge of the penetrance of the disorder (possibly obtained from a segregation analysis). An alternative approach is to assign different liability classes, for example, definitely affected, possibly affected, uncertain, possibly unaffected, and definitely unaffected. Two extreme categories can be used in the primary analysis, while the middle three categories are not utilized until later. An example of this is our algorithm developed for the Dutch asthma family study. Family members were classified as "asthma," presence of BHR and symptoms in the absence of smoking; "possible asthma," for example, BHR but unclear symptoms; "uncertain airway disease," often smoking-confounded BHR, "COPD," smoker with fixed obstruction; and "unaffected," no objective or subjective evidence of airway diseases [2].

Parametric linkage analysis has also been applied successfully in some cases to genetically heterogeneous disorders. Usually, some biologically sound indicators, such as age of onset, severity, and other intermediate variables of a complex disorder, can be used to subdivide a sample into two groups of pedigrees. Families can thus be selected on the basis of a-priori considerations. A good example of this approach is provided by the genetic mapping of a gene for early-onset breast cancer (BRCA1) to chromosome 17q. Families were added to the linkage analysis in order of their average age of onset, resulting in a lod score that rose steadily to a peak of 6.0 with the inclusion of families with onset before age 47 and then fell with addition of late-onset pedigrees [13]. Notwithstanding these successes, many failed linkage studies may result from the presence of a high degree of heterogeneity. It is usually wise to try to define a homogeneous set of families clinically.

Although several simulation studies have suggested that, in a disorder caused by two genes, a single-locus approximation has high power to detect linkage [16], a correctly specified two-locus model can sometimes increase significantly the power to find linkage. An example is the parametric linkage analysis between the locus for IgE and markers on chromosome 5q. A lod score of 3.0 for marker D5S436 was first reported using a one-locus recessive model in a Dutch asthma family study. After a subsequent segregation analysis which suggested that a two-locus recessive model fitted the inheritance pattern significantly better than a one-locus recessive model, parametric linkage analysis using the best two-locus model gave a lod score of 4.6 for the same marker [8].

D. Cautions

Misspecification of marker allele frequencies can cause false-positive linkage results, especially in families where many parents are untyped. This is because underestimation of allele frequencies may lead to spurious linkage information. For example, if cousins share a "rare" allele, this suggests the presence of linkage. However, if the grandparents are deceased, they may have been homozygous for the allele in question and the cousins actually inherited different copies of the allele. Thus, it is important to consider the allele frequencies from both population data and the study sample. The other problem is multiple tests, due mainly to the uncertainty of modes of inheritance. This will inflate the type I error and made lod score results difficult to interpret [9]. Two approaches are very useful in this case. First is a computer simulation method [9]. Marker data with no linkage can be simulated using the same pedigree information (availability of typed persons) and the same characteristics of the marker (heterozygosity) where the highest lod score was observed. Then the simulated data are analyzed using the same approaches (number of models tested) as in the real analysis. An empirical significance level is then obtained. The other approach is to adjust the significance level by the number of models tested [3 + log (number of models tested)] [17]. It is difficult to determine the exact cutpoint for significance in complex disorders. On one hand, it is important to follow up by typing additional markers in any region with a suggestion of linkage. On the other hand, it is important to realize that this may be a false positive result. Replications between studies are very important [18].

III. Allele-Sharing Methods

A. Definition

Unlike parametric linkage analysis, which depends on assuming a genetic model, allele-sharing methods are not based on a specific disease model. One simply tests whether the inheritance pattern of markers for a chromosome region is consistent with random Mendelian segregation. For a qualitative trait, if there is a linkage between a locus for a trait and a chromosomal region, affected relative pairs should share alleles identical by descent (IBD), that is, inherited from a common ancestor within the pedigree, more often than expected under Mendelian expectation. For a quantitative trait, relative pairs should show a correlation between the magnitude of their phenotypic difference and the number of alleles shared IBD. Sib-pair methods are the simplest and most commonly used allele-sharing methods [19].

B. Qualitative Trait: Affected Sib-Pair Analysis

Considering the possible problems in complex disorders, especially incomplete and age-dependent penetrance and misdiagnosis, many researchers focus on affected sib-pair methods, although the theories also apply to unaffected sib pairs. Under no linkage between a disease-predisposing locus and a marker, affected sib pairs sharing marker allele IBD will be independent from their phenotype, and follow Mendelian expectation of sharing IBD 0, 1, 2 with frequencies of 0.25, 0.5, 0.25. This distribution of sharing marker allele IBD can also be expressed as a mean number of alleles IBD = 0.5, $(1*0.5 + 2*0.25)/2$. If, however, there is linkage between the disease-predisposing locus and a marker, the Mendelian expectation of sharing marker allele IBD will deviate from the above distributions. Several statistical methods have been proposed to test this deviance. One of the most powerful methods is a mean test, which tests whether the mean number of a marker allele IBD is significantly different from 0.5 [20].

In an affected sib-pair analysis of BHR to markers on chromosome 5q, mean number of marker alleles IBD were calculated for several markers. Mean number of IBD for most markers was higher than 0.5, however, due to the small number of affected sib pairs, the *p* values were not highly significant, with several markers < 0.05 (Table 2). However, given the relationship between IgE levels and BHR, evidence for linkage to this region may be inferred [21].

Another newly developed affected sib-pair method is the likelihood method [3,22], where a lod score is calculated from the ratio of two likelihoods: the likelihood of observed marker allele IBD of affected sib pairs in the sample and the likelihood of sharing IBD under the null hypothesis of no linkage, that is, Mendelian expectation. Table 2 lists the lod score using this method for the same data, which is consistent with the mean test. However, unlike the lod score in parametric linkage analysis, where one can obtain an estimate of the recombination fraction, the lod score here cannot provide location.

Affected sib-pair allele-sharing methods can also be used to investigate possible parental origin effect for the disorders. One can look at affected sib pairs sharing paternal and maternal alleles IBD separately. This may be useful in the presence of imprinting or mitochondral inheritance. Even though a genetic model is not assumed, information on dominant versus recessive inheritance may be found, since the expected IBD distributions are different. For example, in a situation where a disease is perfectly linked to a marker, if the disease is recessive, the affected sibs will share two alleles IBD (one each from mother and father),

Table 2 Affected Sib-Pair Analysis for the Bronchial Susceptibility Locus and Markers on Chromosome 5q

Markers	No. pairs	Mean IBD	*p* value	Affected pair sharing IBD 2	1	0	lod
I19	10	0.61	0.14	0.55	0.45	0.00	0.78
D5S393	21	0.61	0.04	0.52	0.48	0.00	1.79
D5S500	35	0.58	0.09	0.43	0.38	0.19	0.87
D5S658	34	0.60	0.03	0.46	0.43	0.11	1.29
D5S436	34	0.64	0.009	0.42	0.44	0.14	0.94
FGFA	25	0.62	0.015	0.50	0.50	0.00	1.66
D5S434	32	0.56	0.08	0.41	0.50	0.09	0.68
CSF1R	20	0.60	0.05	0.49	0.50	0.01	0.71
D5S470	35	0.57	0.10	0.34	0.50	0.16	0.31

Adapted from Ref. 21.

while if the disease is dominant, the affected sibs will share only 1.5 (1 + ½), the former is very deviant from the Mendelian expectation of 1 (½ + ½). Thus it is easier to detect linkage of a recessive trait using allele-sharing methods.

C. Quantitative Trait

The basis for the allele-sharing method for a quantitative trait is straightforward: Siblings that share more alleles at a locus IBD should be more similar in phenotypic measurement than siblings that share fewer alleles. Thus, the squared difference of phenotype values between sibs can be regressed on the sharing of marker alleles IBD [19]. If the regression coefficient is significantly negative, it is an evidence of linkage (i.e., siblings with a small difference tend to share two alleles).

An example of this kind of method is the sib-pair analysis for total IgE in the Dutch asthma family study. Significant negative regression coefficients have been seen for several markers, which suggest that the locus regulating IgE levels is linked to chromosome 5q (Table 3).

D. Multipoint Sib-Pair Analysis

Up to now, most allele-sharing method have been based primarily on studying genetic markers one at a time. Such analyses are inadequate for two reasons: (1) The exact IBD status cannot always be inferred at the marker loci [the problem is most acute when parents are unavailable for study, since inferences must be drawn based only on identity by status (IBS) information for the offspring, but it occurs even when parents are available, since some parental mating types are not fully informative]; and (2) the IBD status at locations other than marker loci is not assessed. Kruglyak and Lander [23] proposed a method of complete multipoint

Table 3 Sib-pair Analysis for log (IgE) and Markers on Chromosome 5q

Markers	No. sib pairs	β	p value
I19	132	−1.50	0.07
D5S393	249	−2.17	0.01
FGFA	228	−1.06	NS
D5S436	283	−3.47	0.0003
CSF1R	227	−1.83	0.03
D5S410	239	−0.05	NS
D5S412	253	−0.23	NS
D5S415	231	−0.13	NS

Adapted from Ref. 7.

analysis using the information from all genetic markers to infer the full probability distribution of the IBD status at each point along the genome, which makes it possible to perform the proper maximum likelihood (ML) generalization of any sib-pair method for both qualitative and quantitative traits. Specifically, four types of sib-pair analyses can be performed: (1) ML mapping, to identify loci involved in a qualitative trait; (2) Information-content mapping, to assess the extent to which the available genetic markers have extracted the full inheritance information at each location in the genome; (3) Exclusion mapping, to test specific hypotheses about the degree of allele sharing at each location in the genome; and (4) quantitative-trait-locus (QTL) mapping, to identify loci involved in a quantitative trait.

E. Advantages and Limitations

Allele-sharing methods are nonparametric linkage analyses; that is, they require no prior assumptions about such parameters as mode of inheritance, penetrance, phenocopy rate, and disease allele frequency. In this sense, they are more robust than parametric methods because we are not dependent on many potentially erroneous model assumptions. Moreover, the problem of trying multiple models and correcting for inflation of the lod score (as is often required in such cases) is avoided in these approaches, although we must still correct for multiple diagnostic schemes. The trade-off is that allele-sharing methods are often less powerful than a correctly specified linkage model [9].

Sib-pairs methods are increasingly important tools for linkage studies of complex disorders. Besides the advantages described above, sib pairs are relatively easy to ascertain in large numbers and tend to be more closely matched for age and environment than other relative pairs.

It would be incorrect, however, to conclude that the genetic model of the disease is irrelevant. The fact that a model is not required in the analysis implies only that the model cannot be misspecified. Thus, false negative or false positive findings will not be due to the use of an incorrect model. Instead, the mode of inheritance of the disease influences the power of allele-sharing methods directly. Determining the model of inheritance for major genes for susceptibility to a complex disorder such as asthma may provide useful information on understanding the pathophysiology of the disorder. Once evidence for linkage is obtained, more complex modeling, such as two- and three-locus or MOD score analysis [24] may provide insight into disease mechanisms.

IV. Summary

The approaches of linkage analysis in complex disorders can be summarized as shown in the flowchart of Fig. 1. It is important that clinical, analytical, and molecular investigators be involved in all steps in the process. Mapping genes for

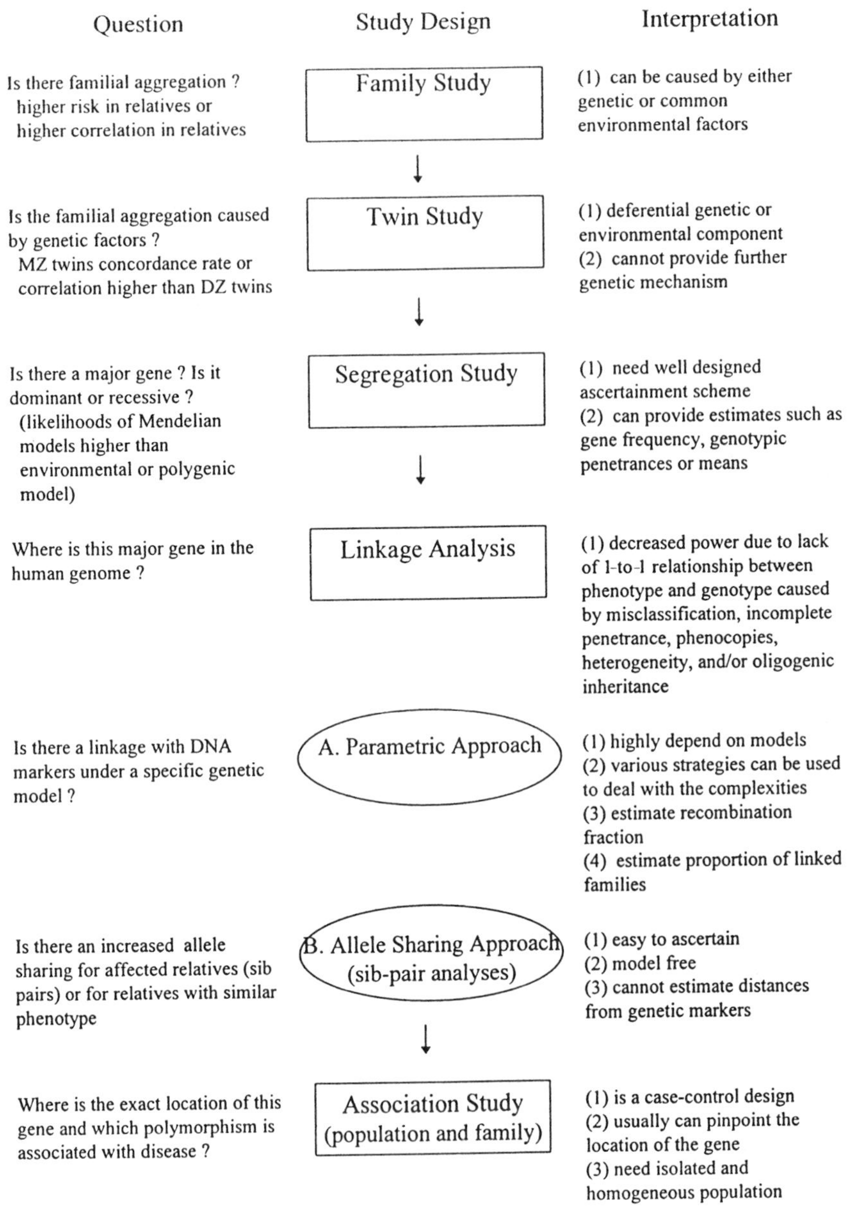

Question	Study Design	Interpretation

Is there familial aggregation ?
higher risk in relatives or
higher correlation in relatives

Family Study

(1) can be caused by either
genetic or common
environmental factors

↓

Is the familial aggregation caused
by genetic factors ?
MZ twins concordance rate or
correlation higher than DZ twins

Twin Study

(1) deferential genetic or
environmental component
(2) cannot provide further
genetic mechanism

↓

Is there a major gene ? Is it
dominant or recessive ?
(likelihoods of Mendelian
models higher than
environmental or polygenic
model)

Segregation Study

(1) need well designed
ascertainment scheme
(2) can provide estimates such as
gene frequency, genotypic
penetrances or means

↓

Where is this major gene in the
human genome ?

Linkage Analysis

(1) decreased power due to lack
of 1-to-1 relationship between
phenotype and genotype caused
by misclassification, incomplete
penetrance, phenocopies,
heterogeneity, and/or oligogenic
inheritance

Is there a linkage with DNA
markers under a specific genetic
model ?

A. Parametric Approach

(1) highly depend on models
(2) various strategies can be used
to deal with the complexities
(3) estimate recombination
fraction
(4) estimate proportion of linked
families

Is there an increased allele
sharing for affected relatives (sib
pairs) or for relatives with similar
phenotype

B. Allele Sharing Approach
(sib-pair analyses)

(1) easy to ascertain
(2) model free
(3) cannot estimate distances
from genetic markers

↓

Where is the exact location of this
gene and which polymorphism is
associated with disease ?

Association Study
(population and family)

(1) is a case-control design
(2) usually can pinpoint the
location of the gene
(3) need isolated and
homogeneous population

Figure 1   Flowchart of linkage analysis in complex disorders.

complex disorders is difficult but may prove to be very important in understanding disease processes and designing new treatments.

References

1. Amelung PJ, Panhuysen CIM, Postma DS, et al. Atopy and bronchial hyperresponsiveness: exclusion of linkage to markers on chromosomes 11q and 6p. Clin Exp Allergy 1992; 22:1077–1084.
2. Panhuysen CIM, Bleecker ER, Van Altena R, Meyers DA, Koeter GH, Postma DS. Results of an algorithm to characterize obstructive airways disease in families of probands with asthma. Am Rev Respir Dis, American Thoracic Society Annual Congress, Boston, 1994.
3. Risch N. Linkage strategies for genetically complex traits. II. The power of affected relative pairs. Am J Hum Genet 1990; 46:229–241.
4. Edfors-Lub M. Allergy in 7000 twin pairs. Acta Allergol 1971; 26:249–285.
5. Hasstedt SJ, Meyers DA, Marsh DG. Inheritance of IgE. Am J Med Genet 1983; 14:61–66.
6. S.A.G.E. Statistical Analysis for Genetic Epidemiology, Release 2.2. Computer program package available from the Department of Biometry and Genetics, LSU Medical Center, New Orleans, 1994.
7. Meyers DA, Postma DS, Panhuysen CIM, et al. Evidence for a locus regulating total serum IgE levels mapping to chromosome 5. Genomics 1994; 23:464–470.
8. Xu J, Levitt RC, Panhuysen CIM, et al. Evidence for two unlinked loci regulating total serum IgE levels. Am J Hum Genet 1995; 57:425–430.
9. Lander ES, Schork NJ. Genetic dissection of complex traits. Science 1994; 265:2037–2048.
10. Elston RC. Segregation analysis. Adv Hum Genet 1981; 11:63–120.
11. Morton NE. Sequential tests for the detection of linkage. Am J Hum Genet 1955; 7:277–318.
12. Tomfohrde J, Silverman A, Barnes R. Gene for familial psoriasis susceptibility mapped to the distal end of human chromosome 17q. Science 1994; 264(1562):1141–1145.
13. Hall JM, Lee MK, Newman B, et al. Linkage of early-onset familial breast cancer to chromosome 17q21. Science 1990; 250(4988):1684–1689.
14. Sears M, Burrows B, Flannery EM, Herbison GP, Hewitt CJ, Holdaway MD. Relation between airway responsiveness and serum IgE in children with asthma and in apparently normal children. N Engl J Med 1991; 325:1967–1071.
15. Panhuysen CIM, Levitt RC, Postma DS, Xu J, Amelung PJ, Holroyd KJ, Altena RV, Koeter GH, Meyers DA, Bleecker ER (1995). Evidence for a susceptibility locus for asthma mapping to chromosome 5q. American Society of Clinical Investigation (Accepted for publication).
16. Greenberg DA, Hodge SE. Linkage analysis under "random" and "genetic" reduced penetrance. Genet Epidemiol 1989; 6:259–264.
17. Ott J. Analysis of Human Genetic Linkage. Baltimore: Johns Hopkins University Press, 1991.

18. Thomson G. Identifying complex disease genes: progress and paradigms. Nature Genet 1994; 8:108–110.

19. Haseman JK, Elston RC. The investigation of linkage between a quantitative trait and a marker locus. Behavior Genet 1972; 2:3–19.

20. Blackwelder WC, Elston RC. A comparison of sib-pair linkage tests for disease susceptibility loci. Genet Epidemiol 1985; 2:85–97.

21. Postma DS, Bleecker ER, Amelung PJ, et al. Genetic susceptibility to asthma—bronchial hyperresponsiveness coinherited with a major gene for atopy. N Engl J Med 1995; 333:894–900.

22. Holman P. Asymptotic properties of affected-sib-pair linkage analysis. Am J Hum Genet 1993; 52:519–527.

23. Kruglyak L, Lander ES. Complete multipoint sib-pair analysis of qualitative and quantitative traits. Am J Hum Genet 1995; 57:439–454.

24. Hodge SE, Elston ER. Lods, Wrods and Mods: the interpretation of lod scores calculated under different models. Genet Epidemiol 1994; 11:329–342.

16

Statistical Considerations for Genetic Analysis of Atopy and Asthma

NEWTON E. MORTON
University of Southampton
and Princess Anne Hospital
Southampton, England

I. Introduction

Human genetics represents a balance between opposing tendencies. On the one hand, reductionist approaches have been amazingly successful, leading to mapping and molecular characterization of hundreds of diseases [1]. On the other hand, most diseases and other traits of interest show complex inheritance, with different major genes in different families and with interaction of multiple genes and environmental factors in some families. An extreme reductionism attempts to fit complex inheritance by a single gene, while extreme holism fits multifactorial models that ignore major genes [2,3]. Genetic epidemiology must avoid both extremes, characterizing major genes against a multifactorial background and providing genetic risks that allow for all sources of variation [4,5]. The search for genetic determinants of atopy and asthma mirrors the history of genetic epidemiology.

II. Environmental Factors

There is overwhelming evidence that environmental factors predispose to atopy and asthma, but disagreement about the relative importance of different mechanisms [6]. Exposure to allergens, especially in early infancy and perhaps prenatally, is a risk factor. Helminth infections are a potent stimulus for IgE. Occupational exposure is a major hazard for late-onset asthma, and environmental air pollutants aggravate asthma. The incidence of childhood respiratory infections is associated with death from chronic obstructive pulmonary disease. Cows' milk in infancy and exposure to tobacco smoke predispose to atopy, although large samples are required to detect these effects. Seasonal trends in aeroallergens influence atopy and clinical allergy.

Attempts by geneticists to characterize allergen exposure in family studies have not been successful. Questionnaire information is soft, and the informant has even less knowledge of exposure in relatives. Genetic epidemiology has many examples of better recall by mothers than fathers, making maternal effects equivocal if based on recall. We have been disappointed in our own work to detect no significant environmental effects by questionnaires addressed to smoking and home environment [7]. Environmental factors are undoubtedly more important than this weak evidence would suggest, but a practical way to characterize the environment has yet to be developed. The same may be said of other complex diseases, making the hope of regressive models elusive [8].

III. Heritability

Early genetic studies were directed to heritability, the proportion of phenotypic variance attributable to genetic factors. This is most easily estimated for quantitative traits such as serum IgE and bronchial reactivity, and it has been argued that at present there is no motive to force an arbitrary dichotomy on quantitative data [4]. However, methods are available to estimate heritability from a dichotomy, assuming an underlying scale of liability on which multiple factors act additively [9].

Table 1 Heritability Estimates

Trait	Heritability, h^2	Reference
Asthma	0.282 ± 0.061	7
Atopy	0.587 ± 0.053	7
Atopy	0.44	44
Atopy	0.49	49
Atopy	0.61	50
Atopy	0.52	51
Atopy	0.59	52
Atopy	0.46	53

A more serious problem is that family environment and genes are confounded in biological families. Monozygous twins share a common placenta and postnatal environment, arguably to a greater extent than dizygous twins, and adopted children provide only partial control over confounding. Estimates of heritability are in rough agreement (Table 1). Given the inherent imprecision of these methods, there does not seem to be a good reason to pursue such studies, at least until better phenotypes are defined.

IV. Single-Locus Models

The early history of human genetics was characterized by attempts to fit single-gene models to everything, with remarkable successes and failures. By inspection of family histories, Cooke and Vander Veer inferred dominant inheritance [10], but recessivity had its advocates during the 1920s and 1930s. A review concluded that "by the 1950s and 1960s most researchers realized that allergy is multifactorially determined" [11].

After a long period in which single-gene models were considered inappropriate, a group at Oxford returned to a dominant model [2,12]. Such oversimplification was encouraged by the most common linkage programs, which did not allow for multifactorial inheritance. However, a linkage program with two disease loci was in use [13], and other multifactorial models were introduced subsequently [14]. Oversimplification tends to inflate apparent recombination, but the effect on power is controversial and has been studied only in special cases.

V. Models of Complex Inheritance

The two-locus disease model is a useful representation of rare major genes, one of which is linked to a marker, and perhaps more generally. This model has been extended to include measures of severity for affection and diathesis for normality, using an ordered polychotomy to minimize distributional assumptions [15]. A model with two unlinked marker loci has been introduced [16]. Other representations of complexity include the mixed model, in which the modifier is polygenic [17], and regressive models, in which modifiers are approximated by regression on relatives [8]. The latter does not correspond with any genetic mechanism except in the special case of a quantitative trait and the class D model, which under certain conditions corresponds to the mixed model. Little is known about how these formulations of complex inheritance perform in practice, and in particular their power to detect linkage and association. All attempts to fit multifactorial models to atopy have rejected a single locus, but they disagree on whether a major locus is present and if so whether it is dominant, recessive, intermediate, or heterogeneous [18].

VI. Candidate Loci and Random Markers

Mapping of disease genes can begin with candidate loci selected through their function as likely to influence the disease process. This leads to tests of allelic association, either by a 2×2 contingency table for case-control studies or in pedigree analysis as coupling frequencies, defined as the probability that a given marker allele carry a given disease allele. Under a realistic model of complex inheritance the recombination value should be zero, but this can be inflated by error in the model. Choice of candidate loci is guided by knowledge of gene action and is therefore more interesting than random markers. However, polymorphism is often less, the optimal conditions for typing candidates often do not coincide, and identification of good candidates is incomplete.

An alternative approach is through highly polymorphic marker loci, chosen to be easily typed and rather uniformly spaced at preassigned distance in males or females. The number of useful markers is very large, making it feasible to multiplex several markers with the same optimal conditions and nonoverlapping fragment sizes. Therefore the number of informative meioses that can be scored with given effort may be larger than with candidate loci. Random markers have been spectacularly successful with major genes, but not in complex inheritance. Association tests on random markers are not promising, as the following argument shows [7]. Suppose that the candidate locus is placed at random between two random markers and that all three loci have n equally frequent alleles. For the candidate locus, one of these alleles, say A', has an additive effect on the trait, the displacement between AA and $A'A'$ being t. Then the covariance between the candidate locus and the trait liability is $t^2(n - 1)/2n^2$. Kinship between the candidate locus and the closer marker is $1/(cw + 1)$, where $c > 1$ is a constant and w is the map distance in morgans, which (to a close approximation) is the recombination fraction between the two loci. The expected value of c is $4N_e$, where N_e is the evolutionary size of the population. Using bioassay of kinship between loci, Morton and Wu [19] estimated that $N_e = 4000$. If D is the distance between markers in morgans (and therefore to a close approximation the recombination rate between them), the expected kinship φ between closer marker and candidate locus is

$$\varphi = \left(\frac{2}{D}\right) \int_0^{D/2} (cw + 1)^{-1} \partial w = \left(\frac{2}{cd}\right) \ln\left(\frac{1 + cD}{2}\right)$$

and the mean covariance between closer marker and trait is $\varphi t^2(n - 1)/2n^2$, which is negligible unless D approaches $1/c$, implying an intermarker distance much less than 1 Mb. This leads us to anticipate observations on the HLA cluster, where a striking association with one allele (for example, between ankylosing spondylitis and B27) is not apparent for other loci in the cluster because the effect is dispersed over many alleles. In general, there is only an infinitesimal probability of detecting an association between a random marker and a complex trait in a population like those that have been bioassayed for kinship between loci. Close inbreeding or recent admixture would increase the probability, but not enough to make this a feasible approach in humans, however appealing it may be in experimental crosses of inbred lines. This confers great value on candidate loci, even if incompletely identified. A compromise is to select a candidate locus and to multiplex with it as many random markers as feasible, chosen to have the same optimal conditions and to be differentiated either by fragment size or fluorescent label.

VII. Association

There is a large literature on association between haplotypes of the major histocompatibility complex (HLA) and response to purified allergens. The haplotypes most implicated have carried DR2, DR3, or DR5 [20]. Responses are Ag-specific, and it is questionable whether total IgE is associated with HLA haplotypes.

Outside the HLA system there is some evidence of association to haplotypes in the interleukin cluster on chromosome 5q. Rosenwasser et al. [21] identified in IL4 a "C to T exchange at position -498 bp that seems to correlate with IgE in atopic asthmatic kindreds." We have found that two low-frequency alleles at the IL9 locus defined by probe RP1 (104 and 116 bp) re significantly associated with atopy as log (total IgE) adjusted for age and sex ($p = 0.00034$). Because of linkage disequilibrium within the interleukin cluster, IL9 may not be causal even if this finding is confirmed. However, the physical distance between IL4 and IL9 suggests that there should be little disequilibrium between them.

Shirakawa et al. [22] published evidence that "an isoleucine to leucine substitution at position 181 of FcεRIβ is found in 10 of 60 (17%) unrelated nuclear families with allergic asymptomatic probands. The sequence variant is strongly associated with atopy and follows the pattern of maternal inheritance previously demonstrated for the 11q12-q13 atopy locus." If the paternal allele is not expressed, this would be the first proof of imprinting in this region. However, questions remain about the definition of atopy, selection of families, and significance of association (discussed in more detail in Chapter 23).

Association may be tested in pedigrees by likelihood analysis using coupling frequencies (as we did with IL9). Since this is model-dependent, there is interest in "nonparametric" sib-pair tests that make strong distributional assumptions but do not specify a genetic model. For many years it has been common to treat all pairs of relatives as if they were independent. This is known to be wrong [23], and it is not sufficient merely to correct the number of degrees of freedom. A set of k relatives generates $k(k-1)/2$ pairs with $k-1$ degrees of freedom, and so each pair may be weighted by $2/k$ using a normalizing transformation

on the squared difference in trait values [24]. More approximate tests of association in pedigrees should not be trusted, since they inflate the type I error.

VIII. Linkage

The hypothesis of a major gene for atopy on proximal 11q has an interesting
history. By inspection of multiplex pedigrees collected through clinics and a
media appeal, Cookson et al. [12] proposed a single dominant gene with high
penetrance and few sporadic cases. An arbitrary definition of atopy that included
total IgE, specific IgE, and skin-prick tests gave a prevalence of 30–40%. Accordingly, Cookson et al. assumed a gene frequency of 0.2, since $1 - 0.8^2 = 0.36$.
Using this model, they reported a lod of 5.58 to the random marker D11S97 at a
recombination frequency of 0.105. A second study, this time of nuclear families,
gave a lod of 3.80 with 0.067 recombination [25]. Pooling these two samples, $Z =$
9.33, $\theta = 0.092$. In a summary paper they reported "over 800 individuals from
over 50 nuclear and 20 extended British families" [26]. Although the probability
they gave ("lod score = 10, $p = 10^{-8}$") is unaccountably conservative, it agrees
substantially with the sum of their two published samples. However, shortly
afterward, recombination was reported to be 0.25 at a maximum lod of 3.88 [27].
This loss of more than 60% of the information has never been explained. Heterogeneity between sexes was not significant. When affected sib pairs were classified
by inspection according to the number of alleles identical by descent, treating all
$s (s - 1)/2$ pairs of s sibs as independent, values of χ^2 corresponding to lods of
1.0 to 1.7 were obtained. However, when maternal and paternal alleles were
distinguished, excess sharing of maternal alleles approached conventional significance ($\chi^2 = 13.4$, $Z = 2.9$), while sharing of paternal alleles was less than expected.
Although a more extreme lod is appropriate to test sex-specific recombination
[28], this suggestive result was ascribed to maternal effect or paternal imprinting.
The former would not be expected to differentiate between alleles transmitted to
the fetus, and the latter is not supported by expression studies or imprinting in the
homologous region of the mouse.

   A number of investigators have failed to replicate these findings [7,29–36].
However, there are two positive results. In a short abstract, Shirakawa et al. [37]
related that families of 274 atopic asthmatic probands were screened for an
extreme definition of atopy and 134 were excluded "because of discrepancies
between measurements." Of the remaining families, 8 contained more than 15
meioses and 4 of these were successfully typed. This highly selected subsample
gave results similar to the first Oxford report ($Z = 4.88$, $\theta = 0.07$). Collee et al. [38]
reported excess sharing of alleles (both maternal and paternal) in a small sample of
affected sib pairs, although this was not significant for the regional candidate locus
FCER1B [39]. Recently, a joint study by researchers in Paris, Australia, and

Oxford was interpreted as favoring a recessive gene with polygenic background for total IgE, which is inconsistent with monogenic dominance, maternal effect, and paternal imprinting [40]. Cautions about distributional assumptions apply to any segregation analysis of a quantitative trait.

Three explanations have been offered for these conflicting results. One is that the "leading factors" [41] are rare and so the evidence for linkage comes from a few families. Significance in the original report depended on one family with 23 meioses. If the altered definition and exclusion of most families in the study of Shirakawa et al. [37] were in ignorance of marker typing, it would favor linkage in a proportion of families with severe atopy, but families suggesting linkage in other studies have been clinically unremarkable. Moreover, this does not explain the lack of significant heterogeneity among the Oxford families, confirmation in a second Oxford sample, and the negative results of most other investigators. Rare genes of large effect could be efficiently detected by combined segregation and linkage analysis of multiplex families, perhaps with random markers.

A second explanation is that genetic factors in atopy may be common and individually of small effect. Then association with polymorphic alleles at candidate loci would be the method of choice, and linkage to random markers would be unpromising.

A third explanation is the occurrence of a type 1 error. It has recently been shown that pairwise independence of multiple sib pairs is not sufficient for control of type 1 errors [23], and other corrections are necessary as with association tests. If there was a type 1 error, interest in the proximal 11q region will have been justified if it leads to more reliable and powerful tests of candidate loci in the rest of the genome. The reported association with a leu 181 allele (22) will give a specific test of linkage.

The search for linkage with other candidate loci has until recently been disappointing. Allowing for allelic association, our evidence for linkage to IL9 is only suggestive ($\chi_1^2 = 3.93$ at $\theta = 0$). Tumor necrosis factor-B (TFNB), a marker for the HLA system, shows no evidence for linkage to atopy as defined by total IgE. Interferon-alpha (IFNA) and the beta chain of the IL2 receptor (IL2RB) are also negative. Marsh et al. [42] have reported evidence of a major gene for IgE regulation in the interleukin cluster of chromosome 5q. This is a strong candidate region, and the sib pair and parametric analyses are concordant. However, several aspects of this report are puzzling. Their results are more significant for individuals without specific IgE to 20 common aeroallergens, the "atopic" sib pairs giving less evidence of linkage. The 119 sibs generated 349 sib pairs, which were analyzed without allowing for dependence and nonnormality of squared differences. The genetic model for parametric tests was a single locus with complete dominance of a high-frequency allele for atopy, the two phenotypic classes having strikingly different variances of log IgE. The maximum-likelihood estimate of sex-averaged recombination was 0, contrary to evidence that an oversimplified model inflates recombination. Finally, the material consisted of 11 large Amish pedigrees with at least one child sensitive to common aeroallergens, and their conclusion may not apply to other populations. If IL4 linkage is confirmed, identification of the responsible sequences may be as difficult as it has been for HLA-association diseases, but detection of linkage would be a strong argument in favor of candidate loci. However, methods are in transition, and little evidence has yet been published. It is too early to assess the utility of candidate loci and random markers.

IX. Maternal Effect and Imprinting

A maternal effect is a direct effect of the maternal genotype or phenotype on the phenotype of the immediate offspring, independent of the genotype of the offspring and therefore giving no evidence of linkage. "Maternal modification of the infants' IgE responses through the placenta or breast milk," as proposed by the Oxford group [43], would not generate linkage to 11q unless it were allele-specific in the infant. That is a rather elaborate hypothesis to rest solely on diminishing evidence of linkage, no longer significant in fathers.

A maternal effect can be simulated in several ways. If the diagnosis of atopy depends on recall and if mothers are informants about spouses, paternal affection

Table 2 The Pericentromeric Region of Chromosome 11

Locus	Bands		Linkage cM	
	Left	Right	Male	Female
D11S905	p13	q13	53.0	75.8
cen	cen	cen	53.0	84.0
D11S429	q13.1	q13.1	53.0	84.0
D11S453	q13.1	q13.1	55.7	86.4
FCER1B	q13	q13	55.7	88.3
D11S451	q11	q12	55.7	92.0
MEN1	q13	q13	55.7	92.7
PGA	q13	q13	55.7	92.9
D11S427	q13.1	q13.1	55.7	96.0
PYGM	q12	q13.2	55.7	96.1
D11S480	q13.1	q13.1	55.7	96.1
SEA	q13	q13	55.7	98.4
D11S913	q13	q13	56.0	98.4
D11S97	q13	q13	56.0	100.0

may be underascertained. Arbitrary classification of smokers and ex-smokers [27] may also make paternal phenotypes less reliable than maternal phenotypes. Mothers and children share home environment more than fathers, and on that account their phenotypes may be more highly correlated [44]. If atopy is dichotomized as affection and if mothers are less frequently affected than fathers, then under genetic or cultural transmission the frequency of affected children will be greater for atopic mothers than for atopic fathers; this has been called the Falconer effect [45]. None of these maternal biases would generate evidence of linkage.

Paternal genomic imprinting means that the allele transmitted by the father is not expressed in some critical tissue or developmental stage of the child. Imprinting can be detected as differential methylation in sperm and embryos and usually persists through life. No locus in the region that includes the FCER1B and CD20 loci is known to be imprinted in any mammal. If atopy is linked to genes in this region, the evidence should not be restricted to maternal transmission. On the contrary, linkage in this centromeric region is much closer in males than females (Table 2).

X. Meta-analysis

In a strict sense, meta-analysis is the quantitative study of published results relating to a particular problem, leading to conclusions about heterogeneity and overall significance [46]. There is insufficient agreement about definitions, genetic models, and statistics to apply this to atopy or asthma. However, quantitative study of results obtained by different collaborators could be useful.

Assuming that definition of atopy and selection of families different among studies, parametric analysis is not feasible. Fortunately, nonparametric tests of association and linkage that conform to distributional assumptions have been developed [47]. Their power has not been investigated, and heterogeneity tests are equivocal because of known differences among studies. Replication remains the only way to validate a claim of association or linkage, and failure of most attempts at replication must be taken as strong evidence against that claim.

XI. Implications for Complex Inheritance

Whereas the search for major genes has been impressively successful, it is too early to evaluate the search for genetic determinants in complex inheritance. Methods developed for genes of large effect are of questionable value, and early attempts to devise special methods for complex inheritance lacked power or rigor [48]. Definitions are in dispute, and basic questions of experimental design have yet to be answered, such as whether to prefer a quantitative trait or a dichotomy, association or linkage, candidate loci or random markers, and parametric or nonparametric tests. Progress in the search for genetic determinants of atopy and asthma will benefit from and contribute to other studies of complex inheritance.

References

1. Cooper ND, Schmidtke J. Molecular genetic approaches to the analysis and diagnosis of human inherited disease: an overview. Ann Med 1992; 24:29–42.
2. Cookson WOCM, Hopkin JM. Dominant inheritance of atopic immunoglobulin E responsiveness. Lancet 1988; i:86–88.
3. Mather K, Jinks JL. Biometrical Genetics. 3d ed. London: Chapman & Hall, 1982.
4. Morton NE. Genetic studies of asthma and allergy: statistical methods. In: Blumenthal MN, Bjorksten B, eds. Genetics of Asthma and Allergy. New York: Marcel Dekker, 1995.
5. Meyers DA. Family analysis and genetic counselling for allergic diseases. In: Marsh DG and Blumenthal MN, eds. Genetic and Environmental Factors in Clinical Allergy. Minneapolis: University of Minnesota Press, 1990:161–173.
6. Lockart A. What is bronchial asthma? The role of genetic and acquired factors. In: Marsh DG, Lockhart A, Holgate ST, eds. The Genetics of Asthma. Oxford: Blackwell 1993:3–14.
7. Lawrence S, Beasley R, Doull I, et al. Genetic analysis of atopy and asthma as quantitative traits and ordered polychotomies. Ann Hum Genet 58:359–368.
8. Bonney G. On the statistical determination of major gene mechanisms in continuous human traits: regressive models. Am J Med Genet 1984; 18:731–749.
9. Rao DC, Morton NE, Gottesman II, Lew R. Path analysis of qualitative data on pairs of relatives: application to schizophrenia. Hum Hered 1981; 31:325–333.
10. Cooke RA, Vander Veer A. Human sensitization. J Immunol 1916; 1:201–305.
11. Marsh DG, Meyers DA, Bias WB. The epidemiology and genetics of atopic allergy. N Engl J Med 1981; 305:1551–1559.
12. Cookson W, Sharp P, Faux J, Hopkin J. Linkage between immunoglobulin E responses underlying asthma and rhinitis and chromosome 11q. Lancet 1989; i:1292–1295.
13. MacLean CJ, Morton NE, Yee S. Combined analysis of genetic segregation and linkage under an oligogenic model. Comput Biomed Res 1984; 17:471–480.
14. Ott J. Recent developments in the theoretical aspects of linkage analysis. In: Majunder PP, ed. Human Population Genetics. New York: Plenum, 1993: 165–179.
15. Morton NE, Shields DC, Collins A. Genetic analysis of complex phenotypes. Ann Hum Genet 1991; 55:301–314.
16. Merette C, Lehner T, Ott J. Two new approaches toward linkage heterogeneity of FAD: two-locus models and age of onset as a discriminator. Genet Epidemiol 1993; 10:455–459.
17. Lalouel JM, Morton NE. Complex segregation analysis with pointers. Hum Hered 1981; 31:12–21.
18. Meyers DA. Genetics of atopic allergy: family studies of total serum IgE levels. In: Marsh DG, Lockart A, Holgate ST, eds. The Genetics of Asthma. Oxford: Blackwell, 1993:153–158.

19. Morton NE, Wu D. Alternative bioassays of kinship between loci. Am J Hum Genet 1988; 42:173–177.
20. Marsh DG. Genetic and molecular analysis of human immune responsiveness to allergens. In: Marsh DG, Lockart A, Holgate ST, eds. The Genetics of Asthma. Oxford: Blackwell, 1993:201–214.
21. Rosenwasser LJ, Eisenberg S, Dresback J, Klemm DK, Borish L. Transcriptional regulation of human IL-4 (abstr). J Allergy Clin Immunol 1994:599.
22. Shirakawa T, Li A, Dubowitz M, et al. Association between atopy and the variants of the β subunit of the high-affinity immunoglobulin E receptor. Nature Genet 1995; 7:125–130.
23. Wilson AF, Elston RC. Statistical validity of the Haseman-Elston sib pair test in small samples. Genet Epidemiol 1993; 10:593–598.
24. Haseman JK, Elston RC. The investigation of linkage between a quantitative trait and a marker locus. Behav Genet 1972; 2:1–19.
25. Young RP, Lathrop GM, Cookson WOCM, Hopkin JM. Confirmation of genetic linkage between atopic IgE response and chromosome 11q13. J Med Genet 1992; 29: 236–238.
26. Hopkin JM, Cookson WOCM, Young RP. Atopy, asthma, and genetic linkage. Ann NY Acad Sci 1991; 629:26–30.
27. Moffatt MF, Sharp PA, Faux JA, Young RP, Cookson WOCM, Hopkin JM. Factors confounding genetic linkage between atopy and chromosome 11q. Clin Exp Allergy 1992; 22:1046–1051.
28. Lander ES, Lincoln SE. The appropriate threshold for declaring linkage when allowing sex-specific recombination rates. Am J Hum Genet 1988; 43:396–400.
29. Inacio F, Perichon B, Desvaux FX, David B, Petre G, Krishnamoorthy R. Genetic transmission study of grass pollen sensitivity in 17 Portuguese families. J Allergy Clin Immunol 1991; 87:204.
30. Amelung PJ, Panhuysen CIM, Postma DS, et al. Atopy and bronchial hyperresponsiveness: exclusion of linkage to markers on chromosomes 11q and 6p. Clin Exp Allergy 1992; 22:1077–1084.
31. Hizawa N, Yamaguchi E, Ohe M, et al. Lack of linkage between atopy and locus 11q13. Clin Exp Allergy 1992; 22:1065–1069.
32. Rich SS, Roitman-Johnson B, Greenberg B, Roberts S, Blumenthal MN. Genetic analysis of atopy in three large kindreds: no evidence of linkage to D11S97. Clin Exp Allergy 1992; 22:1070–1076.
33. Lympany P, Welsh KI, Cochrane GM, Kemeny DM, Lee TH. Genetic analysis of the linkage between chromosome 11q and atopy. Clin Exp Allergy 1992; 22:1085–1092.
34. Coleman R, Trembath RC, Harper JI. Chromosome 11q13 and atopy underlying atopic eczema. Lancet 1993; 341:1121–1122.
35. Brereton HM, Ruffin RE, Thompson PJ, Turner DR. Familial atopy in Australian pedigrees. Adventitious linkage to chromosome 8 is not confirmed, nor is there evidence of linkage to the high-affinity IgE receptor. Clin Exp Allergy 1994; in press.
36. Neely JD, Breazeale D, Schou C, Freidhoff LR, Beaty T, Marsh DG. Sib-pair analysis of total and specific IgE and DNA polymorphisms on chromosome 11q13 in the Amish (abstr). J Allergy Clin Immunol 1994:344. In press.

37. Shirakawa T, Morimoto K, Hashimoto T, Furuyama J, Yamamoto M, Takai S. Linkage between IgE responses underlying asthma and rhinitis (atopy) and chromosome 11q in Japanese families. Cytogenet Cell Genet 1991; 58:1070.

38. Collee JM, ten Kate LP, de Vries HG, Kliphuis JW, Bouman K, Scheffer H. Allele sharing on chromosome 11q13 in sibs with asthma and atopy. Lancet 1993; 342:936.

39. Sandford AJ, Shirakawa T, Moffatt MF, et al. Localization of atopy and β subunit of high-affinity IgE receptor (FceR1) on chromosome 11q. Lancet 1993; 341:332–334.

40. Dizier MH, Hill M, James A, et al. Genetic control of basal IgE level after accounting for specific atopy. Genet Epidemiol 1993; 10:333–334.

41. Wright S. Evolution and the Genetics of Populations. Vol. 1. Genetic and Biometric Foundations. Chicago: University of Chicago Press, 1968:411–417.

42. Marsh DG, Neely JD, Breazeale DR, et al. Linkage analysis of IL4 and other chromosome 5q31.1 markers and total serum immunoglobulin E concentrations. Science 1994; 264:1152–1156.

43. Cookson WOCM, Young RP, Sandford AJ, et al. Maternal inheritance of atopic IgE responsiveness on chromosome 11q. Lancet 1992; 340:381–384.

44. Billewicz WZ, McGregor IA, Roberts DF, Wilson RJM. Family studies in immunoglobulin levels. Clin Exp Immunol 1979; 16:13–22.

45. Falconer DS. The inheritance of liability to certain diseases, estimated from the incidence among relatives. Ann Hum Genet 1965; 29:51–76.

46. Marriott FHC. A Dictionary of Statistical Terms, 5th ed. Singapore: Longman, 1990.

47. Collins A, Lawrence S, Morton NE. Linkage and association between a quantitative trait and a marker locus. In preparation, 1994.

48. Go RCP, Elston RC, Kaplan EB. Efficiency and robustness of pedigree segregation analysis. Am J Hum Genet 1978; 30:28–37.

49. Blumenthal MN, Namboodiri K, Mendell N, Gleich G, Elston RC, Yunis E. Genetic transmission of IgE levels. Am J Med Genet 1981; 10:219–228.

50. Hasstedt SJ, Meyers DA, Marsh DG. Inheritance of immunoglobulin E: genetic model fitting. Am J Med Genet 1983; 14:61–66.

51. Borecki IB, Rao DC, Lalouel JM, McGue M, Gerrard JW. Demonstration of a common major gene with pleiotropic effects on immunoglobulin E levels and allergy. Genet Epidemiol 1985; 2:327–338.

52. Bazaral M, Orgel HA, Hamburger RN. Genetics of IgE and allergy: serum IgE levels in twins. J Allergy Clin Immunol 1974; 54:288–304.

53. Gerrard JW, Rao DC, Morton NE. A genetic study of immunoglobulin E. Am J Hum Genet 1978; 30:46–58.

Part Four

GENETIC STUDIES OF ATOPY AND ASTHMA

17

Genetic Epidemiology of Asthma

STEPHEN S. RICH

Bowman Gray School of Medicine
Winston-Salem, North Carolina

I. Introduction

Asthma is a common clinical disorder characterized by reversible obstruction of the bronchial airways which is an increasingly serious cause of morbidity and mortality in the general U.S. population. Asthma is defined by a spectrum of clinical findings—the presence of a clinical history of coughing, wheezing, and shortness of breath that is intermittent in occurrence; the presence of expiratory wheezes that is episodic; and pulmonary function less than 80% of predicted (based on FEV1 and FEV1/FVC ratio) that is reversed by at least 20% after use of bronchodilators (airflow reversibility). The prevalence of asthma in the population is estimated to range from 3% to 5%, with both sexes equally affected, and African Americans more commonly affected than other ethnic groups. The presence of a genetic component to the susceptibility of asthma has been suggested from evidence of twin, family, and population studies.

Based on the accumulated data, multiple cell types and numerous cellular control mechanisms influence the development of asthma and its response to treatment. Both complex phenotypes (asthma) and intermediate phenotypes (atopy, specific immune responses, serum IgE levels, mediator release, bronchial hyperreactivity) have been used to investigate genetic susceptibility of the observed clinical syndrome of asthma. A central hypothesis is that alleles at multiple single loci are involved in the complex etiology of asthma, either directly (in which asthma is defined as a complex phenotype) or by their action on intermediate phenotypes (where the intermediate phenotypes are each associated with the clinical syndrome).

In the sections that follow, some of the literature concerning the genetics of asthma and its intermediate phenotypes are reviewed. Later sections review the data concerning the genetic influence on serum IgE levels, mediator releasibility, bronchial hyperreactivity, inflammation, asthma, and atopic asthma. Issues related to analytical/statistical concerns are addressed with respect to specific human (patient) resources. Finally, issues relating to data collection and study implementation are discussed.

II. Evidence for Genes

A. Twin Studies

The development of asthma is complex and likely to be a function of genetic susceptibility and environmental exposure. Genetic predisposition has been most clearly demonstrated by a series of twin studies. Using the Swedish twin register [1], a series of 7000 same-sex twin pairs identified over a 40-year period were evaluated with respect to asthma and related symptoms. While the classification of disease was based on a self-administered questionnaire, there was excellent agreement with physician diagnosis for asthma (95%) and hay fever (85%). The prevalence of asthma in the series was 3.8% (3.5% in males, 4.0% in females), and the prevalence of hay fever was 14.8% (15.5% in males, 14.2% in females). Concordance for asthma in monozygotic (MZ) twins was 19.0%, while the concordance in dizygotic twins was 4.8%, consistent with a strong familial (genetic) regulation of asthma. Concordance for hay fever in MZ twins was 21.4%, while the concordance in DZ twins was 13.6%, again consistent with a genetic effect.

A more recent twin study [2] evaluated concordance for asthma/wheezing and hay fever by path analytic methods. Among 3808 pairs of twins from the Australian National Health and Medical Research Council Twin Registry, the cumulative prevalence of asthma or wheezing was 13.2% and of hay fever, 32%, significantly higher than that in the Swedish study. The disease correlation was higher in MZ twin pair ($r = 0.65$) than in DZ pairs ($r = 0.25$); further, the correlation was higher in male MZ twins ($r = 0.75$) compared with female MZ twins ($r = 0.60$). These results are consistent with a genetic factor common to asthma and hay fever. As the twin concordance rates (and the genetic correlation) were less than 100% in both studies, it is clear that both environmental factors and genetic factors must exist which influence susceptibility.

B. Family Studies

Increased rates of asthma in family members of index cases, contrasted to that observed in the general population, are consistent with genetic factors. Family histories relating to asthma were examined in 77 asthmatic and 87 control children, aged between 1 and 12 years [3]. In this study, asthma was defined by the occurrence of wheezy episodes in response to allergens, exercise, or emotion, as well as with symptoms that suggested respiratory infection. The perception of children with at least one asthmatic relative was significantly greater in the asthmatic probands than in the controls; and asthma was more prevalent in the relatives of asthmatic probands than in the relatives of controls. When the histories were partitioned into extrinsic and intrinsic asthma [4], among the relatives of control children, neither the prevalence of asthma nor the atopic status of the asthmatic relatives was influenced by the atopic status of the proband. These findings have been interpreted as supporting the hypothesis that asthma and atopy are inherited independently.

III. Intermediate Phenotypes

Many studies indicate that the genetic control of bronchial asthma is complex. Two major areas of investigation have centered on (1) the components of bronchial asthma and (2) the clinical picture of atopy as a complete clinical entity. The components of bronchial asthma have been more difficult to carry out in a family study setting, since the appropriate clinical measurements often require invasive techniques. On the other hand, studies of atopy can evaluate the immune response to aeroallergens by use of twin, case-control, and family studies. These investigations often center on the determination of associations between specific HLA-D region genotypes and atopy.

A. Atopy

Atopy is thought to be a major component of asthma and, therefore, serves as an intermediate phenotype of asthma. Atopy, defined as a type of hypersensitivity peculiar to humans, appears to have a hereditary influence and present as the characteristic whealing reaction. Atopy further has circulating antibodies and manifests clinical symptoms such as asthma and hay fever. Most patients with atopic allergy are characterized by long-term increased levels of IgE in response to minimal amounts of allergen leading to immediate or type I hypersensitivity. In subjects without atopy, the failure of antigens to produce this rise in IgE may be the result of genetically determined susceptibility or resistance, a different threshold of reactivity (increased amounts of antigen required to elicit a response), or reactivity rapidly replace by tolerance. Most of the features of atopic diseases, however, can be traced to the presence of allergen-specific IgE and the release of inflammatory mediators by cell-bound IgE in patients exposed to an allergen [5].

Complex phenotypes of atopy with respect to their genetic and environmental determinants have been the subject of numerous reports. Earlier studies centered on the relationship between asthma and rhinitis and their association with genes of the human MHC complex. Initial studies of asthmatic cases and controls did not demonstrate any evidence of association between the bronchial asthma and alleles at either HLA class I (A, B, C) or class II (DR) loci. Using family studies, extended HLA-region haplotypes in patients with ragweed pollen allergy (with and without asthma) and in nonatopic controls were contrasted [6]. The mean level of antibodies to a specific allergen, *Amb a* V, was significantly higher in the asthmatic patients than in the allergic patients; further, the HLA haplotype containing the B7, SC31, DR2 haplotype occurred almost exclusively among the patients with IgE anti-*Amb a* V, and the frequency of this haplotype was significantly elevated in patients with asthma. In contrast, the HLA haplotype containing B8, SC01, DR3 was significantly increased in frequency among patients with rhinitis only and patients with minimal IgE anti-*Amb a* V levels. Other families, however, failed to demonstrate a consistent segregation of an HLA haplotype with asthma or rhinitis, thus providing further evidence in favor of a genetically heterogeneous determination of the atopy and its contribution to asthma.

In some populations, the atopy phenotype and its transmission in families have suggested a dominant mode of inheritance [7]. Using this definition, a linkage of atopy with a genetic marker on human chromosome 11 has been reported [8]. The definition of atopy in this analysis included an elevated serum IgE level and/or an elevated specific IgE level as measured by RAST or skin test. On the other hand, several authors found no evidence for linkage in other populations using the same genetic model. Although linkage of atopy to D11S97 could not be confirmed, it remains possible that loci in the region have a contribution to the phenotype in some, but not all, populations.

One interpretation of the immunologic data suggests that the upregulation of IgE synthesis in atopy may be due to the induction of IgE isotype utilization at the DNA level in B cells, rather than to a selective effect on the proliferation of B cells which have already rearranged the IgE heavy-chain sequence [9]. In vivo, IgE response to most allergens is characterized by exposure to extremely low doses of sensitizing antigen. For example, seasonal dosages of inhaled ragweed pollen are on the order of 1 μg over a 6–8 week pollen season [10]. A number of studies have demonstrated that common aeroallergens are composed of multiple components that can be recognized by the IgE and IgG present in the sera of some, but not all, patients [11–13]. Further, each component is likely to have multiple epitopes that can be recognized by B cells. Thus, heterogeneity between patients in response to allergen components likely reflects heterogeneity at the component (epitope) level. This heterogeneity is likely to be a function of genetic factors which are expressed only under certain environmental (exposure) conditions.

B. Specific Immune Response

It has been previously demonstrated that the IgE response to complex antigens (such as *Amb a* I) aggregates in families with moderate heritability. *Amb a* I (antigen E, or AgE) is a 37,800-Da fraction of short ragweed. In several studies, there has been no consistent association of responsiveness to this allergen with any specific HLA antigen [14–16]. Using family data, however, others found that there was significant evidence in favor of linkage of an HLA-linked susceptibility locus ($\theta_m = 0.104$, $\theta_f = 0.5$, lod score = 3.58) in two large pedigrees [17].

Studies using simple purified allergens have supported the hypothesis that one gene that controls the immune response to allergens may reside in the HLA region [18–20]. As indicated previously, much research has centered on the atopic immune response to the purified short ragweed allergen *Amb a* V [6,21]. *Amb a* V is considered a "minor" allergen with molecular weight 5 kDa, to which approximately 10% of ragweed-allergic subjects respond. Although associations between the IgE response to *Amb a* V and HLA-DR2 and HLA-Dw2 was reported [14], many ragweed-sensitive HLA-DR2-positive individuals do not appear to have any significant IgE or IgG *Amb a* V response. There are also patients who do not have the HLA-DR2 allele, yet have a high *Amb a* V response. These studies therefore suggest that factors in addition to the genes in the human MHC region are important to the *Amb a* V response.

The specific immune response in atopy is dependent on a varieyt of different steps leading to the final clinical syndrome. Although much of the interest in the genetic basis of the immune response to specific allergens has focused on genes in the human MHC, studies of elevated IgE levels in response to exposure have also implicated control by HLA genes (*Lol* I, II, and III responses that occur primarily in patients who are HLA-DR3 positive). Increased levels of IgE in response to *Amb a* VI have been associated with HLA-DR5. In order to determine whether specific mutations in the HLA genes are responsible for the differential response, DNA sequencing methods were used. HLA-DRB and DQB genes were sequenced in *Amb a* V-sensitive allergic patients, seven of whom were HLA-DR2 positive; no novel HLA-DRB or -DQB sequences were observed [22]. Although strong associations between IgE response and specific allergens remain with HLA class II genes, there has been no evidence that the presence of specific novel sequences provides susceptibility which is genetically transmitted.

C. Mediator Release

The interaction of IgE with cells and their ability to release mediating substances has not been studied extensively. In a collection of families, histamine releasibility from basophils in response to anti-IgE was investigated, and evidence for a 55–70% heritability was found, independent of serum IgE levels. In children, plasma histamine levels were shown to be normally high at young age and decrease with increasing age [23]; however, atopic children had higher levels than normal children, and there was a significant correlation between plasma histamine levels in atopic children, but not in normal children. Nevertheless, IgE-dependent basophilic histamine release has not been clearly established as being under genetic control in asthma.

Suspensions of leukocytes from patients with allergic and nonallergic asthma were stimulated with Con A and anti-IgE [24]. The basophilic histamine release was greater in asthma patients as compared with normal controls; however, the release to the calcium ionophore A23187 was similar in normal controls and asthmatic patients. These results suggest that basophilic histamine release correlates with disease in an IgE-dependent process. Confirmatory evidence was provided by the existence of a correlation between the provocative dose of inhaled histamine required to produce a reduction in FEV1, the leukocyte histamine release to Con A and to anti-IgE.

A twin study [25] was used to estimate correlations in histamine release from basophils in response to anti-IgE, f-met peptide, and the calcium ionophore A23187. The correlation among MZ twins was significantly greater than among DZ twins for anti-IgE and A23187, but not for f-met peptide. These data suggest that anti-IgE release and calcium ionophore release of histamine are determined in part by genetic factors, while genes likely have little effect on the release of histamine from f-met peptide. Further, the genetic factors which contribute to IgE-mediated release of histamine appeared to be independent of serum IgE levels. Thus, there is potential for genetic factors contributing to IgE-mediated release of inflammatory mediators from mast cell basophils.

D. Bronchial Hyperresponsiveness

Familial factors have been reported to be involved in the development of bronchial hyperresponsiveness, defined principally as bronchial response to methacholine inhalation challenge. An early study compared the methacholine response in normal individuals from families with a history of asthma and normal (control) families [26]. When the response was plotted with respect to family history, two normal distributions were apparent in nonatopic individuals with a family history of asthma, while one distribution appeared in nonatopic individuals without a family history of asthma. The presence of a bimodal distribution for methacholine response is suggestive of a major gene responsible for this measure of bronchial hyperresponsiveness. Bronchial response to methacholine challenge was measured in families in which there was a proband with asthma and in families without a history of atopic disease. The data, after segregation analysis, indicated that pure environmental models could be rejected and that a familial component to the transmission of the bronchial response to methacholine existed [27]. There was no evidence, however, that the observed bimodal response in individuals with a family history of asthma is due to a single major gene.

In a separate study, asthma patients, healthy parents of children with asthma, and normal controls were given carbachol in order to measure bronchial reactivity [28]. Bronchial reactivity index values considered to be in the "asthmatic range" occurred in 10% of controls, in 50% of parents of asthmatic children, and in 100% of currently asthmatic patients. Although bronchial reactivity patterns appear to be consistent with a genetic effect, there was no relationship between bronchial reactivity and serum IgE levels, consistent with the hypothesis of separate genetic control of hyperresponsivity and hyperproduction of IgE.

Recent evidence also supports a role for genetic factors in bronchial hyperreactivity. A study of second-generation Polynesian migrant children, aged 5 to 15 years, used methacholine as an instigator of bronchial hyperreactivity [29]. Bronchial hyperreactivity was present in 25.3% of children tested, while atopy was present in 32% of children. Bronchial hyperreactivity associated with atopy was influenced by a family history of asthma (50% in those with a family history; 34% in those without a family history). Thus, the differences in the frequency of bronchial hyperreactivity and atopy with family history of asthma indicated distinct heterogeneity in the pathogenesis of bronchial hyperreactivity, atopy, and asthma.

E. Inflammation/Cell-Mediated Immune Response

Regulation of IgE synthesis has been shown to be mediated by T cells and T-cell-derived lymphokines. T-cell-derived lymphokines, such as IL-4, IL-5, IFN-α, and IFN-γ, play an important role in the regulation of IgE synthesis. The inflammatory response appears to be a major component in the development of asthma. The role of genetic factors and the relationship among asthma, atopy, hyperreactive airways, and inflammation is not well established, however. Many of the histological and physiological features of asthma are compatible with a mast cell and eosinophil-mediated inflammatory response influenced by T cells. Eosinophilia is a common finding in allergic asthma and may produce many of the mediators responsible for the abnormal airway function in asthma. Mast cells are thought to be the effector cells of the early asthmatic reaction, releasing histamine, neutral proteases, products of arachidonic acid metabolism, as well as products of the 5-lipoxygenase pathway after IgE-mediated activation. Cytokines may also be released, including IL-3, IL-4, IL-5, and GM-CSF. These factors, supplemented by other inflammatory mediators, may serve to perpetuate inflammation and contribute to the development of the late-phase reaction. Increased numbers of T cells that express activation markers are present in the airways and, through the cytokines that they release, may direct the influx of inflammatory cells.

Studies of cloned murine T cells have shown that the helper cells can be divided into two populations that are characterized by their cytokine secretion profile. TH1 clones secrete interferon, GM-CSF, and IL-2. TH2 clones secrete IL-4, IL-5, and IL-6 [30]. Support for an association between IgE secretion and preferential activation of a TH2-like helper T-cell response has been established in humans [31,32]. CD4-positive helper T-cell clones specific for antigens of the house dust mite (*D. pteronyssinus*) were derived from two atopic IgE responders and from one nonatopic subject. In response to a crude extract of dust mite proteins presented by autologous monocytes, all of the dust mite-specific clones from the two atopic subjects secreted significantly increased amounts of IL-4 and undetectable amounts of interferon-gamma; in contrast, all of the dust mite-specific clones from the nonatopic subject produced little or no IL-4 and high levels of interferon-gamma. As a control, clones responsive to tetanus toxoid and candida antigens from an atopic individual secreted high levels of interferon-gamma but no IL-4, indicating that secretion of IL-4 was possibly specific to dust mite and not a general phenomenon for previously encountered antigens.

In both mouse and human systems, it has been shown that IL-4 promotes the synthesis of IgE by B cells, and that the lymphokines IFN-α and IFN-γ reverse the IL-4-mediated IgE syntheses [33–36]. From in-vitro experiments, it is clear that T-cell-derived lymphokines are important in regulating B-cell function. In particular, IL-4 is important because it promotes switching of B cells to expression of IgE synthesis, induces upregulation of B-cell surface CD23 expression, and induces the synthesis of sCD23, which can act to promote B-cell growth. Both IFN-α and IFN-γ can reverse each of these IL-4-mediated events. Bronchoalveolar-lavage fluid from atopic asthma patients have more cells that are positive for mRNA for IL-2, IL-3, IL-4, IL-5, and GM-CSF when compared with cells from normal controls [37], while there was no significant difference in the number of cells expressing mRNA for IFN-γ. This pattern of cytokine profile is compatible with activation of TH2 cones; thus, these regulatory T-cell activities could lead to overproduction of IgE in responses to specific allergens.

F. Serum IgE Level

The genetic mechanism for IgE production has yet to be completely resolved, although several reports suggest a major locus with major gene action [38–41]. Using twins reared together and twins reared apart, it has been shown that total IgE levels have moderate heritability [42]. A reduced model that excluded a genetic effect resulted in a very poor fit, indicating the need for a genetic component (although not necessarily a major gene) to explain IgE-level similarity in twins. There was no significant difference between the similarity in IgE levels in twins reared together and twins reared apart, indicating that familial (common) environmental effects were not critical in determining phenotypic variability. Thus, the accumulated data suggest that a significant genetic component (with 56% heritability) regulates IgE levels.

Several investigators have reported evidence indicating a recessive regulatory locus where an individual with the homozygous recessive genotype has persistently elevated levels of IgE. Based on an earlier hypothesis relating IgE production and genetic liability [43], bivariate segregation analysis of IgE levels and allergy was performed on 173 nuclear families [39]. Using the quantitative family data, the results indicated that an IgE regulatory locus contributed to the familial transmission of allergy, although the mode of inheritance was not clear. In a later study [44], the geometric mean of serum IgE in 363 nonatopic children increased with age. Higher mean values of serum IgE were found for children with a family history of allergy than for children without a history of allergy. Although the mean serum IgE level increased with the degree of air pollution in the living area, the influence of air pollution was smaller than the influence of family history of allergy on the mean values of serum IgE. Thus, genetic factors which influence IgE clearly interact with those factors which control allergy and asthma.

Using segregation analyses, basal total serum IgE levels was investigated in individuals from 42 randomly ascertained nuclear families [45]. The data were analyzed using regressive models, incorporating age, sex, and skin-test responsiveness as covariates. The best-fitting model was one of recessive inheritance of high IgE levels. These results suggest that there may be a rare allele for very low total serum IgE levels that can be detected even after a measurement of allergic responsiveness (skin-test results) is considered as a covariate. From this result, a major gene for basal IgE levels may be independent of any loci controlling atopy, so a search for an IgE locus may not discover an HLA-linked gene.

Recently, sib-pair analysis of 170 individuals from 11 Amish families revealed evidence for linkage of five markers in chromosome 5q31.1 with a gene controlling total serum immunoglobulin E (IgE) concentration [46]. Although no linkage was found between markers in 5q31.1 and specific IgE antibody concentrations, analysis of total IgE within IgE antibody-negative sib pairs suggested linkage to a region that includes IL-4. These analyses suggest that IL-4 or a gene in the 5q31.1 region may regulate basal (nonspecific to allergen) IgE level.

G. Summary

Asthma is a condition in which genetic factors have been shown to play a significant role; genetic factors also play a role in the development of a specific immune response to aeroallergens, IgE production, release of mediators, and the development of a hyperreactive airway. The genetic basis of asthma and its intermediate phenotypes remains unresolved. Whether genes that control basal physiologic responses are important in asthma susceptibility is unclear; however, identification of these genes and their function will facilitate new treatment protocols and will lead to an understanding of the interaction which exists between genes and environment which are relevant to asthma.

IV. Atopic Asthma

The role of specific candidate genes in asthma susceptibility has been equivocal. Older studies have suggested that there were associations between asthma and various HLA antigens; however, these reports could not be reproduced. The phenotype of mite-sensitive allergic asthma has been recently investigated, with an association between the IgE response to *Der p* I and bronchial asthma reported [47]. Studies in two populations [48,49] suggested that specific MHC class II haplotypes segregate with the occurrence of mite-sensitive allergic asthma. In the first study, an affected sib-pair method was used to demonstrate that a significant excess in HLA haplotype sharing occurred in the allergic asthma sib pairs (consistent with linkage of a genetic susceptibility factor to HLA) but not in the intrinsic asthma sib pairs. In the second study, there was a significant decrease of the DPB1*0401 allele in patients with allergic asthma a compared to nonasthmatic controls. These results suggest the presence of an MHC-linked recessive locus that controls the specific-IgE responsiveness to mite allergens and conferring susceptibility to allergic asthma. While the IgE response to specific allergens and atopic asthma may have important HLA-mediated determinants on 6p21.3, the nonspecific IgE response that appears to be near IL-4 on 5q31.1 indicates that many genes spread through the genome may contribute in substantial, and perhaps additive, fashion to asthma genetic susceptibility.

V. Environmental Issues in Asthma

The development of asthma and atopic disease depend on the interaction of genes with an environmental exposure. Genetic factors regulate the specific immune response as well as the IgE responses, mediator release, and end organ response. Clearly, environmental factors influence the clinical outcome and, although not discussed here, complicate the genetic analysis. The most consistent risk factors for asthma include allergen exposure, infection, smoke exposure, temporal exposure, pharmacological agents, air pollution, and occupation. In addition, the intermediate phenotypes of asthma, such as IgE levels, may vary with age and sex, so that recognition of these factors and their influence on the asthma is required in the genetic analysis of molecular markers in ascertained pedigrees. Two of these "environmental" complications, age and time, are addressed briefly.

A. Age

IgE levels at birth are either undetectable or very low, rising rapidly during the first two to three years of life and peaking at puberty [50]. The IgE levels appear to rise more rapidly and to much higher levels in atopic subjects, indicating that atopy plays a role in the increase of IgE. After puberty, levels in the nonatopic individual (already low) remain low and constant over time. In contrast, the IgE levels in the atopic subject begin a slow and steady decline over time. IgE levels begin to decline more rapidly after age 50. Thus, the risk of developing an atopic condition after age 50 (hay fever, bronchial asthma, eczema) or having evidence of specific IgE directed toward an allergen by skin test or RAST decreases to small levels. The sex ratio observed for asthma tends to differ by age. Boys less than 10 years develop asthma and eczema nearly twice as often as girls. Serum IgE levels appear to be higher in males as compared to females at all ages, although when smoking is removed from the analyses (as a covariate), the levels appear to be nearly identical.

B. Time

The time of day, month, and year may influence the atopic and asthmatic condition. It also appears that rhythms for peak flow rates, serum total and specific IgE levels, histamine releasibility, and allergen-specific skin reactivity occur [51]. Thus, a complete medical and exposure history needs to be evaluated when studying family members with respect to asthma and associated (intermediate) phenotypes.

VI. Analytic Issues

Because asthma is a complex genetic disease, any statistical analysis strategy is necessarily more complicated than would be required for mapping a simple Mendelian disorder such as cystic fibrosis or neurofibromatosis. An optimal strategy would include both likelihood-based and nonparametric methods of analysis. Likelihood-based methods offer the advantages of statistical efficiency when the genetic model is known [52] and allow estimation of genetic parameters, including the recombination fraction. Several likelihood-based methods would be appropriate: pairwise linkage analysis for each marker with asthma, multipoint linkage analysis given multiple markers in the region of a putative disease gene, and two-trait-locus methods of linkage analysis. Nonparametric methods of linkage analysis are attractive for mapping complex diseases because they do not require specification of the mode of inheritance. Since the mode of inheritance of asthma is unknown, several nonparametric methods of linkage analysis, including affected sib-pair methods and the affected pedigree member (APM) method [53], may be applied. Finally, other methods (association analysis) can be used to augment these procedures for a gene search.

A. Likelihood Methods

Traditional likelihood-based methods of linkage analysis require specification of a genetic model for the disease. For asthma, the mode of inheritance is unknown, and likely involves multiple genes and environmental factors. Hence, care must be taken in the choice of the (incorrect) models to be used for lod score analysis. A significant concern is that models should be used that have reasonable power to detect linkage even when the mode of inheritance is misspecified.

In the initial linkage analysis, a generalized one-locus, two-allele disease model can be used to test for linkage for asthma for each marker. The parameters of the disease model are the frequency q of the disease susceptibility allele D, and the three genotype-specific penetrances $f(DD)$, $f(Dd)$, and $f(dd)$. Based on a methacholine challenge (for example) as a gold standard of diagnosis, one approach is to make all three disease penetrances low, since there will be greater confidence in the diagnosis of presence of asthma than of no disease; the result is that unaffected individuals will provide relatively little information on the putative disease locus, but still will provide information on the genetic marker. Since correct specification of degree of dominance—that is, whether the disease locus is dominant-acting or recessive-acting—has been shown to have a critical effect on the power to detect linkage [54], two genetic models, a dominant model in which $f(DD) = f(Dd) > f(dd)$, and a recessive model in which $f(DD) > f(Dd) = f(dd)$, can be used. Because other genes and environmental factors almost certainly play a role, the penetrances for the non-disease-susceptibility genotypes can be chosen to be greater than zero and the gene frequency q to be relatively large—say, 25% for the recessive model and 5% for the dominant model. These assumptions allow for sporadic cases and provide alternative explanations for apparent recombinants. The allowance for recombinants is critical, since even a few meioses incorrectly scored as recombinants substantially reduce the evidence for linkage [55].

Once evidence for linkage is obtained in the pairwise analysis, additional markers in the region will be typed for multipoint mapping by the method of location scores [56]. Having information on multiple linked markers can make essentially every meiosis informative for a linked marker, and has the potential to define more precisely the location of the putative disease gene by identifying flanking markers. For the multipoint analysis, one strategy is to continue to employ the same dominant and recessive models described above, since it has been demonstrated that multilocus linkage analysis using these models is robust to a variety of complicating factors, including genetic heterogeneity, epistasis, and phenocopies [57]. As evidence for linkage is obtained with one or more markers/ regions, combined segregation and linkage analysis maximizing the lod score as a function both of the recombination fraction(s) and the genetic model parameters can be used. This approach, under some circumstances, can minimize the problems of ascertainment bias that would be faced in a standard segregation analysis [58].

Once two or more markers/regions have been identified, the combination of likelihood-based and nonparametric-method linkage analysis can be used to attempt to map pairs of trait loci simultaneously. Models in which the trait is determined by two genetic loci ("two-trait-locus models") are a generalization of standard methods that assume a single trait locus, and should be appropriate for mapping complex traits such as asthma [59]. This strategy may be particularly useful for linkage mapping with large asthma pedigrees, pedigrees with bilineal inheritance, and families ascertained on the basis of multiple affected individuals, and may well demonstrate segregation at two or more asthma loci simultaneously. Using information on two trait loci and two tightly linked markers simultaneously may provide more accurate information regarding genetic model using a two-trait-locus combined segregation and linkage analysis.

B. Model-Independent Methods

Nonparametric methods of linkage analysis are attractive for mapping complex diseases such as asthma because they do not require specification of mode of inheritance. Affected sib-pair (ASP) tests compare the proportion of genes shared identical by descent (IBD) at a marker locus to the distribution of 1/4:1/2:1/4 (IBD = 0:IBD = 1:IBD = 2) under the null hypothesis of no linkage. Linkage between the disease and marker results in an increase in the expected number of affected sib pairs sharing two marker alleles and in the mean number of marker alleles shared. Three ASP tests were evaluated [60], and it was shown that the test based on the mean number of marker alleles shared IBD (the mean test) provided a good overall test for linkage, while test based on the number of pairs sharing two alleles IBD (the two-allele test) was often more powerful for recessive-acting loci. It was also noted that multiple affected sib pairs can be constructed and used from sibships with more than two affected siblings. This allows the use of both sib-pair data and all affected sib pairs from pedigree data in the ASP analysis.

Because pedigree data include more than just affected sib pairs, the affected pedigree member (APM) method of linkage analysis [53] is an important tool. APM compares the numbers of alleles shared identical by state (IBS) at the marker locus to its null distribution under the hypothesis of no linkage, using a weighted sum calculated over all affected relative pairs in the pedigree. Linkage between the disease and marker results in an increase in the expected number of marker alleles shared IBS by most affected relative pairs. Weighting is done on the basis of marker allele frequencies, and is useful since the sharing of a rare marker allele by affected relatives, particularly distant ones, is more strongly suggestive of linkage than the sharing of a common allele.

C. Association Approach

Polymorphic genes that are involved in disease etiology or that are in linkage disequilibrium with such disease genes should demonstrate a population associa-tion with disease. Therefore, in parallel to the linkage analysis, a test for associa-tion between asthma and the genetic markers can be employed using allele frequencies for controls and asthma families and sib pairs. This approach recently has been used in identifying an association between familial Alzheimer's disease and apoCII on chromosome 19 [61]. Because of the well-known difficulties with association studies—large numbers of comparisons, and concern about issues of population stratification, even with an apparently well-chosen control group—apparently significant association results need to be interpreted with caution. The difficulties inherent in mapping complex diseases and the need to use multiple strategies is a convincing argument for including the association analysis as part of a mapping strategy, particularly since it requires no additional laboratory anal-yses. Association studies also can be used once evidence is obtained for the existence of an asthma susceptibility gene by linkage analysis. Given multiple tightly linked markers, the strength of the disease-marker associations can provide evidence regarding the location of an asthma susceptibility gene.

D. Summary

The statistical analysis of asthma is complex and can most generally be viewed as a multistage, integrated problem. A unified strategy that incorporates several complementary procedures can proceed in stages for each of the candidate genes and random (anonymous) genetic markers types. Prior to linkage analysis, allele frequency estimation and compatibility testing need to be carried out for the markers in the asthma family data. As necessary, most often for candidate genes, haplotype determination should be carried out for multiple markers detected by the same probe. Gene mapping initially can be performed with two-point methods for asthma and the genetic markers—likelihood-based linkage analysis using lod scores, affected sib-pair and APM linkage analysis, and association analysis. These methods have different strengths and weaknesses, and so a multistage attack is desirable. For chromosomal regions and candidate genes for which suggestive evidence of linkage is obtained, the second level of analysis would include multipoint linkage analysis using location scores, multipoint sib-pair and APM analysis and, given two or more regions/markers of interest, two-trait-locus linkage analysis. By employing both nonparametric and likelihood-based methods, the advantage of employing the strengths of each is gained. By beginning with two-point analyses and moving to multipoint analyses only when suggestive evidence of linkage is obtained, the efficiency of the analysis may be maximized. As with using multiple models, using multiple methods of analysis can increase the probability of falsely concluding linkage; however, since the results for the methods are likely to be highly correlated, a less stringent correction for multiple comparisons may be appropriate. Results obtained should be reported carefully, explicitly stating the different models and methods considered; obviously, any linkage results obtained will require confirmation before they are accepted.

VII. Study Implementation Issues

A number of issues arise prior to the implementation of a study of the genetics of asthma. These issues often revolve around the patient resources [individual clinical patients, sibling pairs, small (nuclear) families, large kindreds, or large pedigrees (such as those in the Amish or Hutterite colonies)]. In many respects, the analytic framework is dependent on the human resources available. In some instances, the families that are studies may have been patients for decades, thereby providing a longitudinal documentation of asthma, as well as clinical and laboratory information, on pedigree members now deceased, members currently with active asthma, members with asthma under remission, and members now demonstrating asthmatic symptoms for the first time. Other families will be presenting with asthma for the first time. Methods for incorporating longitudinal data with prevalence data and incidence data are not clear and need to be carefully developed. This is particularly true when information concerning the diagnosis of asthma is obtained from several sources.

A. Definition of Asthma

Each member of a genetics study will need to be classified as to whether they have asthma using an established set of rules. One approach is to categorize according to the recommendations of the International Consensus Report on Diagnosis and Management of Asthma. In this case, asthma can be defined as having: (1) clinical history of coughing, wheezing, and shortness of breath that is intermittent in nature; (2) physical examination revealing expiratory wheezes which vary in occurrence; (3) pulmonary function studies revealing a FEV1/FVC ratio and FEV1 less than 80% of predicted which reverses at least by 20% after use of bronchodilators and/or on different visits regardless of medication used. All members in all ascertained pedigrees will need to be classified; however, if not all members are local to the study, it may not be possible to evaluate clinically all family members to confirm the disease definition. The confirmation of disease is both time consuming and labor intensive; however, the work is required, since genetic analysis assumes that the phenotype is known without error. Misclassification of phenotype has the effect of mimicking recombination and lowering the evidence for linkage. Since asthma is heterogeneous and may present with signs and symptoms that vary widely between and without patients, the collection and careful documentation of multiple end points that may be important diagnostic indicators is critical to the identification of asthma susceptibility genes.

B. IgE Levels

The determination of the total IgE response to individual allergens as a percentage of the total IgE is difficult, since the allergen preparations are often ill defined, suffer from cross reactivity, and produce results at variance with the season and the relative amounts of allergen present. One approach is to quantitate the levels of IgE against a selected set of highly purified allergens—such as *Amb a* V (from ragweed) and *Der p* I (from mite)—both reported as immunodominant allergens in the case of atopic asthma. The immune response to allergens is not complete, indicating that the B-cell repertoire providing antibodies for defined specificity and affinity is incomplete. Hence, some individuals may recognize one or another epitope preferentially. As a means of reducing potential genetic heterogeneity, the pattern of allergen recognition in individual pedigree members in qualitative terms may need to be evaluated.

C. Historical Information

Historical information can be gathered using a standard questionnaire addressing symptoms, triggering factors, previous treatments, family history of related diseases, and environmental factors. It is important to review all records from previous studies of the families, medical records from hospitals (for the majority of the affected subjects and their relatives), and records obtained from other physicians who may have seen the patient. Issues regarding reliability of patient recall of symptoms, interpretation of questions, and patient report of physician diagnoses are all potential problems. Underreporting and overinterpretation of asthma and its symptoms are additional concerns that affect the genetic analyses.

VIII. Summary

Asthma is a common disorder whose prevalence in the population is estimated to range from 3% to 5%. The presence of a genetic component to the susceptibility of asthma has been suggested from a number of data sources and studies. Studies of the predictors of asthma need to address not only the genetic contributors but also the environmental contributors to the phenotype. It is clear that many in-vitro and in-vivo assay system results are dependent on environmental variables such as time of day and year at which the tests are performed, allergen exposure, and medication effects. Thus, for a complete genetic epidemiologic analysis of asthma susceptibility, an effort should be made to collect environmental exposure data for incorporation into models, stressing geographic locations, type of work (indoor/ outdoor/industrial), heating and cooling systems, smoking status, passive smoking status, and animals at home, in addition to the array of genetic data. For example, the levels of exposure to triggering factors may be determined by daily pollen and mold exposures during the appropriate season, mite exposure in the homes, and air pollution, but only in the presence of a susceptible genotype. These joint effects of genes and environmental exposures need to be addressed in an appropriate design in order to determine their importance and their influence on the appearance and severity of asthma and to allow a rationale approach to risk assessment and application of intervention measures.

Acknowledgments

This work was supported in part by National Institutes of Health grant HL49609.

References

1. Edfors-Bubs ML. Allergy in 7000 twin pairs. Acta Allergol 1971; 26:249–285.
2. Duffy DL, Martin NG, Battistutta D, Hopper JL, Mathews JD. Genetics of asthma and hay fever in Australian twins. Am Rev Respir Dis 1990.
3. Sibbald B, Horn ME, Gregg I. A family study of the genetic basis of asthma and wheezy bronchitis. Arch Dis Child 1980; 55:354–357.
4. Sibbald B, Horn ME, Brain EA, Gregg I. Genetic factors in childhood asthma. Thorax 1980; 35:671–674.
5. Ishizaka K, Ishizaka T. Human reaginic antibodies and immunoglobulin E. J Allergy 1968; 42:330–363.
6. Blumenthal MN, Awdeh Z, Alper C, Yunis E. Ra5 immune responses: HL-A antigens and complotypes. J Allergy Clin Immunol 1985; 75:155.
7. Cookson WOCM, Hopkin JM. Dominant inheritance of atopic immunoglobulin-E responsiveness. Lancet 1988; i:86–88.
8. Cookson WO, Sharp PA, Faux JA, Hopkin JM. Linkage between immunoglobulin E responses underlying asthma and rhinitis and chromosome 11q. Lancet 1989; 1: 1292–1295.
9. Finkelman FD, Holmes J, Katona IM, et al. Lymphokine control of in vivo immunoglobulin isotype selection. Annu Rev Immunol 1990; 8:303–334.
10. Marsh DG, Huang SK. Molecular genetics of human immune responsiveness to pollen allergens. Clin Exp Allergy 1991; 21:168–172.
11. Ishizaka K. Mechanisms of reaginic hypersensitivity. Clin Allergy 1971; 1:9–24.

12. Marsh DG. Molecular studies of human immune recognition of allergens. Allergy 1988; 43:7–9.

13. Ownby DR. Environmental factors versus genetic determinants of childhood inhalant allergies. J Allergy Clin Immunol 1990; 86:279–287.

14. Blumenthal MN, Amos DB, Noreen H, Mendell NR, Yunis EJ. Genetic mapping of Ir locus in man: linkage to second locus of HL-A. Science 1974; 184:1301–1303.

15. Marsh DG, Bias WB. Basal serum IgE levels and HLA antigen frequencies in allergic subjects. II. Studies in people sensitive to rye grass Group I and ragweed antigen E and of postulated immune response (Ir) locus in the HLA region. Immunogenetics 1977; 5:235–251.

16. Blumenthal MN, Yunis E, Gleich G, et al. Lack of association of the immune response to ragweed antigen E, Ra3 and Ra5 with the HLA system. J Immunogenet 1981; 8: 379–386.

17. Mendell NR, Blumenthal MN, Amos DB, Yunis EJ, Elston RC. Ragweed sensitivity: segregation analysis and linkage to HLA-B. Cytogenet Cell Genet 1978; 22:330–334.

18. Marsh DG, Hsu SH, Roebber M, et al. HLA-Dw2: a genetic marker for human immune response to short ragweed pollen allergen Ra5. I. Response resulting primarily from natural antigenic exposure. J Exp Med 1982; 155:1439–1451.

19. Goodfriend L, Choudhury AM, Klapper DG, et al. Ra5G, a homologue of Ra5 in giant ragweed pollen: isolation, HLA-DR-associated activity and amino acid sequence. Mol Immunol 1985; 22:899–906.

20. Freidhoff LR, Ehrlich-Kautzky E, Meyers DA, Ansari AA, Bias WB, Marsh DG. Association of HLA-DR3 with human immune response to Lol p I and Lol p II allergens in allergic subjects. Tissue Antigens 1988; 31:211–219.

21. Marsh DG, Meyers DA, Freidhoff LR. HLA-Dw2: a genetic marker for human response to short ragweed pollen allergen Ra5. II. Response after ragweed immunotherapy. J Exp Med 1982; 155:1452–1463.

22. Zwollo P, Ehrlich-Kautzky E, Scharf SJ, Ansari AA, Erlich HA, Marsh DG. Sequencing of HLA-D in responders and nonresponders to short ragweed allergen, Amb a V. Immunogenetics 1991; 33:141–151.

23. Fujisawa T, Komada M, Iguchi K, Uchida Y. Plasma histamine levels in normal and atopic children. Ann Allergy 1987; 59:303–306.

24. Gaddy JN, Busse WW. Enhanced IgE-dependent basophil histamine release and airway reactivity in asthma. Am Rev Respir Dis 1986; 134:969–974.

25. Marone G, Poto S, Celestino D, Bonini S. Human basophil releasability. III. Genetic control of human basophil releasability. J Immunol 1986; 137:3588–3592.

26. Townley RD, Bewtra AK, Nair NM, Brodkey FD, Burke KM. Methacholine inhalation challenge studies. J Allergy Clin Immunol 1979; 64:569–574.

27. Townley RG, Bewtra A, Wilson AF, et al. Segregation analysis of bronchial response to methacholine inhalation challenge in families with and without asthma. J Allergy Clin Immunol 1986; 77:101–107.

28. Longo G, Strinati R, Poli F, Fumi F. Genetic factors in nonspecific bronchial hyperreactivity. Am J Dis Child 1987; 141:331–334.

29. Crane J, O'Donnell TV, Prior IA, Waite DA. The relationships between atopy, bronchial hyperresponsiveness, and a family history of asthma: a cross-sectional

study of migrant Tokelauan children in New Zealand. J Allergy Clin Immunol 1989.

30. Mosmann TR, Coffman RL. TH1 and TH2 cells: different patterns of lymphokine secretion lead to different functional properties. Annu Rev Immunol 1989; 7:145–174.

31. Wierenga EA, Snoek M, de Groot C, et al. Evidence for compartmentalization of functional subsets of CD2+ T lymphocytes in atopic patients. J Immunol 1990; 144:4651–4656.

32. Wierenga EA, Snoek M, Jansen HM, Bos JD, van Lier RA, Kapsenberg ML. Human atopen specific types 1 and 2 T helper cell clones. J Immunol 1991; 147:2942–2949.

33. Isakson PC, Pure E, Vitetta ES, Krammer PH. T cell derived B cell differentiation factor(s). Effect on the isotype switch of murine cells. J Exp Med 1982; 155:734–748.

34. Vitetta ES, Ohara J, Meyers C, Layton J, Krammer PH, Paul WE. Serological, biochemical, and functional identity of B cell-stimulatory factor 1 and B cell differentiation factor for IgG1. J Exp Med 1985; 161:1726–1731.

35. Coffman RL, Carty J. A T cell activity that enhances polyclonal IgE production and its inhibition by interferon-g. J Immunol 1986; 949–954.

36. Coffman RL, Ohara J, Bond MW, Carty J, Zlotnik A, Paul WE. B cell stimulatory factor-1 enhances the IgE response of lipopolysaccharide-activated B cells. J Immunol 1986; 136:4538–4541.

37. Robinson DS, Hamid Q, Ying S, et al. Predominant TH2-like bronchoalveolar T-lymphocyte population in atopic asthma. N Engl J Med 1992; 326:298–304.

38. Blumenthal MN, Namboodiri K, Mendell N, Gleich G, Elston RC, Yunis E. Genetic transmission of serum IgE levels. Am J Med Genet 1981; 10:219–228.

39. Borecki IB, Rao DC, Lalouel JM, McGue M, Gerrard JW. Demonstration of a common major gene with pleiotropic effects on immunoglobulin E levels and allergy. Genet Epidemiol 1985; 2:327–338.

40. Meyers DA, Bias WB, Marsh DG. A genetic study of total IgE levels in the Amish. Hum Hered 1982; 32:15–23.

41. Meyers DA, Beaty TH, Freidhoff LR, Marsh DG. Inheritance of total serum IgE (basal levels) in man. Am J Hum Genet 1987; 41:51–62.

42. Hanson B, McGue M, Roitman JB, Segal NL, Bouchard TJ, Blumenthal. Atopic disease and immunoglobulin E in twins reared apart and together. Am J Hum Genet 1991; 48:873–879.

43. Willcox HNA, Marsh DG. Genetic regulation of antibody heterogeneity: its possible significance in human allergy. Immunogenetics 1978; 6:209–225.

44. Berciano FA, Crespo M, Bao CG, Alvarez FV. Serum levels of total IgE in non-allergic children. Influence of genetic and environmental factors. Allergy 1987; 42:276–283.

45. Meyers DA, Beaty TH, Colyer CR, Marsh DG. Genetics of total serum IgE levels: a regressive model approach to segregation analysis. Genet Epidemiol 1991; 8: 351–359.

46. Marsh DG, Neely JD, Breazeale DR, et al. Linkage analysis of IL4 and other chromosome 5q31.1 markers and total serum immunoglobulin E concentrations. Science 1994; 264:1152–1156.

47. Sporik R, Holgate ST, Platts-Mills TA, Cogswell JJ. Exposure to house-dust mite

allergen (Der p I) and the development of asthma in childhood. A prospective study. N Engl J Med 1990; 323:502–507.

48. Caraballo LR, Hernandez M. HLA haplotype segregation in families with allergic asthma. Tissue Antigens 1990; 35:182–186.

49. Caraballo L, Marrugo J, Jimenez S, Angelini G, Ferrara GB. Frequency of DPB1*0401 is significantly decreased in patients with allergic asthma in a mulatto population. Hum Immunol 1991; 32:157–161.

50. Stoy PJ, Roitman JB, Walsh G, et al. Aging and serum immunoglobulin E levels, immediate skin tests, RAST. J Allergy Clin Immunol 1981; 68:421–426.

51. Roitman-Johnson B, Sothern RB, Halberg F, Blumenthal MN. Circadian immuno-logic rhythms and their implications in the diagnosis and treatment of atopic dis-orders. In: Smolensky, ed. In: Recent Advances in the Chronobiology of Allergy and Immunology, New York: Pergamon Press, 1980:65.

52. Rao CR. Linear Statistical Inference and Its Applications. New York: John Wiley, 1973.

53. Weeks DE, Lange K. A multilocus extension of the affected-pedigree-member method of linkage analysis. Am J Hum Genet 1992; 50:859–868.

54. Clerget-Darpoux F, Bonaiti-Pellie C, Hochez J. Effects of misspecifying genetic parameters in lod score analysis. Biometrics 1986; 42:393–399.

55. Ott J. Linkage analysis with misclassification at one locus. Clin Genet 1977; 12: 119–124.

56. Lathrop GM, Lalouel JM, Julier C, Ott J. Strategies for multilocus linkage analysis in humans. Proc Natl Acad Sci USA 1984; 81:3443–3446.

57. Risch N, Guiffra L. Model misspecification and multipoint linkage analysis. Hum Hered 1992; 42:77–92.

58. Elston RC. Man bites dog. The validity of maximizing lod scores to determine mode of inheritance. Am J Med Genet 1989; 34:487–488.

59. Schork NJ, Boehnke M, Terwilliger JD, Ott J. Two-trait-locus linkage analysis: a powerful strategy for mapping complex genetic traits. Am J Hum Genet 1993; 53: 1127–1136.

60. Backwelder WC, Elston RC. A comparison of sib-pair linkage tests for disease susceptibility loci. Genet Epidemiol 1985; 2:85–97.

61. Schellenberg G, Boehnke M, Wijsman EM, Moore DK, Martin GM, Bird TD. Genetic association and linkage analysis of the apo CII locus and familial Alzheimer's disease. Ann Neurol 1992; 31:223–227.

18

Issues in Phenotype Assessment in Genetic Studies of Asthma

SCOTT T. WEISS

Channing Laboratory
Boston, Massachusetts

I. Introduction

Asthma is a clinical syndrome that has three essential features: reversible airflow obstruction, increased airway responsiveness, and airway inflammation [1]. This disease definition poses several problems for phenotype assessment in genetic studies. First, the definition is syndromic: It is not based on a definable biochemical or physiologic reaction. Second, the pathophysiology and natural history of the disease are not completely understood, making the assessment of phenotype complex. Finally, alternative disease definitions exist [2]. The extent to which these alternative disease definitions represent the same or different phenotypes as those embodied in the definition given above is unclear. For example, epidemiologic studies have utilized a doctor's diagnosis of asthma, although this has clearly been shown to suffer from bias, particularly as it relates to gender and cigarette smoking status [3]. Epidemiologic studies have also emphasized the operational definition of current wheeze and increased airway responsiveness [4]. The extent to which this definition incorporates the clinical evidence of inflammation is currently unknown. This chapter considers each principal component of the asthma definition (airway responsiveness, reversible airflow obstruction, and airway inflammation) and discusses the physiologic basis for these phenomena as they are currently understand; how they are measured (phenotypically) and the problems with phenotypic measurement; environmental and physiologic differences which may confound the relationship of phenotype to genotype; the relationship to each to asthma as a disease; and existing data that suggest the genetic basis for these conditions.

II. Airway Responsiveness/Reversible Airflow Obstruction

A. Population Genetics of Airway Responsiveness

The degree of heritability of airway responsiveness is not yet established. Brunnerman et al. studied 28 parents of asthmatic children in Tucson, Arizona, to determine the degree of familial aggregation of airway responsiveness, using methacholine challenge [5]. None of the parents smoked. Most subjects (17 of 28, or 61%) had allergic rhinitis defined by clinical history, and atopy defined as skin test positive for environmental antigens. This study suggests significant familial aggregation of the airway responsiveness phenotype, potentially related to genetic or common environmental factors. Townley et al. studied the airway responsiveness phenotype utilizing methacholine challenge test results for 424 family members from 83 families [6]. Ascertainment of families was not uniform, with the majority being ascertained through an affected proband, and approximately one-third of the families through a normal subject. Segregation analysis suggests that a single-gene model could not explain the aggregation of methacholine airway responsiveness within families. Koenig and Godfrey performed an early study of airway responsiveness in 8 monozygotic (MZ) and 7 dizygotic (DZ) pairs of twins utilizing a standard exercise challenge [7]. Six of the MZ pairs had similar levels of airway responsiveness, but only one of the DZ pairs had similar responses to this nonpharmacologic challenge. This study was hampered by the small number of twin pairs, but it does suggest some hereditable component of airway responsiveness. Hopp et al. performed a study in which methacholine challenge tests were used to measure airway responsiveness and questionnaire data on personal history of allergy and asthma, which they obtained from 107 twin pairs (61 MZ and 46 DZ) [8]. The correlation coefficient for area under the dose–response curve for methacholine was 0.67 for the MZ twin pairs, but only 0.34 for the DZ twin pairs. These authors estimated that 66% of airway responsiveness was inherited. No adjustment was made for differences in lung size among subjects in either of these investigations, nor were environmental covariates that might influence the association accounted for. Finally, Longo et al. measured airway responsiveness to carbachol in asthmatic and nonasthmatic subjects obtained via advertisements in a newspaper [9]. No association was found between airway responsiveness and atopy in this study. The authors postulated an autosomal dominant mode of inheritance for airway responsiveness [9]. Ascertainment bias with regard to selection of study subjects creates concerns about the results of this last study. The above data demonstrate that familial aggregation of airway responsiveness occurs. What remains unclear is whether this aggregation is due to shared genes, shared environment, or both. An alternative hypothesis is that the observed aggregation is a result of a separate but linked heritable factor, such as atopy. Additional factors argue for heritability of airway responsiveness. Young et al. studied infants of asthmatic and normal parents, and found that increased airway responsiveness was more often present in the infants of asthmatic parents than in those of normal parents [10]. Although the presence of increased airway responsiveness at birth could be due to genetic causes, this could also be due to in-utero, environmental, or immunologic effects on lung development.

Several studies have documented an increase in airway responsiveness in relatives of patients with lung disease. Bertrand et al. found a fivefold increase in airway responsiveness to methacholine in first-degree relatives of infants born prematurely when compared to control families [11]. Environmental factors such as cigarette smoking were not controlled for in this analysis. Britt et al. found an increase in methacholine airway responsiveness in first-degree relatives of patients with chronic obstructive lung disease [12]. These data also are compatible with heritability or shared environmental changes.

B. Pathophysiology of Airway Responsiveness

Airway responsiveness is a complex, integrated physiologic act which involves epithelium, smooth muscle, and nerves (Fig. 1). The complex nature of the physiology suggests that genes for any or all of these anatomic components may be important in the phenomenon. Mechanistically, a variety of factors are potentially involved in increased airway responsiveness. There can be an increase in smooth muscle shortening, or mass, or contractility; altered or decreased mechanical load against which the smooth muscle must contract; or an increased concentration of contractile agonists for smooth muscle. Many investigators have acknowledged that a decrease in luminal cross-sectional area as a result of inflammatory cell infiltration, edema of the airway wall, vascular or lymphatic engorgement, or proliferation of submucosal connective tissue can all increase airway responsiveness, independent of the other mechanical factors. Although all of these mechanical factors are undeniably important, recent research has focused on the noradrenergic, noncholinergic (NANC) nervous system, and specifically on sensory neurotransmitters and their role in the asthmatic response. Stimulation of these sensory nerves causes the pattern of activity characteristic of airway responsiveness: smooth muscle contraction, vascular dilation, microvascular leakage, submucosal secretion, and epithelial damage. This phenomenon has been termed neurogenic inflammation [13]. Inhibition of neutral endopeptidase can result in an

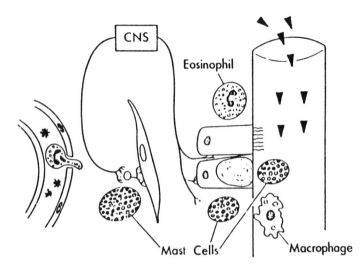

Figure 1   Schematic diagram depicting the basic elements involved in control of bronchomotor tone: 1, nerves; 2, airway epithelium; 3, smooth muscle; 4, cells. Triangles
represent an inhaled stimulus in the airway lumen. (From Shepard D. Mechanisms
of bronchoconstriction from nonimmunologic environmental stimuli. Chest 1986; 90:
584–587.)

increase in sensory neuropeptides in the epithelium, submucosal glands, and
smooth muscle. Environmental events, such as cigarette smoking and viral respiratory illness, have been shown to produce such pathophysiologic changes [14].

C. Phenotypically, How Is Airway Responsiveness Measured in Populations?

Currently, there is no direct test of any of the components of airway responsiveness noted above. The usual methodology is to utilize a nonspecific agonist, such
as methacholine or histamine, and utilize a drop in a measure of pulmonary
function, such as FEV_1, after increasing doses of such a bronchoconstrictor
agonist. The choice of a 20% fall in FEV_1 ($PD_{20}FEV_1$) has been widely accepted
as a clinically useful measure of airway responsiveness. However, expressing
results in this manner does have certain limitations. First the PD_{20} does not
provide a complete description of the dose–response curve. Second, in population
studies, such as will be necessary for phenotyping for linkage analysis, investigators have reported that the majority (66–89%) of study subjects failed to experience a 20% drop in FEV during the bronchial challenge test, and hence the
$PD_{20}FEV_1$ cannot be calculated for these subjects [15]. In statistical terminology,
the $PD_{20}FEV_1$ measure is said to be censored at the lower end of its range. An

additional problem is that because FEV_1 is correlated with airway responsiveness, subjects who have a low initial FEV_1 will be more likely to be responsive, but will also be less likely to be able to perform a test, and thus phenotypic information will not be obtainable on these individuals.

This type of left-censoring is a real concern. Subjects with missing data are uninformative with regard to linkage analysis, and missing phenotype data on family members is likely to be a severe limitation for linkage analysis. The issue of right-censoring of the airway responsiveness distribution can be handled effectively by using continuous measures of airway responsiveness, such as dose–response slope [16]. There is currently no known solution to the issue of left-censoring. An additional concern is that, although techniques are available for measuring airway responsiveness in little children, there is no known comparability of these techniques to the standard measures used in children over the age of 5 years. Thus, missing phenotype information will be enhanced in family pedigrees with children under the age of 5 years.

The conventional approach to avoid missing data on airway responsiveness has been to substitute reversibility or response to a bronchodilator for data on a bronchoconstrictor. It is unclear whether the use of a bronchodilator measures the same physiologic phenomenon as the bronchoconstrictor response. Prior studies suggest that bronchodilator and bronchoconstrictor responses are correlated to the level of approximately 0.6–0.7 [17]. It is unclear whether the strength of this correlation is due to the fact that both are mediated in part by level of FEV_1, or whether they are common physiologic influences on both responses. Clinical data do suggest that both the bronchoconstrictive and the bronchodilatory response may contribute independently to decline in lung function and, hence, outcome in diseased subjects separately [18]. If this is true, there may be separate genetic influences. Finally, the sensitivity, specificity, and repeatability of bronchoconstrictor and bronchodilator tests in the same group of subjects has not been determined. Thus, some degree of misclassification of subjects may occur with the substitution of reversibility for airway responsiveness.

D. Physiologic Influences

A variety of physiologic factors (gender, airway size, level of FEV_1, and age) could all potentially influence airway responsiveness [19]. Of these factors, level of lung function seems to be the most obvious and the most important. There are several reasons why level of lung function or baseline airway caliber may influence airway responsiveness. First, the resistance to flow through a tube is inversely proportional to the radius of the tube raised to the fourth power. Therefore, airway narrowing with a lower FEV_1 would be associated with reduced cross-sectional area. Second, the presence of airflow obstruction results in more central and less peripheral disposition of an inhaled aerosol. Obviously, this may lead to a greater degree of bronchoconstriction upon inhalation of an agent which causes constriction of the central airways. Third, a stimulus causing constriction of the peripheral airways should be expected to cause a relatively greater increase in total airways resistance in individuals with airflow obstruction, as peripheral airways resistance appears to have a greater contribution to total airways resistance in people with low FEV_1 compared to individuals without respiratory disease. Finally, expression of airway responsiveness in terms of percent change from baseline pulmonary function creates an inverse mathematical relationship between responsiveness and level of FEV_1. This purely mathematical relationship can be exaggerated to lower the initial level of FEV_1 [19]. Given these associations, it becomes difficult to disentangle the airway responsiveness phenotype from the phenotypic factors determining level of FEV_1 itself. It appears that different levels of airway responsiveness seen across ages and across genders are in part due to differences in airway size and differences in level of FEV_1.

E. Environmental Influences on Airway Responsiveness

There is no question that individuals who are phenotypically atopic (i.e., have skin test reactivity or elevated total serum IgE levels in conjunction with symptoms) are significantly more likely to have increased airway responsiveness [20]. The strength of this association is greater in children and young adults than in older individuals. Since most of the studies are cross-sectional, current data are uninformative as to whether allergen exposure leads to the development of increased airway responsiveness.

The second major environmental factor is cigarette smoke. Cigarette smoke may be associated with changes in epithelial permeability, cytokine induction, changes in lymphocyte function, direct airway inflammation, and increases in total IgE [20]. Both exposure to environmental tobacco smoke and active cigarette smoking are associated with increased airway responsiveness. Again, the temporal relationship between smoking and the development of airway responsiveness is unclear, as longitudinal studies have not been performed. Finally, human studies have documented that viral respiratory illness, particularly RSV infection, is associated with the development of transient increases in airway responsiveness [21]. It remains unclear whether viral respiratory illness can actually cause asthma, although recent theories have suggested at least two novel mechanisms by which respiratory illness may influence the development of asthma as a disease. Holt and co-workers have postulated that deficiency of viral respiratory illness in the first year of life results in an enhancement of TH2 lymphocyte cell development and the subsequent development of sensitization to environmental allergens and the development of the atopic state [22]. An alternative hypothesis concerning respiratory illness has been proposed by Hogg with regard to adenovirus infections [23]. He postulates an incorporation of adenoviral genes into epithelial cells, such that there is a continued upregulation and enhancement of the inflammatory response as a consequence of subsequent viral exposures. The significance of these environmental factors is twofold. First, they may be etiologic in the development of the disease. Second, even if they are not etiologic, they will increase variability across families, and measurement and control for these factors will enhance linkage analysis.

F. Relationship of Increased Airway Responsiveness to Asthma

Population-based epidemiologic studies have documented a log-normal distribution of airway responsiveness in populations (Fig. 2). These studies have documented that asthmatic subjects tend to be on the left end of the distribution. Epidemiologic studies also clearly demonstrate that the prevalence of airway responsiveness and asymptomatic airway responsiveness far exceeds the prevalence of asthma in cross-sectional population-based studies (Table 1). These data clearly establish that airway responsiveness is present in populations in the absence of asthma. At least three studies document that airway responsiveness precedes and predicts the development of asthma in populations [8]. Hopp and co-

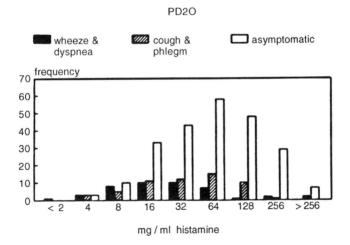

Figure 2 Distribution of PD_{20} by symptom group (Vlaardingen, 1984). The histamine concentration is displayed on a logarithmic scale (log with base 2). Note that the left tail of the distribution is the more responsive tail. (From Rijcken B, Schouten JP, Weiss ST, Meinesz AF, De Vries K, Van Der Lende R. The distribution of bronchial responsiveness to histamine in symptomatic and in asymptomatic subjects. Am Rev Respir Dis 1989; 140:615–623.)

Table 1 Prevalence of Increased Airway Responsiveness in Random Population Samples of Asymptomatic Children and Adults

Author	Population	Criteria for positive response	Percent prevalence of increased airway responsiveness	Prevalence of asymptomatic increased responsiveness	
				Percent of total population	Percent of all responsive subjects
Weiss, 1984 [55]	East Boston, MA, random population, children, young adults ($N = 213$), age range 6–24	$\Delta FEV_1/FVC > 9\%$ to cold air	22	11	51
Salome, 1987 [56]	Australia, random population, children ($N = 2363$), age range 8–11	$PD_{20}FEV_1 \leqslant 7.8$ μmol histamine	17.9	6.7	37
Sears, 1986 [57]	New Zealand, random population sample ($N = 766$), age 9 years	$PD_{20}FEV_1 < 25$ mg/mL methacholine	22	8	30
Woolcock, 1987 [58]	Busselton, Australia, random population, adults ($N = 876$), mean age 49	$PD_{20}FEV_1 \leqslant 3.9$ μmol histamine	11	2	19
Rijcken, 1987 [59]	Netherlands, random population, adults ($N = 1905$), age range 14 to 64+	$PC_{10}FEV_1 \leqslant 16$ mg/mL histamine	24.5	14	58.5
Sparrow, 1987 [60]	Boston, MA, adult males ($N = 458$), mean age 60	$PD_{20}FEV_1 \leqslant 50$ μmol methacholine	29.9	—	—
Burney, 1987 [61]	England, random population, adults ($N = 511$), age range 18–64	$PD_{20}FEV_1 \leqslant 8$ μmol histamine	14	—	—

workers studied a small group of children from asthmatic families with methacholine challenge [24]. In follow-up of these children, none of whom had asthma initially, methacholine challenge was highly predictive of the development of asthma in these high-risk children relative to methacholine values and a comparable age-matched group of controls. Carey and co-workers, studying children and young adults in the East Boston Childhood Respiratory Disease study, found that cold-air challenge test was predictive of the development of wheezing symptoms and recurrent asthma [25].

Zhong and co-workers studied 81 students (age range 11 to 17 years) who were found to have airway hyperresponsiveness and compared them with 88 age-matched controls with normal bronchial responsiveness [26]. In follow-up, there was a sixfold increase in the diagnosis of asthma in subjects with increased airway responsiveness when followed over a two-year period. Coupled with the data on environmental factors, these epidemiologic facts suggest that the appropriate model for this disease is a gene by environment interaction, such that environmental exposure to allergen, cigarette smoke, or respiratory illness enhances airway inflammation and drives airway responsiveness toward the left end of the distribution (Fig. 3). This pathophysiologic formulation is, at present,hypothetical and

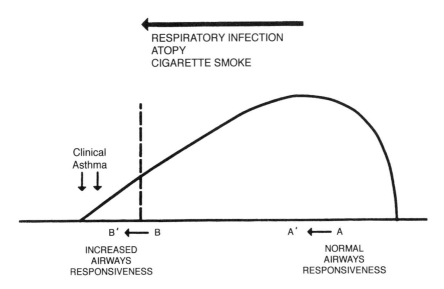

Figure 3 Theoretical population distribution of airway responsiveness and the environmental and host factors responsible for the development of clinical asthma. (From Brown RW, Weiss ST. The influence of lower respiratory illness on childhood asthma: defining risk and susceptibility. Sem Respir Infect 1991; 4:228.)

incomplete. However, an adequate understanding of the relationship of airway responsiveness to the inflammatory stimuli hampers genetic studies by providing an unclear paradigm for the disease.

G. Relationship of Airway Responsiveness to Inflammation

Prevailing paradigms for the relationship of airway responsiveness to inflammation are that inflammation leads to increased airway responsiveness, which leads to asthma (Fig. 4a). Alternative paradigms include the possibility that inflammation and airway responsiveness have independent effects on the development of asthma (Fig. 4b). A third alternative is that there is an interaction between inflammation and airway responsiveness, but that both have independent effects on asthma (Fig. 4c). Clinical studies with inhaled glucocorticoids provide signifi-

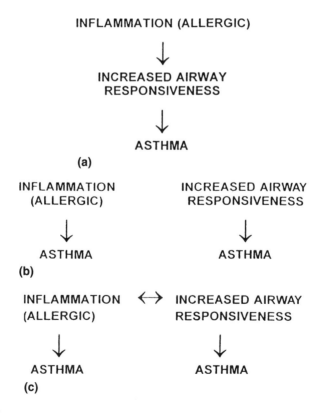

Figure 4

cant information on the relationship of airway responsiveness to inflammation. There is no question that inhaled corticosteroids will reduce baseline airway responsiveness [27]. In this regard, it is useful to examine the actions of glucocorticoids that might influence airway responsiveness, such as inhibition of mediated release from basophils and mast cells, reduction of histamine synthesis, vasoconstriction, inhibition of mucosa edema and mucous secretion, and enhanced beta-adrenergic response to smooth muscle [28]. Inhaled corticosteroids seem to have no effect on the immediate allergic response, but do inhibit the late asthmatic reaction [2]. Although long-term treatment studies do suggest that the effect of corticosteroids on airway responsiveness is duration and dose dependent, steroid treatment does not abolish airway responsiveness [29]. In addition, airway responsiveness can exist in the absence of airway inflammation [30]. These data are most consistent with the concept of a gene by environment interaction, in which the airway responsiveness phenotype interacts with the inflammatory environmental stimuli to produce the development of the disease. If this conceptualization is correct, it will have important implications for the type of family pedigrees chosen for linkage analysis.

III. Allergy, Inflammation, and Altered Immune Function

A. Genetics of Allergy

Significant familial aggregation of skin test reactivity has been demonstrated by Meyers and co-workers in 42 randomly ascertained nuclear families who were not selected for the presence of allergic disease [31]. This work has been confirmed in a population-based study of 344 nuclear families in Tucson, Arizona [32]. Gerrard et al. [33] and Rao et al. [34] performed path and segregation analysis of total serum IgE levels in 173 Canadian nuclear families. Significant polygenic inheritance was found, with heritability estimates of 0.425. Complex segregation analysis provided evidence for polygenic inheritance in a major gene influencing serum total IgE levels. The major gene effect, which appeared to follow other somewhat recessive inheritance, increased serum total IgE levels. In a previously noted Arizona study, in addition to skin test, total IgE levels were studied in the members of 42 randomly ascertained nuclear families [32]. Significant correlations for total IgE levels were seen between both parents and children and among sibling pairs. The mode of inheritance was not discerned. Marsh and Myers have studied the heritability of IgE and have reached varying conclusions about the mode of inheritance, depending on the study [35,36].

Marsh et al. performed a family study of IgE as index of atopy that included segregation and linkage analysis with human leukocyte antigen (HLA) loci [36]. This study, in which families were selected because they had multiply affected members, suggests that an autosomal-dominant major gene for ragweed allergy;

the gene locus was linked to the HLA loci [36]. Other groups have found that a simple autosomal dominant model does not fit the family data for total IgE, although many of these investigations lack adequate statistical power [35]. Recent results from twin studies show the important role of genetics in determining total serum IgE levels, and therefore in determining one specific measure of allergic status. Available data from studies in twins suggest a heritability of approximately 0.6 for total serum IgE levels in several populations studied [37]. Cookson and Hopkins have demonstrated familial inheritance of atopy as defined by a broad definition, which included positive skin prick test and total serum IgE levels in 239 members of 40 nuclear and 3 extended families [38]. The pattern of autosomal-dominant vertical transmission with incomplete penetrance was postulated. These same investigators were later able to establish a DNA polymorphism, defined by p-lambda-m5.51 on chromosome 11Q, with a maximum log score of 5.58 [39]. Several different groups were initially unable to confirm the linkage reported by the Oxford group [40–43]. A Japanese research group has been able to confirm the findings of the Oxford group [44]. It is notable that the negative studies are all based on extended pedigrees, whereas the positive studies are based on multiple different families. Given a high degree of genetic heterogeneity, the latter approach may be preferable, in that a single locus shows a dominant effect in only a few families. An additional concern is that sib-pair analysis, using a large number of unrelated nuclear families, has advantages over linkage analysis for diseases with effects at multiple loci, by allowing the effect of a single locus to be discernible in a complex disorder. Such an analytic approach also does not require prior assumptions about the mode of inheritance, penetrance of the disease, or gene frequency. Two potentially promising candidate genes for the 11Q12–Q13 atopy loci are the $beta_{bn}$ of the high-affinity IgE receptor (FC epsilon RI beta) and CD20, which is found on the surface of all B cells and has a role in B-cell proliferation and differentiation.

B. Description of Pathophysiology

Allergy refers to immediate (type 1) hypersensitivity to an antigen encountered by inhalation, ingestion, or cutaneous contact. Increased production of allergen-specific immunoglobulin (IgE) by sensitized lymphocytes plays an essential role in the pathophysiology of this process. Atopy is a more narrowly defined condition than allergy. It is characterized by clinical manifestations of immediate-type hypersensitivity, immediate wheal-and-flare skin reactions to common environmental antigens, and familial aggregation [45]. Atopic subjects represent a subset of all allergic subjects. Allergy or atopy may be detected in clinical studies by measuring serum total or specific IgE level or by measuring cutaneous immediate hypersensitivity to common environmental aeroallergens. Serum levels of IgE antibody are regulated by two distinct T-cell populations. Helper-inducer T cells induce and enhance IgE synthesis, whereas suppressor T cells inhibit IgE synthesis. These T-cell regulators are controlled by a variety of self-signaling cytokines and by the level and mode of presentation of relevant environmental antigens. The central role of IgE in the pathophysiology of immediate-type hypersensitivity makes serum total and specific IgE measurements useful markers for allergy or atopy in clinical and epidemiologic research.

C. How Is Allergy Measured Phenotypically?

It is well recognized, however, that other potentially nonallergic mechanisms may induce an elevated IgE response. Skin testing, by prick, scratch, or intradermal methods, has been used as a clinical technique to identify the presence of hypersensitivity to allergens. Currently, prick tests are the standard for clinical and epidemiologic investigations, although intradermal tests are more sensitive. To manifest the skin test response to a specific environmental antigen, the following three components must be present: (1) an intact immune system; (2) the presence of a mast cell-basophil complex that can combine with IgE and release mediators when exposed to antigens; and (3) skin that can respond to histamine and the development of an inflammatory response, including erythema and induration.

D. Physiologic Influences

It is clear that skin test reactivity increases with increasing age until early adolescence stabilizes and then declines [46]. Peak age levels for total IgE and skin test reactivity are somewhat different. However, both decline steadily with increasing age after age 35. This creates important problems for genetic studies which span a wide age range, in that the phenotypic markers for older subjects may be absent even if age is clearly controlled for in the analysis. In general, males have higher IgE levels than females, although with appropriate age adjustment and adjustment for environmental influences, these differences narrow. Again, control for these physiologic influences may be important in genetic studies.

E. Environmental Influences

Cigarette smoking may be associated with changes in lymphocyte function, cytokine induction, and direct increases in total serum IgE level [47]. Cigarette smoking is known to be associated with skin test reactivity in children and elevations in serum IgE levels and eosinophils [48]. Environmental tobacco smoke exposure is known to be associated with the development of asthma in early childhood[49]. In those genetically susceptible to develop atopy, the level of allergen may be important in determining the atopic response [50]. Seasonal variation and different distribution of allergens in the home may be important in determining the wheal size or level of total serum IgE. In general, indoor allergens have a greater influence on atopy than outdoor allergens [51]. RSV infection is known to induce elevations in serum IgE level and may be associated with inflammation and altered immune function [52]. The exact relationship of respiratory illness to the development of atopy is unclear.

F. Relationship of Allergy to Asthma

A variety of studies have demonstrated that total serum IgE level is closely correlated with asthma and airway responsiveness [3,18]. However, levels of IgE explain only 60% of the variability in airway responsiveness [53], and cross-sectional studies do not allow clear hypothesis generation as to the temporal sequence of allergen exposure and its relationship to disease development. Roughly 80% of all childhood asthmatics are allergic, although the percentage of allergic asthmatics declines with increasing age. It is unclear whether this issue is a problem of inadequate age adjustment, in that skin test reactivity and IgE levels decline with increasing age, or whether it is a problem of antigen exposure (i.e., lack of the appropriate antigens to detect the presence of atopy in these subjects). Roughly 25–30% of the population has elevated IgE or positive skin test reactivity. The prevalence of asthma is only 5–7%. To date, it is unclear what distinguishes those atopics who develop asthma from those that do not. One hypothesis advanced earlier is that atopy and bronchial hyperresponsiveness represent two common clinical phenotypes, and it is the overlap by chance alone of these tow phenotypes that are independently genetically controlled but related to each other, that determines the development of asthma as a disease. Although allergy itself is not related to asthma severity, the subset of allergic asthmatics that have a late asthmatic response have more severe disease. The clinical determinants of this specific asthma phenotype (i.e., allergic asthmatics with a late asthmatic response) is unclear. One hypothesis is that this is simply a function of dose and duration of exposure. As noted by Cockcroft, response to antigen among allergic asthmatics is a function of three factors: (1) underlying degree of atopy; (2) underlying degree of airway responsiveness; and (3) dose of antigen [54]. Repetitive long-term exposure to antigen in a sensitive individual may lead to the development of a late asthmatic response.

Clearly, allergy is the major source of inflammation in asthma. Two phenotypic problems remain unresolved: (1) the role of other environmental exposures, such as respiratory illness and cigarette smoking, and how they interact with allergen to produce inflammation; and (2) the relationship of inflammation to airway responsiveness in asthma. These phenotypic issues have been outlined above.

IV. Conclusion

Certain problems are clearly identified from a careful review of the phenotypic issues and the assessment of phenotype in studies of asthma genetics. First, there is the problem of censoring and nonspecificity in the assessment of airway responsiveness over age in various pedigrees. Second, there is the lack of clear understanding of the pathophysiologic relationship between inflammation and airway responsiveness. Third, there is the lack of a clear, demonstrable mode of inheritance for either the inflammatory markers or airway responsiveness.

There are two basic approaches to the definition of genetic factors in asthma. The first is to use continuous measures, either with or without a prior segregation analysis. The second approach is more categorical, in attempting to define affected versus unaffected status for segregation or linkage analysis. The advantages of the first approach are that phenotypes can be used as continuous variables and are not categorized based on prior clinical criteria. With regard to genetic analysis, two basic approaches have been attempted. The first is complex segregation analysis followed by linkage analysis, using a predetermined genetic model identified from the segregation analysis. The second approach is linkage analysis performed on affected sib pairs without an underlying genetic model. After reviewing the difficulties with phenotype, it appears that the second approach is the more parsimonious and conservative. Segregation analysis requires unbiased ascertainment through an affected family member, whereas the sib pairs-linkage approach can be performed on a large number of nuclear families in the absence of concerns about ascertainment bias. The recent success of the Oxford group utilizing this latter approach suggests that it has much to recommend it. A third approach, which is currently not practical but may be practical in the near future, is the candidate gene approach, whereby specific genes from mouse or other animal studies may be linked to specific asthma phenotypes and then assessed directly in humans. Recent studies identifying genes for airway responsiveness in mice suggest the viability of this research approach as well.

It is likely that further advances in our understanding of the phenotypic assessment of airway responsiveness, allergy, and inflammation will greatly enhance our ability to perform genetic studies of these complex traits.

Acknowledgments

This work was supported by grants NHLBI HL50811, HL36474, HL36002, HL34645, HL49460, and SCOR HL19170.

References

1. National Asthma Education Program Expert Panel Report. Guideline for the diagnosis and management of asthma. U.S. Department of Health and Human Services publication no. 91-3042, 1991:1.

2.   Samet JM. Epidemiologic approaches to the identification of asthma. Chest 1987; 91:74S–78S.
3.   Weiss ST, Speizer FE. Epidemiology and natural history. In: Weiss E, Stein M, eds. Bronchial Asthma Mechanisms and Therapeutics, 3d ed. Boston: Little, Brown, 1993: 15–25.
4.   Toelle BG, Peat JK, Salome CM, Mellis CM, Woolcock AJ. Toward a definition of asthma for epidemiology. Am Rev Respir Dis 1992; 146:633–637.
5.   Bonnerman I, Cohen R, Shachor J, Horowitz I. Bronchial response to methacholine in parents of asthmatic children. Chest 1987; 91:210–213.
6.   Townley RG, Bewtra M, Wilson AF, et al. Segregation analysis of bronchial response to methacholine inhalation challenge in families with and without asthma. J Allergy Clin Immunol 1986; 77:101–107.
7.   Konig P, Godfrey S. Exercise-induced bronchial lability in monozygotic (identical) and dyzogitic (non-identical) twins. J Allergy Clin Immunol 1974; 54:280–287.
8.   Hopp RJ, Bewtra AK, Watt GD, Nair NM, Townley RG. Genetic analysis of allergic disease in twins. J Allergy Clin Immunol 1984; 73:265–270.
9.   Longo G, Striniati R, Pieli F, Fumi F. Genetic factors in nonspecific bronchial hyperreactivity. Am J Dis Child 1987; 141:331–334.
10. Young S, Le Souef PN, Geelhoed GC, Stick SM, Turner KJ, Landau LI. The influence of a family history of asthma and parental smoking on airway responsiveness in early infancy. N Engl J Med 1991; 324:1168–1173.
11. Bertrand JM, Riley ST, Popkin J, Coates AL. The long-term pulmonary sequelae of prematurity: the role of familial airway hyperreactivity and the respiratory stress syndrome. N Engl J Med 1985; 312:742–745.
12. Britt EJ, Cohen B, Menkes H, Bleecker E, Permutt S, Rosenthal R, Norman P. Airways reactivity and functional deterioration in relatives of COPD patients. Chest 1980; 77(2)(suppl):260–261.
13. Widdicombe J. The contribution of the mucosa to airway responsiveness. In: Page CT, Gardiner PJ, eds. Airway Hyperresponsiveness: Is It Really Important for Asthma? Oxford: Blackwell, 1993:83.
14. Jacobi DB, Tanaoki J, Borson DB, Nadell JA. Influenza infection causes airway hyperresponsiveness by decreasing enkephalinase. J Appl Physiol 1988; 64:2653–2658.
15. Weiss ST. Epidemiologic issues in the study of airways responsiveness. Medicina Thoracica 1988; 10:293–296.
16. O'Connor G, Sparrow D, Taylor D, Segal M, Weiss ST. Analysis of dose-response curves to methacholine: an approach suitable for population studies. Am Rev Respir Dis 1987; 136:1412–1417.
17. Benson MK. Bronchial reactivity. Br J Dis Chest 1975; 69:227–239.
18. Postma DS, DeVries K, Koëter GH, Sluiter HJ. Independent influence of reversibility of airflow obstruction and nonspecific hyperreactivity on a long-term course of lung function in chronic airflow obstruction. Am Rev Respir Dis 1986; 134:276–280.
19. O'Connor G, Sparrow D, Weiss ST. The role of atopy in airways responsiveness in the pathogenesis of chronic airflow obstruction. Am Rev Respir Dis 1989; 140:225–252.
20. Sears MR, Burrows B, Flannery EM, Herbison GP, Hewitt CJ, Holdaway MD.

Relation between airway responsiveness and serum IgE in children with asthma and in apparently normal children. N Engl J Med 1991; 325:1067–1071.

21. Tepper RS, Rosenberg D, Eigen H. Airway responsiveness in infants following bronchiolitis. Ped Pulmonology 1992; 13:6–10.

22. Holt PG, McMenamin C, Nelson D. Primary sensitization to inhalant allergens during infancy. Pediatr Allergy Immunol 1990; 1:3–13.

23. Matsuse T, Hayashi S, Kuwano K, Keunecke H, Jefferies WA, Hogg JC. Latent adenoviral infection in the pathogenesis of chronic airways obstruction. Am Rev Respir Dis 1992; 146:177–184.

24. Hopp RJ, Bewtra AK, Nair NM, Watt GD, Townley RG. Methacholine inhalation challenge studies in a selected pediatric population. Am Rev Respir Dis 1986; 134:994–998.

25. Carey VJ, Weiss ST, Tager IB, Leeder SR, Speizer FE. Airway responsiveness, wheeze onset, and recurrent asthma episodes in young adolescents: East Boston Childhood Respiratory Disease Cohort. Submitted.

26. Zhong MS, Chen RC, Yang MO, Wu ZY, Zheng JP, Li YF. Is asymptomatic bronchial hyperresponsiveness an indication of potential asthma? Chest 1992; 102:1104–1109.

27. Lundgren R, Soderberg M. Effect of chronic steroid treatment on airway inflammation and airway responsiveness. In: Page CP, Gardiner PJ, eds. Airway Hyperresponsiveness: Is It Really Important for Asthma? Oxford: Blackwell, 1993:316.

28. Cockcroft DW, Murdock KY. Comparative effects of inhaled salbutamol, sodium cromoglycate, and beclomethasone dipropionate on allergen-induced early asthmatic responses, late asthmatic responses, and increased bronchial hyperresponsiveness to histamine. J Allergy Clin Immunol 1987; 79:734–740.

29. Kraan J, Koëter GH, Van der Mark THW, et al. Dosage and time effects of inhaled budesonide on bronchial hyperreactivity. Am Rev Respir Dis 1988; 137:44–48.

30. Lundgren R, Soderberg M, Horsted P, Stemling R. Methodologic studies of bronchial mucosal biopsies from asthmatics before and after ten years of treatment with inhaled steroids. Eur Respir J 1988; 1:883–889.

31. Meyers DA, Bias WB, Marsh DG. The genetic study of total IgE levels in the Amish. Hum Hered 1982; 32:15–23.

32. Lebowitz MD, Barbee R, Burrows B. Family concordance of IgE, atopy, and disease. J Allergy Clin Immunol 1984; 73:259–264.

33. Gerrard JW, Rao DC, Morton ME. Genetic study of immunoglobulin-E. Am J Hum Genet 1978; 30:46–54.

34. Rao DC, Vogler GP, Borecki IB, Province MA, Russell JM. Robustness of path analysis of family resemblance against deviations from multivariate normality. Hum Hered 1987; 37:107–112.

35. Hasstedt SJ, Meyers DA, Marsh DG, et al. The inheritance of immunoglobulin-E: genetic model fitting. Am J Med Genet 1981; 14:61–66.

36. Marsh DG, Bias WB, Ishizaka K. Genetic control of basal serum immunoglobulin-E level and its effect on specific reaginic sensitivity. Proc Natl Acad Sci USA 1974; 71:3588–3592.

37. Bazaral M, Orgel HA, Hamburger RN. Genetics of IgE and allergy: serum IgE levels in twins. J Allergy Clin Immunol 1974; 54:288–304.

38. Cookson WOCM, Hopkin JM. Dominant inheritance of atopic immunoglobulin-E responsiveness. Lancet 1988; 1:86–88.

39. Cookson WOCM, Sharp PA, Faux JA, Hopkin JM. Linkage between immunoglobulin-E responses, underlying asthma and rhinitis in chromosome 11Q. Lancet 1989; 1:1292–1295.

40. Lympany P, Welsh J, Cochrane GM, Kemeny DM, Lee PN. Genetic analysis using DNA polymorphisms of the linkage between chromosome 11Q13 and atopy and bronchial hyperresponsiveness to methacholine. J Allergy Clin Immunol 1992; 89: 619–628.

41. Hizawa N, Yamaguchi E, Ore M, et al. Lack of linkage between atopy and locus 11Q13. Clin Exp Allergy 1992; 22:1065–1069.

42. Rich SS, Roitman-Johnson B, Greenberg B, et al. Genetic analysis of atopy in three large kindreds: no evidence of linkage to D11S97. Clin Exp Allergy 1992; 22:1070–1076.

43. Amelung PJ, Panhuxsenli M, Postma DS, et al. Atopy and bronchial hyperresponsiveness exclusion of linkage to markers of chromosomes 11Q and 6P. Clin Exp Allergy 1992; 22:1077–1084.

44. Shirakawa T, Morimoto K, Fumijama J, Yamamoto M, Takai S. Linkage between IgE responses underlying asthma and rhinitis (atopy) and chromosome 11Q in Japanese families. Crytogenet Cell Genet 1992; 58:1970.

45. Coca AF, Cooke RA. On the classification of the phenomena of hypersensitiveness. J Immunol 1923; 8:163–182.

46. Barbee RA, Lebowitz MD, Thompson HC, Burrows B. Immediate skin test reactivity in a general population sample. Am Intern Med 1976; 84:129–133.

47. Holt PG. Immune and inflammatory function in cigarette smokers. Thorax 1987; 42: 241–249.

48. Weiss ST, Tager IB, Muñoz A, Speizer FE. The relationship of respiratory infections in early childhood to the occurrence of increased levels of bronchial responsiveness in atopy. Am Rev Respir Dis 1985; 131:573–578.

49. Ronchetti R, Lucarini N, Lucarelli P, et al. A genetic basis for heterogeneity of asthma syndrome in pediatric ages: adenosine deaminase phenotypes. J Allergy Clin Immunol 1984; 74:81–84.

50. Arshad SH, Matthews S, Gant C, Hide DW. Effect of allergen avoidance on development of allergic disorders in infancy. Lancet 1992; 339:1493–1497.

51. Sporik R, Holgate ST, Platts-Mills TAE, et al. Exposure to house dust mite allergen (der P I) and development of asthma in childhood. N Engl J Med 1990; 323:502–507.

52. Welliver RC, Wong DT, Sun M, et al. The development of respiratory syncytial virus-specific IgE and the release of histamine in nasopharyngeal secretions after infection. N Engl J Med 1981; 305:841–846.

53. Burrows B, Martinez FD, Halonen M, Barbee RA, Cline MG. Association of asthma with serum IgE levels and skin-test reactivity to allergens. N Engl J Med 1989; 320:271–277.

54. Cockcroft DW, Ruffin RG, Frith PA, et al. Determinants of allergen-induced asthma: dose of allergen, circulating IgE antibody concentration, and bronchial responsiveness to inhaled histamine. Am Rev Respir Dis 1979; 120:1053–1058.

55. Weiss ST, Tager IB, Weiss JW, Muñoz A, Speizer FE, Ingram RH. Airways responsiveness in a population sample of adults and children. Am Rev Respir Dis 1984; 129:898–902.

56. Salome CM, Peat JK, Britton WJ, Woolcock AJ. Bronchial hyperresponsiveness in two populations of Australian schoolchildren. I. Relation to respiratory symptoms and diagnosed asthma. Clin Allergy 1987; 17:271–281.

57. Sears MR, Jones DT, Holdaway MD, et al. Prevalence of bronchial reactivity to inhaled methacholine in New Zealand children. Thorax 1986; 41:283–289.

58. Woolcock AJ, Peat JK, Salome CM, et al. Prevalence of bronchial hyperresponsiveness and asthma in a rural adult population. Thorax 1987; 42:361–368.

59. Rijcken B, Schouten JP, Weiss ST, Speizer FE, Van Der Lende R. The relationship of nonspecific bronchial responsiveness to respiratory symptoms in a random population sample. Am Rev Respir Dis 1987; 136:62–68.

60. Sparrow D, O'Connor G, Colton T, Barry CL, Weiss ST. The relationship of nonspecific bronchial responsiveness to the occurrence of respiratory symptoms and decreased levels of pulmonary function. The Normative Aging Study. Am Rev Respir Dis 1987; 135:1255–1260.

61. Burney PGJ, Britton JR, Chinn S, et al. Descriptive epidemiology of bronchial reactivity in an adult population: results from a community study. Thorax 1987; 42:38–44.

Table 1   Asthma Definitions

ATS [3]	1962	Asthma is a disease characterized by an increased responsiveness of the trachea and bronchi to various stimuli and manifested by a widespread narrowing of the airways that changes in severity either spontaneously or as a result of therapy.
Ciba [4]	1959	The condition of subjects with widespread narrowing of the bronchial airways, which changes its severity over short periods of time either spontaneously or under treatment.
World Health Organization [5]	1975	A chronic condition characterized by recurrent bronchospasm resulting from a tendency to develop reversible narrowing of the airway lumina in response to stimuli of a level or intensity not inducing such narrowing in most individuals.
ATS [6]	1987	A clinical syndrome characterized by increased responsiveness of the tracheobronchial tree to a variety of stimuli. Major symptoms are paroxysms of dyspnea, wheezing, and cough, which may vary from mild and almost undetectable to severe and unremitting (status asthmaticus). The primary physiologic manifestation of this hyperresponsiveness is variable airways obstruction. This can take form of fluctuations in the severity of obstruction, following bronchodilators or corticosteroids, or increased obstruction caused by drugs or other stimuli ... evidence of mucosal edema of the bronchi, infiltration of the bronchial mucosa or submucosa with inflammatory cells, especially eosinophils; shedding of epithelium, obstruction of peripheral airways with mucus.
NHLBI/NIH [7]	1991	A lung disease with the following characteristics: (1) airway obstruction that is reversible (but not completely so in some patients) either spontaneously or with treatment; (2) airway inflammation; and (3) increased airway responsiveness to a variety of stimuli.
NHLBI/NIH [8,9]	1993/ 1995	A chronic inflammatory disorder of the airways in which many cells play a role, in particular mast cells, eosinophils, and T lymphocytes. In susceptible individuals this inflammation causes recurrent episodes of wheezing, breathlessness, chest tightness, and cough in early morning. These symptoms are usually associated with widespread but variable airflow limitation that is at least partly reversible either spontaneously or with treatment. The inflammation also causes an associated increase in airway responsiveness to a variety of stimuli.

asthma. Response to bronchodilator inhalation proved to be an inaccurate test for assessing a propensity to bronchoconstriction specific to asthma [11]. Nonspecific airways responsiveness can be readily measured using pharmacologic, physical, or allergen challenge methods [12]; however, it has been shown to be a sensitive but nonspecific test for establishing the presence of asthma [13–15]. As yet, there is no readily applicable and validated biomarker of airways inflammation which can be measured noninvasively, and there is no specific inflammatory hallmark of asthma even if tissue were available [16].

In investigating the genetics of asthma, there is a need to distinguish asthma from other diseases which may have some of the same manifestations. In childhood, cystic fibrosis and bronchiectasis are the principal diseases that might be misdiagnosed as asthma. However, the sweat test provides a highly accurate screening test for cystic fibrosis, and the genetic basis of cystic fibrosis is now well characterized. Bronchiectasis can be detected with sensitive imaging techniques.

In adulthood, the principal disease which overlaps with asthma in its manifestations is chronic obstructive pulmonary disease (COPD). This disease occurs almost exclusively in middle-aged or older persons who have smoked since childhood. The cardinal clinical manifestation is dyspnea, reflecting impairment of ventilatory function due to airflow obstruction produced by airways damage and emphysema. As smokers develop airflow obstruction, they may also have increased airways responsiveness, although not typically to the degree present in asthma [15,17]. However, variable, symptomatic airflow obstruction may lead to a clinical picture consistent with asthma, sometimes referred to as chronic obstructive bronchitis or chronic asthmatic bronchitis [18]. This syndrome overlaps clinically with asthma, and it may be more common in smokers with atopy and a history of asthma. This overlap between asthma and chronic progressive obstructive airways disease led to the "Dutch" hypothesis that these obstructive airways diseases are interrelated and require host susceptibility as well as environmental exposures for their expression. Many other chronic lung diseases in adulthood reflect interstitial inflammation and fibrosis and have a distinctly different clinical picture from asthma.

Studies on the genetics of asthma also need to consider the spectrum of phenotypic manifestations in the population. There is considerable overlap in young individuals among various preclinical conditions and asthma. The mild end of this disease spectrum is characterized by individuals with allergic seasonal rhinitis that may have some evidence of increased lower airway responsiveness. These responses can include bronchospasm after inhalation challenge with antigen and nonspecific agents such as methacholine, histamine, and exercise [19,20]. These individuals often respond positively to specific questions about asthma triggers and meet many of the diagnostic criteria for mild to moderate asthma outlined in recent asthma guidelines. Thus, there is a transition group without a formal physician diagnosis of asthma that is characterized by laboratory and clinical findings associated with asthma. Issues related to classification of preclinical or mild disease are an important but difficult area for classification in studies on the genetics of asthma.

Characterizing the manifestations of asthma as a basis for designating subphenotypes has also proved vexing. The picture of asthma is variable over time and may be altered by medications and environmental stimuli. Moreover, the specific manifestations vary among individuals with asthma; for example, cough predominates in some, whereas exercise-induced bronchospasm may be the sole manifestation in others. The severity of the disease is also highly variable among individuals with a diagnosis of asthma. We lack accepted tools and scales for classifying the disease, although physiologic parameters and symptoms can be readily measured as a basis for such classification. There is a tendency for many individuals with asthma to underestimate the severity of their disease, thus making accurate assessment more difficult [7].

The difficulties of diagnosing asthma and classifying persons with the disease have long been noted, but not satisfactorily solved for either clinical or research purposes. The new search for the genetic basis of asthma has added a further imperative for better understanding the phenotype of asthma and for developing tools to classify the phenotype. Multiple centers are now investigating the genetic basis of asthma and other allergic disorders; some are participating in multicenter collaborative studies, while others are acting on an individual basis. In either instance, there is a need for rigorous and standardized methods for establishing the diagnosis of asthma and also for standardized approaches for characterizing the phenotype. Lacking such standardization, there may be uncertainty as to the comparability of individuals labeled as having asthma in different centers and difficulty in reconciling discrepant findings. The possibilities for pooling studies to gain statistical power may also be constrained by nonstandardized methods and uncertain comparability.

Standardized methods have been developing for conducting epidemiologic research on respiratory diseases including asthma [21,22]. Satisfactory guidelines are available for pulmonary function testing, including spirometry and assessment of airways responsiveness using methacholine or histamine, and for skin testing for establishing the presence of atopy. However, the standardized respiratory symptoms questionnaires developed by the American Thoracic Society and published in 1978 are not appropriate for research on asthma because of their emphasis on chronic and stable symptom patterns rather than episodic symptoms that are more characteristic of asthma [21]. New instruments for asthma have been prepared by the International Union Against Tuberculosis and Lung Disease [23] and by the ISAAC (International Study on Allergy and Asthma in Children) investigative group [24]. However, these questionnaires have not yet been widely and uniformly adopted, and they have not been used in the studies of the genetics of asthma.

Another chapter in this volume addresses the principal components of the definitions of asthma (airway responsiveness, reversible airflow obstruction, and airway inflammation) [25]. Our chapter reviews the approaches that have been used to characterize the asthma phenotype in studies of the genetics of asthma published to date. The picture of asthma is heterogeneous, and a variety of sub-phenotypes of asthma can be specified, although there is no consensus as to classification. Nevertheless, we describe these subphenotypes, as their genetic bases could reasonably be distinct. Misclassification refers to the incorrect categorization of variables, in this instance, the phenotype of asthma. We consider the consequences of misclassifying the phenotype of asthma in the context of research on the genetic basis of asthma. For readers who are not familiar with the methods and terminology of genetic epidemiology, Table 2 [26–30] provides brief definitions and explanations.

II. Phenotype Characterization in Studies of the Genetics of Asthma

Table 3 [31–43] summarizes studies published on the familial aggregation of asthma and its genetic basis. Table 4 [41,42,44–52] provides similar information for studies of atopy.

Review of Table 3 demonstrates an obvious lack of standardization in the approaches used to classify the asthma phenotype. The approaches include reliance on questionnaire reports of symptoms or on a diagnosis by a physician, bronchial responsiveness testing, and the presence of a clinical diagnosis not otherwise documented. Comparability between different studies is lacking. There is less comparability in the approaches used to classify status of relatives and an indication of potential misclassification because of the reliance on questionnaire reports from probands or other persons, and not the relatives themselves.

Atopy was generally not one of the criteria for the classification of persons with asthma. By contrast, the approach to establishing the presence of atopy was more uniform, since these studies primarily used more objective laboratory results such as the results of skin testing or serologic testing (Table 4). This uniformity reflects the unidimensional definition of atopy. By contrast, asthma is a syndrome with multiple and variable components.

III. Asthma Subphenotypes Potentially Relevant to Investigating the Genetic Basis of Asthma

There have long been approaches to classify individuals with asthma into various subphenotypes based on the presence or absence of an obvious atopic component. For clinicians, a number of patterns are evident (Table 5): the atopic child with a

Table 2 Glossary of Terms Used in Genetic Epidemiology

Genetic heterogeneity: Multiple gene causes of the same, or nearly the same, phenotype [26]

Genotype: The precise allelic makeup of an organism or cell [26]

Haplotype: A unique array of closely linked alleles that is usually inherited as a unit [26]

Heritability: The proportion of phenotypic variation that is due to genotypic differences [26]

Linked genes: Two or more genes located on the same chromosome and showing substantially less than 50% recombination [26]

Linkage analysis: A method that uses pedigree data to determine whether two or more loci are linked and to estimate the amount of crossing over between them, i.e., the recombination fraction [27]

Lod score (logarithm of the odds): Summary statistic used in linkage analysis to test the null hypothesis of independent assortment of alleles at different loci [28]

Misclassification: The bias that occurs when there is an error in classifying subjects by disease or risk factor that tends to distort associations between disease and risk factors [29]

Multipoint linkage analysis: Linkage analysis of more than two loci at a time [28]

Penetrance: The proportion of persons known to carry a genotype, who will manifest clinical disease during their lifetime [28]

Phenocopy: An environmentally induced mimic of a genetic condition in an individual who lacks the usual causative gene [26], or an individual with an alternative genetic form of the disease in question

Phenotype: The observed attribute(s) of a cell or individual, brought about by the interaction of genotype and environment [26]

Proband: The affected individual though whom a pedigree is discovered [26]

Segregation analysis: A statistical approach to parameter estimation and hypothesis testing of different modes of inheritance of a disease [30]

Sib-pair analysis (affected sib-pair analysis): A model-free way to test for linkage to one or more marker loci based on the belief that affected sibling pairs who presumably share disease genotypes will also share marker haplotypes more often than by chance [30]

---

family history of asthma and onset of symptoms early in life; the smoker with bronchitis who begins to have intermittent bouts of wheezing and airflow obstruction; the worker exposed to a sensitizing agent in the workplace; and the elderly person who inexplicably develops asthma, having not had the disease previously [53]. One of the first classifications that offered subphenotypes was the proposal by Rackemann in 1918 [54] that asthma could be classified as extrinsic or intrinsic. In extrinsic asthma, allergens "extrinsic" to the individual were considered to determine the expression of the disease, while in "intrinsic" asthma the features were considered to depend on factors internal to the person with symptoms and not triggered primarily by airborne allergen exposures.

The classification of subphenotypes is relevant to investigating the genetic basis of asthma. Asthma is widely acknowledged to be an ill-defined syndrome that may represent the phenotypic expression of multiple genotypes whose expression may be influenced by environmental exposures. Failure to consider this heterogeneity in genetic epidemiology studies of asthma may lead to case groups of mixed subphenotypes and possibly genotypes, with the attendant potential for misclassification. Given the present status of research on the genetics of asthma, it is appropriate to focus on the most homogenous and the most readily classified phenotypes, as well as those subphenotypes for which a genetic basis seems most probable.

Patterns of incidence by age provide some insight concerning relevant subphenotypes. The majority of incident cases of physician-diagnosed asthma occur before age 10 years (Fig. 1) [55]. These early cases often occur in atopic children with a family history [56]. However, some apparent wheezing in childhood may only represent wheezing at the time of lower respiratory illness, particularly during the first two years of life [57,58].

In adulthood, three distinct subphenotypes can be postulated: the previously nonasthmatic worker exposed to a sensitizing agent; the cigarette smoker, often having some degree of fixed airflow obstruction with superimposed symptoms and varying airflow obstruction; and the elderly individual with new onset of wheezing and shortness of breath.

Several hundred agents have now been linked to occupational asthma [59]. Some of these agents act through IgE-dependent mechanisms, whereas others act through mechanisms that do not involve IgE. This subphenotype is estimated to account for approximately 15% of cases. For agents that act through IgE, prior history of atopy and asthma are associated with increased risk. This subphenotype, however, probably should be treated as environmentally induced, and persons with diagnosed occupational asthma should be excluded from studies of the genetics of asthma in general. Such persons are excluded in the current Collaborative Studies on the Genetics of Asthma funded by the National Heart, Lung, and Blood Institute. Studies of the genetic basis of the occupational asthma subphenotype may be warranted as separate studies, since these individuals may have a genetic susceptibility to these agents [60].

In individuals who smoke, there is often an overlapping picture of asthma and COPD. Persistent airflow obstruction consistent with COPD may be associated with increased airways responsiveness and intermittent airflow obstruction with wheezing. Persons having this picture may have a past history of asthma and may often have evidence of atopy. Classification of this picture is problematic in genetic studies, as elements of the COPD and the asthma phenotypes are inextricably linked. There is clearly an issue of susceptibility in cigarette smokers, since only a minority of smokers develop symptomatic obstructive lung disease [17]. Early in the development of their disease, approximately two-thirds of individuals

Table 4 Atopic Phenotype Definitions in Family and Genetic Studies

Reference	Year	Study type	Phenotype definition
Luoma et al. [44]	1982	Familial aggregation	Atopic phenotype-assigned individual had one or more of the following symptoms: (1) past or persistent history of infantile eczema, allergic skin eruptions (flexural) when adult, skin eruptions on cubital or knee folds and (2) past or persistent history of hay fever or asthma.
Cookson et al. [45]	1988	Familial aggregation	Atopic phenotype assigned if one or more of the following criteria were satisfied: (1) one or more positive skin prick tests (a weal more than 1 mm greater than the negative control); (2) a total IgE level more than two standard deviations above the mean for the normal population; (3) one or more positive radioallergosorben IgE tests (RAST).
Cookson et al. [46]	1989	Linkage	Atopy defined by the presence of one or more of the following: (1) positive skin prick test (2 mm greater than a negative control) to one or more allergens; (2) a total serum IgE level more than two standard deviations above the geometric mean for the normal population; (3) raised specific serum IgE levels (> 35 RAST units/mL) to one or more of antigens tested.
Cookson et al. [47]	1992	Affected sib pair	Atopy was defined as the presence of a positive skin-prick test response of 2 mm greater than a negative control, a positive specific IgE, a high concentration of total serum IgE, or any combination of these features.
Lympany et al. [41,48]	1992	Linkage	Atopic phenotype was defined as positive to one or more of the following criteria: (1) a positive skin prick test; (2) a positive RAST score; (3) a raised IgE.
Amelung et al. [42]	1992	Linkage	Atopic phenotype defined as one or more positive skin prick tests ($\geq$ 2 mm), a positive RAST ($\geq$ 35 RU/mL), or elevated total serum IgE levels.

Table 4 Continued

Reference	Year	Study type	Phenotype definition
Hizawa et al. [49]	1992	Linkage segregation analysis	Four definitions of atopy used. **A.** Subjects designated atopic if one more of the following criteria: (1) a raised total serum IgE level; (2) one or more raise antigen-specific serum IgE titers; (3) one or more positive skin prick tests. **B.** Same criteria as definition **A** except that subjects designated atopic only by skin response with a erythema diameter of $\geq$ 15 mm and $<$ 20 mm were judged to be normal. In definitions **C** and **D**, the presence of definite symptoms such as seasonal rhinitis, conjunctivitis, and wheezing was added to the above definitions.
Rich et al. [50]	1992	Linkage sib pair	Atopic phenotype defined as one of the following: (1) a positive skin prick test (5 mm mean weal greater than negative control); (2) a total serum IgE level greater than 87.3 U/mL; (3) specific serum IgE level $>$ 0.35 PRU/mL using common allergens.
Young et al. [51]	1992	Linkage	Atopic phenotype defined as one or more positive skin prick tests ($\geq$ 2 mm), a positive RAST ($\geq$ 35 RU/mL), or elevated total serum IgE levels corrected for age ($>$ 100 kU/L) for persons over 10 years of age and children under 10 years as recommended.
Sandford et al. [52]	1993	Affected sib-pair linkage	Atopy defined as the presence of a positive skin prick test at least 2 mm greater than the negative control, a positive specific IgE titer, a high concentration of total serum IgE, or any combination of these features.

These individuals often have a picture that combines elements of asthma and COPD as well as other conditions that are common in the elderly (cardiovascular disease). These illnesses may complicate diagnosis and management [7]. In the Normative Aging Study, allergic sensitization to house-dust mite was shown to have a role in new onset wheezing in elderly men [61].

Table 5 Proposed Subphenotypes of Asthma in Childhood and Adulthood

Childhood
  Allergic asthma: Onset in childhood, often with a background of atopy and family history
  Lower respiratory illness with wheezing: Onset in early childhood in setting of lower
    respiratory illness
Adulthood
  Occupational asthma: Onset of asthma following exposure to a sensitizing agent
  Chronic obstructive bronchitis: Variable and symptomatic airflow obstruction, typically
    in cigarette smokers, and often overlaid on some permanent loss of ventilatory
    function
  Asthma in the elderly: New onset of wheezing and dyspnea, typically without prior
    history of asthma

IV. Phenotype Misclassification and Its Consequences

A. Introduction

In epidemiologic studies, misclassification can affect the classification of either
the participants' disease or exposure status. For example, persons with COPD may
be incorrectly labeled as having asthma, or persons not having asthma may be
designated as asthmatic. Errors in classification that are random and independent
(with respect to exposure status if one is classifying disease status or the converse
if one is classifying exposure status) will generally tend to diminish the apparent

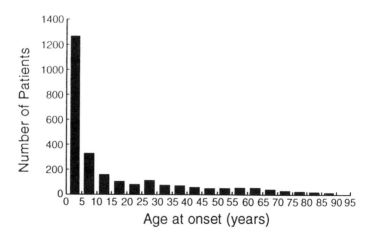

Figure 1 Distribution of ages of onset of asthma among 2499 residents of Rochester,
Minnesota. The bars represent five-year age ranges. (From Ref. 55, with permission.)

degree of association between exposure and disease. This pattern of misclassification is referred to as nondifferential misclassification. Differential misclassification occurs if bias in classification is dependent on either disease or exposure status and can result in positive or negative bias in the estimation of odds ratios or other measures of association [62].

We emphasize misclassification of phenotype, that is, disease status and not exposure status. In studying the genetics of asthma, there is a potential for misclassification by designating asthmatic as nonasthmatic or nonasthmatic as asthmatic. Additionally, phenotypes which may have differing genetic bases may be grouped inappropriately.

In genetic studies, phenotypic misclassification poses several unique problems beyond those of usual etiologic research. Persons with false-positive diagnoses (i.e., persons without the disease being misclassified as affected) cannot be distinguished from phenocopies, individuals who have an environmentally induced form of the disease or an alternative genetic basis for the disease. The phenomenon of multiple genetic causes of the same phenotype is referred to as genetic heterogeneity. Thus, persons with false-positive diagnoses mimic phenocopies and create the impression of genetic heterogeneity.

Furthermore, false-negative diagnoses (i.e., individuals with the disease phenotype are misdiagnosed as unaffected) cannot be distinguished in genetic studies from incomplete penetrance. Penetrance is the probability that a person carrying the gene for a disease will manifest the disease. Incomplete penetrance, therefore, can be viewed as a special form of misclassification [63], since a person who has an incompletely penetrant disease gene will be handled analytically as unaffected.

Simple generalizations concerning the consequences of phenotypic misclassification cannot be made for many of the analytical methods in genetic epidemiology. We consider the effects of such misclassification for the principal approaches applied to asthma; segregation analysis, sib-pair linkage analysis, and likelihood-based linkage analysis (Table 2) [28].

While we focus on phenotype in this review, classification of exposure is also of great importance. Gene–environment interactions may determine the onset of asthma as well as the features of the phenotype. Multiple exposures, in both indoor and outdoor environments, are potentially relevant. Misclassification of exposure is inevitable, and the consequences of this misclassification need further investigation. The topics of exposure assessment for environmental agents and for indoor allergens specifically have been addressed in recent National Research Council reports [64,65].

B. Consequences of Misclassification in Segregation Analysis

Segregation analysis is used to test the consistency of specific models of inheritance with family data. The general approach is to fit genetic and nongenetic models of disease transmission and compare their fit in order to determine which model is most consistent with the data. When misclassification bias is present, the fit of the models can be altered in unpredictable ways depending on the true pattern of inheritance and the pattern of misclassification [28]. For example, as a result of misclassification, a true underlying single-gene dominant inheritance model may be rejected in favor of a recessive-gene model or of a nongenetic environmental causation model. Moreover, phenotypic misclassification will change the heritability estimate, that is, the variance component in segregation analysis expressing the proportion of phenotype variation due to genotype differences [26].

Sources of bias in segregation analysis include misclassification of family members in addition to misclassification of probands. Such misclassification bias may arise from reliance on reported disease status among relatives indirectly classified by interviews with probands or their family members. Similar misclassification bias affecting relatives of cases may also occur if the relatives are still young and there has been insufficient time for disease expression, or if the relatives have developed another phenotype, e.g., COPD [28].

Phenotypic misclassification can be compensated for somewhat in segregation analysis as the penetrance parameters defined in a general model of inheritance. Penetrance parameters specify the relationship between the unobserved genotype and the observed phenotype [28]. For complex diseases such as asthma, reduced penetrance is a reasonable assumption, and as described above, false-negative diagnoses mimic incomplete penetrance. Therefore, by making allowance for incomplete penetrance, false-negative diagnostic errors are absorbed and the correct choice of inheritance model may still be possible. In addition, phenocopy rates can be estimated as a way of compensating for false-positive diagnoses. In the limit, however, high rates of phenotypic misclassification will undermine efforts to identify a genetic mechanism based on segregation analysis.

C. Consequences of Misclassification in Sib-Pair Linkage Analysis

Sib-pair analysis is an alternative nonparametric genetic method that tests for linkage. This robust method examines deviations from the expected Mendelian distribution of shared haplotypes among affected sibling pairs. It is based on the reasoning that if linkage exists, it will be reflected in the *nonrandom* association of two traits (i.e., for a disease and a marker) in independent pairs of affected sibs [66]. Misclassification of phenotype for these type of analyses generally results in a *more random* association of traits than truly exists and therefore less evidence for linkage.

Disease status must be clearly defined in affected sib-pair analysis. For simple Mendelian disorders with clear phenotypes, i.e., cystic fibrosis, it is often easy to classify individuals as affected or unaffected. For complex disorders such as asthma, however, the diagnostic boundary is more uncertain. The decision to use narrow diagnostic criteria, for example, to label only people with severe phenotypes asthmatic (e.g., a high level of bronchial hyperresponsiveness in addition to symptoms, emergency room visits, doctor's diagnosis, use of asthma medication) may be advantageous in selecting a more homogenous subgroup of siblings and fewer phenocopies. This strategy, however, will also decrease the sample size of affected sib pairs and thus the linkage information derived from the population. Broad diagnostic criteria, (e.g., a lesser degree of bronchial hyperresponsiveness, or self-reported asthma on a questionnaire), on the other hand, will increase sample size (which may or may not be the limiting factor), but may not result in more linkage information if some of the "affected" sibs are not truly affected or are phenocopies and therefore do not share marker alleles.

Kendler [67] explored this question of where the diagnostic threshold should be drawn for complex phenotypes in general in order to detect linkage by affected sib-pair analysis most efficiently. Computer simulations were done with varying diagnostic thresholds, assumed true mode of inheritance, and assumed pathogenic allele frequency in a theoretical population for which the underlying genotypic liability for the disease was known. He found that evidence for linkage between marker and disease was highly dependent on the placement of the diagnostic threshold. Moreover, he showed that there was a potential window of diagnostic stringency to be applied for sib-pair analysis, and becoming more strict or lax would result in decreased evidence for linkage. In addition, results indicated that the more common the theoretical pathogenic allele, the broader the diagnostic criteria needed to be to detect linkage by the affected sib-pair method most efficiently. Kendler suggested that this last finding had the potentially unsettling implication that the optimal phenotypic definition may not be constant across populations. For example, in a population isolate with a high pathogenic allele frequency, a broader definition of phenotype would be optimal, whereas in a population in which the pathogenic allele was less common, a narrow definition would be optimal for detecting linkage. Kendler's approach might be informative in addressing diagnostic boundaries for asthma in populations having differing prevalence rates.

D. Consequences of Misclassification in Likelihood-Based Linkage Analysis

Likelihood-based linkage analysis in genetics uses pedigree data to determine whether two or more loci are near each other on a chromosome and if so, the approximate distance that separates them. This distance is termed the recombination fraction and is an estimate of the amount of crossing over between the two loci. The purpose of linkage analysis is to delineate major gene(s) by demonstrat-

taneously increases the information for estimating the recombination fraction and establishing the order of the linked loci [28].

Fine mapping is usually performed after other studies have provided a genetic basis for the disease and two-point linkage analysis has indicated a specific region on a specific chromosome where the disease-causing allele is likely to be located. As shown in the previous linkage example, misclassification may make it extremely difficult to perform fine mapping, as recombinant individuals provide key information of the exact location of the disease gene.

In multipoint mapping, Risch found that when there is evidence for genetic heterogeneity or phenocopies, which will occur when false-positive diagnoses are present, the lod score can become greatly reduced, even negative, even when linkage truly exists. In addition, he showed that when there are a greater number of children, lod scores decrease more dramatically in multipoint mapping in the presence of genetic heterogeneity and phenocopies.

Thus, Risch and Giuffra showed that multipoint linkage analysis was less robust to phenotype misclassification than two-point linkage analysis because errors could not be absorbed into an inflated recombination fraction (since the multiple DNA markers are at a fixed distance from each other). They proposed as a solution, however, estimating high disease allele frequencies. By overestimating the disease allele frequencies in the model, lod scores were minimally reduced from the true value and detection of linkage was still possible. He argued that false exclusion of a true disease chromosomal location is just as serious an error as false conclusion of linkage. Risch and Giuffra therefore concluded that using a liberal genetic model (e.g., high gene frequency) is appropriately conservative when analyzing a complex disease and will make multipoint linkage analysis more robust to phenotype misclassification.

These results also emphasize, however, the necessity of defining an asthma phenotype and subphenotypes more precisely. Although it is important for all genetic analyses, correct phenotype identification of asthma is especially critical for future fine mapping studies in order to avoid spuriously negative lod scores.

V. Implications

The last five years have been a time of explosive research on the genetics of asthma, which should lead to important information on pathogenesis and to new therapeutic possibilities. This research has become possible because of rapid advances in molecular techniques and genome mapping. However, there has not been a parallel advance in our ability to characterize the asthma phenotype. Long-asked questions as to the criteria for establishing the presence of asthma are still unanswered. New insights concerning the inflammatory nature of the disease process have not improved diagnostic validity.

We caution that phenotype misclassification threatens the validity of any study of the genetics of asthma. There has not been consistency in approaches to characterizing the asthma phenotype in studies conducted to date. This lack of consistency constrains comparisons of study findings and may preclude pooling of data. We recommend adherence to standardized methods for characterizing the asthma phenotype. Additionally, we suggest that subphenotypes of interest should be carefully designated in studies of the genetics of asthma.

Acknowledgment

This work was supported by grants from the National Institutes of Health; R01 HL48341 and U01 HL49602.

References

1. Samet JM. Epidemiologic approaches for the identification of asthma. Chest 1987; 91:745s–785s.
2. Ciba Foundation Guest Symposium. Report on the working group on the definition of asthma. Edinburgh: Churchill Livingstone, 1971; 38.
3. American Thoracic Society. Definitions and classification of chronic bronchitis, asthma, and pulmonary emphysema. Am Rev Respir Dis 1962; 85:762–785.
4. Ciba Foundation Guest Symposium. Terminology, definitions and classification of chronic pulmonary emphysema and related conditions. Thorax 1959; 14:286–299.
5. World Health Organization. Epidemiology of chronic and non-specific respiratory diseases. Bull World Health Organ 1975; 52:251–260.
6. American Thoracic Society. Standardization of spirometry—1987 update. Am Rev Respir Dis 1987; 136:1285–1298.
7. National Heart, Lung, and Blood Institute, National Institutes of Health. Guidelines for the diagnosis and management of asthma. Washington, DC: U.S. Government Printing Office, 1991:91-3042.
8. National Heart, Lung, and Blood Institute, National Institutes of Health. Guidelines for the diagnosis and management of asthma. Washington, DC: U.S. Government Printing Office, 1995:95-36S9.
9. National Heart, Lung, and Blood Institute, World Health Organization. Global initiative for asthma. Washington, DC: U.S. Government Printing Office, 1993.
10. Toelle BG, Peat JK, Salome CM, Mellis CM, Woolcock AJ. Toward a definition of asthma for epidemiology. Am Rev Respir Dis 1992; 146:633–637.
11. Brown PJ, Greville HW, Finucane KE. Asthma and irreversible airflow obstruction. Thorax 1984; 39:131–136.
12. Sparrow D, Weiss ST. Methodological issues in airway responsiveness testing. In: Weiss ST, Sparrow D, eds. Airway Responsiveness and Atopy in the Development of Chronic Lung Disease. New York: Raven Press, 1989:103–120.
13. Sparrow D, O'Connor GT, Basner RC, Weiss ST. Predictors of the new onset of

wheezing among middle-aged and older men. The normative aging study. Am Rev Respir Dis 1993; 147:367–371.

14. Pattemore PK, Asher MI, Harrison AC, Mitchell EA, Rea HH, Stewart AW. The interrelationship among bronchial hyperresponsiveness, the diagnosis of asthma, and asthma symptoms. Am Rev Respir Dis 1990; 142:549–554.

15. Woolcock AJ, Anderson SD, Peat JK, et al. Characteristics of bronchial hyperrespon-siveness in chronic obstructive pulmonary disease and in asthma. Am Rev Respir Dis 1991; 143:1438–1443.

16. National Institutes of Health workshop summary and guidelines: investigative use of bronchoscopy, lavage and bronchial biopsies in asthma and other airways disease. J Allergy Clin Immunol 1991; 88:808–814.

17. Tashkin DP, Altose MD, Bleecker ER, et al. The lung health study: airway responsive-ness to inhaled methacholine in smokers with mild to moderate airflow limitation. Am Rev Respir Dis 1992; 145:301–310.

18. Burrows B. Differential diagnosis of chronic obstructive pulmonary disease. Chest 1990; 97:16S–18S.

19. Chatham M, Bleecker ER, Smith PL, Rosenthal RR, Mason P, Norman PS. A comparison of histamine, methacholine, and exercise airway reactivity in normal and asthmatic subjects. Am Rev Respir Dis 1982; 126:235–240.

20. Britt EJ, Cohen B, Menkes H, et al. Airways reactivity and functional deterioration in relatives of COPD patients. Chest 1980; 77:260–261.

21. Ferris BG Jr. Epidemiology standardization project. Part II. Am Rev Respir Dis 1978; 118:1–120.

22. Samet JM. Definitions and methodology in COPD research. In: Hensley M, Saunders N, eds. Clinical Epidemiology of Chronic Obstructive Lung Disease. New York: Marcel Dekker, 1989:1–22.

23. Burney PGJ, Britton JR, Chinn S, et al. Descriptive epidemiology of bronchial reactivity in an adult population: results from a community study. Thorax 1987; 42:38–44.

24. International study of asthma and allergies in childhood. 1992.

25. Weiss ST. Issues in phenotype assessment in genetic studies of asthma. Genet Asthma 1995; in press.

26. Mange EJ, Mange AP. Mange EJ, Mange AP, eds. Basic Human Genetics. Sunder-land, MA: Sinauer Associates, 1994.

27. Lung F. The impact of diagnostic misclassification on linkage analysis in complex disorders: a linkage study by computer simulation in bipolar disorder. D.Sc. thesis. Baltimore, MD: The Johns Hopkins University School of Hygiene and Public Health, 1992.

28. Khoury MJ, Beaty TH, Cohen BH. Fundamentals of Genetic Epidemiology. New York: Oxford University Press, 1993.

29. Flegal KM, Brownie C, Haas JD. The effects of exposure misclassification on estimates of relative risk. Am J Epidemiol 1986; 123:736–751.

30. Weiss KM. Weiss KM, eds. Genetic Variation and Human Disease. Cambridge, New York City, Melbourne: Cambridge University Press, 1993.

31. Edfors-Lubs M. Allergy in 7000 twin pairs. Acta Allergol 1971; 26:249–285.

32. Higgins M, Keller J. Familial occurrence of chronic respiratory disease and familial resemblance in ventilatory capacity. J Chron Dis 1975; 28:239–251.

33. Sibbald B, Turner-Warwick M. Factors influencing the prevalence of asthma among first degree relatives of extrinxic and intrinsic asthmatics. Thorax 1979; 34:332–337.

34. Townley RG, Bewtra A, Wilson AF, et al. Segregation analysis of bronchial response to methacholine inhalation challenge in families with and without asthma. J Allergy Clin Immunol 1986; 77:101–107.

35. Redline S, Tishler PV, Lewitter FI, Tager IB, Munoz A, Speizer F. Assessment of genetic and nongenetic influences on pulmonary function. Am Rev Respir Dis 1987; 135:217–222.

36. Hopp RJ, Bewtra A, Biven R, Nair NM, Townley RG. Bronchial reactivity pattern in nonasthmatic parents of asthmatics. Ann Allergy 1988; 61:184–186.

37. Duffy DL, Nicholas MG, Battistutta D, Hopper JL, Mathews JD. Genetics of asthma and hay fever in Australian twins. Am Rev Respir Dis 1990; 142:1351–1358.

38. Reihsaus E, Innis M, MacIntyre N, Liggett SB. Mutations in the gene encoding for the beta2-adrenergic receptor in normal and asthmatic subjects. Am J Respir Cell Mol Biol 1993; 8:334–339.

39. Martinez FD, Holberg CJ. Segregation analysis of physician diagnosed asthma in Hispanic and non-Hispanic white families. Respir Sci 1995; 14:2–8.

40. Longo G, Strinati R, Poli F, Fumi F. Genetic factors in nonspecific bronchial hyper-reactivity. Am J Dis Child 1987; 141:331–334.

41. Lympany P, Welsh K, MacCochrane G, Kemeny DM, Lee TH. Genetic analysis using DNA polymorphism of the linkage between chromosome 11q13 and atopy and bronchial hyperresponsiveness to methacholine. J Allergy Clin Immunol 1992; 89: 619–628.

42. Amelung PJ, Panhuysen CIM, Postma DS, et al. Atopy and bronchial hyperrespon-siveness: exclusion of linkage to markers on chromosomes 11q and 6p. Clin Exp Allergy 1992; 22:1077–1084.

43. Postma DS, Bleecker ER, Amelung PJ, et al. Genetic susceptibility to asthma: bronchial hyperresponsiveness coinherited with a major gene for atopy. N Engl J Med 1995; in press.

44. Luoma R, Koivikko A. Occurrence of atopic diseases in three generations. Scand J Soc Med 1982; 10:49–56.

45. Cookson WOC, Hopkin JM. Dominant Inheriance of atopic immunoglobulin-E re-sponsiveness. Lancet 1988; i:86–88.

46. Cookson WOCM, Sharp PA, Faux JA, Hopkin JM. Linkage between immunoglobulin E responses underlying asthma and rhinitis and chromosome 11q. Lancet 1989; 1: 1292–1295.

47. Cookson WOCM, Young RP, Sandford AJ, et al. Maternal inheritance of atopic IgE responsiveness on chromosome 11q. Lancet 1992; 340:381–384.

48. Lympany P, Welsh KI, Cochrane GM, Kemeny DM, Lee TH. Genetic analysis of the linkage between chromosome 11q and atopy. Clin Exp Allergy 1992; 22:1085–1092.

49. Hizawa N, Yamaguchi E, Ohe M, et al. Lack of linkage between atopy and locus 11q13. Clin Exp Allergy 1992; 22:1065–1069.

50. Rich SS, Roitman-Johnson B, Greenberg B, Roberts S, Blumenthal MN. Genetic

analysis of atopy in three large kindreds: no evidence of linkage to D11S97. Clin Exp Allergy 1992; 22:1070–1076.

51. Young RP, Sharp PA, Lynch JR, et al. Confirmation of genetic linkage between atopic IgE responses and chromosome 11q13. J Med Genet 1992; 29:236–238.

52. Sandford AJ, Shirakawa T, Moffatt MF, et al. Localisation of atopy and beta subunit of high-affinity IgE receptor on chromosome 11q. Lancet 1993; 341:332–334.

53. Woolcock AJ. Asthma. In: Murray JF, Nadel JA, eds. Textbook of Respiratory Medicine. 2d ed. Philadelphia: W. B. Saunders, 1994:1288.

54. Rackemann FM. A clinical study of one hundred fifty cases of bronchial asthma. Arch Intern Med 1918; 22:517–552.

55. Silverstein MD, Reed CE, O'Connell EJ, Melton LJ III, O'Fallon WM, Yunginger JW. Long-term survival of a cohort of community residents with asthma. N Engl J Med 1994; 331:1537–1541.

56. Coultas DB, Samet JM. Epidemiology and natural history of asthma. In: Tinkelman DG, Naspitz CK, eds. Childhood Asthma. New York: Marcel Dekker, 1993:71–114.

57. Martinez FD, Wright AL, Taussig LM, et al. Asthma and wheezing in the first six years of life. N Engl J Med 1995; 332:133–138.

58. Silverman M. Out of the mouths of babes and sucklings: lessons from early childhood asthma. Thorax 1993; 48:1200–1204.

59. Chan-Yeung M, Malo J. Occupational asthma. N Engl J Med 1995; 333:107–112.

60. Bignon JS, Aron Y, Ju LJ. HLA class II alleles in isocyanate-induced asthma. Am J Respir Crit Care Med 1994; 149:71–75.

61. Ohman JL, Sparrow D, MacDonald MR. New onset wheezing in an older male population: evidence of allergen sensitization in a longitudinal study. J Allergy Clin Immunol 1993; 91:752–757.

62. Rothman KJ. Modern Epidemiology. Boston: Little, Brown, 1986.

63. Ott J, ed. Analysis of Human Genetic Linkage. Rev ed. Baltimore and London: The Johns Hopkins University Press, 1992.

64. National Research Council, Committee on Advances in Assessing Human Exposure to Airborne Pollutants. Human exposure assessment for airborne pollutants. Washington, DC: National Academy Press, 1991.

65. Institute of Medicine, Committee on the Health Effects of Indoor Allergens, Division of Health Promotion and Disease and Disease Prevention. Indoor Allergens: Assessing the Controlling Adverse Health Effects. Washington DC: National Academy Press, 1993.

66. Penrose LS. The general sib-pair linkage test. Ann Eugenics 1953; 18:120–144.

67. Kendler KS. The impact of varying diagnostic thresholds on affected sib pair linkage analysis. Genet Epidemiol 1988; 5:407–419.

68. Martinez M, Khlat M, Leboyer M, Clerget-Darpoux F. Performance of linkage analysis under misclassification error when the genetic model is unknown. Genet Epidemiol 1989; 6:253–258.

69. Ott J. Linkage analysis with misclassification at on locus. Clin Genet 1977; 12: 119–124.

70. Risch N, Giuffra L. Model misspecification and multipoint linkage analysis. Hum Hered 1992; 42:77–92.

20

Approaches to Family Studies of Asthma

D. S. POSTMA

University Hospital
Groningen, The Netherlands

DEBORAH A. MEYERS

Johns Hopkins University School of
Medicine
Baltimore, Maryland

I. Introduction

Determining the role of genetics and environmental factors in common disorders with a heritable component such as asthma and allergy is an area of important research for both geneticists and clinicians. These disorders are not inherited in a simple Mendelian fashion, but there is an increased risk to relatives of affected individuals, suggesting a genetic component. The disorders are also more prevalent in the population than Mendelian disorders, which are relatively rare. Therefore, they are of a greater concern from the public health viewpoint, and delineating the role of genetics in such disorders is expected to have widespread significance. It is expected that further insight into the underlying pathophysiology of the disease will lead eventually to new and better treatment programs.

This chapter reviews the purpose and design of family studies needed to determine the role of genetics in disorders such as asthma. Families as small as two siblings or large extended pedigrees with several hundred members may be studied. The goals of a given study will guide decisions on the type and number of families that will be needed (Table 1). Different sampling schemes have their own advantages and disadvantages and need to be carefully considered before undertaking the expensive and time-consuming task of collecting family data.

Table 1 Examples of Commonly Used Study Designs in Genetic Research

1. Determine relationship of a specific mutation or polymorphism to the disease phenotype
   Study designs:
   Patients ascertained through a clinic versus matched controls
   Patients and DNA samples on their parents to compare the frequency of inherited versus noninherited alleles
2. Estimate proportion of trait due to genetic factors
   Study designs:
   Twins
   Siblings raised apart
   Comparison of case versus control families
3. Determine mode of inheritance of a given trait or disease
   Study designs:
   Nuclear families ascertained through an affected parent (proband)
   Nuclear families ascertained through two affected siblings
   Extended families ascertained through a proband (additional relatives studied according to predetermined criteria)
4. Map susceptibility genes
   Study designs:
   Affected sib pairs
   Nuclear families (often ascertained for multiple affected members)
   Extended pedigrees
   Inbred and/or isolated populations

In general, only limited information can be obtained on the genetics of a disorder by studying a patient population. Therefore, it is necessary to investigate the genetic transmission of the given phenotype from parent to child or, at the very least, to determine the genes shared between two siblings with the disorder. In several other chapters in this volume, there is description and discussion on the "asthmatic" phenotype and the types of subjective (symptoms) and objective (pulmonary function tests, skin tests, and blood analyses) parameters that are useful in defining asthma. Data from all these parameters are useful in genetic studies to determine susceptibility to asthma. The types of data that will be collected are an important aspect of designing a family study. For example, it may be more reasonable and very useful to perform certain studies on siblings of similar ages. This may be the case for atopy and hyperresponsiveness in the expression of the disease. There is an important drawback to these traits in that they are both age and gender dependent [1–3] and can change over time due to exogenous influences such as allergen exposure and viral infection. Whereas bronchial hyperresponsiveness decreases in early childhood and tends to increase at older ages, atopy has an opposite course: It increases from birth to young age and then decreases at older ages.

Studies are furthermore complicated by the fact that clinical features of asthma may change over time and may mirror features of chronic obstructive pulmonary disease (COPD) when asthma has progressed at older age. An example is the study of Panhuysen et al. [3], in which 189 young adult asthmatic individuals were restudied after 25 years. Twelve percent of these asthmatic individuals were no longer asthmatic after 25 years; i.e., they did not have asthmatic symptoms or hyperresponsiveness to histamine and had near normal lung function. In the original study, 93% of these subjects were atopic based on skin tests, but 80% are currently atopic. Some lost evidence of atopy, while others became atopic. These age-related changes may cause problems in cross-sectional investigations of families consisting of children, parents, and grandparents to determine the genetics of asthma.

This problem may be circumvented by selecting families with a proband who is known to have had asthma 25 years ago and who was assessed clinically in a standardized way [4]. Thus, the time component can be ruled out and one is able to compare the initial data set of the probands with the data of their children, who are now in the same age range as their parents were at initial testing. This method of ascertainment has been used successfully for the Dutch asthma study of 92 families, with evidence for linkage of total serum IgE levels, bronchial hyperresponsiveness, and asthma to chromosome 5q [5–8].

II. Ascertainment of Families

For genetic studies, families usually are not ascertained in a random manner. For example, one could ascertain families by studying all children in first grade at the local school as probands and then study their parents and siblings. Many genetic disorders are too rare to use this approach. However, random ascertainment of families is possible for studying allergic disease, since the prevalence of atopy in the population is about 30%. For example, 131 nuclear families with at least three children have been ascertained in a random manner for the study of atopy [9]. However, for the study of asthma, families are being ascertained for having multiple members with the asthma phenotype [9]. For the asthma phenotype, it is unlikely that sufficient numbers of affected individuals would be sampled by random ascertainment of families in the population.

The method of ascertainment of families needs to be clearly specified. If families are being ascertained to determine the mode of inheritance of the disease in question through segregation analysis, the family may not be ascertained in a manner favoring a specific mode of inheritance. For example, if an investigator studies only families with an affected parent and child, the results will be biased in favor of dominant inheritance. If linkage analysis is the aim of the study, families are often ascertained for the presence of multiple affected family members, hopefully "loading" the family in favor of a genetic component to a disease. This is often done after a genetic basis for the disorder has been determined, in order to genotype the most informative families. A compromise situation is to ascertain a family through two affected sibs and to study all parents, other sibs, and possibly additional relatives. Both segregation and linkage analysis can then be performed.

III. Sampling Designs

The purpose of a given study will influence the type of families and data to be collected (Table 1). Association studies may be performed on a sample of unrelated individuals, but, in general, family data are needed. There are several different types of families that may be studied, each with advantages and disadvantages. For any study, it is important to design a database for storage and management of the data collected. Although this is easily done using commercial databases that are available for microcomputers, it is an important step since large amounts of both clinical and molecular data are collected.

A. Unrelated Individuals

Studies of unrelated patients may provide useful genetic information and are often performed before family studies are undertaken. Usually these studies are "association" studies to determine if there is a relationship between a clinical phenotype or a specific measure of the phenotype and a polymorphism or a mutation in a candidate gene. For the asthma phenotype, polymorphisms in the β_2-adrenergic receptor gene on chromosome have been shown to be associated with specific asthma phenotypes [10–11]. For example, patients with severe steroid-dependent asthma or nocturnal asthma have an increased frequency of the Gly16 allele [11].

Once genes that are important in asthma and allergy are mapped, association studies of specific mutations in candidate genes will be needed. However, given the complexity of the phenotype, these studies may not be easy to perform, and the results will need careful interpretation.

B. Twins

Twin studies also provide important information and are useful to perform before studying families. The heritability of the disease in question or components of the disease can be determined by comparing monozygotic twin pairs to dizygotic twin pairs. For example, an intrapair correlation coefficient for total serum IgE of 82% in monozygotic twins compared with 52% in dizygotic twins was found in a study of 107 twins, yielding an overall heritability of 61% [12]. It is usually assumed that twins share a common environment, which lessens the impact of environmental influences. This is important in the investigations of asthma and allergy, since the expression of these disorders is dependent on the environmental exposure to allergens and possibly other pollutants. However, the environment is probably less similar in studies of adult twins living in separate households. For total serum IgE levels, it has been shown that the pairwise concordances for monozygotic twins raised apart were similar to those for monozygotic twins raised together [13]. This suggests a strong genetic control of serum IgE levels. One of the advantages of studying twins is that there are no age differences within a pair of twins. Often, studies are restricted to twins of the same sex, which is appropriate for studies of allergy and asthma since there are reported sex differences in the prevalence of the disorders.

C. Nuclear Families

There are three types of families that may be studied: nuclear families, extended pedigrees, or inbred populations (Table 2). Nuclear families consist of children

Table 2 Different Family Structures That Are Useful in Genetic Studies

Twins	
Advantages:	Provides estimate of familial component by comparing MZ to DZ twins
Disadvantages:	Environment may differ between different types of twins; MZ twins do not provide linkage information
Nuclear families	
Advantages	Likely to be representative of the disease in the general population, easy to ascertain
Disadvantages:	May be difficult to detect major genes if there are multiple genes important in the disorder
Extended pedigrees	
Advantages:	Disease phenotype may be traced through multiple generations, providing important data for segregation and mapping studies
Disadvantages:	Genes present in these families may be relatively rare in the general population; additional genes may be introduced by spouses in some branches of the families
Inbred and/or isolated populations	
Advantages:	Small number of genes may be present for these multifactorial disorders, due to a founder effect
Disadvantages:	These genes may be very rare in the general population

and parents. One may attempt either to phenotype the entire family for the disorder in question, or one may study only affected sibs for the disease in question but draw blood and perform genetic marker studies on the parents also. An advantage of studying nuclear families is that they are probably representative of the disease in the general population.

There are numerous studies of nuclear families, including several multicenter studies underway in several countries, to delineate the genes important in susceptibility to asthma (Table 3). A very large multicenter study is being conducted in France. As of April 1995, data on 350 nuclear families ascertained through a single proband with clinical asthma has been collected [14]. Both segregation and linkage analysis will be performed for asthma, atopy, and associated phenotypes. In Germany, 100 nuclear families are being ascertained through two siblings with asthma from multiple clinical centers [15]. In the U.S. collaborative study on the genetics of asthma, nuclear families from several racial groups, including Caucasians, African Americans, and Hispanics, are being studied. The families are ascertained for two affected siblings, and the parents and other siblings are also studied [16].

An advantage of these multicenter studies is that a large number of families may be collected in a relatively short period of time. Of course, it is important that the same testing and criteria be used at each center. Because of the large number of families being studied, it may be easier to detect linkage in the presence of genetic heterogeneity. If significant heterogeneity exists or if only a proportion of the families have a genetic form of the disorder, it is more difficult to detect linkage, since evidence for linkage will be seen in only a proportion of the families. This disadvantage is also true for affected sib pairs. An advantage of studying only affected sib pairs is that it is likely that the sibs have a similar form of the disorder, and if there are significant age effects, it may be difficult to phenotype the parents. Age effects and the effects of smoking (interfering with a clear-cut diagnosis of asthma versus COPD) are both reasons why one may choose to study affected sib pairs for asthma.

Besides the multicenter studies, several other studies of nuclear families are being performed in different countries (Table 3). Family studies are underway in Western Australia for the purpose of evaluating candidate genes [17]. Fifty families ascertained through a child with asthma and 50 control families are being recruited and characterized. In the United States, there has been a ongoing longitudinal study that includes 906 nuclear Hispanic and non-Hispanic white families [18,19], which has already produced important results on the segregation of total IgE levels and physician-diagnosed asthma in families [19,20]. Another ongoing study that has produced important results is that of Cookson and colleagues, which was originally designed for the study of atopy but now includes families ascertained for asthma [21–23].

Table 3 Examples of Current Family Studies on the Genetics of Asthma

Nuclear families (multicenter studies)

France: 350 nuclear families ascertained through a single proband with clinical asthma have been studied and additional families are being ascertained [14]. Segregation and linkage analyses will be performed for measures of asthma, atopy.

Germany: 100 nuclear families are being ascertained through two siblings with asthma from multiple clinical centers [15].

U.S. collaborative study: Nuclear families from several genetic backgrounds, including African Americans, Caucasians, and Hispanics, are being studied ascertained through two siblings with asthma [16]. A complete genome screen is underway.

Nuclear families

Australia: 50 families with a child with asthma and 50 control families are being studied for candidate genes [17].

The Netherlands: 92 families ascertained through a parent originally studied for asthma approximately 25 years ago. Evidence for linkage of total serum IgE levels, bronchial hyperresponsiveness, and asthma to chromosome 5q has been obtained [5–8].

United States: Large ongoing study of Hispanic and non-Hispanic families. Segregation analyses have been performed for total IgE levels and the asthma phenotype [19,20].

United Kingdom: Random ascertainment of families for studies of atopy as well as ascertainment of multiplex families for asthma [9]. Linkage and association studies are being performed.

United Kingdom: Large ongoing study originally designed to determine genetics factors in atopy but expanded to include the asthma phenotype [21–23].

Extended pedigrees

United States: 262 individuals from five large pedigrees in Minnesota are being studied and a complete genome screen performed [16].

China: 120 members from a four-generation pedigree are being studied; approximately 32% of the family members have airways hyperresponsiveness [25].

Inbred and/or isolated populations

Amish: Evidence has been found for a major locus for total serum IgE levels mapping to 5q [26–27].

Hutterite: 380 individuals from one large pedigree in South Dakota [16] have been studied, and a complete genome screening is being performed.

Tristan da Cunha: All individuals on this small, physically isolated island in the South Atlantic have been studied [25,28]. The population is highly inbred, with a prevalence of 49% of bronchial hyperresponsiveness.

D. Extended Pedigrees

Extended pedigrees are often used for genetic studies, especially for disorders with evidence for a dominantly inherited major gene (Table 2). A family may be ascertained through a single or multiple probands and then extended to aunts, uncles, grandparents, and cousins as available. A single large pedigree may provide evidence for linkage, reducing the problem of genetic heterogeneity. This family may not be representative of most families with this disorder, but if a gene is localized from such a pedigree, it can be tested in other families. Even if it is found to represent a rare form of the disorder, it is still an important step in understanding the genetics of the disorder. For example, the APP mutations on chromosome 21 are now considered to be a "rare" cause of Alzheimer's disease, but they represent the first linkage and gene found for this disorder [24]. For common disorders, a possible disadvantage in studying extended pedigrees is that there may be several genes segregating for the disorder within the pedigree. It is possible that one gene is transmitted through the pedigree but that in another branch of the family, a different gene may be segregating after having been introduced by a spouse marrying into the family. It is important to phenotype all family members (including spouses) to try to determine if multiple genes may be segregating within the pedigree. For example, in a pedigree where a spouse has asthma, additional genes may be brought in by the spouse and transmitted to the children.

Several groups of investigators are studying large extended families to determine the genetics of asthma (Table 3). For example, Blumenthal et al. [16] are studying 262 individuals from five large pedigrees in Minnesota. In china, a large extended family of approximately 120 members from four generations is being studied because of the high reported prevalence of asthma. Approximately 32% of the family members have airways hyperresponsiveness [25].

E. Isolated Populations

Isolated populations with large extended pedigrees and inbreeding are another source of families for genetic studies as long as the disorder being studied is present in the population (Tables 2 and 3). Because of founder effects, a given population may have a low frequency of a trait or disease that is relatively common in the general population. Due to the founder effect, genes mapped in such populations may not be representative of the major genes found in the general population. However, as with studying large pedigrees without inbreeding, such findings are still of importance.

Examples include the Amish population in the United States as well as isolated island populations in other parts of the world. The Amish are a closed community, in which individuals may leave but individuals from the outside community do not marry into Amish families. This represents a closed gene pool with a founder effect; i.e., the genes present and their relative frequency in the current members of the community are derived from the original founding couples. Because of their large family size, known genealogy, and relatively homogeneous environment, such populations are often used for genetic studies. Marsh et al. [26,27] found evidence for a major locus for total serum IgE levels mapping to 5q from studying 11 Amish pedigrees consisting of 20 nuclear families. Currently, as part of a multicenter collaborative U.S. study, Ober and colleagues have clinically characterized 380 individuals from one large Hutterite pedigree in South Dakota [16]. Complete genome screening is underway.

Other examples of closed populations include those that are physically isolated, such as island populations. A well-studied island population is that of the Tristan da Cunhas from an island in the South Atlantic. In 1961, the population of approximately 268 members was removed because of a volcano eruption. Almost of the individuals except young children were studied while in the United Kingdom. They have returned to the island and are still of interest to geneticists, since it remains a small, closed, and isolated population. Again, results from such studies may or may not be directly applicable to families in the general population, but the results could provide useful insights into studies of noninbred families. All inhabitants on this island can be traced back to 15 ancestors, and the population is highly inbred. The prevalence of hyperresponsiveness is 49% [18,28]. The high incidence of asthma on Tristan probably derives from two or three asthmatics among the original founders, representing a clear founder effect. This population offers a unique opportunity to study why some children of two parents with asthma do not develop asthma themselves. Detection of protective mechanisms for development of asthma are as interesting as provoking factors, certainly in view of gene therapy. It may also be that a local factor affects the outcome of asthma. Although it is never possible to define all possible environmental factors, at least these families are all exposed to the same environmental influences. There is little industry or resulting air pollution on this island. However, viral infections come to Tristan on visiting ships and occur usually in well-defined epidemics, at which time the incidence of wheeze increases. Possibly the timing of the encounter of viral infections may be of crucial importance in the development of asthma. Therefore, even in isolated populations, an important role for environment influences may exist [18,28].

IV. Summary

In summary, various sample designs are useful for genetic studies of complex genetic disorders such as asthma and allergy. The goals (both short term and long term) of a given study will determine the types of individuals and families to be studied. It is important for the investigator to consider carefully the types of families available for study and the manner in which the families will be ascertained. These decisions should be based on the aims of the study as well as the availability of various populations (Table 1). Generally, it is important to study family members as completely and accurately as possible. Since there is usually a large and expensive effort involved in genotyping families for mapping genes, it is important that the clinical data as well as the molecular data be of the highest quality.

Acknowledgment

This work was supported by a grant from the Dutch Asthma Foundation (90.39) and grants from the National Institutes of Health; R01 HL48341 and U01 HL49602.

References

1. O'Connor GT, Sparrow D, Weiss ST. The role of allergy and nonspecific airway hyperresponsiveness in the pathogenesis of chronic obstructive pulmonary disease. Am Rev Respir Dis 1989; 140:225–252.
2. Postma DS, De Vries K, Koeter GH, Sluiter HJ. Independent influence of reversibility of air-flow obstruction and non-specific hyperreactivity on the long-term course of lung function in chronic air-flow obstruction. Am Rev Respir Dis 1986; 134:276–280.
3. Panhuysen CIM, Vonk JM, Schouten JP, Van Altena R, Koeter GH, Postma DS. Do adult patients outgrow their asthma? Am J Respir Crit Care Med 1995; 151(4):A472.
4. Panhuysen CIM, Bleecker ER, Koeter GH, Meyers DA, Postma DS. Dutch approach to the study of the genetics of asthma. Clin Exper Allergy 1995; 25(S2):35–38.
5. Meyers DA, Postma DS, Panhuysen CIM, et al. Evidence for a locus regulating total serum IgE levels mapping to chromosome 5. Genomics 1994; 23:464–470.
6. Postma DS, Bleecker ER, Amelung PJ, et al. Genetic susceptibility to asthma—bronchial hyperresponsiveness coinherited with a major gene for atopy. N Engl J Med 1995; 333:894–900.
7. Bleecker ER, Amelung PJ, Levitt RC, Postma DS, Meyers DA. Evidence for linkage of total serum IgE and bronchial hyperresponsiveness to chromosome 5q: a major regulatory locus important in asthma. Clin Exp Allergy 1994; 25(S2):84–88.
8. Panhuysen CIM, Levitt RC, Postma DS, et al. Evidence for a susceptibility locus for asthma mapping to chromosome 5q. J Invest Med 1995; 43:281A.
9. Morton NE. Genetic studies on atopy and asthma in Wessex. Clin Exp Allergy 1995; 25(S2):107–109.
10. Reishaus E, Innis M, MacIntyre N, Liggett SB. Mutations in the gene encoding for the β_2-adrenergic receptor in normal and asthmatic subjects. Am J Respir Cell Mol Biol 1993; 8:334–339.
11. Liggett SB. Genetics of β_2-adrenergic receptor variants in asthma. Clin Exp Allergy 1995; 25(S2):89–94.

12. Hopp RJ, Bewtra AK, Watt GD, Nair NM, Townley RG. Genetic analysis of allergic disease in twins. J Allergy Clin Immunol 1984; 73:265–270.

13. Blumenthal MN, Bonini S. Immunogenetics of specific immune responses to allerfens in twins and families. In: Marsh DG, Blumenthal Mn, eds. Genetic and Environmental Factors in Clinical Allergy. Minneapolis, MN: University of Minnesota Press, 1990:132–139.

14. Kauffmann F, Dizier M-H, on behalf of the EGEA Co-operative Group. Design issues. Clin Exp Allergy 1995; 25(S2):19–22.

15. Wjst M, Wichmann HE. Collaborative studies on the genetics of asthma in Germany. Clin Exp Allergy 1995; 25(S2):23–25.

16. Blumenthal MN, Banks-Schlegel S, Bleecker ER, Marsh DG, Ober C. Collaborative studies on the genetics of asthma—NHLBI. Clin Exp Allergy 1995; 25(S2):29–32.

17. Le Souef PN. Asthma genetics studies in Western Australia. Clin Exp Allergy 1995; 25(S2):26–28.

18. Taussig LM, Wright AL, Morgan WJ, Harrison MR, Ray CG, and the GHMA Pediatricians. The Tucson Children's Respiratory Study. I. Design and implementation of a prospective study of acute and chronic respiratory illness in children. Am J Epidemiol 1989; 129:1219–1231.

19. Martinez FD, Holberg CJ. Segregation analysis of physician-diagnosed asthma in Hispanic and non-Hispanic white families. Clin Exp Allergy 1995; 25(S2):68–70.

20. Martinez FD, Holberg CJ, Halonen M, Morgan WJ, Wright AL, Taussig LM. Evidence for Mendelian inheritance of serum IgE levels in Hispanic and non-Hispanic white families. Am J Hum Genet 1994; 55:555–564.

21. Cookson WOCM, Hopkin JM. Linkage between immunoglobulin E responses underlying asthma and rhinitis and chromosome 11q. Lancet 1989; 23:957–963.

22. Moffatt MF, Hill MR, Cornelis F, et al. Genetic linkage of T-cell receptor α/γ complex to specific IgE responses. Lancet 1994; 343:1597–1600.

23. Cookson WO. 11q and high-affinity of igE receptor in asthma and allergy. Clin Exp Allergy 1995; 25(S2):71–73.

24. Tanzi RE, Vaula G, Romano DM, et al. Assessment of amyloid B-protein precursor gene mutations in a large set of familial and sporadic Alzheimer disease cases. Am J Hum Genet 1992; 51:273–282.

25. Slutsky AS, Zamel N, and the University of Toronto Genetics of Asthma Research Group. Genetics of asthma: University of Toronto. Clin Exp Allergy 1995; 25(S2): 33–34.

26. Marsh DG, Neely JD, Breazeale DR, et al. Linkage analysis of IL4 and other chromosome 5q31.1 markers and total serum immunoglobulin E concentrations. Science 1994; 264:1152–1156.

27. Marsh DG, Neely JD, Breazeale DR, et al. Total serum IgE levels and chromosome 5q. Clin Exp Allergy 1995; 25(S2):79–83.

28. Zamel N, McClean PA, Sandell PR, Slutsky AS, and the University of Toronto Genetics of Asthma Research Group. Asthma in Tristan da Cunha. Am J Respir Crit Care Med 1994; 149:A1051.

21

The Genetics of β_2-Adrenergic Receptor Polymorphisms

Relevance to Receptor Function and Asthmatic Phenotypes

STEPHEN B. LIGGETT

University of Cincinnati College of Medicine
Cincinnati, Ohio

The human β_2-adrenergic receptor (β_2AR) exists in several variant forms in the population due to polymorphisms in the gene encoding for the receptor. The β_2AR is localized to a number of cell types in the lung which are relevant to asthma (see Chapter 4). Due to its expression on bronchial smooth muscle, the receptor participates in establishing bronchomotor tone and is the target for the most rapid-acting and effective class of bronchodilating drugs: βAR agonists. The genetics, molecular biology, pharmacology, and clinical importance of these polymorphic forms of the receptor in asthma are reviewed in this chapter.

I. β_2AR Signaling Defects in Asthma

An early hypothesis of Szentivanyi suggested that the pathogenesis of asthma was centered around an imbalance between bronchodilating and bronchoconstrictive neurogenic pathways leading to airway obstruction [1]. A defective β_2AR was considered a potential candidate. In a broader sense, this scenario is essentially true; that is, pathways leading to obstruction in asthma are not effectively counteracted by other mechanisms, resulting in the physiologic manifestations of the disease. However, pro-obstructive and anti-obstructive factors are clearly not

455

limited to (and indeed their contribution may be small as compared to others) neurogenic pathways. Further, a defective β_2AR does not appear to be the primary cause of the disease. Nevertheless, altered β_2AR expression or function has been demonstrated to accompany asthma by a number of different investigators using various models and techniques. Early studies utilized circulating lymphocyte or neutrophil β_2AR acting as potential surrogates for lung receptors. Some of these studies showed depressed expression or function of these β_2AR, and in some cases correlations with the severity of obstruction, while in other studies no differences were found, or the receptor alterations were attributed to concomitant use of certain medications [2–8]. In the guinea pig ovalbumin-sensitized model of asthma, β_2AR expression has been shown to be depressed [9,10]. One study has shown βAR responses to infused agonist to be depressed in asthmatics [11]. The Basenji-greyhound dog has been used as an animal model of bronchial hyperreactivity, and studies using both in-vivo and ex-vivo responses, and tissue radioligand binding, have indicated a partially uncoupled β_2AR [12]. In a viral model of asthma, β_2AR responsiveness has been reported to be depressed [13,14]. Human macrophage cAMP responses in asthma have been demonstrated to be decreased, although this defect did not appear to be confined to the β_2AR [15]. Studies of autopsy-derived tissues from normal subjects and from those who died of asthma have shown varied results, including increases and decreases in expression, and no changes or decreased function of the receptor [16–21]. These latter studies are particularly difficult to control for the effects of pharmacologic agents administered prior to death. Taken together, the above studies suggest that dysfunctional β_2AR may have some as yet not clearly defined role in the pathogenesis of human asthma or accompanies asthma in some individuals contributing to some asthmatic phenotypes. It is also clear that there appears to be a certain degree of interindividual variation between patients with regard to β_2AR function. Also, it has been difficult to assess receptor function at the level of pertinent lung cells in humans. And finally, the effects of therapeutic agents such as β-agonists and corticosteroids make assessing receptor function in human subjects who require such treatment somewhat problematic.

We have considered that β_2AR dysfunction in asthma could arise from three basic mechanisms: (1) acquired from β-agonist use; (2) acquired from intrinsic factors in the lung (such as cytokines) which are present in asthma; or (3) mutations of the β_2AR gene. The signal transduction pathway of β_2AR and the mechanisms by which function is altered by the first two mechanisms are discussed in Chapter 4. As is also discussed in that chapter, structure/function studies using site-directed mutagenesis and recombinant expression of adrenergic receptors by our group and others have delineated a number of key portions of these receptors responsible for their function and regulation [22–24]. Small mutations in these regions can result in significant changes in these parameters. We thus undertook studies to determine if genetic variation of β_2AR structure occurred in humans, whether such variations resulted in any changes in receptor function, and whether these had physiologic relevance with regard to the pathogenesis or treatment of asthma.

At the time of our original studies, only one other G-protein-coupled receptor, rhodopsin, had been studied with regard to genetic variation [25,26]. It had been shown that patients with autosomal-dominant retinitis pigmentosa had mutations of the rhodopsin gene within the coding region. Control subjects (i.e., age-matched subjects with normal vision and normal ophthalmic examinations) showed no variation in sequence from wild type. Subsequently, several mutations resulting in increased coupling, decreased coupling, or altered folding of the receptor protein have been implicated in the disease [27,28]. Over the past 5 years, mutations of several G-protein-coupled receptors have been implicated in various diseases (Table 1). For example, in X-linked nephrogenic diabetes insipidus [29], a point mutation of the V2 vasopressin receptor results in a receptor which is not capable of coupling to its G protein (G_s). This is consistent with the observed pathology and clinical findings of the disease: an inability to concentrate the urine despite a normal or increased level of endogenous vasopressin, and a lack of responsiveness to exogenously administered vasopressin. In contrast to this type of mutational defect, where the receptor is unable to couple, some diseases are associated with mutations resulting in constitutive activation of the receptor (i.e., coupling to the G protein even in the absence of agonist). For example, in one form

Table 1 Human Diseases Caused by Mutations of G-Protein-Coupled Receptors

Disease	Gene	Coupling pathway	Effect
Retinitis pigmentosa	Rhodopsin	G_T	↓ and ↑ coupling, improper folding
X-linked nephrogenic diabetes insipidus	V2 vasopressin receptor	G_S	Absent coupling
Hyperthyroidism (hyperfunctioning adenoma)	TSH receptor	G_S	Constituitively active
Familial male precocious puberty	LH receptor	G_S	Constituitively active
Familial glucocorticoid resistance	ACTH receptor	G_S	Inactive (mechanism unknown)
Familial hypocalciuric hypercalcemia	Ca^{++} sensing receptor	G_q	Inactive (mechanism unknown)
Neonatal severe hyperparathyroidism	Ca^{++} sensing receptor	G_q	Inactive (mechanism unknown)
Color blindness, monochromatism, spectral perception variation	Opsins	G_T	Inactive "fusion" red–green opsins, improper folding?

of hyperthyroidism, the thyroid-stimulatory hormone (TSH) receptor has a mutation which renders it constituitively activated [30], thus constantly activating G_s and stimulating cAMP production, resulting in excess thyroid hormone secretion even in the presence of depressed endogenous TSH.

II. Determining β_2AR Polymorphisms

To investigate whether mutations of the β_2AR gene occurred in asthma, we developed a screening technique for identification of variations from wild-type DNA sequence [31]. For these initial studies, we utilized temperature gradient gel electrophoresis (TGGE) for such screening [32]. For verification of the technique, we constructed plasmids containing mutations throughout the coding block using site-directed mutagenesis. These included point mutations, deletions, and insertions. In addition, we developed techniques to directly sequence products from polymerase chain reactions (PCR) representing all regions of the receptor using biotinylated PCR primers and a magnetic steptavadin bead separation technique, followed by dideoxy sequencing. The approach for TGGE was to amplify β_2AR coding block sequence using genomic DNA derived from blood samples using five overlapping PCRs. Individual PCR products from patients were then mixed with PCR products derived from the cloned β_2AR in a plasmid, denatured at 98° and then renatured at 50°. The complex was then electrophoresed over a temperature gradient (which varied depending on the region being assessed), and mismatches between wild-type were identified by multiple bands on the silver stained gel. As can be seen in Fig. 1, the heteroduplex migrates as a single band when

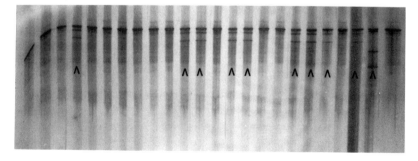

Figure 1   Delineation of β_2-adrenergic receptor gene polymorphisms using temperature gradient gel electrophoresis (TGGE). Genomic DNA was extracted from lymphocytes from 24 patients and a portion of the β_2AR coding block was amplified by PCR. These products were annealed to authentic wild-type β_2AR sequence and electrophoresed over a temperature gradient. Arrows highlight samples which deviate from wild-type sequence as indicated by multiple bands.

there is an exact match between the products derived from patient samples and the products derived from plasmid containing wild-type β_2AR sequence. Deviations (indicated by the arrows in Fig. 1) are identified by the multiple bands. For these initial studies, all products which screened positive for a deviation from wild type by TGGE were subsequently sequenced to identify the mutation. It should be noted that the most 5' portion of the coding block was not amenable to TGGE, and all PCR products from this region were directly sequenced. As is shown in Fig. 2, the quality of this sequencing was such that deviations could be clearly identified and the homozygous versus heterozygous state ascertained. For rapid assessment of sequence variation, single nucleotide tracking can be utilized, where products from each nucleotide sequencing reaction from all samples are run in adjacent lanes. Using the above approach, deviation from wild-type sequence was identified at nucleic acids 46, 79, 100, 252, 491, 523, 1053, 1098, and 1239. These corresponded to triplet codons at positions 16, 27, 34, 84, 164, 175, 351, 366, and 413 (Fig. 3). Most of these were common and henceforth will be termed polymorphisms. In some cases, the polymorphisms at the nucleotide level did not result in a change in the encoded amino acid (i.e., these were degenerate; darkened circles of Fig. 3). However, at codons 16, 27, 34, and 164, the nucleotide changes resulted

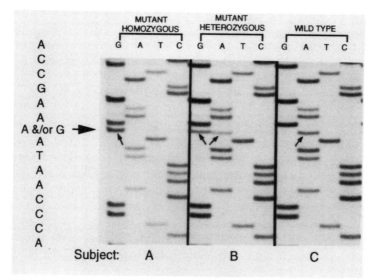

Figure 2 Direct sequencing of PCR derived β_2AR DNA from genomic. Genomic DNA prepared from blood samples from three patients was used as templates for PCRs generating products containing the β_2AR coding block. These were subjected to dideoxy sequencing. Shown are results from three subjects illustrating the homozygous and heterozygous states of two polymorphismic alleles (A or G) at nucleic acid position 46.

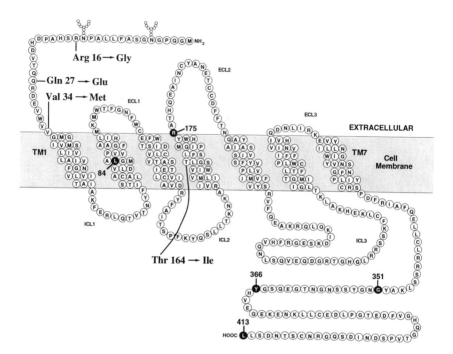

Figure 3 Primary amino acid sequence and polymorphic sites of the human β$_2$-adrenergic receptor. Darkened circles indicate codons where nucleic acid changes were identified (as compared to "wild-type" sequence), but the encoded amino acid was not altered. The four nondegenerate polymorphisms, two in the transmembrane spanning regions and two in the extracellular domain, are shown.

in a change in the encoded amino acids and are indicated as Arg16→Gly, Gln27→Glu, Met34→Val, and Thr164→Ile. (In subsequent publications, these have also been indicated simply as Arg16, Gly16, etc.) No deletions, insertions, or altered termination sites were identified. As will be discussed, the frequency of some of these polymorphisms is fairly high, suggesting that designation of a "wild-type" sequence is probably inappropriate. However, to maintain a common frame of reference with prior mutagenesis studies, wild-type sequence will continue to be considered that reported with the original cloning of the receptor [33] with Arg in position 16, Gln in position 27, Met in position 34, and Thr in position 164.

The results from initial studies of normal subjects and asthmatics will be discussed below. In the context of this section, other techniques for identification of these polymorphisms which we have subsequently utilized will be described. Polymorphisms at position 16, 27, and 164 result in alterations of receptor phenotypes, as will be discussed further. We therefore developed techniques specifically to assess the presence of the different alleles at these three positions [34]. For this, we utilized allele-specific PCR [35], also called amplification refractory mutation detection system or ARMs. The approach is based on the fact that the PCR is most efficient when there is a match between the 3'-most nucleotide of the primer and the analogous nucleotide of the template. Depending on the conditions of the PCR, a mismatch in this position results in no product. Thus by using primers whose 3' nucleotide matches the known polymorphic forms of the gene, the absence or presence of products indicates the absence or presence of the given allele. To develop the appropriate conditions to detect these β$_2$AR polymorphisms, we first utilized templates which consisted of plasmids containing the coding block cDNA which had been mutated by site-specific techniques to mimic these polymorphisms. Then, genomic DNA was used as template, with direct sequencing used to verify the results of the allele-specific PCR. The results from these types of studies are shown in Fig. 4. As can be seen, using primers for one allele provides for one product specific for the appropriate template. When templates are mixed together (simulating the heterozygous state), products are obtained with both sets of primers. Note the approximate same level of intensity of the products under the heterozygous condition. The bottom portion of Fig. 4 shows results using genomic DNA derived from blood samples. Again, an unambiguous signal of the appropriate molecular weight is obtained from each subject, which correlated with the results of sequencing. Finally, we have also used an oligonucleotide hybridization technique for identification of polymorphisms at positions 16 and 27 [36].

There are several points to be made concerning the above techniques that are applicable to any candidate gene study. First, techniques involving restriction-fragment length polymorphisms (RFLP), which are dependent on the polymorphism creating or ablating a restriction endonuclease site, may be of little utility in delineating genetic variance of a specific sequence. For the β$_2$AR, none of the polymorphisms which resulted in the amino acid changes is detectable with RFLP. Nevertheless, a polymorphic marker identified with RFLP could be in linkage disequilibrium with the true genetic defect distant from the RFLP site (see Chapters 13 and 16). In this regard, a Ban I RFLP is present in the β$_2$AR [37], probably representing the silent polymorphism at nucleic acid 523, and has recently been shown to be associated with asthmatic phenotypes [38]. Second, the use of screening techniques such as TGGE or single-stranded conformation polymorphism analysis (SSCP) must be carried out using optimized conditions established using positive and negative controls. Useful positive controls include cDNAs with mutations constructed along the sequence using site-directed techniques. Regardless of such controls, ultimately, sequencing of the PCR products needs to be carried out to verify the sensitivity and specificity of the screening technique. Techniques such as allele-specific PCR are useful when the polymorphic sites are

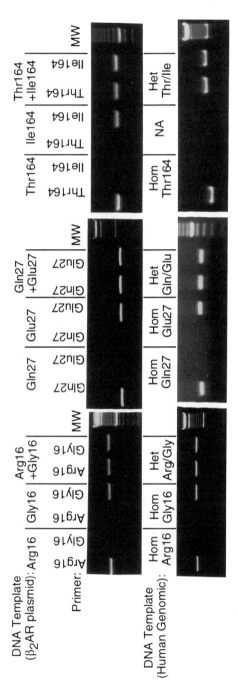

Figure 4 Identification of β$_2$AR polymorphisms with allele-specific PCR. PCRs were carried out using sense primers that matched at the most 3′ nucleotide of the various known polymorphisms of the β$_2$AR. The upper portion of the figure shows the specificity of the method when plasmids containing β$_2$AR cDNA with the indicated mutations were used as templates. Note that products were obtained only when template matched primer. The lower portion shows typical results obtained with genomic DNA derived from blood samples. NA = not available.

already known and provide for rapid genotyping at these loci. The conditions for successful allele-specific PCR are highly template dependent. Appropriate controls must be utilized in establishing these conditions, and once again sequencing needs to be carried out to establish unequivocally the specificity of the approach.

III. Molecular Consequences of β_2AR Structural Variability

Our initial study examined the frequency of β_2AR polymorphisms in a heterologous group of unrelated asthmatics and normal controls [31]. Polymorphisms were found to be germline (i.e., they occurred in all cells in the body) and were inherited in a classic Mendelian manner. The distribution of these polymorphisms in the normal and asthmatic groups from this study is shown in Table 2. Succinctly stated, there was no association between any polymorphism and asthma found. As can be seen in the upper portion of Table 1, the frequencies of heterozygous or homozygous polymorphisms at the degenerate sites were virtually identical between the two groups. Concerning polymorphisms that resulted in amino acid changes (bottom portion of Table 2), again the frequencies of polymorphisms were similar between the two groups except at codons 34 and 164, which were rare and the number of subjects too small for analysis. It should be noted that the polymorphisms at positions 16 and 27 can occur together, but again the frequencies were the same between the two groups. We were concerned about the possibility that some of our normal subjects had clinically inapparent bronchial hyperreactivity, which obviously would have affected interpretation of the results. We therefore performed pulmonary function tests and methacholine challenges on 10 of the subjects in the normal group who had the combination of polymorphisms at positions 16 and 27. All 10 had normal pulmonary function, and 9 of the 10 displayed no reactivity to methacholine. Thus we felt confident that the normal group was without asthma. Finally, we assessed within the asthmatic group whether polymorphisms were associated with a particular clinical characteristic. This study was not originally designed to address this, and such an analysis was carried out for exploratory purposes only. Indeed, the cohort had not been extensively phenotyped. Nevertheless, we noted that most (75%) of the asthmatics who were chronic oral steroid dependent were homozygous for the Arg16→Gly polymorphism. In addition, 100% of patients who were receiving allergic desensitization therapy were homozygous for the same polymorphism independent of steroid usage. β-Agonist use was similar between groups with or without the various polymorphisms.

At this juncture we proceeded to determine the functional consequences of these polymorphisms [39–41]. If there were no consequences, then we would have been reticent to pursue further clinical studies. To approach this, the cDNA for the wild-type β_2AR sequence was mutated using oligonucleotide-directed site-

Table 2 Distribution of β_2AR Gene Polymorphisms in Normal and Asthmatic Subjects[a]

Designation	Mutated nucleic acid	Asthmatic (n = 51)		Nonasthmatic (n = 56)	
		Heterozygous	Homozygous	Heterozygous	Homozygous
No amino acid change					
Codon 84	252	18	2	18	4
Codon 175	523	15	2	16	4
Codon 351	1053	19	3	22	5
Codon 366	1098	0	0	1	0
Codon 413	1239	21	6	26	7
Amino acid changes					
Arg16→Gly	46	19	27	16	33
Gln27→Glu	79	26	12	23	16
Val34→Met	100	1	0	0	0
Thr164→Ile	491	0	0	3	0
Arg16→Gly + Gln27→Glu	46 + 79	0	12	16	16

[a]Shown are the number of asthma patients or normal subjects who had each of the indicated polymorphisms.

specific techniques and subcloned into the mammalian expression vector pcDNA 1/Neo. These constructs were then used to transfect Chinese hamster fibroblasts (CHW 1102 cells). These cells do not express β_2AR, but do express other G-protein-coupled receptors and other components of the signal transduction cascade (i.e., G_s, adenylyl cyclase, etc.). Cells resistant to the neomycin analog G418 (conferred by a neomycin resistance gene in the expression vector) were isolated and permanent cell lines expressing wild-type and mutant β_2AR were established. Morphologically, the cells from the various lines were indistinguishable, as were their growth characteristics. In addition, cells harboring various mutant β_2AR displayed the same basal, forskolin (a direct activator of adenylyl cyclase), and NaF (an activator of G_s) stimulated adenylyl cyclase activities. Thus there were no apparent artifacts induced in the cell lines by the transfection and selection process.

The receptors were then studied with regard to expression, affinities for agonists and antagonists, physical and functional coupling to G_s, and receptor regulation and trafficking by agonist. The Val34→Met receptor was indistinguishable from wild type and will not be discussed further. On the other hand, the other three polymorphic forms of the receptor imparted distinct properties. The Thr164→Ile receptor displayed a number of abnormalities [39]. In agonist competition studies using the radioligand [^{125}I]cyanopindolol, the affinities for epinephrine, norepinephrine, and isoproterenol were found to be lower (~ fourfold) for the mutant receptor as compared to wild type. It has been postulated that the β-hydroxyl group of catecholamines forms a hydrogen bond with Ser165. We considered that the mutation at the 164 position, substituting Ile for Thr, may have disrupted this milieu. To test this, two agonists without such β-hydroxyl groups, dopamine and dobutamine, were studied. The affinities for these two agonists were the same for both receptors, consistent with the above hypothesis. Also, the (+) stereoisomer of propranolol, which has the β-hydroxyl group pointing in the opposite direction (i.e., away from Ser165), showed an equal affinity for both receptors, in contrast to the (−) stereoisomer, which displayed a lower affinity for the Thr164→Ile receptor. This further supports the notion that the mutation disrupts the milieu for interaction between Ser165 and the β-hydroxyl groups of ligands. However, the (+) and (−) stereoisomers of isoproterenol both displayed lower affinities for the mutants, suggesting that the effect of the mutation is not confined to this region alone. Indeed, several structurally distinct antagonists, all of which have β-hydroxyl groups, also showed lower affinities for Thr164→Ile as compared to wild-type β_2AR. In general, antagonists without aromatic-ring polar substituents displayed lower affinities for the mutant receptor. In functional studies, the mutant receptor displayed a decreased maximal stimulation of adenylyl cyclase (~50% of wild-type receptor) and an ~threefold higher EC_{50} (lower potency) for epinephrine-mediated stimulation (Fig. 5). Thus agonist-mediated coupling to G_s was also impaired in this receptor, which we considered to be due to an impaired ability to

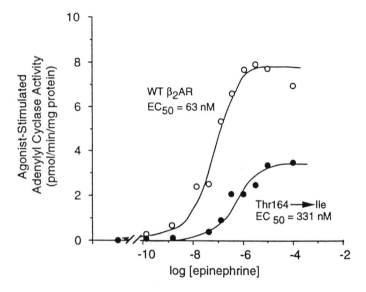

Figure 5 Functional properties of the Thr164→Ile β₂-adrenergic receptor polymorphism. Membranes were prepared from Chinese hamster fibroblasts expressing the wildtype or the mutated β_2AR and adenylyl cyclase activities determined. The response to increasing concentrations of epinephrine in the assay indicates that the Thr164→Ile receptor displays depressed coupling to G_s as indicated by a decreased maximal responses and a decreased potency.

form the agonist–receptor–G_s ternary complex. In agonist competition studies conducted in the absence of guanine nucleotide, this hypothesis was confirmed. With the wild-type receptor, two affinity states (K_L and K_H) could be observed, with the loss of the high-affinity state occurring with addition of the GTP analog GppNHp to the assay. In contrast, the Thr164→Ile receptor displayed a single class of receptors of low affinity, which was not altered by guanine nucleotide. In addition to impaired agonist-mediated coupling to G_s, this receptor also displayed depressed basal (nonagonist) coupling. Also, basal adenylyl cyclase increases with receptor expression for both receptors. However, for any given level of receptor expression, the activity is less for the mutant receptor as compared to wild type. Finally, we also found that agonist-promoted sequestration is depressed with the Thr164→Ile mutant. Taken together, it appears that this mutation has affected both agonist dependent and independent functions. With regard to asthma, we have considered that patients harboring this polymorphism may express a more severe form based on a depressed basal coupling of the receptor or a depressed response to endogenous catecholamines; or such patients may display a depressed responsiveness to administered β-agonists. To date, we have not encountered a sufficient number of patients with this polymorphism to explore these hypotheses.

In contrast to what was found with the Thr164→Ile receptor, the amino-terminal polymorphisms, Arg16→Gly and Gln27→Glu, displayed wild-type affinities for agonists and antagonists, and coupled normally to G_s [40]. Since the amino terminus has been shown to play a role in receptor trafficking, we proceeded to study agonist-promoted sequestration and downregulation of these receptors. In transfected CHW cells expressing each of these, we found that agonist-promoted downregulation was clearly different between the receptor variants (Fig. 6). After 24 h of agonist exposure, wild-type receptor displayed a 26 ± 3% loss of receptor. The Arg16→Gly variant, however, underwent enhanced downregulation, amounting to 41 ± 3%. In contrast, the polymorphism at position 27, Gln27→Glu, failed to undergo downregulation under these conditions. The downregulation pattern of the combination polymorphism was also enhanced compared to wild type. These differences were explored along several lines. First, we assessed the relative levels of cellular β_2AR mRNA in the basal state to the levels of receptor protein and found no differences in this parameter between wild

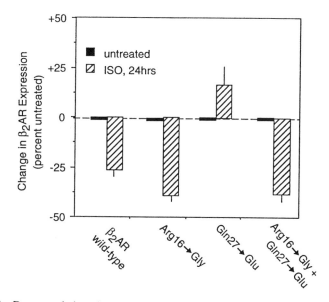

Figure 6   Downregulation phenotypes of β_2AR polymorphic variants expressed recombinantly in Chinese hamster fibroblasts. Treated cells were exposed to 10 μM isoproterenol for 24 h.

type and the different variants. We also examined the rate of new receptor synthesis and found no significant differences. In addition, the basal distribution of receptor protein (i.e., cell surface versus intracellular) was the same between wild type and the different polymorphic forms. These results all suggested that there were no differences in the efficiencies of transcriptional and translational processes leading up to expression of receptor protein at the cell surface. Next, we assessed whether there were any differences in agonist-promoted regulation of β_2AR mRNA levels. In CHW cells expressing wild-type receptor being driven by elements in the pcDNA 1/Neo vector, we found that agonist exposure up to 24 h resulted in no significant decrease in mRNA levels. Studies with cells expressing the different receptor variants showed no deviation from this pattern. Thus it appeared that under these conditions downregulation is due primarily to degradation of receptor protein. Receptor sequestration (also termed internalization), which may act as an initial step in agonist-promoted downregulation of β_2AR, amounted to ~59% after 30 min of agonist exposure to wild-type β_2AR. The extent and rate of sequestration, however, was virtually identical between wild type and the polymorphic forms of the receptor. We considered then that the downregulation differences may be due to steps distal to this process. To begin to explore this, the electrophoretic mobility of the receptors on SDS-PAGE was examined. The Arg16→Gly and wild-type receptor migrated at the same molecular weights, with bands at 91, 72, 67, and 53 kDA as determined by Western blots using a carboxy-terminal antibody. Gln27→Glu, on the other hand, did not appear to reach the fully mature form, with bands at 62, 58, and 46 kDa. We have considered that this immature form of the receptor may be resistant to the degradation process. As to why the Arg16→Gly variant has enhanced downregulation is unclear to date but is being pursued.

We have recently also assessed polymorphic β_2AR downregulation in human bronchial smooth muscle cells [41]. This was pursued for several reasons. First, in our recombinant studies, β_2AR expression was being driven by promoter elements in the expression vector. Thus, the effects of polymorphisms on downregulation when expression was under control of the natural promoter was unknown. Second, it was not clear that events in fibroblasts accurately reflected similar events in smooth muscle. Because the fibroblasts used in the recombinant studies do not natively express βAR, we also considered that they may lack cell-specific components involved in receptor regulation. Bronchial smooth muscle cells were harvested by rapid autopsy from subjects without lung disease, and primary cultures were established. These could be passaged 8–10 times and expressed ~70 fmol/mg of β_2AR. The genotype of the receptor in each line was then determined by allele-specific PCR [41]. The pharmacologic properties of these different receptors were no different than wild-type receptor. As with the recombinant cells, though, agonist-promoted downregulation was different among the variants (Fig. 7). With the bronchial smooth muscle cells, after 24 h of

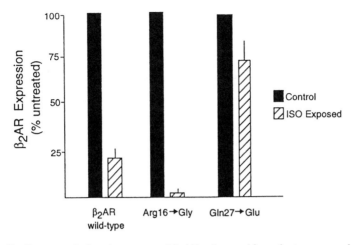

Figure 7 Downregulation phenotypes of β₂AR polymorphic variants expressed natively on human bronchial smooth muscle cells. Treated cells were exposed to 10 μM iso-proterenol for 24 h. * = $p < 0.05$ as compared to wild-type (Gly16).

exposure wild-type receptor underwent ~77% downregulation. The Gly 16 variant underwent a greater degree of downregulation which amounted to ~96%. The Glu27 form of the receptor displayed substantially less downregulation (~30%). The results from these studies with bronchial smooth muscle cells, i.e., that Gly16 has enhanced agonist-promoted downregulation and Glu27 has less downregulation compared to wild type, was consistent with what was observed in the recombinant system.

IV. Potential Relevance of β₂AR Polymorphisms in Asthma

Having delineated the phenotypes of the different receptor polymorphisms, we have recently begun to assess their roles in asthma, as have several other groups. Based on the importance of other pathways such as inflammation in the pathogenesis of asthma, and the fact that β₂AR polymorphisms are frequent in non-asthmatic populations (Table 2), it seems unlikely that these are a major cause of the disease. A study to address this specifically, however, has not been carried out with a large population of well-phenotyped asthmatics. Interestingly, the β₂AR gene is located on chromosome 5, near the D5S436 marker which has been found to be in linkage with total IgE levels and bronchial hyperreactivity (see Chapters 24 and 25). It seems more likely that β₂AR polymorphisms represent only one component of a multigenetic disease and that their impact may be centered primarily around defining subphenotypes of asthma or the response of the disease to therapy.

Based on the results from these studies in cells, which have also been reviewed elsewhere [42–44], a number of potential implications in asthma can be considered. If one assumes that β_2AR expression is constantly under control by circulating catecholamines, then the Gly16 variant, which undergoes the greatest degree of agonist promoted downregulation, would be expected to display an overall reduced level of expression as compared to wild-type receptor. Under this scenario, basal bronchomotor tone might be decreased or bronchial hyperreactivity increased. Also, if nocturnal asthma is due to an enhanced nocturnal downregulation of β_2AR (induced by an earlier diurnal increase in catecholamines), then the Gly16 polymorphism may predispose to this asthmatic phenotype. Responsiveness to β-agonist may also be depressed in asthmatics harboring this polymorphism. In the case of the acute response in the absence of prior exposure, the response may be blunted due to the lower expression as described above. During chronic agonist therapy, the potential for tachyphylaxis would appear to be greatest with the Gly16 variant. It should be noted here that whether clinical tachyphylaxis to the bronchodilating effects of β-agonist occurs is a matter of some debate. Such tachyphylaxis has been shown in some studies but not others [45–53]. Recently, inhaled β-agonists in standard doses have clearly been shown to result in substantial receptor desensitization of epithelial and macrophage β_2AR in humans [54]. Given reports that suggest a relationship between "overuse" of β-agonists and adverse outcomes in asthma [55–57], it seems prudent to consider that tachyphylaxis may occur in some individuals. Indeed, in most studies, there is a range of tachyphylatic responses. It is interesting to consider whether these responses (i.e., those that do and those that do not display tachyphylaxis) segregate based on their β_2AR genotypes. Patients harboring the Glu27 polymorphism, on the other hand, might have higher β_2AR expression and thus exhibit less bronchial hyperreactivity and a greater response to β-agonists, and less pronounced or absent tachyphylaxis to chronic β-agonist therapy.

To date, only a few clinical studies to address these possibilities have been carried out. Initially, we focused our attention as to whether the Gly16 polymorphism was associated with nocturnal asthma [34]. In patients with this phenotype, it has been reported that β_2AR undergo a nocturnal decrease in expression [58]. Such downregulation was not observed in normal subjects or in those with non-nocturnal asthma. We therefore genotyped 45 patients with asthma at the β_2AR polymorphic loci 16, 27, and 164 [34]. Twenty-three patients were defined as having nocturnal asthma and 22 patients had non-nocturnal asthma. The assignment to the two groups was based on nocturnal variation in peak expiratory flow rates. To be included in the nocturnal asthmatic group, subjects were required to have five consecutive bedtime-to-morning peak expiratory flow rate decrements of greater than 20%. Subjects in the non-nocturnal asthmatic cohort had less than

10% decrements for five consecutive days. Those not fulfilling these criteria were excluded from the study altogether. The nocturnal asthmatic group had peak expiratory flow rate decrements of 34 ± 2%, while the non-nocturnal asthmatic group had decrements of 2.3 ± 0.8%. All were atopic by history. Resting daytime pulmonary function testing revealed a depressed predicted forced expiratory volume in 1 sec (FEV1) for the nocturnal asthmatic group (70.9 ± 3.1% predicted) as compared to the non-nocturnal asthmatic group (85.1 ± 3.0% predicted). The distribution of β₂AR polymorphisms in the two groups is shown in Table 3. As indicated in the upper portion of Table 3, where the allele frequencies are shown, there is a clear overrepresentation of the Gly16 allele in the nocturnal asthmatic group. This was significant at $p = 0.007$ with an odds ratio of 3.8. The allele frequencies of the two polymorphisms at position 27 were not different between the two groups. The substitution of Ile for Thr at position 164 occurred only twice, both in the non-nocturnal asthmatic group. A comparison of the homozygous and the heterozygous states at position 16 is shown in the lower portion of Table 3. If one examines only the homozygous state, there were 16 of 18 patients who were homozygous for Gly16 and only 2 of 18 who were homozygous for Arg16 in the nocturnal asthmatic group. On the other hand, there was about an

Table 3 Distribution of β₂AR Polymorphisms in Nocturnal and Non-nocturnal Asthma

| Allele | Number of alleles | | p value | Odds ratio |
	Nocturnal asthma	Non-nocturnal asthma		
Gly16	37	23	0.007	3.8
Arg 16	9	21		
Glu27	23	23	>0.05	NA
Gln27	23	21		
Thr164	46	42	>0.05	NA
Ile164	0	2		

Genotype	Number of patients			
Homozygous Gly16	16	8	0.046	7.0
Homozygous Arg16	2	7		
Homozygous Gly16	16	8		7.0
Heterozygous Arg/Gly16	5	7	0.017	2.5
Homozygous Arg16	2	7		1.0
Homozygous Gly16	16	8	0.038	4.0
Not homozygous Gly16	7	14		

equal distribution of homozygous Arg 16 and homozygous Gly16 subjects in the non-nocturnal group. This association of homozygous Gly16 with nocturnal asthma was significant at p = 0.046, with an odds ratio of 7.0. Inclusion of heterozygous patients in this comparison did not alter these results. We also show a comparison based on the model that only the homozygous form of Gly16 imparts the nocturnal phenotype, with heterozygosity or homozygosity for Arg16 being insufficient. Such a comparison of homozygous Gly16 or "not homozygous Gly16" again shows an overrepresentation of Gly16 in the nocturnal asthmatic cohort. Of the 23 patients with nocturnal asthma, 16 (69.6%) were homozygous for Gly16, while 8 of 22 (36.4%) of the non-nocturnal cohort were homozygous for Gly16. Further support that the Gly16 polymorphism is associated with nocturnal asthma is noted when patients are segregated based on a history of frequent nocturnal asthma rather than the more strict peak expiratory flow rate decrement criteria. Of the 31 asthmatics with histories of nocturnal worsening, 23 (74.2%) had the homozygous Gly16 polymorphism, while among those without nocturnal histories only 1 of 14 (7.1%) was homozygous for Gly16 (p < 0.0001, odds ratio = 33). We have interpreted these results as consistent with the Gly16 polymorphism predisposing patients with asthma to having the nocturnal phenotype. The basis of this association is the observation that the Gly16 polymorphism expressed in either recombinant cells or in human bronchial smooth muscle cells undergoes an enhanced downregulation. We also explored whether the Gly16 polymorphism was merely a reflection of more severe asthma, since the nocturnal group had evidence of greater obstruction on pulmonary function tests. The percent predicted FEV1 for those patients who did or did not have the homozygous Gly16 polymorphism (regardless of their nocturnal versus non-nocturnal phenotype) were compared. These values, although clearly trending toward a lower predicted FEV1 for the nocturnal group, were not statistically different, being 73.9 ± 3.2% versus 82.5 ± 3.5% predicted, respectively. In addition, we assessed the prevalence of Gly16 in these asthmatics based on whether they are defined as mild (FEV1 >70% predicted) or moderate, and did not find an over-representation of the polymorphism in the moderately severe group. Of the 13 moderate asthmatics as so defined, 61% had the Gly16 polymorphism; and of the 32 mild asthmatics, 50% had the polymorphism. Finally, of those originally assigned to the nocturnal cohort by peak expiratory flow rate criteria, but who had the homozygous Gly16 polymorphism, 7 of 8 (87.5%) had positive histories of nocturnal asthma, whereas in this same group in those without homozygous Gly16, only 1 of 14 (7.1%) had positive nocturnal histories.

Two studies have explored potential relationships between specific β_2AR polymorphisms and bronchial hyperreactivity. Hall and colleagues determined methacholine responsiveness and β_2AR genotype at loci 16 and 27 in 65 asthmatic subjects [36]. Based on our studies in cells expressing these polymorphisms, we predicted that the Glu27 polymorphism would provide a protective effect against

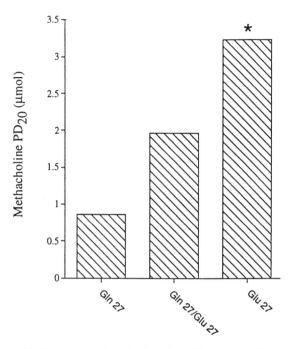

Figure 8 Bronchial hyperreactivity of asthmatics with polymorphisms of the β_2AR at amino acid position 27. Shown are the geometric means of the PD_{20} values for methacholine. The patients with the homozygous Glu27 polymorphism had higher PD_{20} values (i.e., lower bronchial reactivity to methacholine) as compared to those who were homozygous for Gln27. Heterozygotes had an intermediate value. See text for actual values and 95% confidence levels.

bronchial hyperreactivity as compared to the wild-type form of the receptor. As shown in Fig. 8, this was indeed the case. The geometric mean PD_{20} values for those who were homozygous for Gln27 was 0.86 μmol (95% confidence interval, 0.25–2.15). In contrast, those homozygous for Glu27 had mean PD_{20} values of 3.23 μmol (1.25–7.04). Those who were heterozygous had an intermediate PD_{20} value. The methacholine PD_{20} values for subjects with the different alleles at locus 16 were not different. These data suggests that the β_2AR genotype at position 27 may be important in establishing the extent of bronchial hyperreactivity in patients with asthma. Holroyd et al. [59] have reported in abstract form studies examining the relationship between histamine bronchial hyperresponsiveness and β_2AR polymorphisms at position 16. In this study, 64 asthmatics with high IgE levels (IgE >100 IU/mL) were genotyped at locus 16. Subjects were segregated based on the presence or absence of bronchial hyperreactivity to histamine. The Gly16 allele was found to be strongly associated with bronchial hyperreactivity with a reported odds ratio of 6. The frequencies of allelic variants at position 27 were not reported.

Kawakami and colleagues [38] recently reported an association between a β_2AR Ban I RFLP and asthma and the airway response to β-agonists. The Ban I RFLP in this report probably identifies the polymorphism at nucleic acid 523 (codon 175, Fig. 3), which does not result in a change in the encoded amino acid. In four families consisting of 58 members, the 2.1-kb and the 2.3-kb Ban I RFLP alleles were assessed. Associations were found between this RFLP and the presence of asthma (defined as an individual given the diagnosis by a physician) and responsiveness to inhaled salbutamol. No association with the RFLP and atopy or the responsiveness to methacholine was found. Since this RFLP probably represents a polymorphism which does not change the amino acid, the relevance of these findings to structural variation of the β_2AR is unclear. This marker may be in linkage disequilibrium with polymorphisms of the β_2AR at amino acids 16, 27, or 164, or another gene altogether.

V. Conclusion

The β_2AR displays an unexpectedly high degree of genetically based structural variance in the population. Some of these polymorphic receptors display unique properties, including altered affinities for ligands, defective coupling, and enhanced or depressed agonist-promoted regulation. It appears unlikely that any of these represents a major cause of asthma. However, the fact that these receptors do differ in certain properties suggests that β_2AR polymorphisms may play roles in establishing the severity of the disease or the degree of bronchial hyperreactivity, expression of certain asthmatic phenotypes, or how patients respond to therapy. Studies to address such possibilities are underway, and to date published results support these concepts.

References

1. Szentivanyi A. The beta adrenergic theory of the atopic abnormality in bronchial asthma. J Allergy 1968; 42:203–232.
2. Gillespie E, Valentine MD, Lichtenstein LM. Cyclic AMP metabolism in asthma: studies with leukocytes and lymphocytes. J Allergy Clin Immunol 1974; 53:27–33.
3. Parker CW, Smith JW. Alternations in cyclic adenosine monophosphate metabolism in human bronchial asthma. Leukocyte responsiveness to beta-adrenergic agents. J Clin Invest 1973; 52:48–59.
4. Kariman K. β-Adrenergic receptor binding in lymphocytes from patients with asthma. Lung 1980; 158:41–51.

5. Galant SP, Duriseti L, Underwood S, Allred S, Insel PA. Beta-adrenergic receptors of polymorphonuclear particulates in bronchial asthma. J Clin Invest 1980; 65:577–585.

6. Conolly ME, Greenacre JK. The lymphocyte β-adrenoreceptor in normal subjects and patients with bronchial asthma. J Clin Invest 1976; 58:1307–1316.

7. Tashkin DP, Conolly ME, Deutsch RI, et al. Subsensitization of beta-adrenoceptors in airways and lymphocytes of healthy and asthmatic subjects. Am Rev Respir Dis 1982; 125:185–193.

8. Sano Y, Watt G, Townley RG. Decreased mononuclear cell beta-adrenergic receptors in bronchial asthma: parallel studies of lymphocyte and granulocyte desensitization. J Allergy Clin Immunol 1983; 72:495–503.

9. Barnes PJ, Dollery CT, MacDermot J. Increased pulmonary α-adrenergic and reduced β-adrenergic receptors in experimental asthma. Nature 1980; 285:569–571.

10. Gatto C, Green TP, Johnson MG, Marchessault RP, Seybold V, Johnson DE. Localization of quantitative changes in pulmonary beta-receptors in ovalbumin-sensitized guinea pigs. Am Rev Respir Dis 1987; 136:150–154.

11. Kaliner M, Shelhamer JH, Davis PB, Smith LJ, Venter JC. Automonic nervous system abnormalities and allergy. Ann Intern Med 1982;96:349–357.

12. Emala CW, Black C, Curry C, Levine MA, Hirshman CA. Impaired β-adrenergic receptor activation of adenylyl cyclase in airway smooth muscle of the basenji-greyhound dog model of airway hyperresponsiveness. Am J Respir Cell Mol Biol 1993; 8:668–675.

13. Buckner CK, Clayton DE, Ain-Shoka AA, Busse WW, Dick EC, Shult P. Para-influenza 3 infection blocks the ability of a beta adrenergic receptor agonist to inhibit antigen-induced contraction of guinea pig isolated airway smooth muscle. J Clin Invest 1981; 67:376–384.

14. Busse WW. Decreased granulocyte response to isoproterenol in asthma during upper respiratory infections. Am Rev Respir Dis 1977; 115:783–791.

15. Bachelet M, Vincent D, Havet N, et al. Reduced responsiveness of adenylate cyclase in alveolar macrophages from patients with asthma. J Allergy Clin Immunol 1991; 88: 322–328.

16. Sharma R, Jeffery P. Airway β-adrenoceptor number in cystic fibrosis and asthma. Clin Sci 1990; 78:409–417.

17. Goldie RG, Spina D, Henry PJ, Lulich KM, Paterson JW. *In vitro* responsiveness of human asthmatic bronchus to carbachol, histamine, β-adrenoceptor agonists and the-ophylline. Br J Clin Pharmacol 1986; 22:669–676.

18. Spina D, Rigby PJ, Paterson JW, Goldie RG. Autoradiographic location of beta-adrenoceptors in asthmatic human lung. Am Rev Respir Dis 1989; 140:1410–1415.

19. Goldie RG, Spina D, Henry PJ, Lulich KM, Paterson JW. *In vitro* responsiveness of human asthmatic bronchus to carbachol, histamine, β-adrenoceptor agonists and theophylline. Br J Clin Pharmacol 1986; 22:669–676.

20. Barnes PJ. Muscarinic receptor subtypes in airways. Life Sci 1993; 52:521–527.

21. Bai TR, Mak JC, Barnes PJ. A comparison of beta-adrenergic receptors and *in vitro* relaxant responses to isoproterenol in asthmatic airway smooth muscle. Am J Respir Cell Mol Biol 1992; 6:(6)647–651.

22. Liggett SB, Lefkowitz RJ. Regulation of receptor function by phosphorylation,

sequestration and downregulation. In: Sibley D, Houslay M, eds. Regulation of Cellular Signal Transduction Pathways by Desensitization and Amplification. London: John Wiley, 1993:71–97.

23. Liggett SB, Raymond JR. Pharmacology and molecular biology of adrenergic receptors. In: Bouloux PM, ed. Catecholamines. London: W. B. Saunders, 1993:279–306.

24. Liggett SB. G-protein coupled receptors in the lung. In: Crystal R, West JB, Weibel ER, Barnes PJ, eds. The Lung: Scientific Foundations. New York: Raven Press, 1996; in press.

25. Sung CH, Davenport CM, Hennessey JC, et al. Rhodopsin mutations in autosomal dominant retinitis pigmentosa. Proc Natl Acad Sci USA 1991; 88:6481–6485.

26. Dryja TP, McGee TL, Lauri BA, et al. Mutations within the rhodopsin gene in patients with autosomal dominant retinitis pigmentosa. N Engl J Med 1990; 323:1302–1307.

27. Robinson PR, Cohen GB, Zhukovsky EA, Oprian DD. Constitutively active mutants of rhodopsin. Neuron 1992; 9:725.

28. Min KC, Zvyaga TA, Cypress AM, Sakmar TP. Characterization of mutant rhodopsins responsible for autosomal dominant retinitis pigmentosa. J Biol Chem 1993; 268:9400–9404.

29. Rosenthal W, Antaramian A, Gilbert S, Birnbaumer M. Nephrogenic diabetes insipidus: a V2 vasopressin receptor unable to stimulate adenylyl cyclase. J Biol Chem 1993; 268:13030–13033.

30. Parma J, Duprez L, Van Sande J, et al. Somatic mutations in the thyrotropin receptor gene cause hyperfunctioning thyroid adenomas. Nature 1993; 365:649–651.

31. Reihsaus E, Innis M, MacIntyre N, Liggett SB. Mutations in the gene encoding for the β_2-adrenergic receptor in normal and asthmatic subjects. Am J Respir Cell Mol Biol 1993; 8:334–339.

32. Wartell RM, Mosseini SH, Moran CP Jr. Detecting base pair substitutions in DNA fragments by temperature-gradient gel electrophoresis. Nucleic Acids Res 1990; 18: 2699–2706.

33. Kobilka BK, Dixon RA, Frielle HG, et al. cDNA for the human β_2-adrenergic receptor: a protein with multiple membrane-spanning domains and encoded by a gene whose chromosomal location is shared with that of the receptor for platelet-derived growth factor. Proc Natl Acad Sci USA 1987; 84:46–50.

34. Turki J, Pak J, Green S, Martin R, Liggett SB. Genetic polymorphisms of the β_2-adrenergic receptor in nocturnal and non-nocturnal asthma: evidence that Gly16 correlates with the nocturnal phenotype. J Clin Invest 1995; 95:1635–1641.

35. Newton CR, Graham A, Hepinstall LE, et al. Analysis of any point mutation in DNA. The amplification refractory mutation system (ARMS). Nucleic Acids Res 1989; 17: 2503–2516.

36. Hall IP, Wheatley A, Wilding P, Liggett SB. Association of the Glu27 β_2-adrenoceptor polymorphism with lower airway reactivity in asthmatic subjects. Lancet 1995; 345:1213–1214.

37. Lentes KU, Berrettini WH, Hoehe MR, Chung FZ, Gershon ES. A biallelic DNA polymorphism of the human beta-2-adrenergic receptor detected by Ban I-Adrbr-2. Nucleic Acids Res 1988; 16:2369.

38. Ohe M, Munakata M, Hizawa N, et al. Beta$_2$ adrenergic receptor gene restriction fragment length polymorphism and bronchial asthma. Thorax 1995; 50:353–359.

39. Green SA, Cole G, Jacinto M, Innis M, Liggett SB. A polymorphism of the human β₂-adrenergic receptor within the fourth transmembrane domain alters ligand binding and functional properties of the receptor. J Biol Chem 1993; 268:23116–23121.

40. Green SA, Turki J, Innis M, Liggett SB. Amino-terminal polymorphisms of the human β₂-adrenergic receptor impart distinct agonist promoted regulatory properties. Biochemistry 1994; 33:9414–9419.

41. Green SA, Turki J, Bejarano P, Hall IP, Liggett SB. Influence of β₂-adrenergic receptor genotypes on signal transduction in human airway smooth muscle cells. Am J Respir Cell Mol Biol 1995; 13:25–33.

42. Green SA, Turki J, Hall IP, Liggett SB. Implications of genetic variability of human β₂-adrenergic receptor structure. Pulmonary Pharmacol 1995; in press.

43. Liggett SB. Functional properties of human β₂-adrenergic receptor polymorphisms. News Physiol Sci 1995; in press.

44. Liggett SB. Genetics of β₂-adrenergic receptor variants in asthma. Clin Exp Allergy 1995; in press.

45. Cockroft DW, McPharland CP, Britto SA, Swystun VA. Regular inhaled salbutamol and airway responsiveness to allergen. Lancet 1993; 342:833–836.

46. Newnham DM, Grove A, McDevitt DG, Lipworth BJ. Tolerance of bronchodilator and systemic beta-2 adrenoceptor responses after regular twice daily treatment with eformoterol dry powder in asthmatic patients. Eur Respir J 1994; 7:235s.

47. Newnham DM, McDevitt DG, Lipworth BJ. Bronchodilator subsensitivity after chronic dosing with eformoterol in patients with asthma. Am J Med 1994; 97:29–37.

48. Repsher LH, Anderson JA, Bish RK, et al. Assessment of tachyphylaxis following prolonged therapy of asthma with inhaled albuterol. Chest 1984; 85:34–38.

49. Vathenen AS, Knox AJ, Higgins BG, Britton JR, Tattersfield AE. Rebound increase in bronchial responsiveness after treatment with inhaled terbutaline. Lancet 1988; 1:554–558.

50. Weber RW, Smith JA, Nelson HS. Aerosolised terbutaline in asthmatics: development of subsensitivity with long term administration. J Allergy Clin Immunol 1982; 70: 417–422.

51. Larsson S, Svedmyr N, Thiringer GJ. Lack of bronchial beta adrenoceptor resistance in asthmatics during long term treatment with terbutaline. J Allergy Clin Immunol 1977; 59:93–100.

52. O'Connor BJ, Aikman S, Barnes PJ. Tolerance to the non-bronchodilator effects of inhaled beta-2 agonists in asthma. N Engl J Med 1992; 327:1204–1208.

53. van Wheel E, van Herwaarden CLA. Increased bronchial hyperresponsiveness after inhaling salbutamol during 1 year is not caused by subsensitization to salbutamol. J Allergy Clin Immunol 1990; 86:793–800.

54. Turki J, Green SA, Newman KB, Meyers MA, Liggett SB. Lung cell β₂-adrenergic receptors desensitize in response to *in vivo* administered β-agonist in humans. Am J Physiol: Lung Cell Mol Physiol 1995; in press.

55. Spitzer WO, Suissa S, Ernst P, et al. The use of β-agonists and the risk of death and near death from asthma. N Engl J Med 1992; 326:501–506.

56. Ernst P, Habbick B, Suissa S, et al. Is the association between inhaled beta-agonist use and life-threatening asthma because of confounding by severity? Am Rev Respir Dis 1993; 148:75–79.

57. Grainger J, Woodman K, Peace N, et al. Prescribed fenoterol and death from asthma in New Zealand, 1981–7: a further case-control study. Thorax 1991; 46:105–111.

58. Szefler SJ, Ando R, Cicutto LC, Surs W, Hill MR, Martin RJ. Plasma histamine, epinephrine, cortisol, and leukocyte β-adrenergic receptors in nocturnal asthma. Clin Pharmacol Ther 1991; 49:59–68.

59. Holroyd KJ, Levitt RC, Dragwa C, et al. Evidence for β$_2$-adrenergic receptor (ADRB2) polymorphism at amino acid 16 as a risk factor for bronchial hyperresponsiveness (BHR). Am J Respir Crit Care Med 1995; 151:A673 (abstr).

22

Overview of Genetic Factors in the Allergic Response

MALCOLM N. BLUMENTHAL

Medical School
University of Minnesota
Minneapolis, Minnesota

I. Introduction

Allergies are conditions which have been noted for many years [1], but the importance of genetics in these conditions was not recognized until rather recently. The definition of a condition such as allergy is relatively new. The original data on which a definition was based were provided by Portier and Richet [2] for anaphylaxis, by Arthus [3] for the local Arthus reaction, and by Clemens von Pirquet with Bela Schick [4] for serum sickness syndrome, all reported at the beginning of the twentieth century. It was von Pirquet who coined the word "allergy" in 1906 [5]. He wrote: "For this general concept of changed reactivity, I propose the term Allergy. 'Allos' implies deviation from the original state, from the behavior of the normal individual." Allergy was defined as an adverse immune reaction, and the formal study of allergy as a discipline began. The term atopy was proposed by Coca and Cooke in 1923 to identify what was commonly known as clinical allergies. These were said to involve reaginic or skin-sensitizing antibodies and are subject to hereditary influences [6]. Atopy is derived from the Greek word meaning "out of place" or "strange disease." It has been used to refer to a variety of allergic conditions (i.e., those defined clinically, regardless of whether an antibody could be demonstrated, to those conditions where there is

479

only the occurrence of a specific skin-sensitizing antibody, regardless of clinical history). In this chapter, I will define atopy as an adverse immune reaction involving IgE antibodies. The connection between atopy and the immune system was suggested by work of Blackley, who reported skin reactivity to grass pollen [7]. Alfred Wolff-Eisner, in 1906, provided further evidence of skin-sensitizing antibodies being related to hayfever [8]. Samuel Meltzer, in 1910, demonstrated a similar relationship between reaginic antibodies and asthma [9].

Early studies stressed the familial component in allergy; however, it was not until Cooke et al. performed a systematic study of these conditions that it was first established that there are genetic factors involved in their development [10]. Since these studies suggesting a familial and genetic component to the development of asthma and allergies, progress has been slow. However, with the improved techniques developed to study of the genetics of complex human diseases, much new information has been reported regarding allergy and IgE (reviewed in other chapters).

A better understanding of the pathogenesis of atopic conditions is allowing us to characterize the phenotype of asthma and allergies. This has consisted of the characterizations of IgE by Ishizaka [11,12] and Johanssen [13] in the 1960s, followed by further definitions of T cells and cytokines [14,15]. Other advances have been made in the field of molecular genetics. These include the techniques for isolation of recombinant DNA, the cloning of DNA fragments, the discovery that DNA fragments can be separated by electrophoresis, and the development of the polymerase chain reaction, which allows the rapid amplification of regions of DNA with ease [14].

Statistical methods have also improved, permitting the analysis of the genetics of complex diseases such as allergies [16]. These include methods such as likelihood analysis using lod scores, regressive models of segregation analysis taking into account environmental factors, the transmission/disequilibrium test (TDT), affected sib-pair analysis, and affected-pedigree-member analysis. All these advances are allowing researchers to define the molecular basis of diseases such as asthma and allergies.

Understanding the molecular basis of an inherited disease ultimately requires us to know everything about its gene(s): their chromosomal location, the DNA sequence, how expression is controlled, and the function of the gene product. For a given disease, there are several routes to this knowledge, as discussed in other chapters. The main ones are called forward and reverse or positional genetics. Another approach is that of looking at candidate genes, or genes already identified which may be involved in the condition being studied. An example of this would be investigating the genes on chromosome 5 which are known to be involved in the regulation of IgE.

Using these newer methodologies, the study of allergy and IgE has progressed. These investigations have typically involved either population or family studies [17]. Families are groups of individuals that may consist of sibling pairs including twins, sibships, nuclear families, extended pedigrees, or inbred populations. As discussed in other chapters, there are problems of ascertainment of families, definition of parameters to be measured (i.e., phenotypes), and methods of statistical analysis. Family studies, although difficult to perform, are needed to evaluate the genetics of allergy and IgE.

II. Rationale for Asthma and Atopy Genetic Studies

Allergic conditions, because they are such common diseases, are a good model for studying complex diseases resulting from the interaction of genetic with environmental factors [18]. It is estimated that approximately 30% of the total population have atopic diseases such as asthma rhinitis. The clinical picture has been well defined. In addition, the causative allergens can be identified and characterized, and the immune response (i.e., the specific IgE antibody) to them can be identified. Lastly, a suggested pathogenesis is available to use as a model.

Based on the accumulated data, it appears that multiple cell types and numerous cellular control mechanisms influence the development of asthma and the allergies and their response to treatment. According to current understanding, the following model is being used for the investigation of the genetics of the atopic conditions [19–21].

> *Sensitization*: Exposure to the allergen (antigen) occurs, following which it is taken up by an antigen-presenting cell (APC) such as a dendritic or B cell. Afterwards the allergen (antigen) will, through intracellular processing, be broken down into a specific peptide which becomes associated with a class II MHC (major histcompatibility complex) molecule selected from an MHC library. The allergen (antigen) peptide–MHC complex then moves to the surface of the APC, where it can interact with TH clones which have T-cell receptors (TCRs) specific for the class II peptide complex chosen from a TCR library. In atopic individuals there appears to be the preferential development of a disproportionate number of TH2 as opposed to TH1 cells which interact with the allergen (antigen)-binding B-cell clones, either through the production of cytokines and/or directly through action on B cells. This interaction results in signals for the B cells to differentiate and produce antigen-specific antibodies whose Ig has been chosen from a V(h) library for its ability to bind the allergen (antigen). This step may result in two major effects: (1) B cells mature to plasma cells. In the allergen-specific response, isotope switching occurs, followed by the production of allergen-specific IgE. (2) New virgin B and T cells are stimulated, further diversifying the immune response. After the specific IgE is formed, it will interact with a cell containing an IgE receptor.

Reexposure: Upon reexposure, the allergen (antigen) will interact with allergen-specific IgE on the surfaces of cells, which will initiate the release of inflammatory mediators. The end-organ responses to the released mediators will result in the clinical picture of asthma and atopy.

It appears that these activities must be coordinated in order to produce asthma and allergic responses. In addition, there are a multitude of steps by which the process can be enhanced or attenuated. Many of these steps are under genetic control, and many involve environmental interactions. While the specificity of each step may be relatively low, the overall specificity is much greater as a result of sequential gating of independent points of recognition. By studying this proposed mechanism, we should be able to further define the biology of asthma and allergies and develop an understanding of the genetics involved.

III. Methodology Used for the Determination of the Genetics of Asthma and Allergies

Asthma and allergies are conditions which involve an interaction of host and genetic factors with environmental factors. Studies have been performed to determine their mode of inheritance, whether a major gene is involved, and the characteristics of the gene. The adequate study of these complex diseases requires a proper definition of the phenotype under study. A decision regarding the presence of one or multiple phenotypes for a particular disease is needed. In addition, one has to consider environmental factors which will influence the phenotype, factors such as age, sex, time and type of exposure to allergens, infections, air pollutants, and emotional variables.

Determination of heritability, mode of inheritance, and characterization of the gene(s) is information which is needed to be defined for the phenotype under study. They can be obtained using population and family studies. Is there heritability? Is the phenotype a dominant, codominant, or recessive trait? Characterization of the gene(s) involved can be performed using a variety of methods. Asthma and allergies are complex phenotypes. As we do not know an exact mechanism or the gene products involved, positional genetics rather than forward genetics or the candidate gene approaches have been used to characterize the gene(s) involved. To identify the gene(s) involved with a particular phenotype, genotyping needs to be performed in order to do positional cloning or to use the candidate gene approach. Microsatellite repeat sequences can be used as the primary type of markers to be analyzed. Supplementary information may be obtained using minisatellite (VNTR) and/or RFLP markers, if required. Data analysis will include segregation and linkage analysis to determine the mode of inheritance and characterization of the gene(s) involved. It should be stressed that the results need to be replicated. Using these methodologies, researchers are beginning to understand the role that both genetic and environmental factors play in the development of allergies. In this chapter we review family studies of asthma, allergy, and IgE involving sib pairs, twins, nuclear families, extended families, and inbred populations.

Using data from family studies, positional cloning and the candidate gene approach are being used to investigate conditions such as asthma and allergies, because we do not know enough about their biology to do forward genetics. It is therefore important to identify and characterize the phenotype under study. The genetic control of asthma and allergies has been studied using intermediate phenotypes such as specific immune responses, serum IgE levels, and more complex phenotypes such as clinical atopy [22].

IV. Specific Immune Response

The overall mechanics of the specific immune response is one of the earliest phenotypes to be defined genetically. Allergens which are well defined with regard to size, structures, sequence, epitopes, and binding capacity to T- and B-cell sites are needed for such studies. The smaller and fewer are the epitopes, the better the allergen is for study. The ragweed model has been used. It is an identifiable allergy which is well characterized, and there is an identifiable IgE immune response to it. Ragweed contains at least 55 allergens, of which approximately 22 are important clinically and bind to IgE [23,24]. *Ambrosia artemisiaefolia* I (*Amb a* I) is the major purified allergen of short ragweed, with a molecular weight of 35,000. *Amb a* V, the smallest ragweed allergen identified, has a molecular weight of 4500. It has been sequenced and shown to have 45 amino acids [25]. Its structure is known, and at least three epitopes have been identified which bind to immunoglobulin E [26]. The binding capacities for *Amb a* V IgE antibodies range from 0.9×10^{-10} to 26×10^{-10}, compared to 1×10^{-7} for *Amb a* V IgG. It has also been demonstrated that, in the same individual, different epitopes can bind to different immunoglobulin groups (i.e., the epitope for binding IgE may be different from that for IgG in the same individual). The immune response to *Amb a* I was first reported to be associated with the HLA system by Levine et al. [27]. Work in our laboratory demonstrated that *Amb a* I was linked with the HLA system [28]. Because of its large size and multiple epitopes, *Amb a* V has subsequently been used to study the immune response in the ragweed model. This purified allergen has been noted to be strongly associated with HLA DR2 *1500 [29]. The β chain appears to be the chain needed for presentation [30]. Although *Amb a* V is highly associated with DR1500, there is no correlation between the particular B cell epitopes of *Amb a* V with the HLA class II allergen [26]. *Amb a* V derived from short, giant, and false ragweed has been demonstrated to be associated with HLA DR2, even though they are immunologically different [25]. Furthermore, atopic *Amb a* V-sensitive and *Amb a* V-nonsensitive DR2-positive individuals do not differ with regard to their sequence. This suggests that *Amb a* V responders do not have unique sequences with regard to the HLA DR2 locus [30–32]. The immune response to *Amb a* V appears to require the involvement of the HLA DR system, but other factors are also involved. Other purified allergens which have been found to be associated with HLA class II allergens include Olive (*Ole* I), giant ragweed (*Amb t* V), and rye grass (*Lol p* I) [29].

There is growing evidence that the specific immune response is associated with the HLA system, specifically the DR region. The presence of a particular DR-associated class II molecule appears to provide a necessary, but not the only, condition needed for responsiveness to a particular epitope.

The next step to develop an immune response, after interaction of a peptide of the allergen with the HLA class II allergen, is to have this HLA class II allergen complex from the APC interact with the T-cell receptors (TCRs). The antigen specificity of the T cell appears to be determined by the arrangement of TCR elements on the α and β chains. Renz et al. demonstrated in mice that the specific V β-expressing T-cell subpopulations in mice influences the stimulation of IgE/ IgG1 production and increased airways responsiveness [33]. Using 66 nuclear families and five extended pedigrees, Moffatt et al. presented evidence indicating genetic linkage of T-cell receptor α/δ complex to specific IgE responses [34]. These studies suggest that chromosome 14 may be important in the specific atopic response.

V. IGE Regulation

In view of the apparent importance of IgE regulation in the development of allergic conditions, this phenotype has been investigated genetically. The up-regulation of IgE synthesis in atopy appears to be due to the induction of IgE isotope utilization at the DNA level in B cells [20]. IgE synthesis appears to involve signals following direct T cell–B cell interaction. One of the major ones is delivered by an IgE isotope-specific signal, provided by the activated CD4 T cell or TH2 cell-derived IL-4. Other IgE-promoting cytokines possibly involved include IL-5, IL-9, and TNF-α. Cognate signals which require the engagement of the TCRs with antigenic fragments (peptides) that are recognized on MHC class II molecules on APC are also involved in IgE production. These include CD40 ligand (CD40-L) and FcεRII B-cell activation signal. Other cytokines, such as interferon-gamma (IFN-γ), interferon-alpha (IFN-α), and probably IL-8, IL-10, and IL-14, inhibit IgE production.

Twin and family studies have demonstrated the heritability of serum IgE levels [22]. Twin studies have demonstrated that monozygotic twins are more concordant than dizygotic twins for total serum IgE levels. Hanson et al. studied twins raised apart and compared them with those raised together [35]. This offered an opportunity to examine the effect of different environments on identical genotypes. Intraclass correlations for log-transformed serum IgE, with one exception, showed significantly greater than zero and higher for monozygotic twins as compared to the dizygotic twins. Biometric modeling indicated that the results did not support the existence of a common familial environmental effect, because the reared-apart twins who did not share a familial environment were more similar than the reared-together twins, who did. The data suggests that common breeding environment has very little effect on IgE levels, and that there is a significant genetic component regulating IgE levels.

Family studies are also consistent with a significant genetic regulatory effect. We have investigated the genetic aspects of IgE levels in three large pedigrees, many of which had atopy [36]. Based on data from 184 individuals, the environmental model was significantly rejected, suggesting a strong hereditary involvement in IgE control. The best-fitting single model was that high IgE levels are determined by a dominant allele. However, when the families were analyzed separately, there was evidence of heterogeneity. Further studies of extended pedigrees were performed regarding the inheritance of IgE [37]. In these studies, both nongenetic and purely environmental experimental models were rejected when evaluating the pooled data. However, when the pedigrees' inheritance models were evaluated individually, two families showed a better fit with a dominant model and five a close fit with the recessive model of inheritance. Additional studies found evidence of a recessive model of inheritance, while others have shown significant heterogeneity [38,39]. A major gene appears to be involved in the regulation of serum IgE levels. These studies are described further in Chapter 24.

Several studies have examined markers on chromosome 5 with the IgE response [40–42]. Evidence for linkage with markers in chromosome 5q3.1 with a gene controlling total serum IgE level concentrations was reported by Marsh et al. They performed sib-pair analysis of 170 individuals from 11 Amish families [40]. Evidence for a locus regulating total serum IgE levels mapping to chromosome 5 was reported by Meyers et al. in families ascertained through a parent with asthma [41].

VI. IGE Receptors

Atopic or IgE-associated reaction requires the attachment of the IgE to a cell receptor. High-affinity receptors on basophil and mast cells and low-affinity receptors on eosinophil and lymphocytes have been identified and characterized. These genes for these receptors are being used as candidate genes. Sandford et al. reported that the gene regulating the β chain of the high-affinity receptor for IgE

(FcεRI-β) is on chromosome 11q [43]. Shirakawa et al., of the same group, subsequently reported findings from their analysis of 60 untreated nuclear families with allergic asthmatic probands. They found an association between atopy and variants of the β subunit of the high-affinity immunoglobulin IgE receptor [44]. Other candidate genes for study include those for the low-affinity IgE receptor (FcεRII-β), and its ligand CD40.

VII. IGE Receptor/IGE Interaction/Mediator Release

The mechanisms of the IgE receptor–IgE and allergen–IgE interactions and the regulation of the release of mediators and cytokines are just being characterized. The genetics of the regulation of the release of mediators or cytokines involving the interaction of IgE cells and their ability to release mediating substances also has not been extensively investigated. Heritability of the phenotype of histamine release following the anti-IgE challenge of peripheral blood basophils has been reported in a twin study by Marone et al. [45], and in a nuclear family study by Roitman-Johnson et al. [46].

VIII. Atopy, Asthma, Allergic Rhinitis and Hay Fever

The general expression of the complex phenotypes of allergic diseases has been noted for many years to be familial and to have a genetic basis [21]. It is fairly well established that there is heritability of certain allergic conditions including some cases of asthma, rhinitis, urticaria, angioedema, and eczema. Depending on the study, as many as 40–80% of patients with allergic rhinitis or bronchial asthma have been noted to have a positive family history of allergy, as opposed to 20% or less of the nonallergic subjects. Some studies suggest that the incidence of allergic disease in children roughly doubles with each parent who is allergic or has asthma. The problems of definition of phenotypes in these early studies is apparent. Recently, investigators have been attempting to restudy the phenotypes of the complex diseases such as atopy, allergic rhinitis, and asthma using updated parameters to define the phenotypes and more sophisticated molecular, genetic, and statistical approaches to their analysis.

A. Atopy and Asthma

It has been estimated that between 10% and 30% of the general population has some form of atopic disease [47]. There have been problems regarding how to define atopy. It may be characterized using a variety of different parameters, including historical items as well as IgE responses [47]. Hopkin and Cookson investigated families by looking at total serum IgE levels as well as the specific IgE response to allergens as determined by skin testing and RAST in families with asthma and allergic rhinitis [48]. They defined atopy as an elevated serum IgE level and/or an elevated specific IgE as measured by RAST or skin test. They suggested that atopy, as defined by the ability to produce IgE response using these parameters, is inherited as an autosomal dominant character and is linked to C 11q. Rich et al. investigated in three extended families the same complex phenotypes of atopy with respect to their genetic and environmental determinants [49]. No evidence for linkage was found in three large pedigrees using the dominant mode of inheritance using their phenotype, as well as several others. Lympany et al. [50,51], Hizawa et al. [52], and Amelung et al. [53], in separate studies, also could not confirm linkage of atopy and C 11q. Cookson et al. also suggested that the 11q13-linked atopy gene is inherited preferentially from the maternal side, possibly due to either paternal genetic imprinting or maternal modification of the infants' IgE responses through the placenta or breast milk [54]. These studies have not been confirmed by other groups.

Bronchial asthma and mite-sensitive allergic asthma have been investigated in relationship with HLA antigens. Carabello et al. studied HLA haplotype segregation in families with mite-sensitive allergic asthma [55]. Twenty families with allergic asthma and *D. farniae* sensitivity and eight families with intrinsic or no allergic asthma were studied genetically using the affected sib-pair method. The existence of a HLA-linked recessive gene controlling the IgE immune responsiveness to mite allergens and conferring susceptibility to allergic asthma is suggested by their study. Association of other specific triggers, such as aspirin-induced asthma, has been reported with antigens of the HLA system [56]. The general expression of certain diseases has been noted to be associated with the presence of the extended HLA haplotypes. Different extended haplotypes appear to contain a different pattern of chromosomal deletions and insertions, some of which may influence the level of gene expression. As a result, certain combinations of alleles, especially of the D/DR and complement loci, are seen to be highly associated with a disease. The association of ragweed allergic rhinitis and bronchial asthma with the extended HLA haplotype has been investigated in nuclear families [57]. The frequencies of HLA-DR2 and the extended MHC haplotype B7, SC31, DR2 were significantly increased among the patients with asthma and high titers of IgE anti-*Amb a* V. Conversely, this group had decreased frequencies of HLA-DR3 and the extended haplotype HLA B8, SC01, DR3 compared with patients with only rhinitis. This rhinitis group had an increased number of individuals with the extended haplotype HLA B8, SC01, DR3 and low levels of IgE *Amb a* V. It appears from this investigation that there may be a dominant MHC-linked gene or genes on HLA B7, SC31, DR2 controlling the IgE immune response to *Amb a* V and predisposing to asthma.

B. Allergic Rhinitis/Hay Fever

Allergic rhinitis is defined as inflammation of the nasal mucous membrane involving an IgE mechanism and characterized by periods of nasal discharge, sneezing,
and congestion. Epidemiologic studies estimated that between 10% and 41% of
the general population have allergic rhinitis [58]. It has been noted to be associated
with asthma and atopic dermatitis. A hereditary diathesis for allergic rhinitis was
reported in families by many early investigators, including Bostock, Elliotson,
Wyman, and Mackenzie as well as Cooke and VanderVeer [1,59]. Few family
studies of the genetics of allergic rhinitis have been performed using newer
methodology. The HLA system in relationship to allergic rhinitis has been studied
without any definite conclusions.

IX. Eczema/Atopic Dermatitis

Eczema has never been satisfactorily defined and has different interpretations in
different areas [60]. As a result, the term has gradually lost its medical significance. It is in general used to refer to a variety of chronic as well as acute derma-
tites. Eczema has been defined as a cutaneous response to various noxious stimuli.
It is characterized in its acute stages by erythema and vesiculation and in its
chronic stages by scaling and thickening of the skin.

   Atopic dermatitis is a chronic dermatitis which possesses distinctive features with respect to localization of the lesion, personal and family history of
allergy, and a characteristic—though often erratic—course [60]. It is defined as
a chronic, heritable, distinctive, especially pruritic form of eczema frequently
associated with asthma and allergic rhinitis. In addition, most but not all atopic
dermatitis patients have elevated serum IgE levels. Atopic dermatitis has a variety
of clinical manifestations, including those seen in infants, teens, and adults. Terms
used for atopic dermatitis include atopic eczema, eczema, dermatitis, Besnier
prurigo, and neurodermatitis. Ten percent of patients with atopic dermatitis do not
have a family history of allergy. Associations between atopic dermatitis and the
HLA system have been suggested in population studies, but no definitive family
studies have been reported at the present time.

X. Contact Dermatitis

Allergic contact dermatitis is a result of sensitization to a wide variety of different
contactant material. It has been found to be mediated by a cellular, nonatopic
immune mechanism. Common antigens include poison ivy, metals such as nickel,
and cosmetics, as well as medications. Genetic factors are probably involved as

shown in the guinea pig by Chase, Geczy, and de Weck [61,62]. There does not appear to be more allergic contact dermatitis in atopic as compared to nonatopic populations. In humans there are no family studies which define the genetics of the condition.

XI. Urticaria/Angioedema

Urticaria is characterized by a cutaneous elevation that typically presents as a wheal with erythema and which blanches with pressure. It is frequently associated with itching. Angioedema is thought to involve a similar process but involves the deep dermal and subcutaneous tissue. Their pathogenesis is thought to involve a variety of complex cellular and humoral factors. Although many etiological factors have been reported, the majority of the cases are idiopathic [63]. Family reports by Quincke, Dinkelacher, Valentin, Strubing, and Osler in the latter part of the nineteenth century revealed that some cases of angioedema had a hereditary factor [64–67]. Hereditary angioedema (HAE) is probably the best defined of the genetic syndromes of this type [67]. This condition is associated with an autosomal dominant deficiency of C1 esterase inhibitor activity. The C1-INH gene, comprised of 7 exons and at least 7 introns, is located on chromosome 11 region q11-q13. Several copies of Alu sequences that are highly repetitive DNA sequences dispersed throughout the human genome are contained in the C1-INH gene. It is thought that Alu sequences predispose the gene to deletions and insertions as a result of unequal crossover during meiosis. Two different types of HAE have been identified on the basis of apparent protein abnormalities. HAE type I is characterized by a decreased level of functionally normal C1-INH in the plasma. Approximately 85% of patients with HAE exhibit this type. It appears that it results from the apparent lack of function of one C1-INH allele in the genome. Analysis of the genomic sequence indicates the partial deletions or insertions within the C1-INH gene. Repetitive Alu sequences in the C1-INH gene has been suggested to play a primary role in this process. Polymorphism, however, is not seen in the majority of patients with type I HAE. These cases may have small mutations in the regions of the C1-INH gene which are required for either proper transcription or translation. The remaining 15% of cases of HAE are of the type II variety, which is characterized by normal or increased levels of C1-INH, but the protein has reduced functional activity. In these cases the underlying molecular changes responsible for the functional defects are of two varieties: mutation in the reactive 100 p of the C1-INH molecules and mutation outside the reactive 100 p. Seventy percent of cases of type II HAE may be due to point mutations affecting the nucleotides that code for Arg. A less well defined syndrome is familial cold urticaria [63], which is thought to be an autosomal dominant syndrome of cold intolerance. Other defined hereditary syndromes which appear to be autosomal dominant conditions are hereditary vibratory angioedema [68,69] and urticaria associated with amyloidosis [70]. Both appear to be autosomal dominant conditions.

XII. Modulation of the Genetic Factors and Clinical Picture by Environmental Factors

The ultimate clinical picture of an allergy and IgE responses depend on genetic factors interacting with those of the environment. It has been suggested that environmental factors may modulate the genetic factors as well as the resulting clinical picture. Nongenetic factors which may influence the ultimate clinical picture are age, infections, psychological factors, air pollutants including tobacco smoke, and allergen exposure. The conditions under which allergen exposures occur will affect the ultimate clinical picture. There is increasing evidence that factors which an individual encounters before the age of one year, including during fetal life, may have consequences for the rest of his or her life [71].

XIII. Summary

The search for the genes involved in the control of allergy and IgE is just beginning. Researchers are starting to sort out the genetic control of these conditions. Many steps are hypothesized for the development of allergies and IgE. It is evident that the specific immune response to certain aeroallergens is genetically determined by a gene (or genes) located on chromosome 6 at the DR loci. The T-cell receptors may play a role in the specific IgE response. Regulation of IgE is heritable and due to at least one major gene. The IgERII has been suggested in one study to be under genetic control and related to the development of atopy. The genetics of more complex phenotypes such as allergic rhinitis, atopy, eczema, urticaria, and angioedema are being investigated using the newer methodologies. In addition, environmental factors may modulate both the genes and the ultimate clinical picture. The identification of these genetic and environmental controls has many implications for the management of asthma and allergic diseases. This includes a better understanding of their pathogenesis; redefinition of asthma and allergic conditions; improved diagnostic measures; and more specific modes of managing these conditions, including genetic manipulation, avoidance of environmental risk factors, and manipulation of pathways involved in their production. In addition, studies with regard to the genetics of the phenotypes of asthma, allergic diseases, and IgE will give us basic knowledge regarding factors which determine the type of health we all enjoy during our lifetimes.

References

1. Silverstein A. The History of Immunology. San Diego, CA: Academic Press, 1989.
2. Portier P, Richet C. Chapter de l'action anaphylactique de certains benins. C R Soc Biol Paris, 1902; 54:170.
3. Arthus M. Injections repetees de serum de cheval chez le pain. C R Soc Biol Paris, 1903; 55:817.
4. Von Pirquet, Schick CF, Didia B. Serum Krankheit. Leipzig: Franz Deuticke, 1905.
5. Von Pirquet, Clemens, Munch. Med Wochenschr 1906; 53:1457. Prausnitz C, trans. Gell PGH, Coombs RRA, eds. Clinical Aspects of Immunology. Philadelphia: F. A. Davis, 1963.
6. Coca AF, Cooke RA. On the classification of the phenomena of hypersensitiveness. J Immunol 1923; 8:163.
7. Blackley CH. Experimental Researches on the Causes and Nature of *Catarrhus aestivus* (hay fever or hay asthma). London: Balliere, Tindall and Cox, 1873.
8. Wolff-Eisen A. Das Heufieber. Munich, 1906.
9. Maltzer SJ. Bronchial asthma as a phenomenon of anaphylaxis. JAMA 1910; 55: 1021.
10. Cooke RA, Vander Veer A. Human sensitization. J Immunol 1916; 1:201–305.
11. Ishizaka K, Ishizaka T. Physiochemical properties of reaginic antibody. I. Assiciation of reaginic activity with an immunoglobulin other than γA- or γG-globulin. J Allergy 1966; 37:169.
12. Ishizaka K, Ishizaka T. Physiochemical properties of reaginic antibody. III. Further study on the reaginic antibody in γA-globulin preparation. J Allergy 1966; 38:108.
13. Johansson SG, Bennich H. Immunological studies of an atypical (myeloma) immuno-globulin. Immunol 1967; 13:381–394.
14. Blumenthal MN. Genetics of asthma, allergy, and related conditions. In: Blumenthal MN, Björkstén B, eds. Genetics of Asthma and Allergy. New York: Marcel Dekker. In press.
15. Lee T, Lympany P. Inflammation. In: Blumenthal MN, Björkstén B, eds. Genetics of Asthma and Allergy. New York: Marcel Dekker. In press.
16. Morton N. Statistical methods. In: Blumenthal MN, Björkstén B, eds. Genetics of Asthma and Allergy. New York: Marcel Dekker. In press.
17. Meyers, D. Tools for the study of genetics. In: Blumenthal MN, Björkstén B, eds. Genetics of Asthma and Allergy. New York: Marcel Dekker. In press.
18. Marsh DG, Blumenthal MN. Genetic and environmental factors in clinical allergy. Minneapolis: University of Minnesota Press, 1990.
19. Abbas, et al. Cellular and molecular immunology. Philadelphia: W. B. Saunders, 1991: 186–203.
20. Sutton BJ, Gould HJ. The human IgE network. Nature 1993; 66:421.
21. Blumenthal MN. Family, twin and population studies of allergic responsiveness. In: Marsh DG, Lockhart A, Holgate S, eds. The Genetics of Asthma. Oxford: Blackwell, 1993:133–141.
22. Blumenthal MN, Boninis S. Immunogenetics of specific immune responses to aller-

gens in twins and families. In: Marsh DG, Blumenthal MN, eds. Genetic and Environmental Factors in Clinical Allergy. Minneapolis: University of Minnesota Press, 1990:132–142.

23. Lowenstein H, Marsh DG. Anitgens of *Ambrosia elatior* (short ragweed) pollen. I. Cross immunoelectrophoretic analysis. J Immunol 1981; 126:943.

24. Lowenstein H, Marsh DG. Anitgens of *Ambrosia elatior* (short ragweed) pollen. I. Cross immunoelectrophoresis of ragweed and allergic patients' sera with special attention to quantifications of IgE response. J Immunol 1983; 130:727.

25. Marsh DG. Immunogenetic and immunochemical factors determining immune responsiveness to allergens: studies in unrelated subjects. In: Marsh DG, Blumenthal MN, eds. Genetic and Environmental Factors in Clinical Allergy. Minneapolis: University of Minnesota Press, 1990:97–123.

26. Kim KE, Rosenberg A, Blumenthal MN. Regulation of IgE response to Amb a V by a gating mechanism (abstr). J Allergy Clin Immunol 1994; 93:252–535.

27. Levine B, Stember R, Fontino M. Ragweed hayfever: genetic control and linkage to HLA haplotypes. Science 198:1201–1203.

28. Blumenthal MN, Amos DB, Noreen H, Mendell NR, Yunis EJ. Genetic mapping of Ir locus in man: linkage to second locus of HLA. Science 1974; 184:1301–1303.

29. Marsh DG, Blumenthal MN, Ishikawa T, et al. HLA and specific immune responsiveness to allergens. In: Tsuji K, Aizawa M, Sasazuki T, eds. HLA 1991: Proc 11th Int Histocompatibility Workshop. New York: Oxford University Press, 1992:765–771.

30. Huang S, Zwollo P, Marsh DG. Class II major histocompatibility complex restriction of human T cell responses to short ragweed allergen *Amb a* V. Eur J Immunol 1991; 21:1469–1473.

31. Dalan D, Rich S, Blumenthal MN. IgE *Amb a* V response and Class II HLA polymorphism (abstr). J Allergy Clin Immunol 1991; 87:198–237.

32. Zwollo P, Erlich Kautzky E, Scharf S, et al. Sequences of HLA D in responders and nonresponders to short ragweed *Amb a* V. Immunogenetics 1991; 33:141–151.

33. Renz H, Saloga J, Bradley KL, et al. Specific V β T cell subsets mediate the immediate hypersensitivity response to ragweed allergy. J Immunol 1993; 151:1907–1917.

34. Moffatt M, Mill M, Cornelis F, et al. Genetic linkage of T cell receptors and α/δ complex to specific IgE response. Lancet 1994; 343:1597–1600.

35. Hanson B, McGue M, Roitman-Johnson B, et al. Atopic disease and immunoglobulin E in twins reared apart and together. Am J Hum Genet 1991; 48:873–879.

36. Blumenthal MN, Namboodiri M, Gleich G, et al. Genetic transmission of serum IgE levels. Am J Hum Genet 1981; 10:219.

37. Blumenthal MN, Yunis E, Mendell N, Elston RC. Preventative allergy: genetics of IgE-mediated diseases. J Allergy Clin Immunol 1986; 78:962–968.

38. Rao DC, Lalonel JM, Morton NE, Gerrard JW. Immunoglobulin E revisited. Am J Hum Genet 1980; 32:620–625.

39. Gerrard JW, Rao DC, Morton NE. A genetic study of immunoglobulin E. Am J Hum Genet 1978; 30:46–58.

40. Marsh DG, Needly J, Breazeale D, et al. Linkage analysis of IL4 and other chromo-

somes Sq31, 1 markers and total serum immunoglobulin E concentration. Science 1994; 264:1152.

41. Meyers DA, Postma DS, Panhuysen CIM, et al. Evidence for a locus regulating total serum IgE mapping to chromosomes. Genomics 1994; 23:464.

42. Blumenthal MN, Weber N, Rich S. Unpublished observations.

43. Sandford AO, Shirakawa TS, Moffatt M. Localization of atopy and the β sub-unit of the high-affinity IgE receptor (FcεR1) on chromosome 11q. Lancet 1993; 341: 332–334.

44. Shirakawa TS, Airong L, Dubowiitz M, et al. Association between atopy and variants of the β sub-unit of the high-affinity IgE receptor. Nature Genet 1994; 7:125.

45. Marone G, Poto S, Celestino D, Bonini S. Human basophil releasability. III. Genetic controls of the humAN basophil releasabilty. J Immunol 1986; 137:3588–3592.

46. Roitman-Johnson B, Blumenthal MN. Family analysis of histamine release (abstr). J Allergy Clin Immunol 1988; 81:232.

47. Friedhoff L. Epidemiology of atopic allergy. In: Marsh DG, Blumenthal MN, eds. Genetic and Environmental Factors in Clinical Allergy. Minneapolis: University of Minnesota Press, 1990; 53–72.

48. Cookson WO, Sharp PA, Faux JA, Hopkin JM. Linkage between immunoglobulin E responses underlying asthma and rhinitis and chromosome 11q. Lancet 1989; 1: 1292–1295.

49. Rich SS, Roitman-Johnson B, Greenberg B, et al. Genetic analysis of atopy in three large kindreds: no evidence of linkage to D11S97. Clin Exp Allergy 1992; 22:1070–1076.

50. Lympany P, Welsh K, MacCochrane G, et al. Genetic analysis using DNA polymorphism of the linkage between chromosome 11q13 and atopy and bronchial hyper-responsiveness to methacholine. J Allergy Clin Immunol 1992; 89:619–628.

51. Lympany P. Welsh KI, Cochrane GM, et al. Genetic analysis of the linkage between chromosome 11q and atopy. Clin Exp Allergy 1992.

52. Hizawa N, Yamaguchi E, Ohe M, et al. Lack of linkage between atopy and locus 11q13. Clin Exp Allergy 1992; 22:1065–1069.

53. Amelung PJ, Panhuysen CIM, Postma DS, et al. Atopy and bronchial hyperrespon-siveness: exclusion of linkage to markers on chromosomes 11q and 6q. Clin Exp Allergy 1992; 22:1077–1084.

54. Cookson WOCM, Young RP, Sandford AJ, et al. Maternal inheritance of atopic responsiveness on chromosome 11q. Lancet 1992; 340:381–384.

55. Caraballo LR, Hernandez M. HLA haplotype segregation in families with allergic asthma. Tissue Antigens 1990; 35:182–186.

56. Lympany P, Welsh KI, Christie PE, et al. Analysis with sequence-specific oligo-nucleotide probes of the association between aspirin-induced asthma and antigens of the HLA system. J Allergy Clin Immunol 1993; 92:114.

57. Blumenthal MN, Marcus-Bagley D, Adweh Z, et al. Extended major: HLA-DR2, [HLA-B7, SC31, DR2] and [HLA-B8, SC01, DR3] haplotypes distinguish subjects with asthma from those with only rhinitis in ragweed pollen allergy. J Immunol 1992; 148:411–416.

58. Smith J. Epidemiology and natural history of asthma, allergic rhinitis and atopic dermatitis (eczema). In: Middleton E, Reed, Ellis E, eds. Allergy Principles and Practice. 2d ed. St. Louis: C. V. Mosby, 1983.

59. Blumenthal MN. Historical perspectives. In: Blumenthal MN, Björkstén B, eds. Genetics of Asthma and Allergy. New York: Marcel Dekker. In press.

60. Rasmussen J, Provost T. Atopic dermatitis. In: Middleton E, Reed C, Ellis E, eds. Allergy: Principles and Practice. 2d ed. St. Louis: C. V. Mosby, 1983:1297.

61. Chase MW. Inheritance in guinea pigs of the susceptibility to skin sensitizations with simple compounds. J Exp Med 1941; 73:711–729.

62. Geczy A, de Weck A. Genetic control of sensitization to chemically defined antigens and its relationship to histocompatible antigens in guinea pigs. In: Contact Hypersensitivity in Experimental Animals. Basel: S. Karger, 1974:83–88.

63. Kaplan AP. Urticaria and angioedema. In: Middleton E, Reed C, Ellis E, eds. Allergy Principles and Practices. 3d ed. St. Louis: C. V. Mosby, 1988:1377–1406.

64. Quincke H. Über akutes umschreibenes H-autoderm. Monatsshrifte für Praktische Dermatologie 1992; 1:129.

65. Osler W. Hereditary angioedema. Am J Med Sci 1888; 95:362.

66. Major R. Classic description of disease. Springfield, IL: Charles C Thomas, 1945.

67. Oltvai ZN, Wong E, Atkinson J, Tung K. C-1 inhibitor deficiency: molecular and immunologic basis of hereditary and acquired angioedema. Lab Invest 1991; 65:381.

68. Metzger W, Kaplan A, Beaven M, et al. Hereditary vibratory angioedema: confirmation of histamine release in a type of physical hypersensitivity. J Allergy Clin Immunol 1976; 57:605.

69. Patterson R, Mellus C, Blankenship M, Pruzansky J. Vibratory angioedema: a hereditary type of physical hypersensitivity. J Allergy Clin Immunol 1972; 50:174.

70. Black JT. Amyloidosis, deafness, urticaria and limb pain: a hereditary syndrome. Ann Intern Med 1969; 70:989–994.

71. Björkstén B. Epidemiology of factors influencing the development of asthma and allergy. In: Blumenthal MN, Björkstén B, eds. Genetics of Asthma and Allergy. New York: Marcel Dekker. In press.

23

Genetic Components of Atopy and Asthma

WILLIAM O. C. M. COOKSON

John Radcliffe Hospital
Oxford, England

I. Introduction

A. Asthma

Asthma is the most common disease of childhood in the United Kingdom, with one in seven children now suffering from the illness [1]. Asthma costs $£400,000,000 per annum to treat, and a similar amount is wasted through lost production. There are approximately 2000 asthma deaths per year in Great Britain. Ninety-five percent of childhood asthma is atopic. The prevalence of childhood asthma rises to a peak in the early teens, and is more common and earlier in onset in boys than in girls. The clinical course in many children is that of gradual improvement as they enter adulthood. Many individuals, unfortunately, remain disabled throughout their lives.

In adults most cases of asthma are also atopic, but many individuals with adult-onset asthma have no evidence of underlying atopy. In these cases, cigarette smoking is often, but not invariably, a contributing cause. Other asthma syndromes are also recognized, including aspirin–sensitive asthma and industrial asthma. These kinds of asthma may operate through nonatopic mechanisms.

Atopic asthma is clinically easily recognized and defined, and has the most obvious familial clustering. For this reason, in our laboratory most effort toward elucidating the genetic causes of asthma has been directed at asthma in children and in young adults, and at the underlying condition of atopy.

B. Atopy

Atopy is distinguished by immunoglobulin E (IgE) responses to inhaled proteins, known as allergens. Typical allergen sources include house dusts mites (HDM), grass pollens, and animal danders (sheddings from skin and fur). The total annual exposure to allergens is small, often of the order of micrograms. IgE binds by its high-affinity receptor (FcεRI), most notably to mast cells in the skin and in mucosal surfaces of the lung and intestines. Mast cells contain dense granules, which contain histamine and other inflammatory mediators, in addition to pro-inflammatory cytokines. In sensitized individuals, exposure to allergen produces cross-linking of IgE, triggering of high-affinity receptors, and release of mast cell granules. The subsequent inflammation is in two waves, the first immediate and the second some hours later. Inflammation produces airway narrowing, with wheeze when occurring in the lung, and sneezing and obstruction when in the nose. The regulation of IgE and of some components of early and late inflammation are under the control of antigen-specific T cells.

The atopic state is detected most easily by skin-prick tests. In these, allergen in dilute solution is placed on the skin, and a superficial prick is made to introduce minute amounts of allergen below the dermis. Sensitization and mast cell degranulation is detected by a wheal which is maximal after 10–15 min. A significant wheal is judged to be between 2 and 4 mm greater than a negative control. Ninety-five percent of individuals who are atopic will react either to HDM or to grass pollen or to both.

Atopy may also be detected by elevation of the total serum IgE, or by elevation of serum IgE titres against common allergens. Elevation of antigen-specific IgE is detected by RAST or ELISA techniques. In the affluent populations of the West, there is a close correlation between prick skin tests, specific IgE titers (RASTs), the total serum IgE, and symptoms of wheeze or rhinitis. Despite these close correlations, the relationships among the variables are complex.

Atopy, defined by skin tests, is very common, and has been shown in several large Western population samples to affect between 40% and 50% of young adults [2–4]. Any trait as common as atopy cannot be considered abnormal, and it is obvious that the atopic state gives some advantage to those who carry it. The most likely evolutionary reason for atopy to exist is that IgE is particularly important in handling parasite infestations [5,6].

C. Factors Confounding Genetic Studies of Atopy

The high population prevalence of atopy may seriously confound genetic studies [7]. If atopy is present in 40–50% of the population, then a fifth of marriages may be between two atopics. Any large pedigree is therefore likely to contain several atopy genes introduced through different individuals, instead of a single abnormal gene introduced through one progenitor. If atopy was due to a single gene disorder, then many of the population would be homozygous. If, as is the case, more than one gene predisposes to the syndrome, then many individuals will carry two or more of these genes.

The substantial prevalence of atopy means that great care has to be taken in the recruitment of families for genetic studies. Ascertainment by public appeals for families with asthma [8] or with eczema [9] produced samples in which 70% and 80%, respectively were atopic, with considerable loss of power to detect linkage [8]. For this reason, we now recruit families either from population samples (i.e., complete ascertainment), or through a defined proband with atopic disease.

For the purposes of genetic investigations, it is necessary to decide which measures of the atopy or asthma phenotype should be studied. The total serum IgE is an attractive parameter for genetic study, as it has well-established normal values, and in large population surveys correlates well with the presence of asthma. However, about 45% of the variation in the total serum IgE is attributable to the specific IgE (RAST) to HDM or grass pollen [10]. When multiple regressions are carried out on population data, asthma and bronchial hyperresponsiveness are found to relate to variation in the specific IgE, most notably to HDM [10,11]. Once specific IgE is taken into account, the residual total IgE does not correlate with the presence of asthma. The specific IgE, either detected indirectly by skin tests or directly in the serum by RAST or ELISA techniques may therefore be suitable for genetic analysis. Bronchial hyperresponsiveness is a further intermediate phenotype which is currently being investigated.

It is also possible to study asthma as the principal phenotype. If this is done, care needs to be taken that the asthma being investigated is as clinically homogeneous as possible, which will usually mean the asthma of children and young adults. As there is no clear-cut division between normal and abnormal individuals, studies of asthma should exclude marginal phenotypes, and concentrate on "barn door" affected and unaffected subjects.

Selection will affect the type of genetic effects found in particular samples of subjects or families. Even if total or specific IgE is used as a phenotype, the factors influencing the IgE in asthmatics may be different from those affecting the IgE in children with eczema, or in subjects selected for the presence of positive skin tests rather than for symptoms.

The behavior of atopy with age presents a particular problem for geneticists. While many diseases have increasing penetrance throughout life, atopy has a low penetrance in infancy, which rises to a maximum from 15 to 25 years of age. Thereafter the serum IgE and skin-prick test responses decline steadily, until at the age of 45 the serum IgE may be half of its value at the age of 15 [2].

D. The Inheritance of Atopy

Diverse models have been proposed for the inheritance of atopy at different times, with varying definitions of atopy, and different methods of analysis [12–24]. It is perhaps as a result of the diversity of approaches that dominant, dominant with incomplete penetrance, recessive, and polygenic modes of inheritance have all been suggested. None of these hypotheses explains the results of many studies which have shown that the risk of atopy is much higher in the children of atopic mothers than in the children of atopic fathers. That asthmatic mothers had more asthmatic children than asthmatic fathers was reported 60 years ago [25], and large studies have shown a similar maternal pattern to the inheritance of elevations of the cord blood IgE [26,27], atopic symptoms [28,29], and skin-prick test responses to common allergens [30]. This finding may be due to interactions between the mother and her child in utero through the placenta, or postpartum through the breast milk. Genomic imprinting, in which a paternal "atopy gene" may be suppressed during spermatogenesis, is also possible [31].

One new approach to the problem of a complex phenotype has been the application of regressive models to segregation analysis. Despite the close correlations among symptoms, the total serum IgE, and the specific IgE, genetic effects independently modifying these different variables can be dissected out with these models. This type of segregation analysis has been applied to the total serum IgE. The results demonstrate that the total IgE is influenced by at least one gene which is independent of genes affecting skin tests or positive RAST tests [32].

The failure to show a simple consistent model of inheritance means that the most likely possibility is that of several genes interacting with a strong environmental component. For the purpose of identifying genes causing atopy, an eclectic approach to phenotype definition is necessary, allowing for potential differences in the genes influencing skin tests and RASTs, the total serum IgE, or disease states such as asthma.

II. Finding Genes

As with other complex diseases, genes that contribute to atopy may be found either by examining candidate genes, or by genetic linkage. The most obvious candidate genes for atopy include *IL4*, *γ-interferon*, *IL10*, *G-CSF*, and the genes making up the high- and low-affinity receptors for IgE. Also included in this list should be the corresponding ligands or receptors. The enormous increase in understanding of the complex cytokine networks that influence atopy has meant, however, that a plausible case could be made for as many as 20 different candidates. The role of candidate genes may be assessed by defining polymorphisms within the respective genes, and testing for associations with disease. At the moment, a systematic search through the various candidates has not yet been

Table 1 The Power to Detect Linkage

Fraction linked	Recessive inheritance	Dominant inheritance
0.80	22	69
0.50	62	181
0.30	181	508
0.20	412	1152
0.10	1662	4637

The table shows the number of affected sibling pairs required to detect loci at $p = 0.05$ with 90% power at $\theta = 0.005$, with different proportions of families linked to the putative locus. The required numbers of sib pairs are estimated for three modes of inheritance. The table assumes 70% marker informativeness.

carried out. Two candidates, *IL-4*, and the beta chain of the high-affinity receptor for IgE (*FcεRIβ*), have been implicated by genetic linkage studies.

Genetic linkage relies on the demonstration of co-inheritance of disease and genetic markers of known chromosomal localization. This approach has the advantage of not requiring any preexisting knowledge of the pathophysiology of the disease. However, the power to detect linkage in multigenic diseases is very limited (Table 1), so several hundred families may be necessary to detect linkage to a gene affecting a third of subjects with disease. A further problem with complex diseases is that of replication of linkage [33]. Linkage to a heterogeneous trait will normally be found only fortuitously, in samples which contain an exceptional proportion of individuals or families influenced by that particular gene. Simulation experiments have shown that, in these circumstances, many studies may be necessary before replication occurs.

III. Genes Influencing Atopy

A number of genes have now been identified which influence atopy. These may be divided into genes which predispose in general to atopy, and those which influence the particular allergens to which atopic individuals react. Genes predisposing to generalized atopy have been identified on chromosome 11 and chromosome 5, by a combination of genetic linkage and candidate gene approaches.

A. Generalized Atopy

Chromosome 11q12-13

The first suggested linkage of atopy was to the marker d11s97 on chromosome 11q13 [34,35]. Following enormous controversy [36], which was the result of unrealistic expectations about detecting linkage to a complex trait with limited sample sizes, this linkage has been replicated several times [37,38] (Marsh DG, personal communication). The linkage was confounded by the high prevalence of atopy, and because the linkage was seen predominately in maternal meioses [37,39]. In the largest study described, linkage was exclusively maternal [39]. The reasons for the maternal linkage are not known, and it is not clear that this maternal phenomenon corresponds to the phenotypic maternal inheritance of atopy which has been previously noted.

Recognition of the maternal linkage allowed better localization of the atopy locus, known as *APY1*, to within a 7-centiMorgan one-lod unit support interval [40,41]. This interval was centromeric to and excluded the original d11s97 marker to which linkage was first observed. A lymphocyte surface marker, *CD20*, was noted to be within the interval. *CD20* shows sequence homology to the beta chain of the high-affinity receptor for IgE (*FcεRIβ*), and has been localized close to that gene on mouse chromosome 19 [42]. The human *FcεRIβ* was subsequently found to be on chromosome 11q13, in close genetic linkage to atopy [40]. Two coding polymorphisms have now been identified within the gene, *FcεRIβ Leu 181*, and *FcεRIβ Leu181/Leu183* [43]. These both show strong associations with atopy, when inherited maternally. The population prevalence of *FcεRIβ Leu181/Leu183* is about 4% [44], and *FcεRIβ Leu181* has been reported in 15% of asthmatics [43].

These results with *FcεRIβ* variants have not been replicated outside of the Oxford group, and a reliable assay system for the variants has not yet been established. *FcεRIβ Leu181* does not show functional differences from the wild-type receptor (Kinet JP, personal communication). A third homologous gene, *Htm4*, is in close proximity to *FcεRIβ* and *CD20* [45], so that it is not clear how many members of the gene family are present. As it stands, it is therefore not yet established if *APY1* is *FcεRIβ*, or if it is some other gene in linkage disequilibrium with the *FcεRIβ* variants. Nevertheless, it remains most likely that *FcεRIβ* is indeed *APY1*.

FcεRIβ Leu 181 and *FcεRIβ Leu181/Leu183* cannot explain all the chromosome 11 effect. *FcεRIβ* is a large gene with 7 exons and a 3-kb untranslated region, which together span 11 kb. The upstream and downstream controlling elements have not yet been identified. We propose to find the sequences that vary between atopic and nonatopic individuals by linkage disequilibrium mapping, and we have now begun to identify further polymorphisms in and around *FcεRIβ*. The definition of a disease-associated haplotype will be an important step in finding the DNA variants that influence atopy from this locus.

Chromosome 5

Linkage of the total serum IgE to markers near the cytokine cluster on chromosome 5q31-33 has been demonstrated by Marsh et al. [46]. Marsh and his colleagues studied Amish pedigrees, selected to contain members with positive skin-prick tests. Linkage to this locus, *APY2*, was strongest, however, in families with the lowest serum IgE and absent skin-test responses. The result was replicated by Myers et al. [47] in Dutch asthmatic families. Linkage has not been found in other studies of extended families (Rich S, personal communication). My group has tested 1500 individuals from 300 nuclear families, and find no evidence for linkage either by sib-pair or by lod-score methods. However, in order to test the claim that linkage is seen predominantly with the low-IgE phenotype, we have used class D regressive models to account for the specific IgE response. The residual IgE shows strong evidence of linkage to a microsatellite repeat found in IL-4, but not to the other polymorphic markers studied by Marsh or Myers and their colleagues (Dizier et al., in preparation).

The region contains a number of cytokines, the most important of which, from the point of view of atopy, are *IL-4, IL-13,* the p40 subunit of *IL-12,* and *IL-5.* Other cytokines include *IL-9* and granulocyte-colony stimulating factor (*G-CSF*). A substantial amount of work is now required to establish which of these various candidates accounts for the linkage.

B. Specific Atopy

Atopic individuals differ in the particular allergens to which they react. This difference is of clinical significance, as asthma and bronchial hyperresponsiveness are associated with allergy to house dust mites (HDM) but not grass pollens [10,11]. It is therefore of interest to examine whether particular genes influence the IgE response to specific allergens. In addition, study of these genes may give an insight into the inheritance of normal variation within the immune system, and the functional consequences of such variation.

There are two classes of genes which are likely candidates for constraining specific IgE reactions. These are the genes encoding the human leukocyte antigen (HLA) proteins, and the genes for the T-cell receptor (TCR). These molecules are central to the handling and recognition of foreign antigen.

Inhaled allergen sources such as HDM are complex mixtures of many proteins. A number of "major allergens," to which IgE responses are consistently found in most individuals, have been identified from each allergen source. It is likely that genetic associations will be better detected with reactions to purified major allergens, rather than with complex allergen sources. Major allergens include *Der p* I (25.4 kDa) and *Der p* II (14.1 kDa) from the house dust mite *Dermatophagoides pteronyssinus, Alt a* I (28 kDa) from the mold *Alternaria alternata, Can f* I (25 kDa) from the dog *Canis familiaris, Fel d* I (18 kDa) from the cat *Felis domesticus,* and *Phl p* V (30 kDa) from Timothy grass, *Phleum pratense.*

C. HLA

The human major histocompatibility complex (MHC) includes genes that code for HLA class II molecules (HLA-DR, DQ and DP), which are involved in the recognition and presentation of exogenous peptides.

An HLA influence on the IgE response was first noted by Levine et al. [48]. This locus may be known as *ASE1* (antigen-specific E 1). Levine found an association between HLA class I haplotypes and IgE responses to antigen E derived from ragweed allergen (*Ambrosia artemisifolia*). This association has been subsequently found to be due to restriction of the response to a particular component of ragweed antigen (*Amb a* V) by HLA-DR2 [49]. To date the association of *Amb a* V (molecular weight 5000) and HLA-DR2 is the only HLA association to have been consistently confirmed [48–50]. Other suggested associations are of the rye grass antigens *Lol p* I, *Lol p* II, and *Lol p* III with HLA-DR3 (in the same 53 allergic subjects) [51,52], American feverfew (*Parthenium hysterophorus*) and HLA-DR3 in 22 subjects from the Indian subcontinent [53], the IgE response to *Bet v* I, the major allergen of birch pollen, and HLA-DR3 in 37 European subjects [54], and an HLA-DR5 association with another ragweed antigen, *Amb a* VI, in 38 subjects [55].

Other authors have reported negative associations with particular allergens. These include HLA-DR4 and IgE responses to mountain cedar pollen (37 subjects) [56] and HLA-DR4 and melittin (from bee venom) (22 subjects) [57]. Nonresponsiveness to Japanese cedar pollen may be associated with HLA-DQw8 [59].

There is to date no confirmation of many of these results, and the number of subjects has generally not approached that required to establish an unequivocal HLA association. In addition, there has not been recognition of the problems of reactivity to multiple allergens: Significant relationships between HLA-DR alleles and five antigens (*Amb a* V, *Lol p* I *Lol p* II, *Lol p* III, and *Amb a* 6) have been claimed from the same pool of approximately 200 subjects [49,51,52,55].

In order to test more definitively if HLA class II gene products have a general influence on the ability to react to common allergens, we have genotyped for HLA-DR and HLA-DP in a large sample of atopic subjects from the British population [59]. The subjects were tested for IgE responses to the most common British major allergens.

Four hundred and thirty-one subjects from 83 families were genotyped at the HLA-DR and HLA-DP loci and serotyped for IgE responses to six major allergens from common aero-allergen sources. Three hundred subjects were used as controls. The subjects and the controls have come from the same relatively homogeneous population. In the United Kingdom and Europe, allergens other than *Bet v* I and those tested for in our study are uncommon causes of sensitization and IgE-mediated allergy.

The results showed only weak associations between HLA-DR allele frequencies and IgE responses to common allergens. A possible excess of HLA-DR1 was found in subjects who were responsive to *Fel d* I compared to those who were not [odds ratio (OR) = 2, *p* = 0.002], and a possible excess of HLA-DR4 was found in subjects responsive to *Alt a* I (OR = 1.9, *p* = 0.006). Increased sharing of HLA-DR/DP haplotypes was seen in sibling pairs responding to both allergens. *Der p* I, *Der p* II, *Phl p* V, and *Can f* I were not associated with any definite excess of HLA-DR alleles. No significant correlations were seen with HLA-DP genotype and reactivity to any of the allergens.

Of the possible associations, that of *Alt a* I with HLA-DR4 and of *Fel d* I with HLA-DR1 were supported by a finding of excess sharing of a HLA haplotype in affected sibling pairs. Regression analysis shows the apparent association of *Phl p* V with HLA-DR4 is due to the presence of many individuals who have reacted with an IgE response both to *Alt a* I and *Phl p* V. The association of HLA-DR1 and *Fel d* I is the strongest statistically, and is significant even taking the multiple comparisons into account.

The study was the first to investigate HLA-DP alleles and reactivity to common allergens. As no definite correlation was found between any antigen response and HLA-DP genotypes with substantial numbers of subjects, HLA-DP genes are unlikely to have a major role in restricting IgE responses to these allergens.

The results suggest that HLA-DR alleles do modify the ability to mount an IgE response to particular antigens. However, the odds ratio for the association of *Alt a* I with HLA-DR4 was only 1.9, and that of *Fel d* I with HLA-DR1 was 2.0. Thus class II HLA restriction seems insufficient to account for individual differences in reactivity to common allergens. It is therefore likely that environmental factors or other loci such as T-cell-receptor genes may also determine an individual's susceptibility to specific allergens.

D. The T-Cell Receptor

The T-cell receptor (TCR) is usually made up of α and β chains, although 5% of receptors consist of γ and δ chains. The β-chain locus is on chromosome 7, and the α-chain locus is on chromosome 14. The δ-chain genes are found within the α-chain locus.

An enormous potential for TCR variety follows from the presence of many variable (V) and junctional (J) segments within the TCR loci. However, the usage of the TCR Vα and Vβ segments by lymphocytes is not random, and may be under genetic control [60–63].

In order to examine if the TCR genes influence susceptibility to particular allergens, we have therefore tested for genetic linkage between IgE responses and microsatellites from the TCR-α/δ and TCR-β regions [64]. Two independent sets of families, one British and one Australian, were investigated. Because the mode of inheritance was unknown, and because of interactions from the environment and other loci, affected sibling-pair methods were used to test for linkage.

No linkage of IgE serotypes to TCR-β was detected, but significant linkage of IgE responses to the house dust mite allergens *Der p* I and *Der p* II, the cat allergen *Fel d* I, and the total serum IgE to TCR-α was seen in both family groups. The results show that a locus in the TCR α/δ region, which may be called *ASE2*, is modulating IgE responses. The close correlation between total and specific IgE makes it difficult to determine if the locus controls specific IgE reactions to particular allergens or confers generalized IgE responsiveness. Nevertheless, linkage was strongest with highly purified allergens, suggesting that the locus primarily influences specific responses. The pattern of allele sharing seen with some serotypes suggests a recessive genetic effect, making it possible that this linkage corresponds to the recessive atopy locus implied by previous segregation analyses [32,65].

Replication of positive results of linkage in a second set of subjects is important in interpreting this study. Differences between the populations for the serotypes showing TCR-α allele sharing may be due to different allergen exposures, as grass pollen responses were much more common in Australian subjects. In addition, British subjects were recruited through clinics, whereas Australian subjects were not selected by symptoms.

No strong association was seen between particular IgE responses and specific TCR-α microsatellite alleles, implying that the microsatellite is not in immediate proximity to the IgE-modulating elements. The degree of linkage disequilibrium across the TCR-α/δ locus seems low [66], and the microsatellite has only been localized within a 900-kb yeast artificial chromosome [67]. The observed linkage may therefore be with any elements of TCR-α or TCR-δ, or with other genes in the locality.

Several Vα genes have been recognized to be polymorphic, [68], and limitation of the response to an allergen may correspond to these polymorphisms. Particular TCR-Vα usage may induce IL-4 dominant (Th2) helper T cells, which enhance IgE production [69]. A reported nonrandom usage of Vα13 usage in *Lol p* I specific T-cell clones supports independently the possibility of Vα genes controlling IgE responses [70].

The TCR-δ locus is also a candidate for *ASE2*. The function of TCR-γ/δ cells is not known, but their location on mucosal surfaces, where allergens initiate IgE responses, could suggest a role in IgE regulation [71].

This study has therefore identified a further genetic locus affecting atopy. The genetic restriction of specific IgE responses may be of clinical significance, and may be of general interest in understanding the control of humoral immunity. Further localization of *ASE2* requires the identification of TCR α/δ elements showing allelic associations with specific IgE responses. Studies are also needed to investigate the interactions between *ASE2* and the HLA class II genes (*ASE1*).

E. A Genome Screen for Atopy and Asthma

The four loci described above do not account for all atopy. Segregation analysis is unable to predict with any accuracy the number and nature of genes contributing to atopy and asthma. In order to discover if atopy is a genuine polygenic disorder, my group has carried out a complete genome screen in 80 nuclear families, with 260 markers spaced at approximately 10% recombination. Using sib-pair analysis we have discovered three probable new linkages and several possible linkages. Before releasing these localizations, we are now attempting to confirm each linkage in 300 further asthmatic families. We intend to complete a screen in a final total of 250 families, in three groups ascertained for atopy, asthma, and eczema, respectively.

Large-scale genome scans are currently to be carried out in the United States and Canada, in addition to Oxford. It is likely that extensive cooperation among all groups will be necessary for mapping and identification of the many loci causing atopy.

References

1. Strachan DP, et al. A national survey of asthma prevalence, severity, and treatment in Great Britain. Arch Dis Childhood 1994; 70:174–178.
2. Cline MG, Burrows BB. Distribution of allergy in a population sample residing in Tuscon, Arizona. Thorax 1989; 44:425–432.
3. Holford-Strevens V, et al. Serum total immunoglobulin E levels in Canadian adults. J Allergy Clin Immunol 1984; 73:516–522.
4. Peat JK, Britton WJ, Salome CM, Woolcock AJ. Bronchial hyperresponsiveness in two populations of australian school children III. Effect of exposure to environmental allergens. Clin Allergy 1987; 17:271–281.
5. Ogilvie BM, Jones VE. Protective immunity in helminth diseases. Proc R Soc Med 1969; 62:298.
6. Capron M, Capron A. Immunoglobulin E and effector cells in schistosomiasis. Science 1994; 264:1876–1877.
7. Cookson WOCM. Atopy: a complex genetic disease. Ann Med 1994; 26:351–353.
8. Moffatt MF, Sharp PA, Faux JA, Young RP, Cookson WOCM, Hopkin JM. Factors confounding genetic linkage between atopy and chromosome 11q. Clin Exp Allergy 1992; 22:1046–1051.
9. Coleman R, Trembah RC, Harper JI. Chromosome 11q13 and atopy underlying atopic eczema. Lancet 1993; 341:1121–1122.
10. Cookson WOCM, et al. Relative risks of bronchial hyperresponsiveness associated

with skin-prick test responses to common antigens in young adults. Clin Exp Allergy 1991; 21:473.

11. Sears MR, et al. The relative risks of sensitivity to grass pollen, house dust mite and cat dander in the development of childhood asthma. Clin Allergy 1989; 18:419.

12. Cooke RA, van der Veer A. Human sensitisation. J Immunol 1916; 1:201.

13. Schwartz M. Heredity in bronchial asthma. Acta Allergol 1952; 5(suppl 2).

14. Weiner A, Zieve I, Fries J. The inheritance of allergic diseases. Ann Eugen 1936; 7:141.

15. Sibbald B, Turner-Warwick M. Factors influencing the prevalence of asthma in first degree relatives of extrinsic and intrinsic asthmatics. Thorax 1979; 34:332.

16. Edfors-Lubs ML. Allergy in 7000 twin pairs. Acta Allergol 1971; 26:249.

17. Bazaral M, Orgel HA, Hamburger RN. IgE levels in normal infants and mothers and an inheritance hypothesis. J Immunol 1971; 107:794.

18. Bazaral M, Orgel HA, Hamburger RN. Genetics of IgE and allergy: serum IgE levels in twins. J Allergy Clin Immunol 1974; 54:288.

19. Hanson B, et al. Pulmonary function, serum IgE levels and specific IgE responses in monozygotic twins reared apart. J Allergy Clin Immunol 1985; 75:155.

20. Marsh DG, Meyers DA, Bias WB. The epidemiology and genetics of atopic allergy. N Engl J Med 1981; 305:1551–1559.

21. Gerrard JW, Horne S, Vickers P, et al. Serum IgE levels in parents and children. J Pediatr 1974; 85:660.

22. Blumenthal •, et al. Genetic transmission of serum IgE levels. Am J Med Genet 1981; 10:219.

23. Boreki I, et al. Demonstration of a common major gene with pleiotrophic effects on immunoglobulin E and allergy. Genet Epidemiol 1985; 2:327–328.

24. Cookson WOCM, Hopkin JM. Dominant inheritance of atopic immunoglobulin-E responsiveness. Lancet 1988; i:86–88.

25. Bray GW. The hereditary factor in hypersensitiveness anaphlaxis and allergy. J Allergy 1931; II:205–224.

26. Magnusson CG. Cord serum IgE in relation to family history and as predictor of atopic disease in early infancy. Allergy 1988; 43:241–251.

27. Halonen M, Stern D, Taussig LM, Wright A, Ray CG, Martinez FD. The predictive relationship between serum IgE levels at birth and subsequent incidences of lower respiratory illnesses and eczema in infants. Am Rev Respir Dis 1992; 146:866–870.

28. Arshad SH, Matthews S, Grant C, Hide DW. Effect of allergen avoidance on development of allergic disorders in infancy. Lancet 1992; 339:1493–1497.

29. Åberg N. Familial occurrence of atopic disease: genetic versus environmental factors. Clin Exp Allergy 1994; 23:829–834.

30. Kuehr J, Karmaus W, Forster J, et al. Sensitisation to four common inhalant allergens within 302 nuclear families. Clin Exp Allergy 1993; 23:600–605.

31. Hall JG. Genomic imprinting. Arch Dis Childhood 1990; 65:1013–1016.

32. Dizier MH, Hill M, James A, et al. Genetic control of IgE level after accounting for specific atopy. Genet Epidemiol 1993; 10:333–334.

33. Suarez BK, Hampe CL, Van Eerdewegh P. Problems of replicating linkage claims in psychiatry. In: Gershon ES, Cloninger CR, eds. Genetic Approaches to Mental Disorders. Washington, DC: American Psychiatric Press, 1994:23–46.

34. Cookson WOCM, Sharp PA, Faux JA, Hopkin JM. Linkage between immunoglobulin E responses underlying asthma and rhinitis and chromosome 11q. Lancet 1989; i: 1292–1295.

35. Young RP, Lynch J, Sharp PA, Faux JA, Cookson WOCM, Hopkin JM. Confirmation of genetic linkage between atopic IgE responses and chromosome 11q13. J Med Genet 1992; 29:236–238.

36. Marsh DG, Myers DA. A major gene for allergy—fact or fancy? Nature Genetics 1992; 2:252–254.

37. Shirakawa T, Morimoto K, Hashimoto T, Furuyama J, Yamamoto M, Takai S. Linkage between severe atopy and chromosome 11q in Japanese families. Clin Genet 1994; in press.

38. Collée JM, ten Kate LP, de Vries HG, et al. Allele sharing on chromosome 11q13 in sibs with asthma and atopy. Lancet 1993; 342:936.

39. Cookson WOCM, Young RP, Sanford AJ, et al. Maternal inheritance of atopic IgE responsiveness on chromosome 11q. Lancet 1992; 340:381–384.

40. Sanford AJ, Shirakawa T, Moffatt MF, et al. Localisation of atopy and the β subunit of the high affinity IgE receptor (FcεRI) on chromosome 11q. Lancet 1993; 341:332–334.

41. Sandford AJ, Moffatt MF, Daniels SE, et al. A genetic map of chromosome 11q, including the atopy locus. Eur J Hum Genet 1995; in press.

42. Hupp K, Siwarski D, Mock BA, Kinet JP. Gene mapping of the three subunits of the high affinity FcR for IgE to mouse chromosomes 1 and 19. J Immunol 1989; 143: 3787–3791.

43. Shirakawa TS, Li A, Dubowitz M, et al. Association between atopy and variants of the β subunit of the high-affinity immunoglobulin E receptor. Nature Genet 1994; in press.

44. Hill MR, Daniels SE, James AL, et al. A coding polymorphism for FcεRIβ in a random population sample: associations with atopy. Genet Epidemiol 1994; 11:297.

45. Adra CN, Lelias J-M, Kobayashi H, et al. Cloning of the cDNA for a haemopoietic cell-specific protein related to CD20 and the beta subunit of the high-affinity IgE receptor: evidence for a family of proteins with four membrane spanning regions. Proc Natl Acad Sci USA 1994; 91:10178–10182.

46. Marsh DG, Neely JD, Breazeale DR, et al. Linkage analysis of IL4 and other chromosome 5q31.1 markers and total serum IgE concentrations. Science 1994; 264: 1152–1155.

47. Myers DA, Postma DS, Panhuysen CIM, et al. Evidence for a locus regulating total serum IgE levels mapping to chromosome 5. Genomics 1994; 23:464–470.

48. Levine BB, Stember RH, Fontino M. Ragweed hayfever: genetic control and linkage to HLA haplotypes. Science 1972; 178:1201–1203.

49. Marsh DG, Meyers DA, Bias WB. The epidemiology and genetics of atopic allergy. N Engl J Med 1981; 305:1551–1559.

50. Blumenthal MN, et al. Immune response genes of ragweed sensitive individuals. J Allergy Clin Immunol 1988; 81:307.

51. Freidhoff LR, Ehrlich-Kautzky E, Meyers DA, Ansari AA, Bias WB, Marsh DG. Association of HLA-DR3 with human immune response to Lol p I and Lol p II allergens in allergic subjects. Tissue Antigens 1988; 31:211–219.

52. Ansari AA, Freidhoff LR, Meyers DA, Bias WB, Marsh DG. Human immune responsiveness to Lolium perenne pollen allergen Lol p III (rye III) is associated with HLA-DR3 and DR5 [published erratum appears in Hum Immunol 1989; 26:149]. Hum Immunol 1989; 25:59–71.

53. Sriramarao P, Selvakumar B, Damodaran C, Rao BS, Prakash O, Rao PV. Immediate hypersensitivity to *Parthenium hysterophorus*. I. Association of HLA antigens and *Parthenium rhinitis*. Clin Exp Allergy 1990; 20:555–560.

54. Fischer GF, Pickl WF, Fae I, et al. Association between IgE response against Bet v I, the major allergen of birch pollen, and HLA-DRB alleles. Hum Immunol 1992; 33: 259–265.

55. Marsh DG, Freidhoff LR, Ehrlich-Kautzky E, Bias WB, Roebber M. Immune responsiveness to *Ambrosia artemisiifolia* (short ragweed) pollen allergen Amb a VI (Ra6) is associated with HLA-DR5 in allergic humans. Immunogenetics 1987; 26(4–5): 230–236.

56. Reid MJ, Nish WA, Whisman BA, et al. HLA-DR4-associated nonresponsiveness to mountain cedar allergen. J Allergy Clin Immunol 1992; 89:593–598.

57. Lympany P, Kemeny DM, Welsh KI, Lee TH. An HLA-associated nonresponsiveness to mellitin: a component of bee venom. J Allergy Clin Immunol 1990; 86:160–170.

58. Sasazuki T, Nishimura Y, Muto M, Ohta N. HLA-linked genes controlling immune response and disease susceptibility. Immunol Rev 1983; 70:51–75.

59. Young RP, Dekker JW, Wordsworth BP, et al. HLA-DR and HLA-DP genotypes and immunoglobulin E responses to common major allergens. Clin Exp Allergy 1994; 24: 431–439.

60. Loveridge JA, Rosenberg WMC, Kirkwood TBL, Bell JI. The genetic contribution to human T-cell receptor repertoire. Immunology 1991; 74:246–250.

61. Moss PAH, Rosenberg WMC, Zintzaras E, Bell JI. Characterization of the human T cell receptor α-chain repertoire and demonstration of a genetic influence on Vα usage. Eur J Immunol 1993; 23:1153–1159.

62. Gulwani-Akolar B, Posnett DN, Janson CH, et al. T cell receptor V-segment frequencies in peripheral blood T cells correlate with human leukocyte antigen type. J Exp Med 1991; 174:1139–1146.

63. Robinson MA. Usage of human T-cell receptor V beta, J beta C beta and V alpha gene segments is not proportional to gene number. Hum Immunol 1992; 35:60–67.

64. Moffatt MF, Hill MR, Cornélis F, et al. Genetic linkage of the TCR-α/δ region to specific immunoglobulin E responses. Lancet 1994.

65. Gerrard JW, Rao DC, Morton NE. A genetic study of Immunoglobulin E. Am J Hum Genet 1978; 30:46–58.

66. Robinson MA, Kindt TJ. Genetic recombination within the human T-cell receptor alpha-chain complex. Proc Natl Acad Sci USA 1987; 84:9089–9093.

67. Cornélis F, Hashimoto L, Loveridge J, et al. Identification of a CA repeat at the TCRA locus using yeast artificial chromosomes: a general method for generating highly polymorphic markers at chosen loci. Genomics 1992; 13:820–825.

68. Cornélis F, Pile K, Loveridge J, Moss P, Harding C, Julier C, Bell JI. Systematic study of human αβ T-cell receptor V segments shows allelic variations resulting in a large number of distinct TCR haplotypes. Eur J Immunol 1993; 23:1277–1283.

69. Heinzel FP, Sadick MD, Mutha SS, Locksley RM. Production of interferon gamma, interleukin 2, interleukin 4, and interleukin 10 by CD4+ lymphocytes in vivo during healing and progressive murine leishmaniasis. Proc Natl Acad Sci USA 1991; 88: 7011–7015.

70. Mohapatra SS, Mohapatra S, Yang M, et al. Molecular basis of cross-reactivity among allergen-specific human T Cells. T-cell receptor Vα gene usage and epitope structure. Immunology 1994; 81:15–20.

71. Holt PG, McMenamin C. IgE and mucosal immunity: studies on the role of intra-epithelial Ia+ dendritic cells and δ/γ T-lymphocytes in regulation of T-cell activation in the lung. Clin Exp Allergy 1991; 21(suppl):148–152.

72. Charpin D, Birnbaum J, Haddi E, et al. Altitude and allergy to house dust mites. A paradigm of the influence of environmental exposure on allergic sensitisation. Am Rev Respir Dis 1991; 143:983–986.

73. Holt PG, McMenamin C, Nelson D. Primary sensitisation to inhalant allergens during infancy. Pediatr Allergy Immunol 1990; 1:3–15.

74. Sporik R, Holgate S, Platts-Mills TAE, Cogswells JJ. Exposure to house dust mite allergen der P1 and the development of asthma is children. N Engl J Med 1990; 323:502–507.

75. von Mutius E, Fritzsch C, Weiland SK, Roell G, Magnussen H. Prevalence of asthma and allergic disorders among children in united Germany: a descriptive comparison. Br Med J 1992; 305:1395–1399.

76. von Mutius E, Martinez FD, Fritzsch C, Nicolai T, Roell G, Thiemann HH. Prevalence of asthma and atopy in two areas of west and East Germany. Am J Respir Crit Care Med 1994; 149:358–364.

77. Bråzbäck L, Breborowicz A, Dreborg S, Knutsson A, Pieklik H, Björkstén B. Atopic sensitization and respiratory symptoms among Polish and Swedish school children. Clin Exp Allergy 1994; 24:826–835.

78. von Mutius E, Martinez FD, Fritzsch C, Nicolai T, Reitmer P, Thiemann HH. Skin test reactivity and number of siblings. Br Med J 1994; 308:692–695.

79. Lynch NR, Hagel I, Perez M, Di Prisco MC, Lopez R, Alvarez N. Effect of antihelmintic treatment on the allergic reactivity of children in a tropical slum. J Allergy Clin Immunol 1993; 92:404–411.

24

Genetic Regulation of Total Serum IgE Levels

CAROLIEN I. M. PANHUYSEN

University of Maryland School of Medicine
Baltimore, Maryland

DEBORAH A. MEYERS

Johns Hopkins University School of
Medicine
Baltimore, Maryland

I. Introduction

As described in other chapters, family studies on asthma may be complicated by problems in defining the "affected" phenotype. However, compared to many other disorders (such as mental illness), there are quantitative measures that reflect the clinical expression. For example high total serum IgE levels correlate with the clinical expression of both allergy and asthma [1–4], and epidemiological studies have shown a relationship between IgE levels and BHR, a major component of the asthma phenotype [3,5,6]. Approximately 30% of the variance in bronchial responsiveness is explained by an individual's total serum IgE levels [2,3]. Therefore, the results from segregation and linkage studies on total serum IgE levels will be important for mapping genes for the allergic and asthmatic phenotypes.

A. Genetic Epidemiology

Total serum IgE levels are known to change with age. After a rapid increase in infancy, there is a gradual increase until puberty, when total serum IgE levels tend slowly to decrease [7–11]. IgE levels are also affected by other factors, including

gender, ethnicity, environmental factors such as parasitic infections, recent allergen exposure, and smoking [12–16]. Magnussen [17] reported that cord-blood
IgE concentrations were elevated in smoking mothers, and that maternal smoking
after birth is associated with an increased risk of allergy in infants, although
different studies could not confirm this finding [9,18]. Other studies reported an
influence of the month of birth on the infant's risk of atopy and high serum IgE
levels [19–21].

B. Genetic Component

Significant familial aggregation of the phenotypes associated with asthma and
allergy has been described in numerous studies, but this does not always imply a
genetic basis. Familial aggregation can be caused by common environmental
factors or by an interaction of environmental and genetic factors that can influence
the perceived pattern of inheritance. The presence of familial aggregation for high
serum IgE levels, after adjusting for all known environmental factors, provides
evidence for a genetic component. Meyers et al. [22] investigated the association
of total serum IgE levels in 278 individuals of 42 random families, and showed a
significant correlation between parents and offspring ($p < 0.05$), and an even
stronger correlation among siblings ($p < 0.001$).

The excess risk for relatives can also be expressed as the risk ratio (lambda),
which is the relative's risk compared to the prevalence within the population.
These risk ratios can be used to postulate the number of loci involved in the
disorder [23,24]. However, they are very sensitive to accurate estimates of the
population prevalence, which often differ significantly between studies and populations. In addition, they are usually used for qualitative measures (presence or
absence of disease) and not for quantitative measures such as total serum IgE
levels. Although it may be possible to define "high" levels as a phenotype, it is
probably better to utilize heritability estimates instead.

C. Twin Studies

Twin studies showed that total serum IgE levels are under strong genetic control.
Heritability, the ratio of genetic variance to the total variance, is often used to
express how much of the familial aggregation is due to a genetic component. In
twin studies with monozygotic (MZ) and dizygotic (DZ) twin pairs, the difference
between the disease frequency in MZ and DZ twins provides an indication for
heritability, while the difference within MZ twins is an indication of environmental influence. In a twin study by Hopp et al., the intrapair correlation coefficient
for IgE levels was 82% in the 61 MZ twins and 52% in the 46 DZ twins, showing
an overall heritability of 61% [25].

II. Segregation Analyses

Segregation analysis is used to determine whether there is evidence for at least one major gene regulating the trait of interest. Data on the segregation pattern of the trait, here total serum IgE levels, from parents to children is tested for the fit of several genetic models and nongenetic models. The method of ascertainment of families is very important in segregation analysis. For example, the selection of families with an affected child and parent could bias the results of the analysis in favor of a dominant model of inheritance. Thus, one needs to correct for ascertainment bias in this analytical method.

Segregation analysis on total serum IgE levels is usually performed to test whether the segregation of IgE levels is consistent with a major gene model with two alleles, "*L*" for "low" levels (gene frequency $= q_L$) and "*H*" for "high" levels. For each model, the means (μ_{LL}, μ_{LH}, μ_{HH}) and variances for the three distributions representing the three types of individuals (LL, LH, HH) are estimated. Individuals of type LL, LH, HH transmit the L allele with probability τ_{LL}, τ_{LH}, τ_{HH} respectively. Under a Mendelian model, these parameters are restricted to $\tau_{LL} = 1.0$, $\tau_{LH} = 0.5$, $\tau_{HH} = 0.0$. The parent–offspring (ρ_{po}) and sib–sib (ρ_{ss}) correlations may be constrained to be equal, since this represents the conventional "mixed model" [26]. The likelihood ratio test is used to compare hierarchical models and approximates a χ^2 distribution. To compare nonhierarchical models, Akaike's information criterion (AIC) [27] is used ($-2 \ln L + 2k$, where k is the number of parameters estimated in the model).

Several models should be tested. The first is a general model—a model without restrictions for any of the previously mentioned parameters. Because all parameters are estimated without restrictions, this model, per definition, gives the best fit to the data, and the best likelihood. There are three Mendelian models, a recessive, a dominant, and a codominant model, testing for a single locus model. In a dominant and recessive model the μ_{LH} is fixed to be the same as μ_{LL} or μ_{HH}, respectively; in the codominant model, however, the three means are estimated. In a polygenic model, we hypothesize that there are many genes involved, which makes it impossible to estimate the separate distributions. In the environmental, or sporadic model, the transmission probability (τ) is the same as the gene frequency, while the means (μ) are not restricted.

The best-fitting model can be determined by comparing the likelihoods from the several models tested with the likelihood of the general model. Models that significantly differ from this general model can be rejected. Estimates of gene frequency, and mean values for "high" and "low" IgE phenotypes are obtained. The best-fitting model and its estimates can be used in subsequent linkage analysis.

Our analyses on data from 92 Dutch families will be described as an example of this type of analysis. We tested 92 families ascertained through a parent, the proband, with asthma diagnosed approximately 25 years ago in Holland [28]. During the last three years, the probands and their families have been reevaluated. Total serum IgE (IU) was measured by solid-phase immunoassay (Pharmacia IgE EIA, Pharmacia Diagnostics AB, Sweden). The mean of duplicate tests was used for the IgE level. The test was repeated if the difference between duplicates was > 5%.

The log[IgE} data were analyzed by fitting the class D regressive models of Bonney [29] as implemented in SAGE [30]. Age was included as a covariate, since there was a significant correlation between age and total serum IgE levels in the overall sample. There was no significant correlation between gender and log[IgE] levels in this sample, and similar results were obtained when the segregation analysis was repeated including gender as a covariate. An ascertainment correction was not used because the families were ascertained through one parent with asthma, and not through affected offspring. Since individuals with asthma may have an increased IgE level, this may bias the estimate of the gene frequency but should not affect the segregation pattern observed in the offspring. The results of the segregation analysis are shown in Table 1 [28]. It shows six different genetic models with their estimates for the parameters described in a previous paragraph. It shows clearly that the AIC (a measure of likelihood) for the recessive model is the lowest, marking it as the most parsimonious model for inheritance of serum IgE levels. The estimates of the mean levels for the "low" and "high" phenotypes in this study appear clinically relevant (38 IU and 437 IU, respectively). In this study, only recessive inheritance of "high" levels gave a good fit to the data; the other genetic and nongenetic models could be rejected. The codominant model had a similar likelihood, but since an additional parameter was estimated, similar results to the recessive model were obtained but not significantly better (AIC).

A. Other Segregation Analysis Studies

In several other studies, evidence for recessive inheritance of "high" total serum IgE levels has been found with different estimates for gene frequency and for mean levels in the "low" and "high" phenotypes [31–33]. Blumenthal studied several large pedigrees and reported evidence for genetic heterogeneity in the mode of inheritance [34]. In an inbred Amish population, evidence for codominant inheritance has been reported [35]. In another study on large Mormon families, however, evidence for polygenic inheritance was found [36].

In a recent, large study of 50 Hispanic families, and 241 non-Hispanic white families, Martinez et al. showed significant familial correlation coefficients between mother and offspring, between father and offspring, and between sibs, all p values < 0.0001 [37]. The results of their segregation analyses showed evidence for a codominant mode of inheritance, as shown in Table 2. For their analyses,

Table 1 Results of Segregation Analysis for Serum IgE Levels in 92 Dutch Asthma Families[a,b]

Model	q_L	τ_{LL}	τ_{LH}	τ_{HH}	μ_{LL}	μ_{LH}	μ_{HH}	δ_{sp}	δ_{po}	$-2\ln(L)$	AIC	χ^2	d.f.	p Value
General	0.60	[1.0]	0.30	[0.0]	1.26	1.60	2.65	−0.19	0.07	1040.7	1062.7			
Codominant	0.39	(1.00)	(0.50)	(0.00)	1.66	1.49	2.53	−0.02	0.29	1046.6	1062.6	5.9	4	>0.05
Dominant	0.84	(1.00)	(0.50)	(0.00)	1.62	(2.55)	2.55	−0.07	0.18	1065.7	1079.7	25.0	3	<0.05
Recessive	0.46	(1.00)	(0.50)	(0.00)	1.58	(1.58)	2.64	0.03	0.27	1047.6	1061.6	6.9	3	>0.05
Polygenic	(1)				1.89			−0.01	0.30	1069.2	1079.2	28.5		<0.05
Sporadic	0.31	q_L	q_L	q_L	1.43	1.65	2.11	−0.02	0.36	1061.6	1077.6	20.9	3	<0.05

[a] [ ], Estimate meet boundary; ( ), estimate fixed.
[b] Results from Ref. 28.

Table 2 Results of Segregation Analysis for Serum IgE Levels in 241 Non-Hispanic White Families[a,b]

Model	q_L	τ_{LL}	τ_{LH}	τ_{HH}	μ_{LL}	μ_{LH}	μ_{HH}	δ_{sp}	δ_{po}	$-2\ln(L)$	AIC	χ^2	d.f.	p Value
General	0.27	[1.00]	0.48	[0.00]	1.49	0.46	−0.74	(0.00)	(0.00)	2,426.3	2448.3			
Environment	0.37	q_L	q_L	q_L	0.34	0.53	−0.71	(0.00)	(0.00)	2498.2	2512.2	71.9	2–4	<0.0001
Codominant	0.37	(1.00)	(0.50)	(0.00)	1.19	0.34	−0.76	(0.00)	(0.00)	2428.4	2442.4	2.1	2–4	<0.3
Dominant	0.71	(1.00)	(0.50)	(0.00)	0.62	(−0.60)	−0.60	(0.00)	(0.00)	2449.2	2461.2	20.8	1	<0.0001
Recessive	0.29	(1.00)	(0.50)	(0.00)	0.63	(0.63)	−0.60	(0.00)	(0.00)	2445.7	2457.7	19.4	1	<0.0001
Sporadic	(1)	q_L	q_L	q_L	0.02	0.02	0.02	(0.00)	(0.00)	2500.7	2508.7	74.4	6–7	<0.0001

[a] [ ], Estimate meet boundary; ( ), estimate fixed.
[b] Results from Ref. 37.

they used the logarithm of the total serum IgE levels, corrected for age and gender, by obtaining Z scores, and normalized the distribution using the standardized Box-Cox transformation. Their analyses show the same codominant model in both ethnic groups separately, and when analyzed together. A test for genetic heterogeneity across the ethnic groups was not significant, meaning that there is no evidence for a difference in mode of inheritance between the two groups.

It is important to note that the difference in the best-fitting models of inheritance in the studies mentioned do not necessarily represent conflicting results. Rather, it reflects the inability to distinguish between two or three underlying distributions of the mode of inheritance of total serum IgE levels, which display substantial overlap. In the smaller study of Meyers et al., the recessive model was the best-fitting model although the codominant model was not rejected [28]. However, in the larger study of Martinez et al., they were able to obtain evidence for three distributions fitting a codominant model of inheritance [37]. It is simply a question of whether it is possible to distinguish "gene carriers" from "unaffected" family members.

B. Two-Locus Segregation Analysis

Although evidence for a major gene maybe obtained from segregation evidence, this does not mean that there is necessarily only one locus involved. In the Dutch asthma family data, there was evidence for significant residual variance from the segregation analysis, suggesting an additional genetic influence. Therefore, two-locus segregation and linkage analysis was performed to determine whether a portion of this residual variance was due to a second major locus [38]. The log[IgE] data were analyzed by fitting two-locus models using the computer package PAP [39]. Analysis was performed to determine whether the segregation of IgE levels was consistent with two loci (D1, D2) each with two alleles (A,a and B,b). For each model, the following parameters were estimated: gene frequency for the alleles at each locus (q_A, $q_a = 1 - q_A$; q_B, $q_b = 1 - q_B$), the recombination fraction between the two loci (q), the means (μ's) for the nine possible distributions representing the nine types of individuals (AABB, AABb, AAbb, AaBB, AaBb, Aabb, aaBB, aaBb, aabb) with a common standard deviation (σ), and heritability (h^2), which is a measure of the residual variance. Different two-locus models were tested by constraining various means to be equal. Although multiple tow-locus models including dominant models were tested, the two-locus recessive models with epistasis were the most parsimonious (Table 3). Five different recessive models (II–VI) were tested and had similar AICs (all between 1054.3 and 1056.1). Models IV and V were the most parsimonious. Both of these models and a heterogeneity model (model VI) had relatively high residual variances ($h^2 = 0.40$, 0.42, and 0.46, respectively) compared to models II and III ($h^2 = 0.15$ and 0.13, respectively). These five models were more likely, based on their AICs, than

Table 3 Two-Locus Analysis for log[total serum IgE] Levels[a]

			Mean (μ)						D5S436
Model	q_A	q_B	AABB AABb AAbb	AaBB AaBb Aabb	aaBB aaBb aabb	σ	h^2	$-2\ln L$ (AIC)	LOD (θ)
Two-locus									
I. Codominant	0.54	0.36	1.31	0.45	1.89	0.30	0.09	1031.3	4.86
			1.04	1.39	2.63			(1057.3)	(0.08)
			1.71	2.05	2.82				
Recessive inheritance of "high" levels with epistasis									
II.	0.54	0.36	1.34	0.46	1.97	0.31	0.15	1032.1	4.64
			1.05	1.40	(2.73)			(1056.1)	(0.08)
			1.71	2.05	(2.73)				
III.	0.56	0.31	1.37	0.42	(2.71)	0.32	0.13	1033.6	4.67
			0.96	1.40	(2.71)			(1055.6)	(0.09)
			1.57	2.02	(2.71)				
IV.	0.44	0.72	1.45	1.29	[2.09]	0.36	0.40	1034.3	1.99
			0.56	1.59	(2.68)			(1054.3)	(0.10)
			[2.09]	(2.68)	(2.68)				
V.	0.74	0.43	1.47	0.54	(2.68)	0.37	0.42	1034.4	1.61
			1.27	1.60	(2.68)			(1054.4)	(0.10)
			2.08	(2.68)	(2.68)				
Heterogeneity									
VI.	0.50	0.76	1.48	0.66	(2.52)	0.41	0.46	1037.6	0.41
			1.46	1.60	(2.52)			(1055.6)	(0.04)
			(2.52)	(2.52)	(2.52)				
One-locus									
VII. Recessive	0.41		(1.36)	(1.36)	2.38	0.51	0.49	1046.2	3.00
								(1056.2)	(0.10)

[a] ( ), [ ] represent means that were constrained to be equal under the given model.

the two-locus codominant (general) model. The two-locus model was significantly more likely than the one-locus recessive model, model I versus model VII, ($\chi^2 = 14.9$, d.f. = 7, $p < 0.05$). No evidence for linkage between the two loci was observed for any of the models.

The first locus explains 50.6% of the variance in total IgE levels, and the second locus explains 19% of the variance. Considered jointly, the two loci account for 78.4% of the variance in total serum IgE levels. However, this may represent an overestimate, since the families were ascertained through an asthmatic parent. This study provides evidence that there are at least two loci involved in regulation of total serum IgE levels.

III. Linkage Analyses

The purpose of linkage analysis is to delineate major gene(s) by demonstrating co-segregation of the disease with polymorphic DNA markers. A polymorphic marker is usually not a specific disease-related gene but is a chromosomal marker with multiple alleles that can be characterized in all family members and followed through different generations. For example, one can test the hypothesis that children with high total serum IgE levels inherited the same marker allele from their parent with a high level, and that the unaffected offspring inherited the other allele. The results of linkage analyses are expressed in LOD scores, which are the logarithm of the odds ratio. A LOD score of 3 represents odds of 1000:1 favoring linkage between the marker and the trait. To perform this analysis, it is necessary to have a segregation model for the disease or trait. In the Dutch families, two-point LOD scores were calculated using the best-fitting genetic model from the segregation analysis.

In the Dutch asthma family study, linkage analysis was also performed using the sib-pair method [28,40]. In sib-pair analysis, we test whether two siblings with the same affection status (of similar levels of total serum IgE) inherited the same marker alleles. This method is based on sharing of marker alleles identical by descent from each parent and is not dependent on the genetic model from the segregation analysis. Basically, a regression analysis is performed for the squared difference in log[IgE] levels between sibs and the estimated proportion of marker alleles identical by descent. In the presence of linkage, sibs who are identical by descent for the marker would be expected to have similar IgE levels, and those not sharing marker alleles would be expected to have a bigger difference in their IgE levels.

A. Mapping to Chromosome 5q

There are several genes on chromosome 5q that may be important in the regulation of IgE and the development or progression of inflammation associated with allergy and asthma. They include interleukin-3 (IL-3), IL-4, IL-5, IL-9, IL-13, granulocyte macrophage colony-stimulating factor (GM-CSF), a receptor for macrophage colony-stimulating factor (CSF-1R), and fibroblast growth factor acidic (FGFA) [41]. The genes for the IL-4-related cytokines stimulate B-cell growth and regulate specific immunoglobulin synthesis [42,43].

In the Dutch study, sib-pair analysis showed significant evidence for linkage with the highly polymorphic marker D5S436 and with the flanking loci, D5S393 and CSF-1R [28]. The FGFA polymorphism that was typed was not very informative in these families (both parents were homozygous in approximately one-third of the families), resulting in little evidence for or against linkage (Fig. 1).

The results of the LOD score analyses for IgE show a similar result as the

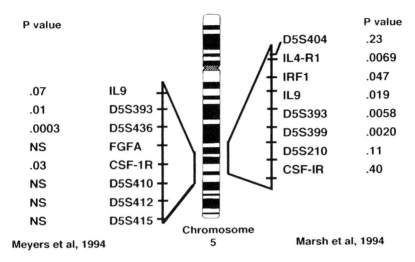

Figure 1   Results of sib-pair analysis on log[total serum IgE levels].

sib-pair results. The highest LOD (3.56) was obtained for D5S436 with 9% recombination. Lower LOD scores were observed for the flanking markers: D5S393 and CSF-1R. The IL-9 polymorphism is very close to the other interleukin gene candidates, and resulted in a LOD of 0.98 (Fig. 2).

Marsh et al. described the results of linkage analysis for a major gene for total serum IgE levels and markers on chromosome 5q in 170 individuals of 11 Amish families [44]. They performed segregation analyses and reported that a Mendelian model fitted the data better than a non-Mendelian model, although there was not significant evidence favoring a single model for the inheritance of total serum IgE levels.

In testing for linkage to 5q, sib-pair analysis was performed and resulted in a p value of 0.002 with D5S399, a marker tightly linked to D5S393, one of the markers typed in the Dutch study (Figure 1). They performed LOD score analysis assuming dominant inheritance of "high" serum IgE levels. For D5S399 a LOD score of 1.3 at 0.0 recombination was obtained. The highest LOD score reported was 1.84 for the marker D5S210 with a recombination fraction of 0.0 (Fig. 2). Five other markers spanning over 20cM also showed 0.0 recombination with total serum IgE levels, probably because of the marked overlap between the distributions of low and high IgE levels in this inbred population. Thus, although both studies reported evidence for linkage to 5q, the results do not appear to specify one gene candidate within this large region containing multiple candidate genes.

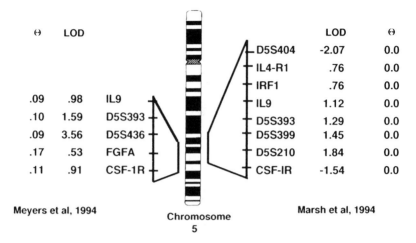

Figure 2   Results of two-point linkage analysis on log[total serum IgE levels].

B.   Two-Locus Linkage Analysis

After performing two-locus segregation analyses on the Dutch asthma families, two-locus linkage analyses was used to test the hypothesis that there are two unlinked loci, only one of which maps to chromosome 5q [38]. Although there was significant evidence favoring two-locus models, it was not possible from the segregation analysis alone to determine the best two-locus model. Therefore, LOD scores were calculated for D5S436 (the marker with the highest LOD from the previous one-locus analysis [28]) for the most likely two-locus models. This procedure is described as the MOD score method, maximizing the LOD score over several genetic models [45]. Except for the general model, where more parameters were estimated, one of all the models had the highest LOD (4.67 at 9% recombination compared to 3.00 at 10% recombination obtained from the one-locus analysis), increasing the evidence for linkage to this region. An increase in the LOD was also observed for D5S393 and FGFA. No positive LODs were obtained when the second locus was tested for linkage to 5q. Therefore, it appears that only the locus accounting for the highest percentage of the variability in the total serum IgE levels maps to this candidate region, and there is at least one additional locus mapping elsewhere in the genome.

IV.   Summary

Since total serum IgE levels are correlated with the clinical expression of allergy, bronchial hyperresponsiveness, and asthma, it represents an important quantitative parameter that can be used to map genes for these complex disorders. From segregation analyses it appears that there are at least two major loci involved in determine an individual's total serum IgE level in addition to environmental factors.

The locus with the strongest influence on total serum IgE levels has been mapped to chromosome 5q, a region with multiple candidate genes. Fine mapping studies are underway; multiple genes on 5q may be involved. In addition, genome searches are being performed to map additional genes. Once these studies are completed, the relationships between these loci and other measures of the asthma phenotype can be investigated. All these studies are important in investigating the complex nature of the genetics of asthma and atopic disease.

Acknowledgment

This work was supported by a grant from the Dutch Asthma Foundation (90.39) and grants from the National Institutes of Health; R01 HL48341 and U01 HL49602.

References

1. Johansson SG, Bennich HH, Berg T. The clinical significance of IgE [review]. Prog Clin Immunol 1972; 1:157–181.
2. Burrows B, Martinez FD, Halonen M, Barbee RA, Cline MG. Association of asthma with serum IgE levels and skin-test reactivity to allergens. N Engl J Med 1989; 320: 271–277.
3. Sears MR, Burrows B, Flannery EM, Herbison GP, Hewitt CJ, Holdaway MD. Relation between airway responsiveness and serum IgE in children with asthma and in apparently normal children. N Engl J Med 1991; 325:1067–1071.
4. Halonen M, Stern D, Taussig LM, Wright A, Ray CG, Martinez FD. The predictive relationship between serum IgE levels at birth and subsequent incidences of lower respiratory illnesses and eczema in infants. Am Rev Respir Dis 1992; 146:866–870.
5. Hopp RJ, Townley RG, Biven RE, Bewtra AK, Nair NM. The presence of airway reactivity before the development of asthma. Am Rev Respir Dis 1990; 141:2–8.
6. Burrows B, Sears MR, Flannery EM, Herbison GP, Holdaway MD. Relationships of bronchial responsiveness assessed by methacholine to serum IgE, lung function, symptoms, and diagnoses in 11-year-old New Zealand children. J Allergy Clin Immunol 1992; 90:376–385.
7. Barbee RA, Lebowitz MD, Thompson HC, Burrows B. Immediate skin-test reactivity in a general population sample [review]. Ann Intern Med 1976; 84:129–133.
8. Gerrard JW, Brook D. Serum IgE levels in forty families studied for two or three years. Ann Allergy 1977; 38:396–399.
9. Halonen M, Stern D, Lyle S, Wright A, Taussig L, Martinez FD. Relationship of total

serum IgE levels in cord and 9-month sera of infants. Clin Exp Allergy 1991; 21: 235–241.

10. Stoy PJ, Roitman-Johnson B, Walsh G, et al. Aging and serum immunoglobulin E levels, immediate skin tests, RAST. J Allergy Clin Immunol 1981; 68:421–426.

11. Kjellman NI. Epidemiology and prevention of allergy. Allergy 1988; 43(suppl)8: 39–40.

12. Halonen M, Barbee RA, Lebowitz MD, Burrows B. An epidemiologic study of interrelationships of total serum immunoglobulin E, allergy skin-test reactivity, and eosinophilia. J Allergy Clin Immunol 1982; 69:221–228.

13. Croner S, Kjellman NI. Predictors of atopic disease: cord blood IgE and month of birth. Allergy 1986; 41:68–70.

14. Freidhoff LR, Meyers DA, Bias WB, Chase GA, Hussain R, Marsh DG. A genetic-epidemiologic study of human immune responsiveness to allergens in an industrial population: I. Epidemiology of reported allergy and skin-test positivity. Am J Med Genet 1981; 9:323–340.

15. Marsh DG, Meyers DA, Bias WB. The epidemiology and genetics of atopic allergy [review]. N Engl J Med 1981; 305:1551–1559.

16. Burrows B, Halonen M, Barbee RA, Lebowitz MD. The relationship of serum immunoglobulin E to cigarette smoking. Am Rev Respir Dis 1981; 124:523–525.

17. Magnusson CG. Maternal smoking influences cord serum IgE and IgD levels and increases the risk for subsequent infant allergy. J Allergy Clin Immunol 1986; 78: 898–904.

18. Bjerke T, Hedegaard M, Henriksen TB, Nielsen BW, Schiotz PO. Several genetic and environmental factors influence cord blood IgE concentration. Pediatr Allergy Immunol 1994; 5:88–94.

19. de Groot H, Stapel SO, Aalberse RC. Statistical analysis of IgE antibodies to the common inhalant allergens in 44,496 sera. Ann Allergy 1990; 65:97–104.

20. Aalberse RC, Nieuwenhuys EJ, Hey M, Stapel SO. "Horoscope effect" not only for seasonal but also for non-seasonal allergens. Clin Exp Allergy 1992; 22:1003–1006.

21. Backer V, Ulrik CS, Hansen KK, Laursen EM, Dirksen A, Bach-Mortensen N. Atopy and bronchial responsiveness in random population sample of 527 children and adolescents. Ann Allergy 1992; 69:116–122.

22. Meyers DA, Beaty TH, Freidhoff LR, Marsh DG. Inheritance of total serum IgE (basal levels) in man. Am J Hum Genet 1987; 41:51–62.

23. Risch N. Linkage strategies for genetically complex traits. III. The effect of marker polymorphism on analysis of affected relative pairs [published erratum appears in Am J Hum Genet 1992; 51(3):673–675]. Am J Hum Genet 1990; 46:242–253.

24. Risch N. Linkage strategies for genetically complex traits. II. The power of affected relative pairs. Am J Hum Genet 1990; 46:229–241.

25. Hopp RJ, Bewtra AK, Watt GD, Nair NM, Townley RG. Genetic analysis of allergic disease in twins. J Allergy Clin Immunol 1984; 73:265–270.

26. Demenais FM, Bonney GE. Equivalence of the mixed and regressive models for genetic analysis. I. Continuous traits [published erratum appears in Genet Epidemiol 1990; 7(1):103]. Genet Epidemiol 1989; 6:597–617.

27. Akaike H. A new look at the statistical model identification. IEEE Trans Automatic Control 1974; 19:716–723.

28. Meyers DA, Postma DS, Panhuysen CI, et al. Evidence for a locus regulating total serum IgE levels mapping to chromosome 5. Genomics 1994; 23:464–470.

29. Bonney GE. Regressive logistic models for familial disease and other binary traits. Biometrics 1986; 42:611–625.

30. SAGE. Statistical Analysis for Genetic Epidemiology. (2.1) Department of Biometry and Genetics, LSU Medical Center, New Orleans, LA: 1992.

31. Marsh DG, Bias WB, Ishizaka K. Genetic control of basal serum immunoglobulin E level and its effect on specific reaginic sensitivity. Proc Natl Acad Sci USA 1974; 71:3588–3592.

32. Gerrard JW, Rao DC, Morton NE. A genetic study of immunoglobulin E. Am J Hum Genet 1978; 30:46–58.

33. Meyers DA, Hasstedt SJ, Marsh DG, et al. The inheritance of immunoglobulin E: genetic linkage analysis. Am J Med Genet 1983; 16:575–581.

34. Blumenthal MN, Namboodiri K, Mendell N, Gleich G, Elston RC, Yunis E. Genetic transmission of serum IgE levels. Am J Med Genet 1981; 10:219–228.

35. Meyers DA, Bias WB, Marsh DG. A genetic study of total IgE levels in the Amish. Hum Hered 1982; 32:15–23.

36. Hasstedt SJ, Meyers DA, Marsh DG. Inheritance of immunoglobulin E: genetic model fitting. Am J Med Genet 1983; 14:61–66.

37. Martinez FD, Holberg CJ, Halonen M, Morgan WJ, Wright AL, Taussig LM. Evidence for Mendelian inheritance of serum IgE levels in Hispanic and non-Hispanic white families. Am J Hum Genet 1994; 55:555–565.

38. Xu J, Levitt RC, Panhuysen CI, et al. Evidence for two unlinked loci regulating total serum IgE levels. Am J Hum Genet 1995; 57:425–430.

39. PAP: Pedigree Analysis Package, Rev. 4, Hasstedt SJ. Department of Human Genetics, University of Utah, Salt Lake City, UT: 1994.

40. Amelung PJ, Panhuysen CI, Postma DS, et al. Atopy and bronchial hyperresponsiveness: exclusion of linkage to markers on chromosomes 11q and 6p. Clin Exp Allergy 1992; 22:1077–1084.

41. Chandrasekharappa SC, Rebelsky MS, Firak TA, Le Beau MM, Westbrook CA. A long-range restriction map of the interleukin-4 and interleukin-5 linkage group on chromosome 5. Genomics 1990; 6:94–99.

42. Kelley J. Cytokines of the lung [see comments] [review]. Am Rev Respir Dis 1990; 141:765–788.

43. Boulay JL, Paul WE. The interleukin-4-related lymphokines and their binding to hematopoietin receptors [review]. J Biol Chem 1992; 267:20525–20528.

44. Marsh DG, Neely JD, Breazeale DR, et al. Linkage analysis of IL4 and other chromosome 5q31.1 markers and total serum immunoglobulin E concentrations. Science 1994; 264:1152–1156.

45. Hodge SE, Elston RC. Lods, wrods, and mods: the interpretation of LOD scores calculated under different models. Genet Epidemiol 1994; 11:329–342.

25

Genetics of Bronchial Hyperresponsiveness

PAMELA J. AMELUNG

University of Maryland School of Medicine
Baltimore, Maryland

EUGENE R. BLEECKER

University of Maryland School of Medicine
Baltimore, Maryland

ALAN F. SCOTT

Johns Hopkins University School of
 Medicine
Baltimore, Maryland

I. Introduction

Asthma is an obstructive pulmonary disease that develops because of both a genetic predisposition as well as exposure to inciting agents such as allergens, respiratory infections, and environmental pollutants. Since there appears to be a worldwide increase in its prevalence and severity [1], the etiology and pathophysiology of asthma is under intensive study. Thus, the investigation of the genetic mechanisms that are responsible for susceptibility to asthma, as well as associated phenotypes such as bronchial hyperresponsiveness, will improve our understanding of the underlying mechanisms responsible for its development. This approach will ultimately lead to improved therapies and new methods for disease identification [2].

Asthma is a complex genetic disorder that is not inherited in a simple Mendelian fashion. More than one gene is thought to interact with environmental or other exposures to produce the clinical manifestation of this disorder. One of the principal obstacles to studying the genetics of asthma is difficulty in the development of accurate and precise methods to diagnose asthma and characterize the features of this disorder. Characterization of phenotype and genetic epidemiology in asthma are the subjects of separate chapters in this book [3,4]. The definition of asthma has changed dramatically throughout the years. Recently, inflammation has become the central feature of most definitions of asthma; however, there is no readily available validated marker for airways inflammation in asthma [5]. Clinical asthma is also a variable disease process that can remit or progress over time. In addition, it may be altered by medications, exposure to environmental stimuli, and viral infections. Furthermore, there is a wide spectrum of specific phenotypic manifestations among individuals with asthma that often makes this disease difficult to differentiate from other obstructive pulmonary diseases [6].

II. Bronchial Hyperresponsiveness and Clinical Asthma

Because of the complexity in defining asthma, investigators have begun to study individual physiologic responses that are closely associated with the development and progression of asthma, such as allergic parameters or bronchial hyperresponsiveness (BHR). These critical components of asthma can be defined more objectively. BHR is the most common physiologic abnormality associated with bronchial asthma [7]. This increased bronchoconstrictor response to a variety of stimuli is found in virtually all individuals with asthma, and many patients with other obstructive airways disease, such as chronic obstructive pulmonary disease (COPD) or cystic fibrosis [7–10]. It is a useful parameter to study because airways responsiveness can be readily measured using pharmacologic, physical, or allergen challenge methods [7,8].

The mechanisms responsible for BHR in asthma include individual susceptibility and the effects of environmental exposures to proinflammatory stimuli [7,9,11]. Therefore, one can focus on the genes that predispose an individual to the development of BHR as a logical method to investigate the hereditary factors that cause asthma. This approach allows dissection of individual aspects of asthma which may have a simpler, more definable genetic component compared with genetic studies on the more complicated heterogeneous disease process. In addition, BHR is a trait that can be measured objectively either as a qualitative (positive or negative) or as a quantitative [slope, provocative dose (PD), or provocative concentration (PC)] measure in most individuals [12]. The advantage of this latter approach is that phenotypic information is available on the majority of individuals in a given population sample, making genetic analytic approaches including both segregation and linkage analysis more feasible [13].

The limitations inherent in the use of BHR as a sensitive marker for asthma is that other conditions that may not reflect genetic susceptibility to asthma, such as COPD, cystic fibrosis, or viral upper respiratory infections [10,14], are associated with BHR. In addition, there are several different methods for assessing BHR that may measure different responses. In general, responses to methacholine and histamine are correlated closely [8], but responses to exercise and inhalation challenge with specific allergens may be less sensitive, and may not differentiate asthma from allergic disorders (specific allergen challenge) or may not include all asthmatics (exercise challenge) [8,15,16]. More recently, adenosine challenge has been proposed as a method to assess asthmatic responses more precisely and to better reflect disease severity [17,18]. Despite these issues, use of associated or intermediate phenotypes is an important strategy that should be successful in dissecting some of the complex genetic factors responsible for asthma [19,20]. Although this approach has limitations, the recent identification of major genetic loci important in essential hypertension [21] and diabetes [22] supports the use of methods utilizing associated phenotypes (diastolic blood pressure levels and treatment for hypertension; age of onset and HLA haplotype for diabetes). When an associated phenotype can be measured as a quantitative trait, additional useful information for investigating the pathogenesis of common complex genetic disorders is gained. Thus, studies that explore the genetic component of BHR are important in understanding basic physiologic processes that lead to the development and progression of asthma and may lead to more effective therapeutic interventions.

III. Mechanisms of Bronchial Hyperresponsiveness

Several factors are related to BHR in asthma. These include geometric factors related to airway caliber, the role of the autonomic neural pathways, and the degree of airways inflammation [7,23,24]. Important links between markers of inflammation and BHR in asthma are based on studies using investigative bronchoscopic techniques that have demonstrated migration and activation of inflammatory cellular elements in the airways of asthmatics [25–27]. Biochemical mediators that include regulatory cytokines produced by these airway inflammatory cells provide a local mechanism to modulate or amplify the inflammatory response in the airways. Interleukin-4 (IL-4) has been promoted as the major regulator of IgE production [28]. In addition, it stimulates MHC Class II antigens and upregulates Fc receptor expression for IgE (CD23) on B cells and monocytes [29], resulting in enhanced antigen-presenting capacity of these cells. IL-13 shares many of IL-4's biological activities and is also important in IgE isotype switch [30]. IL-5 is the most important stimulus for eosinophil production. It has also been shown to induce degranulation, the respiratory burst, and the generation of hypodense eosinophils [31]. IL-5 is chemotactic for eosinophils and activates mature eosinophils, inducing eosinophil secretion and enhanced antibody-dependent cytotoxicity. IL-3 and GM-CSF share with IL-5 the ability to generate active, hypodense eosinophils and to prolong eosinophil survival [32]. IL-3 is also a macrophage-activating factor which induces low-affinity IgE receptors on monocytes [33] and can function as a mast-cell differentiating factor [34]. IL-9 was

for macrophage colony-stimulating factor (CSF-1R), interferon regulatory factor-1 (IRF-1), and fibroblast growth factor acidic (FGFA) [72]. In addition, there is a β-adrenergic receptor (ADRB2) and a lymphocyte-specific glucocorticoid receptor (GRL1) in this region. The genes for IL-4 related cytokines stimulate B-cell growth and regulate specific immunoglobulin synthesis [73,74]. IL-9 and IL-13 enhance IL-4-dependent immunoglobulin synthesis and expression of CD23, an IgE surface binding factor, respectively. GM-CSF as well as other cellular growth factors such as FGFA also reside in this area of chromosome 5q, and these factors stimulate proliferation of granulocytes, macrophages, and eosinophils. Thus, this region of 5q contains genes that regulate a large number of factors that appear to be important regulatory factors in the inflammatory processes in BHR, atopy, and asthma.

There is a strong association between airway responsiveness and serum IgE levels [75–78]. Population studies have not identified patterns of inheritance or the number of genes involved, the magnitude of their effect, or in most cases, their location. To explain the close interrelationship between BHR and atopy, family studies are needed to investigate whether these traits are coinherited.

VII. Susceptibility Loci for Bronchial Hyperresponsiveness

Molecular genetic studies that have attempted to localize BHR to a specific area of the genome are summarized in Table 1. Clearly, this phenotype is not inherited in a simple Mendelian fashion, and multiple genes are more likely to regulate this response. To date, only one study has demonstrated positive linkage results for

Table 1 Genetic Studies of Bronchial Hyperresponsiveness

Reference	Year	Study
Lympany (83)	1992	With BHR defined as $PD_{20}FEV_1 \leq 8$ umol methacholine, this study found no linkage of BHR with D11S97, a marker on chromosome 11q.
Amelung (84)	1992	Potential linkage of BHR to markers on chromosomes 6p and 11q was studied. BHR, defined as $PC_{20}FEV_1 \leq 32$ mg/ml histamine, was not found to be linked to either area.
Postma (19)	1995	Using a definition of BHR as $PC_{20}FEV_1 \leq 16$ mg/ml histamine, evidence for linkage of this phenotype to markers on chromosome 5q was found, near an area where linkage of IgE levels has previously been described.

BHR. In this analysis, BHR was localized to chromosome 5q [19], a region rich in cytokine genes. Previously, three groups of investigators have demonstrated linkage of serum IgE levels to this same general region of 5q [13,71,79]. Meyers and co-workers found evidence for linkage of a gene for IgE production to this area of chromosome 5q by performing sib-pair analysis on the quantitative measure of total serum IgE levels in a population of Dutch families ascertained for a parent with asthma. In addition, lod score analysis provided evidence for linkage based on the recessive model of high IgE levels obtained from their segregation analysis [13]. Further, two-locus segregation linkage analysis showed that two separate loci are important in the regulation of total serum IgE levels [80]. Because these studies were performed in families with asthma, this model may overestimate the role of each locus in a random population; however, the locus on 5q accounted for approximately 50% of the variance in total serum IgE levels. In 11 Amish families, Marsh and co-workers have found evidence for linkage of markers on chromosome 5q with a gene controlling total serum IgE levels, but not specific IgE antibody concentrations [71]. More recently, Doull and co-workers have reported linkage of IgE levels (allelic association) with polymorphisms in interleukin-9 in a random population, further replicating this linkage [79]. These studies indicate the presence of a regulatory gene for control of IgE levels. Recently, a susceptibility gene for BHR on 5q has been reported; this linkage and approaches to finding genes for these traits are the subjects of the remainder of this chapter. In addition, several groups of investigators are performing genome-wide searches to detect additional regions with susceptibility loci for BHR [81].

VIII. Linkage Studies for Bronchial Hyperresponsiveness to Chromosome 5q

In the study by Postma and co-workers, BHR was determined to be linked to markers on chromosome 5q [19]. This study involved the ascertainment of Dutch asthmatic probands and their family members. Between 1962 and 1970, over 1000 patients with obstructive airways disease were evaluated while clinically stable at Beatrixoord, a regional asthma and airways disease referral center hospital near Groningen, the Netherlands. Beginning in 1962, families were selected through a proband with symptomatic asthma, including BHR to histamine, at the time of this first study [83]. All probands were reexamined, and spouses, children, and in some cases grandchildren were examined with the following tests: (1) standardized respiratory questionnaire, (2) pulmonary function testing, (3) bronchial responsiveness to inhaled histamine, (4) intradermal skin tests, (5) total serum IgE, (6) specific IgE levels to house dust mite and grass mix and (7) total peripheral blood eosinophil counts. Total serum IgE (IU) was measured by solid phase immunoassay (Pharmacia IgE EIA, Pharmacia Diagnostics AB, Sweden). The mean of duplicate tests was used for the reported IgE level. Phenotypic data on 84 complete families is summarized in Table 2 [19].

A major component of this family evaluation was a measurement of bronchial responsiveness to histamine. Testing of bronchial responsiveness was performed using the method of DeVries and co-workers [84] that was used for the initial assessment of the probands approximately 25 years ago. The bronchial reactivity testing protocol consists of having each subject inhale increasing concentrations of histamine for 30 s of tidal breathing starting with a diluent control and continuing until the FEV_1 falls by $\geq 20\%$ or the highest concentration of histamine (32 mg/mL) is reached. The raw data were used to calculate the provocation concentration (PC) of histamine that produced a 20% fall in FEV_1 ($PC_{20}FEV_1$) by extrapolation from the dose-response curve. This value was used for analysis of BHR as a quantitative trait. For analysis of BHR as a qualitative trait, individuals were considered to have bronchial hyperresponsiveness if they had a $\geq 20\%$ decrease in FEV_1 at ≤ 32 mg/mL histamine. Because a major gene-regulating serum IgE has been previously mapped to chromosome 5q31-q33 [13], these investigators sought to determine whether genetic susceptibility to BHR, provoked by histamine, is coinherited with markers from this region. In other words, chromosome 5q31-q33 may also represent a candidate region for the genetic regulation of BHR. Earlier studies by these investigators had excluded linkage to regions of chromosomes 6 and 11 with this phenotype [83]. To explore further the relationship between BHR and allergy (total serum IgE levels), the hypothesis that BHR would map to the same chromosomal region as a locus that regulates total serum IgE on chromosome 5q [19] was tested.

Serum total IgE levels were strongly correlated ($r = 0.65$, $p < 0.01$) in pairs of siblings concordant for BHR, suggesting that these traits are coinherited. However, there was no significant association ($r = 0.04$, $p > 0.10$) between

Table 2. Clinical and Physiologic Characteristics of Asthma Families

Characteristic	Probands ($N = 84$)	Spouses[a] ($N = 113$)	First-degree offspring ($N = 247$)	Second-degree offspring ($N = 56$)
Gender (%M/%F)	56/44	50/50	49/51	50/50
Mean age (yrs)	51	48	25	14
Bronchial hyperresponsiveness % ($PC_{20} \leq 32$mg/mL)	89[b]	20	34	36
Percent predicted FEV_1	68	98	95	97

[a]This category includes 29 spouses of the proband's children (first-degree offspring).
[b]All probands (100%) had bronchial hyperresponsiveness at the time of first study.

$PC_{20}FEV_1$ values (histamine threshold value ≤ 32 mg/mL) in pairs of siblings concordant for elevated serum total IgE levels. This implies that serum total IgE levels can be influenced by other genetic and environmental factors that may not be common to the development of bronchial hyperresponsiveness.

Linkage analyses were performed by estimating the proportion of alleles shared at each marker between siblings with BHR, an established approach for the investigation of the genetic basis of complex traits such as BHR, atopy, and asthma. In this approach, the clinical characteristics of the parents are not used in testing for linkage; the pertinent observation is how often two affected offspring share copies of the same parental marker allele. If the same copy of a marker allele is observed in each sibling, the alleles are said to be inherited in a manner that is termed "identical by descent." There is evidence for linkage when pairs of siblings with BHR are identical by descent for a marker allele more often than expected by chance (50%). The transmission of the same allele to each sibling with BHR suggests that the marker locus is located physically close enough on the same chromosomal region to the susceptibility locus that they cosegregate during meiosis. Analysis of affected pairs of siblings demonstrated statistically significant evidence of linkage between BHR and D5S436, D5S658 and several other markers located nearby on chromosome 5q31-q33. These data strongly support the hypothesis that one or more closely spaced genes on chromosome 5q31-q33 are important in the regulation of bronchial hyperresponsiveness. These results are summarized in Table 3 and Fig. 1.

Bronchial hyperresponsiveness was also analyzed as a quantitative trait using a regressive approach to identify the relationship between siblings for actual $PC_{20}FEV_1$ values and the proportion of marker alleles identical by descent. When linkage between BHR as a quantitative trait and the marker D5S436 was evaluated, the p value was 0.0002. This relationship remained significant even when

Table 3 Linkage Results for IgE and BHR

	Log [IgE] Sib-pair p value	Log [IgE] LOD score (θ)	BHR Sib-pair p value
IL-9	0.05	0.58 (0.13)	0.012
D5S393	NS	1.14 (0.14)	0.084
D5S500	0.006	1.41 (0.16)	0.102
D5S658	0.04	1.05 (0.16)	0.001
D5S436	0.0008	3.63 (0.09)	0.0002
FGFA	NS	0.33 (0.20)	0.198
D5S470	0.02	0.76 (0.16)	0.189
DSF1R	0.03	0.82 (0.13)	0.118
D5S410	NS	0.00 (0.50)	0.025

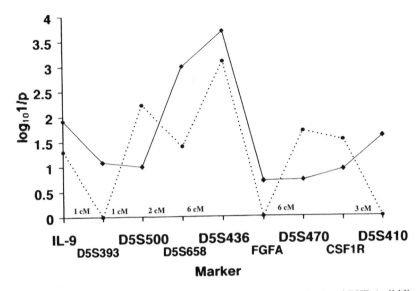

Figure 1   Sib-pair analysis results for total serum IgE (dashed line) and BHR (solid line) with markers on chromosome 5q, expressed as $\log_{10} 1/p$. Significance at the level of $p = 0.05$ corresponds to a value of 1.3 on the ordinate; significance at the level of $p = 0.01$ corresponds to a value of 2.

$\log_{10}$ serum total IgE levels were included as a covariate ($p < 0.002$). These data confirm the close genetic relationship between IgE and BHR, but suggest a strong heritable component to BHR apart from the genetic regulation of total serum IgE levels. This study demonstrates that an elevated level of total serum IgE is coinherited with BHR and more than 50% of the offspring in this study with elevated IgE levels had physiologic evidence of BHR. The evidence of coinheritance of these traits in this family study provides a potential genetic mechanism to explain the strong relationship between these responses in epidemiologic studies [53,54]. These results can be interpreted as suggesting that there are one or more than one closely associated susceptibility genes on chromosome 5q that are important in producing susceptibility to asthma. These data represent an important step toward understanding the interrelationship between allergy (IgE) and BHR. Specifically, the coinheritance and colocalization of essential components of asthma generates major questions about the molecular basis for susceptibility to this disorder.

The results of this study cannot determine whether total serum IgE and BHR are linked to the same gene(s) or to different genes in this chromosomal region. It is likely that several of the candidate loci on chromosome 5q may be linked to the asthmatic and allergic phenotypes, especially since there was still evidence for linkage of BHR after controlling for total serum IgE levels. Specific localization will be difficult to determine, since the allergic and asthmatic phenotypes are closely related and the candidate loci are linked to each other. It will be important to distinguish between the effects of a locus involved in BHR production compared with other measures such as total serum IgE. Future studies should include fine mapping of the region of chromosome 5q31-33 where there is evidence for a susceptibility locus for total serum IgE levels and BHR, and the examination of known cytokine gene candidates on 5q for genetic mutations that determine the biologic variability observed in total IgE and bronchial responsiveness. The mutations of the gene(s) on chromosome 5q which control total IgE levels and BHR in families with asthma are as yet unknown. However, chromosome 5q was examined for evidence of linkage because a number of candidate genes for allergy and asthma are known to exist in this area of the genome. Moreover, linkage in the 5q region for similar subphenotypes has been suggested by other investigators [71,85]. In addition, using an algorithm based on BHR to histamine, respiratory symptoms, smoking, atopy, percent predicted FEV_1, and reversibility with bronchodilators to characterize obstructive airways diseases, one group of investigators found linkage of the asthma phenotype to markers on chromosome 5q [86]. Thus, it is now essential to examine the known candidate genes for the presence of mutations. This is an important first step because fine mapping is much more difficult in complex genetic disorders and a localization cannot be anticipated from the inspection of critical recombinants as in Mendelian disorders [20]. Indeed, the combination of linkage, physical mapping, and candidate gene analyses optimize the likelihood for success in identifying genes important in allergic asthma.

IX. Identification of Susceptibility Genes for Bronchial Hyperresponsiveness and Atopy

Now that one potential chromosomal localization of a disease locus for BHR and allergic responsiveness (total serum IgE levels) has been identified on chromosome 5q, studies to identify susceptibility genes and characterize their biologic function are indicated (Fig. 2). This linkage to chromosome 5q has been replicated for serum IgE levels and appears to represent a major regulatory locus for both IgE levels and BHR [19,13,71,87]. The presence of a number of appropriate candidate genes makes this area a logical choice for study, but the presence of a number of relevant candidates also complicates gene localization. Therefore, although the search for the gene (or genes) involved in BHR and its mutations is relatively straightforward, it is potentially quite laborious. Two general strategies can be used to find genes for allergy, bronchial hyperresponsiveness, and asthma. The

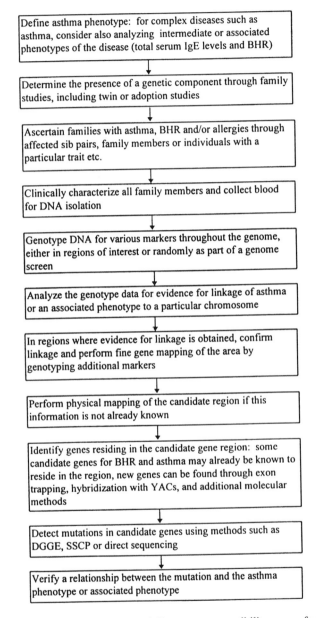

Figure 2   Methods for identification of disease or susceptibility genes for asthma.

first is to characterize known genes from normal and affected individuals in the region identified by genetic analysis, if this fails, the second is to identify new genes in the region of interest. Biologic studies in relevant animal models as well as studies in patients with allergic diseases and asthma will be necessary to determine the relative importance of these gene products in these disorders.

Often one can identify possible candidate genes that have been mapped to a region based on inferences about the biology of the disorder. As noted earlier, certain cytokines are produced to a greater or lesser extent in asthmatics when compared to normal individuals. Consequently, it is not unreasonable to consider these genes and their promoter regions as candidates [88–90]. If candidate gene sequences are known, PCR primers can be designed to screen for mutations, the majority of which produce changes in the protein coding regions and result in reduced levels of protein or a functionally altered protein product. Mutations in PCR products can be screened indirectly by gel based methods such as denaturing gradient gel electrophoresis (DGGE) or single-strand conformation polymorphism (SSCP). For each of these methods, differences in the sequences of the normal and mutant DNAs result in mobility shifts during gel electrophoresis. Confirmation is made by DNA sequencing. In order to confirm the association of a specific mutation found with a disorder or trait (BHR), a collection of "normal" and "affected" individuals can then be screened for the specific mutation by a variety of methods [e.g., hybridization with allele-specific oligomers (ASO), restriction enzyme analysis (if a restriction site is altered by the mutation), oligomer ligation assays (OLA), etc.]. Alternatively, sequencing of PCR products can be used to identify base changes in DNA directly. The latter method has the advantage that all substitutions should be identifiable but is less economical if many exons from a large number of people are to be screened. This method has been used successfully by a variety of investigators [91].

Unfortunately, linkage analysis for complex disorders such as BHR and asthma is unlikely to be able to define regions of interest with a resolution of less than several megabases, and the number of potential genes that will need to be screened will be extensive. Furthermore, the number of currently identified genes in regions of interest is likely to be a small percentage of the actual number of genes present. To find additional candidates in a region, various strategies have been used, including exon trapping, a method that can screen genomic DNA for sequences that are flanked by splice donor and acceptor sites (i.e., as in intron–exon junctions) [92]. Exon trapping is a useful technique for positional cloning strategies to isolate candidate genes. It has been used to isolate, among others, the gene for Huntington's disease [93]. Exon trapping results in the direct isolation of gene sequences from the cloned genomic DNA without prior knowledge of a gene's structure or pattern of expression.

An alternative approach to detecting coding regions in genomic DNA is to use genomic clones such as yeast artificial chromosomes (YACs) or cosmids to select cDNAs directly by hybridization [94]. More recently, there has been a concerted effort to identify partial cDNAs or expressed sequence tags (ESTs) from a variety of tissue cDNA libraries. Expressed sequences tags are partial cDNA clones obtained from a variety of tissue mRNAs. By early 1996 over 317,000 human ESTs were listed in the dbEST collection of Genbank. This number far exceeds the anticipated number of human genes (75,000–100,000) because of redundancy and the fact that ESTs can be derived from separate regions of a longer cDNA. The "Unigene" Project (Ref. 95 or URL:http://www.ncbi.nlm.nih.gov/ Schuler/Papers/ESTtransmap/) is attempting to identify ESTs with overlapping sequences as representatives of a single genes and to map these genes. As of January 1996, there were 171 expressed sequences listed for chromosome 5 by the National Center for Biotechnology Information (NCBI), and 84 of these were ESTs. Because relatively few ESTs have yet to be assigned to a chromosome, let alone regionally mapped, it is likely that the total number of expressed sequences on this chromosome will quickly far exceed the number of characterized genes. Recently, Hudson and co-workers [96] published a map of the human genome with over 15,000 sequenced tagged sites (STSs), some of which are expressed genes or ESTs. These STSs were mapped either by genetic linkage to the Centre d'Etude du Polymorphisme Humaine (CEPH) reference pedigrees [97], by radiation hybrid analysis [98], or by hybridization to the Genethon mega-YACs [99]. The integration of these three methods produced a detailed integrated map with markers spaced approximately every 200 kb. As additional ESTs and expressed sequences are added to the integrated map, the ability to identify candidate genes will become relatively simple. The ESTs that are mapped to a region can then be used to "trap" full-length cDNAs or as starting points for genomic sequencing.

Unfortunately, one can never know if all ESTs represent all expressed genes. NCBI presents on their Web site (see URL:http://www.ncbi.nlm.nih.gov/ dbEST/dbEST_genes/) a list of positionally cloned genes which are represented as ESTs. As of January 1996, 81% of positionally cloned genes were represented. This implies that approximately 20% of genes remain to be "tagged" with an EST. There may be many reasons that certain genes are not included in the current database. Genes expressed during very narrow developmental windows or in tissues not represented by currently used cDNA libraries might not be represented. Further, genes which are transcribed at low levels or which lack polyadenylated tails would be disproportionately represented.

For this and other reasons, an increasingly feasible and desirable alternative for gene identification is direct genomic DNA sequencing. Already large blocks of genomic DNA have been sequenced by several groups, including 700 kb from the cytokine-rich region of 5q, by the Human Genome Center of the Lawrence Berkeley National Laboratory (see URL:http://www.hcg.lbl.gov/DirSeq.html). The advantage of genomic sequencing, and the principle rationale for sequencing the human genome, is that all of the genes, promoters, and other control elements will be found. However, a problem that confounds large-scale direct sequencing is that it is necessary to have a physical map of the region and overlapping P1 clones, cosmids, or other mapping reagents. Fortunately, the process demonstrated by Hudson and co-workers [96] means that many of the obstacles to genomic sequencing have been met. There are still organizational, computational, and engineering issues that need to be addressed before efficient and cost-effective genomic sequencing can be performed. For example, with the current method of "shotgun" sequencing, a large region such as a 50-kb cosmid is subcloned as "random" 1- or 2-kb fragments, and, simply by chance, some subclones will be sequenced more often than others. Thus, a sufficient number of sequences must be acquired so that no regions are missed. This inflates the cost and time needed to complete such a project. Different directed sequencing strategies such as "primer walking" and insertional mutagenesis [100] are being evaluated by various groups, but none has emerged as a clearly superior approach to efficient large-scale sequencing. Nevertheless, the cost and efficiency of large-scale sequencing continue to improve, and the availability of sequence data for all genes in regions of biological interest may ultimately be the fastest and most cost-effective way to unravel the genetic components of complex genetic conditions or disorders such as allergic diseases, BHR, and asthma.

X. Summary

Studies have demonstrated that bronchial hyperresponsiveness is related to the development of inflammation in the airways, which is an important determinant of the development and progression of asthma. The level of BHR to nonspecific stimuli has been shown to correlate with asthmatic symptoms and responses to treatment. BHR, a critical component of asthma, can therefore be used as a marker of the asthmatic phenotype in genetic studies. Measures of airway responsiveness have previously been used in family and twin studies to establish a genetic basis of asthma. Data from these studies support a strong genetic predisposition to BHR. This is an important step toward elucidating the genetic basis of asthma, a complex disease. While few molecular genetic analyses have been performed to localize genetic loci responsible for bronchial responsiveness, BHR has been shown to map to one area of the genome, chromosome 5q, using linkage analysis in asthma families. This chromosomal region needs to be investigated further, with evaluation of known candidate genes in this area for mutations or polymorphisms that may be important in BHR, as well as identification of and subsequent evaluation of additional candidate genes in this area. Molecular methods to identify and characterize these candidate genes continue to become more refined. In addition, several studies are currently underway to localize additional major genetic loci responsible for the development of BHR and asthma.

Acknowledgment

This work was supported by grants from the National Institutes of Health; R01 HL48341 and U01 HL49602 and American Lung Association Research Award.

References

1. Gergen PJ, Weiss KB. The increasing problem of asthma in the United States. Am Rev Respir Dis 1992; 146:823–824.
2. Meyers DA, Bleecker ER. Approaches to mapping genes for allergy and asthma. Am J Respir Crit Care Med 1995; 152:411–413.
3. Weisch DG, Meyers DA, Bleecker ER, Samet JM. Classification of the asthma phenotype in genetic studies. In: Liggett S, Meyers DA, eds. Lung Biology in Health and Disease, Genetics of Asthma. New York: Marcel Dekker, 1996; 421–442.
4. Weiss ST. Issues in phenotype assessment in genetic studies of asthma. In: Liggett S, Meyers DA, eds. Lung Biology in Health and Disease, Genetics of Asthma. New York: Marcel Dekker, 1996; 401–419.
5. National Heart, Lung and Blood Institute, National Institutes of Health. Guidelines for the diagnosis and management of asthma. 1995. Washington, DC: U.S. Government Printing Office 95-36S9.
6. Orie NGM, Sluiter HJ, de Vries K, Tammeling GJ, Witkop J. The host factor in bronchitis. In: Orie NGM, Sluiter HJ, eds. Bronchitis. Assen: Royal van Gorcum, 1961:43–59.
7. Boushey HA, Holtzman MJ, Sheller JR, Nadel JA. Bronchial hyperresponsiveness. Am Rev Respir Dis 1980; 121:389–413.
8. Chatham M, Bleecker ER, Smith PL, Rosenthal RR, Mason P, Norman PS. A comparison of histamine, methacholine and exercise airways reactivity in normal and asthmatic subjects. Am Rev Respir Dis 1982; 126:235–240.
9. Holgate ST, Beasley R, Twentyman OP. The pathogenesis and significance of bronchial hyperresponsiveness in airway disease. Clin Sci 1987; 73:561–572.
10. Tashkin DP, Murray DA, Bleecker ER, et al. The lung health study: airway responsiveness to inhaled methacholine in smokers with mild to moderate airflow limitation. Am Rev Respir Dis 1992; 145:301–310.
11. O'Connor GT, Sparrow D, Weiss ST. The role of allergy and nonspecific bronchial hyperresponsiveness in the pathogenesis of chronic obstructive pulmonary disease. Am Rev Respir Dis 1989; 140:225–252.
12. O'Connor GT, Sparrow D, Segal MR, Weiss ST. Smoking, atopy, and methacholine airway responsiveness among middle-aged and elderly men. The normative aging study. Am Rev Respir Dis 1989; 140:1520–1526.
13. Meyers DA, Postma DS, Panhuysen CIM, et al. Evidence for a locus regulating total serum IgE levels mapping to chromosome 5. Genomics 1994; 23:464–470.
14. Empey DW, Laitinen LA, Jacobs L, Gold WM, Nadel JA. Mechanisms of bronchial hyperreactivity in normal subjects after upper respiratory tract infection. Am Rev Respir Dis 1976; 113:131–139.

15. Permutt S, Rosenthal RR, Norman PS, Menkes HA. Bronchial challenge in ragweed sensitive patients. In: Lichtenstein LM, Austen KF, eds. Asthma. New York: Academic Press, 1977:266–277.

16. Bascom R, Bleecker ER. Bronchoconstriction induced by distilled water: sensitivity in asthmatics and relationship to exercise-induced bronchospasm. Am Rev Respir Dis 1986; 134:248–253.

17. Cushley MJ, Tattersfield AE, Holgate ST. Inhaled adenosine and guanosine on airway resistance in normal and asthmatic subjects. Br J Clin Pharm 1983; 15: 161–165.

18. Holgate ST, Church MK, Polosa R. Adenosine; a positive modulator of airway inflammation in asthma. Ann NY Acad Sci 1991; 629:227–236.

19. Postma DS, Bleecker ER, Amelung PJ, et al. Genetic susceptibility to asthma-bronchial hyperresponsiveness coinherited with a major gene for atopy. N Engl J Med 1995; 333:894–900.

20. Lander ES, Schork NJ. Genetic dissection of complex traits. Science 1994; 265: 2037–2048.

21. Caufield M, Lavender P, Martin F. Linkage of the angiotensinogen gene to essential hypertension. N Engl J Med 1994; 330:1629–1633.

22. Davies JL, Kawaguchi Y, Bennett ST. A genome-wide search for human type I diabetes susceptibility genes. Nature 1994; 371:130–136.

23. Sheffer AL, Bailey WC, Bleecker ER, et al. Guidelines for the diagnosis and management of asthma. J Allergy Clin Immunol 1991; 88:425–534.

24. Djakanovic R, Roche WR, Wilson JW. Mucosal inflammation in asthma. Am Rev Respir Dis 1990; 142:434–457.

25. Bousquet J, Chanez P, Lacoste JY, et al. Eosinophilic inflammation in asthma. N Engl J Med 1990; 323:1033–1039.

26. Lui MC, Hubbard WC, Proud D, et al. Immediate and late inflammatory responses to ragweed antigen challenge of the peripheral airways in allergic asthmatics: cellular, mediator and permeability changes. Am Rev Respir Dis 1991; 144:51–58.

27. Wenzel SE, Fowler AA, Schwartz LB. Activation of pulmonary mast cells by bronchoalveolar allergen challenge: in vivo release of histamine and tryptase in atopic subjects with and without asthma. Am Rev Respir Dis 1988; 137:1002–1008.

28. Romagnani S. Regulation and deregulation of human IgE synthesis. Immunol Today 1990; 11:316.

29. Vercelli D, Jabara HH, Lee BW, Woodland N, Geha RS, Leung DY. Human recombinant interleukin-4 induces Fc epsilon R2/CD23 on normal human monocytes. J Exp Med 1988; 167;1406–1416.

30. de Vries JE, Zurawski G. Immunoregulatory properties of IL-13: its potential role in atopic disease. Int Arch Allergy Immunol 1995; 106:175–179.

31. Lopez AF, Sanderson CJ, Gamble JR, Campbell HD. Recombinant human interleukin-5 is a selective activator of human eosinophil function. J Exp Med 1988; 167:219–224.

32. Warringa RA, Koenderman L, Kok PT, Kreukniet J, Bruijnzeel PL. Modulation and induction of eosinophil chemotaxis by granulocyte-macrophage colony-stimulating factor and interleukin-3. Blood 1991; 77:2694–2700.

33. Alderson MR, Tough TW, Ziegler SF, Armitage RJ. Regulation of human monocyte cell-surface and soluble CD23 (FCεRII) by granulocyte-macrophage colony-stimulating factor and IL-3. Immunology 1992; 149:1252–1257.

34. Kirshenbaum AS, Goff JP, Dreskin SC, Irani SC, Schwartz LB. IL-3 dependent growth of basophil-like cells and mastlike cells from human bone marrow. J Immunol 1989; 142:2427.

35. Hultner L, Druez C, Moeller J, et al. Mast cell growth-enhancing activity (MEA) is structurally related and functionally identical to the novel mouse T cell growth factor P40/TCGFIII (interleukin-9). Eur J Immunol 1990; 20:1413.

36. Murray HW. Interferon-gamma, the activated macrophage and host defense against microbial challenge. Ann Intern Med 1988; 108:595–608.

37. Berman JS, Beer DJ, Theodore AC. Lymphocyte recruitment to the lung. Am Rev Respir Dis 1990; 142:238–257.

38. Snapper CM, Paul WE. Interferon-gamma and B cell stimulatory factor-1 reciprocally regulate Ig isotype production. Science 1987; 236:944–947.

39. Fiorentino DF, Bond MW, Mosmann TR. Two types of mouse T helper cell. IV. Th2 clones secrete a factor that inhibits cytokine production by Th1 clones. J Exp Med 1989; 170:2081.

40. Chan SH, Kobayashu M, Santoi D, Perussia B, Trinchieri G. Mechanisms of interferon-gamma induction by natural killer cell stimulatory factor (NKSF/IL-12). Role of transcription and mRNA stability in the synergistic interaction between NKSF and IL-12. J Immunol 1992; 148:92–98.

41. Kiniwa M, Gately M, Gubler U, Chizzonite R, Fargeas C, Delespesse G. Recombinant interleukin-12 suppresses the synthesis of IgE by interleukin-4 stimulated human lymphocytes. J Clin Invest 1992; 90:262–266.

42. MacDonald HR, Nabholz M. T cell activation. Ann Rev Cell Biol 1986; 2:231–253.

43. Rubin LA, Kurman CC, Fritz ME. Soluble interleukin-2 receptors are released from activated human lymphoid cells in vitro. J Immunol 1985; 135:3172–3177.

44. Broide DH, Lotz M, Cuomo AJ, Coburn DA, Federman EC, Wasserman SI. Cytokines in symptomatic asthma airways. J Allergy Clin Immunol 1992; 89:958–967.

45. Brown PH, Crompton GK, Greening AP. Proinflammatory cytokines in acute asthma. Lancet 1991; 338:590–593.

46. Robinson DS, Ying S, Bentley AM, et al. Relationships among numbers of bronchoalveolar lavage cells expressing messenger ribonucleic acid for cytokines, asthma symptoms, and airway methacholine responsiveness in atopic asthma. J Allergy Clin Immunol 1993; 92:397–403.

47. Ackerman V, Marini M, Vittori E, Bellini A, Vassali G, Mattoli S. Detection of cytokines and their cells sources in bronchial biopsy specimens from asthmatic patients. Relationship to atopic status, symptoms, and level of airway hyperresponsiveness. Chest 1994; 105:687–696.

48. Bleecker ER, McCrea KA, Meltzer SS, Hasday JD. Inflammatory abnormalities in the airways of asthmatics and asymptomatic cigarette smokers. Bronchitis V 1994; 106–116.

49. Hargreave FE, Ryan G, Thomson NC, et al. Bronchial responsiveness to histamine or methacholine in asthma. J Allergy Clin Immunol 1981; 68:347–355.

50. Cockcroft DW, Ruffin RE, Dolovich J, Hargreave FE. Allergen-induced increase in non-allergic bronchial reactivity. Clin Allergy 1977; 7:503–513.

51. Laitinen LA, Laitinen A, Haahtela T. A comparative study of the effects of an inhaled corticosteroid, budesonide, and a beta2-agonist, terbutaline, on airway inflammation in newly diagnosed asthma: a randomized, double-blind, parallel-group controlled trial. J Allergy Clin Immunol 1992; 90:32–42.

52. Kerrebijn KF, van Essen-Zandvliet EE, Neijens HJ. Effects of long-term treatment with inhaled corticosteroids and beta-agonists on the bronchial responsiveness in children with asthma. J Allergy Clin Immunol 1987; 79:653–659.

53. Burrows B, Sears MR, Flannery EM, Herbison GP, Holdaway MD. Relationship of bronchial responsiveness assessed by methacholine to serum IgE, lung function, symptoms, and diagnoses in 11-year-old New Zealand children. J Allergy Clin Immunol 1992; 90:376–385.

54. Sears M, Burrows B, Flannery EM, Herbison GP, Hewitt CJ, Holdaway MD. Relation between airway responsiveness and serum IgE in children with asthma and in apparently normal children. N Engl J Med 1991; 325:1067–1071.

55. Liu MC, Bleecker ER, Lichtenstein LM, et al. Evidence for elevated levels of histamine, prostaglandin D2, and other bronchoconstricting prostaglandins in the airways of subjects with mild asthma. Am Rev Respir Dis 1990; 142:126–132.

56. Kay AB. Mediators and inflammatory cells in allergic disease. Ann Allergy 1987; 59(6):35–42.

57. Cartier A, Thomsom NC, Frith PA, Roberts R, Hargreave FE. Allergen-induced increase in bronchial responsiveness to histamine: relationship to the late asthmatic response and changes in airway caliber. J Allergy Clin Immunol 1982; 70(3): 734–740.

58. Cockroft DW, Murdock KY. Comparative effects of inhaled salbutamol, sodium cromoglycate, and beclomethasone dipropionate on allergen-induced early asthmatic responses, late asthmatic responses, and increased bronchial responsiveness to histamine. J Allergy Clin Immunol 1987; 79:734–740.

59. Kerstjens HAM, Brand PLP, Hughes MD, et al. A comparison of bronchodilator therapy with or without inhaled corticosteroid therapy for obstructive airways disease. N Engl J Med 1992; 327:1413–1419.

60. Haahteka T, Larvinen M, Kava T, et al. Comparison of a beta-2 agonist, terbutaline, with an inhaled corticosteroid, budesonide, in newly detected asthma. N Engl J Med 1991; 325:388–392.

61. Bel EH, Timmers MC, Hermans J, Dijkman JH, Sterk PJ. The long-term effects of nedocromil sodium and beclomethasone dipropionate on bronchial responsiveness to methacholine in nonatopic asthmatic subjects. Am Rev Respir Dis 1990; 141:21–28.

62. Schleimer RP. Effects of glucocorticoids on inflammatory cells relevant to their therapeutic applications in asthma. Am Rev Respir Dis 1990; 141(suppl):S59–S69.

63. Burrows B, Martinez FD, Halonen M, Barbee RA, Cline MG. Association of asthma with serum IgE levels and skin-test reactivity to allergens. N Engl J Med 1989; 320:271–277.

64. Burrows B, Sears MR, Flannery EM, Herbison GP, Holdaway MD. Relationship of bronchial responsiveness to allergy skintest reactivity, lung function, respiratory

symptoms, and diagnosis in 13-year-old New Zealand children. J Allergy Clin Immunol 1995; 95:548–556.

65. Sunyer J, Anto JM, Sabria J, et al. Respiratory pathophysiologic responses. Relationship between serum IgE and airway responsiveness in adults with asthma. J Allergy Clin Immunol 1995; 95:699–706.

66. Hopp RJ, Bewtra AK, Watt GD, Nair NM, Townley RG. Genetic analysis of allergic disease in twins. J Allergy Clin Immunol 1984; 73:265–270.

67. Hopp RJ, Townley RG, Biven RE, Bewtra AK, Nair NM. The presence of airway reactivity before the development of asthma. Am Rev Respir Dis 1990; 141:2–8.

68. Hopp RJ, Bewtra AK, Biven R, Nair NM, Townley RG. Bronchial reactivity pattern in nonasthmatic parents of asthmatics. Ann Allergy 1988; 61(3):184–186.

69. Townley RG, Bewtra MD, Wilson AF, et al. Segregation analysis of bronchial response to methacholine inhalation in families with and without asthma. J Allergy Clin Immunol 1986; 77:101–107.

70. Longo F, Strinati R, Poli F, Fumi F. Genetic factors in non-specific bronchial hyperreactivity. Am J Dis Children 1987; 141:331–334.

71. Marsh DG, Neely JD, Breazeale DR, et al. Linkage analysis of IL4 and other chromosome 5q31.1 markers and total serum immunoglobulin E concentrations. Science 1994; 264:1162–1166.

72. Chandrasekharappa SC, Rebelsky MS, Firak TA, LeBeau MM, Westbrook CA. A long-range restriction map of the interleukin-4 and interleukin-5 linkage group on chromosome 5. Genomics 1990; 6:94–99.

73. Kelley J. Cytokines of the lung. Am Rev Respir Dis 1991; 141:765–788.

74. Boulay JL, Paul WE. The interleukin-4-related lymphokines and their binding to hematopoietin receptors. J Biol Chem 1992; 297:20525–20528.

75. Sears MR, Burrows B, Flannery EM, Herbison GP, Holdaway MD. Atopy in childhood. I. Gender and allergen related risks for development of hayfever and asthma. Clin Exp Allergy 1993; 23:941–948.

76. Sears MR, Burrows B, Herbison GP, Holdaway MD, Flannery EM. Atopy in childhood. II. Relationship to airway responsiveness, hayfever and asthma. Clin Exp Allergy 1993; 23:949–956.

77. Sears MR, Burrows B, Herbison GP, Flannery EM, Holdaway MD. Atopy in childhood. III. Relationship with pulmonary function and airway responsiveness. Clin Exp Allergy 1993; 23:957–963.

78. Grainger DN, Stenton SC, Avery AJ, Duddridge M, Walters EH, Hendrick DJ. The relationship between atopy and non-specific bronchial responsiveness. Clin Exp Allergy 1990; 20:181–187.

79. Doull IJM, Lawrence S, Watson M, et al. Allelic association of gene markers on chromosomes 5q and 11q with atopy and bronchial hyperresponsiveness. Am J Respir Crit Care Med. In press.

80. Xu J, Levitt RC, Panhuysen CIM, et al. Evidence for two unlinked loci regulating total serum IgE levels. Am J Hum Genet 1995; 57:425–430.

81. Recent advances in the genetics of asthma and allergy. Clin Exp Allergy 1995; 25(suppl 2):1–125.

83. Amelung PJ, Panhuysen CIM, Postma DS, et al. Atopy and bronchial hyperrespon-

siveness: exclusion of linkage to markers on chromosome 11q and 6p. Clin Exp Allergy 1992; 22:1077–1084.

84. DeVries K, Goei JT, Booy-Noord H, Orie NGM. Changes during 24 hours in the lung function and histamine hyperreactivity of the bronchial tree in asthmatic and bronchitic patients. Int Arch Allergy 1962; 20:93–101.

85. Borish LC, Mascall JJ, Klinnert M, Leppert M, Rosenwasser L. Polymorphisms in the chromosome 5 gene cluster. J Allergy Clin Immunol 1994; 93(1):abstr 345.

86. Panhuysen CIM, Levitt RC, Postma DS, et al. Evidence for a susceptibility locus for asthma mapping to chromosome 5q. Clin Res 1995; 43:281A.

87. Watson M, Lawrence S, Collins A, et al. Exclusion from proximal 11q of a common gene with megaphenic effect on atopy. Ann Hum Genet 1995; 59:403–411.

88. Rossenwasser LJ, Klemm DJ, Dresback JK, et al. Promoter polymorphisms in the chromosome 5 gene cluster in asthma and atopy. Clin Exp Allergy 1995; 25(suppl 2): 74–78.

89. Atamas SP, Choi J, Yurovsky VV, White B. An alternative splice variant of human IL-4, IL-4δ2, inhibits IL-4-stimulated T cell proliferation. J Immunol 1996; 156: 435–441.

90. Song Z, Casolaro V, Chen R, Georas SN, Monos D, Ono SJ. Polymorphic nucleotides within the human IL-4 promoter that mediate overexpression of the gene. J Immunol 1996; 156:424–429.

91. Jabs EW, Li X, Scott AF, et al. Weiss and Crouzon syndromes are allelic with mutations in fibroblast growth factor receptor 2. Nature Genet 1994; 8:275–279.

92. Wallace MR, Marchuk DA, Anderson LB, et al. Type I neurofibromatosis gene: identification of a large transcript disrupted in three NF1 patients. Science 1990; 249:181–186.

93. Huntington's Disease Collaborative Research Group. A novel gene containing a trinucleotide repeat that is expanded and unstable on Huntington's disease chromosomes. Cell 1993; 72:971–983.

94. Lovett M. Fishing for complements: finding genes by direct selection. Trends Genet 1994; 10:352–357.

95. Boguski MS, Schuler GD. ESTablishing a human transcript map. Nature Genet 1995; 10:369–371.

96. Hudson TJ, Stein LD. An STS-based map of the human genome. Science 1995; 270: 1945–1952.

97. Dausset J, Cann H, Cohen D, Lathrop M, Lalouel JL, White R. Centre d'etude du polymorphisme humaine (CEPH): collaborative genetic mapping of the human genome. Genomics 1990; 6:575–577.

98. Cox DR, Burmeister M, Price ER, Kim S, Myers RM. Radiation hybrid mapping: a somatic cell genetic method for constructing high resolution maps of mammalian chromosomes. Science 1990; 250:245–250.

99. Cohen D, Chumakov I, Weissenbach J. A first generation physical map of the human genome. Nature 1993; 366:698–701.

100. Devine SE, Boeke JD. Efficient integration of artificial transposons into plasmid targets in vitro: a useful tool for DNA mapping, sequencing and genetic analysis. Nucleic Acids Res 1994; 22:3765–3772.

AUTHOR INDEX

Italic numbers give the page on which the complete reference is listed.

McCaslin, D.R., 166, *176*
Macchia, D., 189, *202*
McClean, P.A., 449, 451, *453*
MacCochrane, G., 425, 429, 430, *441*, 487, *493*
McCombie, W.R., 319, 322, *348*
McCoy, K.L., 134, *144*
McCrea, K.A., 528, *542*
MacDermott, J., 124, 129, *140*, 345, *349*, 456, *475*
McDevitt, D.G., 470, *477*
McDevitt, H.O., 131, 135, *144*
MacDonald, H.R., 528, *542*
McDonald, J.R., 263, *278*
MacDonald, M.R., 431, *442*
MacDonald, N.E., 48, *62*
MacDonald, R.J., 166, *176*
MacDonald, S.M., 128, *143*
McFarlane, C.S., 221, *231*
McGee, T.L., 75, *87*
McGee, T.T., 457, *476*
MacGlashan, D.W., Jr., 4, *12*, 128, *143*, 187, *202*
McGregor, I.A., 368, 375, *378*
McGue, M., 368, *378*, 388, 389, *399*, 485, *492*
McGuire, J.C., 323, *349*
Mcintosh, K., 39, 42, 43, 47, 48, *57*, *58*, *59*, *60*
MacIntyre, N., 75, 80, *87*, 347, *350*, 425, 429, *441*, 446, *452*, 458, 463, *476*
McKenzie, A.N.J., 183, *200*
MacKenzie, T., 196, *206*
McKersey, M., 28, *36*
McKiernan, B.C., 213, *229*
Macklem, P.T., 228, *233*
McKnight, S.L., 195, *205*
McLaughlin, F.J., 18, *31*
MacLean, C.J., 369, *376*
MacLennan, I.C.M., 184, 185, *200, 201*
Maclouf, J., 6, *13*
McLoughlin, L., 75, *87*
McMenamin, C., 24, 28, *35*, *36*, 406, *417*, 504, *509*
McMichael, A.J., 48, *61*

McNeil, H.P., 164, 165, 166, 167, 168, 169, 170, 171, *175, 176, 177*
McNish, R.W., 4, 7, 9, *12*
McPhaden, A.R., 125, *141*
McPharland, C.P., 470, *477*
McPherson, E.A., 212, *229*
McQuillin, J., 48, 52, *61*
Macri, F., 18, *31*
Macri, P., 242, 250, 251, *257*
Madtes, D.K., 243, *255*
Maggi, E., 189, 190, *203*
Magnussen, H., *509*
Magnusson, C.G., 498, *506*, 512, *522*
Major, R., 489, *494*
Majuri, M.L., 46, *60*
Mak, J.C., 78, 79, 80, *88*, 456, *475*
Makuch, R., 101, *114*
Malabarba, M.G., 195, *205*
Malaviya, R., 8, *14*
Malbon, C.C., 74, *86*
Malefyt, R.d.W., 126, *141*
Malek, D., 71, *85*
Malencik, D.A., 94, *111*
Mallet, A.E., 20, *34*
Malley, A., 260, *276*
Malo, J., 427, *442*
Malo, J.L., 6, *13*
Maltzer, S.J., 480, *491*
Manara, G.C., 135, *144*
Mancini, J.A., 9, *15*
Manetta, J., 4, 7, 8, *12, 14*
Manetti, R., 152, *161*, 189, 190, *203*
Mange, A.P., 425, 426, 434, *440*
Mange, E.J., 425, 426, 434, *440*
Maniatis, T., 309, *316*
Mann, T.N., 49, 51, 56, *62*
Mannervik, B., 9, *15*
Manning, P.J., 6, *13*
Manogue, K.R., *145*
Marabini, A., 126, *141*
Marchuk, D.A., 537, *545*
Marcus-Bagley, D., 487, *493*
Margolskee, D.J., 6, *13*
Marini, M., 251, *257*, 528, *542*
Marker, O., 45, *60*
Markham, A.F., 296, *314*

SUBJECT INDEX